Hematology in the Adolescent Female

Lakshmi V. Srivaths
Editor

Hematology in the Adolescent Female

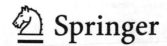

Springer

Editor
Lakshmi V. Srivaths
Department of Pediatrics
Baylor College of Medicine
Houston, TX
USA

ISBN 978-3-030-48448-4   ISBN 978-3-030-48446-0   (eBook)
https://doi.org/10.1007/978-3-030-48446-0

This Springer imprint is published by the registered company Springer Nature Switzerland AG
The registered company address is: Gewerbestrasse 11, 6330 Cham, Switzerland

Contents

Part VI   Bone Marrow Failure Disorders in the Adolescent Female

Part VII   Blood Disorders in the Pregnant Adolescent

About the Author

Lakshmi V. Srivaths, MD is a Professor of Pediatrics in the Section of Hematology at Baylor College of Medicine. She is the Director of the Young Women's Hemostasis and Thrombosis Program at Texas Children's Hospital.

She is a member of the Medical Advisory Council for the Foundation for Women and Girls with Blood Disorders, and Chair for the Education/Advocacy Sub-Committee for the Women and Girls with Blood Disorders-Learning Action Network. As chair of the committee, Dr. Srivaths is in charge of the subcommittee's organization and ongoing activities, which include creating education for clinic staff, referring providers, providers outside of primary institution, and organized/informal education opportunities.

Dr. Lakshmi V. Srivaths is the recipient of Women of Excellence Award, 2020, Norton Rose Fulbright Faculty Excellence Award, "Teaching and Evaluation" category, 2016, Rising Star Clinician Award, Baylor College of Medicine, 2015, Fulbright & Jaworski L. L. P. Faculty Excellence Award, "Teaching and Evaluation" category, 2011, and Fellow's Education Award, Texas Children's Cancer and Hematology Center, 2011.

Contributors

Suchitra S. Acharya, MD Hemostasis and Thrombosis Center, Northwell Health Bleeding Disorders and Thrombosis Program Cohen Children's Medical Center, Northwell Health Zucker School of Medicine at Hofstra/Northwell, Hempstead, NY, USA

Enitan Adegite, MD, MPH Section of Adolescent Medicine, St Christopher's Hospital for Children, Drexel University, Philadelphia, PA, USA

Sanjay P. Ahuja, MD UH Rainbow Hemostasis & Thrombosis Center, Rainbow Babies & Children's Hospital & Case Western Reserve University, Cleveland, OH, USA

Lauren E. Amos, MD Division of Hematology/Oncology/BMT, Children's Mercy Kansas City, Kansas City, MO, USA

Irmel A. Ayala, MD Hemophilia and Bleeding Disorders Treatment Center, Johns Hopkins All Children's Hospital, Cancer and Blood Disorders Institute, St. Petersburg, FL, USA

Maureen K. Baldwin, MD, MPH Department of Obstetrics and Gynecology, Oregon Health & Science University, Portland, OR, USA

Shannon M. Bates, MDCM, MSc, FRCPC Thrombosis and Atherosclerosis Research Institute and Department of Medicine, McMaster University, Hamilton, ON, Canada

Jennifer L. Bercaw-Pratt, MD Department of Obstetrics and Gynecology, Baylor College of Medicine, Houston, TX, USA

Neha Bhasin, MD Department of Pediatrics, University of Arizona, Tucson, AZ, USA

Brian Branchford, MD Children's Hospital Colorado, University of Colorado School of Medicine, Aurora, CO, USA

Vicky R. Breakey, MD, MEd, FRCPC McMaster University, Division of Pediatric Hematology/Oncology, Hamilton, ON, Canada

James B. Bussel, MD Weill Cornell Medicine, Department of Pediatrics, New York, NY, USA

Weill Cornell Medicine, Internal Medicine, New York, NY, USA

Weill Cornell Medicine, Obstetrics and Gynecology, New York, NY, USA

Shannon L. Carpenter, MD, MSCI, FAAP University of Missouri Kansas City, Kansas City, MO, USA

Meera Chitlur, MD Wayne State University, Children's Hospital of Michigan, Detroit, MI, USA

Clay T. Cohen, MD Department of Pediatrics, Section of Hematology-Oncology, Baylor College of Medicine, Texas Children's Hospital, Houston, TX, USA

Jennifer Davila, MD Hemophilia and Thrombosis Center at Montefiore, The Children's Hospital at Montefiore, Albert Einstein College of Medicine, Bronx, NY, USA

Candice M. Dersch, MD Tuft University School of Medicine, Maine Medical Center, Portland, ME, USA

Tazim Dowlut-McElroy, MD, MS Department of Obstetrics and Gynecology, University of Missouri-Kansas City School of Medicine, Kansas City, MO, USA

Stephanie A. Fritch Lilla, MD Children's Hospitals and Clinics of Minnesota, Minneapolis, MN, USA

Anna Griffith, MD Division of Hematology Oncology, University of North Carolina at Chapel Hill, Chapel Hill, NC, USA

Amanda B. Grimes, MD Baylor College of Medicine, Texas Children's Cancer and Hematology Centers, Houston, TX, USA

Shveta Gupta, MD Arnold Palmer Hospital for Children, Orlando, FL, USA

Sweta Gupta, MD Indiana Hemophilia and Thrombosis Center, Indianapolis, IN, USA

Patricia Huguelet, MD University of Colorado Anschutz Medical Campus, Aurora, CO, USA

Children's Hospital Colorado, Aurora, CO, USA

Nelda Itzep, MD Department of Pediatrics, University of Texas MD Anderson Cancer Center, Department of Pediatric Hematology Oncology, Houston, TX, USA

Amanda E. Jacobson-Kelly, MD Department of Pediatrics, Division of Hematology/Oncology/BMT, Nationwide Children's Hospital/The Ohio State University College of Medicine, Columbus, OH, USA

Julie Jaffray, MD Children's Hospital Los Angeles, University of Southern California Keck School of Medicine, Los Angeles, CA, USA

Shilpa Jain, MD, MPH Division of Pediatric Hematology-Oncology, Women and Children's Hospital of Buffalo and Hemophilia Center of Western New York, Buffalo, NY, USA

Maissa Janbain, MD, MSCR Tulane School of Medicine, New Orleans, LA, USA

Sue Kearney, MD Medical Director CHCMN Hemophilia and Thrombosis Center, Children's Hospital and Clinics of Minnesota, Minneapolis, MN, USA

Taylor Olmsted Kim, MD Baylor College of Medicine, Department of Pediatrics, Houston, TX, USA

Texas Children's Hematology Center, Houston, TX, USA

Christine Knoll, MD Department of Child Health, Phoenix Children's Hospital, Phoenix, AZ, USA

Barbara Konkle, MD Bloodworks Northwest and Department of Medicine, University of Washington, Seattle, WA, USA

Peter A. Kouides, MD University of Rochester School of Medicine and Dentistry, Rochester Regional Health, Rochester, NY, USA

Roshni Kulkarni, MD Michigan State University Center for Bleeding and Clotting Disorders, Emerita Pediatric Hematology/Oncology, Department of Pediatrics and Human Development, B216 Clinical Center, East Lansing, MI, USA

May Lau, MD, MPH Department(s) of Pediatrics, The University of Texas Southwestern Medical Center, Dallas, TX, USA

The University of Texas Southwestern Medical Center, Dallas, TX, USA

Division of Developmental and Behavioral Pediatrics, The University of Texas Southwestern Medical Center, Dallas, TX, USA

Alice D. Ma, MD, FACP Division of Hematology Oncology, University of North Carolina at Chapel Hill, Chapel Hill, NC, USA

Arash Mahjerin, MD Children's Hospital Orange County, University of California – Irvine, Irvine, CA, USA

Kelley McLean, MD Department of Obstetrics, Gynecology and Reproductive Medicine, University of Vermont, Burlington, VT, USA

Genevieve Moyer, MD, MSc University of Colorado Anschutz Medical Campus, Aurora, CO, USA

Children's Hospital Colorado, Aurora, CO, USA

University of Colorado Anschutz Medical Campus Hemophilia and Thrombosis Center, Aurora, CO, USA

Trinh Nguyen, DO Department of Pediatrics, Section of Hematology, Baylor College of Medicine, Houston, TX, USA

Anjali Pawar, MD University of California Davis, Hemostasis and Thrombosis Center, Professor Department of Pediatrics, Hematology Oncology, Sacramento, CA, USA

Claire Philipp, MD Rutgers Robert Wood Johnson Medical School, New Brunswick, NJ, USA

Jacquelyn M. Powers, MD, MS Department of Pediatrics, Baylor College of Medicine, Texas Children's Cancer and Hematology Center, Houston, TX, USA

Michael Recht, MD, PhD The Hemophilia Center at Oregon Health & Science University and American Thrombosis and Hemostasis Network, Orgeon, OR, USA

Sarah E. Sartain, MD Department of Pediatrics, Section of Hematology-Oncology, Baylor College of Medicine, Texas Children's Hospital, Houston, TX, USA

Ghadir S. Sasa, MD Department of Pediatrics, Section of Hematology-Oncology, Baylor College of Medicine, Houston, TX, USA

Mukta Sharma, MD, MPH, FAAP University of Missouri Kansas City, Kansas City, MO, USA

Ruchika Sharma, MD Department of Pediatrics, Medical College of Wisconsin, Milwaukee, WI, USA

Vivien Sheehan, MD, PhD Department of Pediatrics, Baylor College of Medicine, Division of Hematology/Oncology, Houston, TX, USA

Robert F. Sidonio, MD, MSCI Aflac Cancer and Blood Disorders, Emory University, Department of Pediatrics, Atlanta, GA, USA

Sylvia T. Singer, MD UCSF Benioff Children's Hospital Oakland, Oakland, CA, USA

Tammuella Chrisentery Singleton, MD Pediatric Hematology, Mississippi Center for Advanced Medicine, Madison, MS, USA

Leslie M. Skeith, MD Department of Medicine, University of Calgary, Calgary, Alberta, Canada

Lakshmi V. Srivaths, MD Department of Pediatrics, Section of Hematology, Baylor College of Medicine, Houston, TX, USA

Janice M. Staber, MD Division of Hematology, Oncology, and BMT, Stead Family Department of Pediatrics, University of Iowa Carver College of Medicine, Iowa City, IA, USA

Pamela Trapane, MD University of Florida Health, Gainesville, FL, USA

Maria C. Velez-Yanguas, MD Hemophilia Treatment Center, Hemostasis and Thrombosis Program, Louisiana State University Health Sciences Center and Children's Hospital of New Orleans, New Orleans, LA, USA

Elliott P. Vichinsky, MD UCSF Benioff Children's Hospital Oakland, Oakland, CA, USA

Adrianna Vlachos, MD Zucker School of Medicine at Hofstra/Northwell, Division of Hematology/Oncology and Stem Cell Transplantation, Cohen Children's Medical Center, New Hyde Park, NY, USA

Feinstein Institutes for Medical Research, Manhasset, NY, USA

Deepti Warad, MD Mayo Clinic, Rochester, MN, USA

Angela C. Weyand, MD Division of Hematology and Oncology, Department of Pediatrics, University of Michigan Medical School, Ann Arbor, MI, USA

Allison P. Wheeler, MD, MSCI Vanderbilt University Medical Center, Department of Pathology, Microbiology & Immunology, Nashville, TN, USA

Kalinda Woods, MD, FACOG Department of Gynecology and Obstetrics, Emory University School of Medicine, The Emory Clinic, Atlanta, GA, USA

Ayesha Zia, MD Division of Pediatric Hematology-Oncology, The University of Texas Southwestern Medical Center, Dallas, TX, USA

Department(s) of Pediatrics, The University of Texas Southwestern Medical Center, Dallas, TX, USA

The University of Texas Southwestern Medical Center, Dallas, TX, USA

Part I

Bleeding Disorders and Heavy Menstrual Bleeding

Evaluation of the Adolescent with Heavy Menstrual Bleeding

Ayesha Zia and May Lau

Introduction

Adolescence is a time of change, and this change is often reflected in their menstrual bleeding. Heavy menstrual bleeding (HMB) is common in adolescents [1]. In a large insurance claims database of more than 200,000 females aged 10–17 years in the United States, 27% had an outpatient diagnostic code consistent with HMB at least once during the study period [2]. The complaint of HMB is subjective. Beliefs derived from personal experience and cultural, social, and educational influences give rise to a sense of what constitutes "normal" blood loss during menses. HMB is qualitatively defined as blood loss that interferes with a woman's physical, social, emotional, and/or material quality of life, irrespective of the volume lost [3]. School absenteeism and interruption in sports or social activities frequently occur in adolescents with HMB [4]. Given the consequences of HMB, physicians and other healthcare providers should be able to evaluate an adolescent presenting with HMB competently.

Normal Menstruation and Terminologies

The median age of menarche is 12 years old, with a range of 10–15 years [5]. Typically menstrual cycles should occur every 21–45 days and last ≤7 days [6, 7]. Average blood loss during menses for an adolescent female is approximately 30–40 ml, which translates to six menstrual pads/tampons on the heaviest day of bleeding [8]. Many terms have been used to describe abnormal uterine bleeding. The International Federation of Gynecology and Obstetrics (FIGO) recommends against using terms such as menorrhagia, dysfunctional uterine bleeding, or hypermenorrhea [9]. Abnormal uterine bleeding is the umbrella term to describe menstrual bleeding that is abnormal with regard to frequency, volume, duration, and cycle regularity [9]. While blood loss of >80 mL is broadly used in clinical studies and trials to define HMB, this measurement (involving

A. Zia (✉)
Division of Pediatric Hematology-Oncology, The University of Texas Southwestern Medical Center, Dallas, TX, USA

Department(s) of Pediatrics, The University of Texas Southwestern Medical Center, Dallas, TX, USA

The University of Texas Southwestern Medical Center, Dallas, TX, USA
e-mail: Ayesha.zia@utsouthwestern.edu

M. Lau
Department(s) of Pediatrics, The University of Texas Southwestern Medical Center, Dallas, TX, USA

The University of Texas Southwestern Medical Center, Dallas, TX, USA

Division of Developmental and Behavioral Pediatrics, The University of Texas Southwestern Medical Center, Dallas, TX, USA

© Springer Nature Switzerland AG 2020
L. V. Srivaths (ed.), *Hematology in the Adolescent Female*,
https://doi.org/10.1007/978-3-030-48446-0_1

extracting hemoglobin from sanitary wear) is impractical outside of research settings; therefore, a requirement to change sanitary pads or tampons more often than hourly, clots at least 1 inch in diameter, and a low ferritin level are clinical predictors of heavy periods [10]. FIGO recommends that HMB in women be classified according to the PALM–COEIN system: polyp, adenomyosis, leiomyoma, malignancy and hyperplasia, coagulopathy, ovulatory dysfunction, endometrial, iatrogenic, and not otherwise classified [11].

The Association of HMB and Bleeding Disorders

The frequency of bleeding disorders in the general population is approximately 1–2%, but bleeding disorders are found in about ~30% of adolescent girls who are referred for evaluation of HMB to a specialty [12]. Low von Willebrand factor (VWF) levels or von Willebrand disease (VWD) and platelet functional disorders (PFD) are the most common type of bleeding disorders encountered in adolescents [12]. Importantly, bleeding disorders coexist with anovulation and non-hemostatic disorders (Table 1.1). HMB confers a significantly lower perceived quality of life in terms of the ability to fully participate in school, work, and athletic and social activities [13]. It is, therefore, imperative that bleeding disorders resulting in HMB are diagnosed without delay. Additional key points in history taking and screening tools for HMB in adolescents that point toward an underlying bleeding disorder are discussed in Chap. 2.

Laboratory Evaluation of the Adolescent with HMB: The Hematology Perspective

General Perspectives on Laboratory Evaluation of Bleeding Disorders The laboratory evaluation of an underlying bleeding disorder in an adolescent with HMB does not differ from the assessment in any patient presenting with unusual

Table 1.1 Frequency of non-hemostatic and concomitant disorders in adolescents with heavy menstrual bleeding

	Anovulatory HMB		Ovulatory HMB	
	BD ($n = 31$)	No BD ($n = 69$)	BD ($n = 36$)	No BD ($n = 64$)
PCOS	3	3	0	0
BJH[a]	3	7	6	4
Uterine structural ab.	1[f]	1[g]	3[h]	0
Systemic disorders	6[b]	10[c]	1[d]	4[e]
VWF exon 28 polym.	0	1	0	3

Table adapted from Zia et al. [12]
Ab. abnormalities, BD bleeding disorder, PCOS polycystic ovarian syndrome, BJH benign joint hypermobility, polym. polymorphism. [a]BJH assessment was performed only on 100 participants
No differences in the prevalence of bleeding disorders according to menstrual bleeding pattern (31% in anovulatory pattern bleeding vs. 36% ovulatory pattern bleeding; $p = 0.45$)
Systemic or medical disorders = [b]depression ($n = 4$), remote history of cancer ($n = 1$) and hypothyroidism ($n = 1$); [c]depression ($n = 3$), asthma requiring medications ($n = 3$), remote history of cancer ($n = 3$), hypothyroidism ($n = 1$); [d]one had juvenile rheumatoid arthritis; [e]depression ($n = 1$), diabetes mellitus ($n = 2$), celiac disease ($n = 1$)
Uterine structural abnormalities: [f]One had endometriosis; [g]one had erosive vaginitis from tampon use; [h]two were diagnosed with endometriosis, and one was diagnosed with uterine polyps

bruising or bleeding. Table 1.2 reviews the estimated sensitivity and specificity of various hemostasis assays in the evaluation of a bleeding phenotype. There are certain caveats specific to the testing approach in adolescents due to acute HMB and concomitant hormonal use that we will highlight below. There is no simple diagnostic strategy or testing algorithm that can adequately cover all possible bleeding disorders when the presenting complaint is HMB, but a proposed algorithm that the authors have used prospectively to diagnose bleeding disorders in HMB is covered elsewhere [14, 15]. As an educational book chapter, this work does not reflect a systematic review methodology but instead serves as an overview of laboratory evaluation of bleeding disorders in adolescents with HMB. While efforts

Table 1.2 Estimated sensitivities and specificities of hemostasis assays used to evaluate bleeding problems

	Estimated sensitivity (%)	Estimated specificity (%)
PTT	2.1	98
PT	1.0	>99
TT	1.0	86
Clauss fibrinogen	1.0	>99
VWD screen	6.7	>98
Light transmission aggregometry	26	96
Factor assays	Not reported	Not reported

Table adapted from Hayward and Moffat [37]. The estimated sensitivities and specificities reported in this table for a bleeding problem have not been tested specifically in the setting of HMB. PTT indicates partial thromboplastin time; *PT* prothrombin time, *TT* thrombin time, *VWD* von Willebrand disease

were taken to highlight pertinent evidence without bias, the interested reader is encouraged to conduct an additional review of the literature.

The initial laboratory evaluation of patients with a suspected bleeding disorder should include a complete blood count, a review of peripheral blood smear for platelet morphology, prothrombin time, partial thromboplastin time (PTT), and either fibrinogen or thrombin time [16]. These routine coagulation studies can suggest whether a severe coagulation factor deficiency or thrombocytopenia might be the reason for clinical bleeding but will neither rule in nor rule out VWD or PFD, the most common bleeding disorders encountered in adolescents with HMB. When using the PTT in the diagnosis of VWD, the results of this test are abnormal only if the coagulation factor (F) VIII is sufficiently reduced [17]. Some centers add a platelet function analyzer (PFA-100) assay to their initial laboratory screening tests to "loosely" screen for either VWD or PFD. A clinician, faced with an individual with a personal and family history of bleeding, should not use the results of a normal PFA-100 to influence his/her decision to undertake more specific laboratory testing. Thus, irrespective of an abnormal or normal PFA-100 result, VWF and platelet function testing are still warranted to assess the possibility of these disorders in patients with HMB; so in this context, the PFA-100 has a limited utility [18].

VWD Testing in HMB The laboratory diagnosis of VWD can be complicated. The initial tests commonly used to detect VWD or low VWF are determinations of plasma levels of (i) VWF:Antigen (Ag); (ii) VWF:Ristocetin Co-factor activity (RCo); and (iii) FVIII [17]. These three tests, readily available in most larger hospitals, measure the amount of VWF protein present in plasma (VWF:Ag), the function of the VWF protein that is present as VWF:RCo, and the ability of the VWF to serve as the carrier protein to maintain normal FVIII survival. New options for laboratory assessment of VWF activity include a new platelet-binding assay, the VWF:GPIbM, which is subject to less variability than VWF:RCo assay, and collagen-binding (CB) assays that provide insight into a different function of VWF. Because the VWF:RCo uses the nonphysiologic agonist ristocetin to bridge VWF and platelet glycoprotein (GP) Ibα, there is the potential for false results due to defects in VWF's ability to bind ristocetin. The most common of these is the p.D1472H variant, which affects ristocetin binding but not VWF function [19]. The VWF:GPIbM assay introduces gain-of-function mutations into GPIbα, allowing it to bind VWF spontaneously in vitro without the requirement for ristocetin [20]. The VWF:GPIbM allows higher precision, with a reported lower limit of detection of 2 IU/dL and a coefficient of variation of 5.6% [21]. There is a reasonable correlation between VWF:RCo and VWF:GPIbM results [20].

VWF also binds to exposed collagen at sites of injury, which requires specific testing. Collagen binding is dependent on the presence of high-molecular-weight VWF multimers [22]. There may be a dual role for collagen-binding assays in VWD diagnosis, to evaluate multimer status and to screen for a possible collagen-binding defect. Assays using either type I, type III, or a combination of the two will suffice to detect specific A3 domain collagen-binding variants [23]. Specific A1 binding defects are more common, although binding to types IV and VI collagen is rarely assessed in clinical practice [24]. Research from the Zimmerman Program, a large multicenter

US study on patients with all types of VWD, has shown a relatively high incidence of type IV and VI collagen-binding defects in patients with both type 1 (5%) and type 2 M VWD (27%) [24]. The presence of a collagen-binding variant was associated with an increased bleeding score compared with similar subjects without a collagen-binding defect in this cohort. Adolescents with HMB and other unexplained bleeding symptoms or a strong family history of HMB may benefit from collagen-binding testing to explore the possibility of an undiagnosed collagen-binding defect in VWF.

The increased availability and lower cost of genetic testing enable increased use in the diagnosis of VWD. An impediment to the routine use of genetic analysis for VWD is the weak correlation between VWF sequence variants and type 1 VWD, the most common VWD type. A large study of VWD subjects in the United States showed a relatively low rate of probably causative VWF variants in those subjects with VWF:Ag >30 IU/dL [25]. Genetic analysis is most useful in type 2 VWD. Genetic analysis either specifically for the p.D1472H variant or of VWF exon 28 is helpful when the VWF:RCo/VWF:Ag ratio is decreased in the setting of a normal multimer distribution. Sequencing can either verify that the low ratio is caused by p.D1472H or, in patients with suspected type 2 M VWD, reveal a causative variant [26].

VWF levels will increase in the setting of stress, inflammation, and illness and are often found to be quite elevated when measured in adolescents hospitalized for severe HMB [17]. Recent data suggest that VWF levels >100 IU/dL in the pediatric population may not need repeat testing to rule out the diagnosis of VWD [27]; however, a relatively small proportion (18%) of the included patient population in this study tested for VWD had HMB. Patients with blood group type O have VWF levels that are approximately 25% lower than non-O blood group individuals [28]; however, current guidelines recommend against using blood-type-specific reference values and suggest instead using either absolute cutoffs or population-based reference ranges in conjunction with personal and family history of bleeding in making a diagnosis of VWD [17, 29]. High-dose estrogen therapy also elevates VWF levels, but the influence of standard dose (30–35 mcg) estrogen is less clear and unlikely to affect the laboratory diagnosis of VWD. The majority of studies in healthy women who use standard dose combined hormonal contraceptives have shown no significant increase in VWF [30, 31]; however, there have been no studies in women with VWD or low VWF levels at baseline. Patients on a taper of combined hormonal contraceptives or a high-dose pill (estrogen dose >50 mcg) should not undergo testing for VWD until the patient has been tapered down to standard dose for ~3 months [32]. To avoid continued or recurrent HMB, treatment with combined hormonal contraceptives should not be delayed or withheld to complete testing for VWD [32].

PFD Testing in HMB PFD are clinically important bleeding disorders that are particularly challenging for clinical laboratories to diagnose. Many PFD are associated with increased bleeding scores and increased risks for bleeding. Often, laboratory testing for PFD is done after VWD is excluded [33], although testing for PFD and VWD at the same time may improve the evaluation of suspected bleeding disorders. Most PFD tests require rapid processing and testing of freshly collected, hand-delivered blood samples, using assays with validated reference intervals, derived from an adequate number of female and male healthy control samples [34]. The performance characteristics of PFD tests, and the control of pre-analytical, analytical, and post-analytical factors (including ingestion of drugs that inhibit platelet function) and procedures, influence their overall diagnostic usefulness [34].

Beyond complete blood count to assess disorders of platelet numbers and peripheral smear for platelet morphology for platelet storage pool and membrane deficiencies, platelet aggregation is the gold-standard platelet function testing method. It began with light transmittance aggregometry in 1965 and continues to be used extensively [35]. In light transmittance aggregometry, the operator prepares platelet-rich plasma, adds a platelet agonist to the platelet-rich plasma, and records the rise in light transmission as platelets aggregate and the suspension clears [34, 36]. Whole blood impedance lumiaggregometry represents an updated methodology and is technically more straightforward, wherein the operator prepares a whole blood suspension, adds an agonist, and records the rise in impedance as platelets coat electrodes suspended in the blood. Both whole blood and light transmission aggregation may be enhanced with a luminescence channel to measure and detect platelet-dense granule ATP secretion after in vitro platelet activation [34, 36].

Inherited PFD include platelet membrane receptor abnormalities, secretion disorders related to internal enzyme deficiencies, and storage pool defects, whereas acquired defects are seen with medications and liver and renal disease [36]. Abnormalities on platelet aggregation should be repeated to help rule out false positives, particularly if the findings suggest a drug-induced defect, and should be reproducible. Single agonist abnormalities are usually a false positive and are much less predictive of a bleeding disorder than multiple agonist abnormalities. Many PFD encountered in practice are uncharacterized inherited disorders with abnormal aggregation responses to multiple agonists that do not fit a well-described pattern of abnormal findings [37]. A lack of standardized reference ranges for delta granules/platelets in children and adolescents limits the upfront utilization of platelet electron microscopy in the workup of HMB at this time. Recent strides, however, have been made to establish references and ranges and validate the methodology [38]. Newer technologies such as high-throughput DNA sequencing are low yield unless the clinical picture suggests a probable etiology [33]. The most recent guidance, from the SSC of the ISTH, recommends many tests for the diagnosis of inherited PFD, including assays validated for diagnostic purposes and assays predominantly used for research investigations [33].

Coagulation Factor Deficiencies in HMB Coagulation factor assays may be considered in the presence of a significant bleeding phenotype if the tests mentioned above are normal, but a suspicion of a bleeding disorder remains high. Evidence of abnormal bleeding in factor XI deficiency not confined to severely deficient patients and a previously reported 26% prevalence of HMB in FXIII-deficient women with FXIII levels <70 IU dL justify testing FXI and FXIII levels in select patients [39, 40].

Laboratory Evaluation for "Bleeding Tendencies" It is not infrequent for hematologists to care for adolescents with HMB and other bleeding tendencies such as easy bruising but for whom available hemostatic testing does not reveal a diagnosis [41]. For such patients, it is important to consider a bleeding tendency that may result from a benign joint hypermobility syndrome and to assess for hypermobility [42]. Joint hypermobility is more common in females, and patients with joint hypermobility syndromes (Ehlers-Danlos syndrome being the most common) may bleed because of increased capillary fragility, alterations in collagen protein interactions in platelet function, or changes in the interaction between exposed collagen in endothelial walls and platelet receptors or VWF [43]. Prolonged menses, irregular menses, and dysmenorrhea are all commonly reported by women with Ehlers-Danlos syndrome [44]. Although many of these patients will have prolonged bleeding times [45], results from hemostatic tests are typically normal [46].

Identifying and Managing Iron Deficiency in HMB Hematologists play a key role in diagnosing and managing concomitant iron deficiency or iron deficiency anemia in adolescents with HMB. A CBC and iron panel should be part of the diagnostic evaluation of adolescents with

HMB. This aspect of assessment in HMB is discussed in Chap. 17.

Laboratory Evaluation of the Adolescent with Heavy Menstrual Bleeding: The Adolescent Medicine and Gynecology Perspective

The most frequent cause of HMB in an adolescent medicine or gynecology practitioner's office is anovulatory bleeding. This is a diagnosis of exclusion. Two years post-menarche, over half of menstrual cycles are anovulatory, whereas by 5 years, about one-tenth of menstrual cycles are anovulatory [47]. Anovulation cannot be based on cycle frequency, given that despite irregularity in their cycle frequency, most adolescent females are ovulating [48]. Polycystic ovarian syndrome (PCOS) is an important diagnosis to consider when anovulatory cycles are present. It occurs when hyperandrogenism results in anovulatory cycles. Approximately 1/3 of adolescent female patients admitted for HMB and anemia were diagnosed with PCOS in one study [49]. It is important to remember that either hypothyroid or hyperthyroid states can cause HMB [50].

An often-overlooked reason for HMB is combined hormonal contraceptives due to medication adherence issues, prolonged menstrual suppression, inadequate estrogen dose [51, 52], or the inability of progesterone to regulate shedding of the endometrium [53, 54]. Trauma and foreign bodies are additional causes of HMB [55]. There are a few essential non-hematological tests to evaluate for HMB [56]. These include urine pregnancy test to rule out any pregnancy-related causes, urine for sexually transmitted diseases such as gonorrhea and chlamydia, thyroid studies including thyroid-stimulating hormone and free T4 to evaluate for thyroid disease, and free testosterone to assess for PCOS.

Speculum and pelvic examinations depend on the age of the patient, diagnostic suspicion, and the clinician's judgment [57]. Papanicolau test, endometrial biopsy, or endocervical/vaginal swab for *Chlamydia* and gonorrhea depends on

the age of the patient and other features in history. In a virginal adolescent, an abdominal ultrasound may be substituted for the pelvic examination. The transabdominal approach is the procedure of choice for any nonsexually active female, and the transvaginal approach is the procedure of choice for those females who are emotionally mature and sexually active [58]. Intrauterine saline instillation at the time of transvaginal ultrasound (sonohysterography) increases the sensitivity for abnormalities of the uterine cavity but is usually reserved for the evaluation of acquired uterine abnormalities in perimenopausal bleeding [59].

A systematic review examined the use of ultrasound, sonohysteroscopy, and hyteroscopy in the setting of HMB [60]. This review found a wide variation in published results on the accuracy of the various imaging modalities. Ultrasound is an accurate method for identifying uterine pathology with sensitivity ranging from 48% to 100% and specificity 12% to 100% in the setting of HMB. Furthermore, ultrasound is better at identifying fibroids than hysteroscopy but is less accurate for identifying polyps or endometrial disease when compared with hysteroscopy. Saline infusion sonography accurately identifies uterine pathology, with a sensitivity of 85–100% and a specificity of 50–100%. For hysteroscopy, the sensitivity was 90–97% and the specificity was 62–93%. MRI has no advantage over ultrasound as the firstline investigation for HMB but may be reserved for problem-solving where ultrasound provides indeterminate results.

References

1. Friberg B, Orno AK, Lindgren A, Lethagen S. Bleeding disorders among young women: a population-based prevalence study. Acta Obstet Gynecol Scand. 2006;85(2):200–6.
2. Jacobson AE, Vesely SK, Koch T, Campbell J, O'Brien SH. Patterns of von Willebrand disease screening in girls and adolescents with heavy menstrual bleeding. Obstet Gynecol. 2018;131(6):1121–9.
3. National Collaborating Centre for Women's and Children's Health (UK). Heavy menstrual bleeding. London: RCOG Press; 2007.
4. Nur Azurah AG, Sanci L, Moore E, Grover S. The quality of life of adolescents with menstrual problems. J Pediatr Adolesc Gynecol. 2013;26(2):102–8.

5. ACOG Committee Opinion No. 651: Menstruation in girls and adolescents: using the menstrual cycle as a vital sign. Obstet Gynecol. 2015;126(6):e143–6.
6. Screening and management of bleeding disorders in adolescents with heavy menstrual bleeding: ACOG Committee Opinion, Number 785. Obstet Gynecol. 2019;134(3):e71–e83.
7. World Health Organization multicenter study on menstrual and ovulatory patterns in adolescent girls. II. Longitudinal study of menstrual patterns in the early postmenarcheal period, duration of bleeding episodes and menstrual cycles. World Health Organization Task Force on Adolescent Reproductive Health. J Adolesc Health Care. 1986;7(4):236–44.
8. Bennett AR, Gray SH. What to do when she's bleeding through: the recognition, evaluation, and management of abnormal uterine bleeding in adolescents. Curr Opin Pediatr. 2014;26(4):413–9.
9. Fraser IS, Critchley HO, Broder M, Munro MG. The FIGO recommendations on terminologies and definitions for normal and abnormal uterine bleeding. Semin Reprod Med. 2011;29(5):383–90.
10. Warner PE, Critchley HO, Lumsden MA, Campbell Brown M, Douglas A, Murray GD. Menorrhagia I: measured blood loss, clinical features, and outcome in women with heavy periods: a survey with follow-up data. Am J Obstet Gynecol. 2004;190(5):1216–23.
11. Munro MG, Critchley HO, Fraser IS. The FIGO systems for nomenclature and classification of causes of abnormal uterine bleeding in the reproductive years: who needs them? Am J Obstet Gynecol. 2012;207(4):259–65.
12. Zia A, Jain S, Kouides P, Zhang S, Gao A, Salas N, et al. Bleeding disorders in adolescents with heavy menstrual bleeding in a multicentre prospective US cohort. Haematologica. 2019 Oct 17:haematol.2019.225656. https://doi.org/10.3324/haematol.2019.225656. Online ahead of print. PMID: 31624107.
13. Shankar M, Chi C, Kadir RA. Review of quality of life: menorrhagia in women with or without inherited bleeding disorders. Haemophilia. 2008;14(1):15–20.
14. Zia A, Lau M, Journeycake J, Sarode R, Marshall J, De Simone N, et al. Developing a multidisciplinary young women's blood disorders program: a single-centre approach with guidance for other centres. Haemophilia. 2016;22(2):199–207.
15. Zia A, Rajpurkar M. Challenges of diagnosing and managing the adolescent with heavy menstrual bleeding. Thromb Res. 2016;143:91–100.
16. James AH, Kouides PA, Abdul-Kadir R, Edlund M, Federici AB, Halimeh S, et al. Von Willebrand disease and other bleeding disorders in women: consensus on diagnosis and management from an international expert panel. Am J Obstet Gynecol. 2009;201(1):12e1–8.
17. Nichols WL, Hultin MB, James AH, Manco-Johnson MJ, Montgomery RR, Ortel TL, et al. von Willebrand disease (VWD): evidence-based diagnosis and management guidelines, the National Heart, Lung, and Blood Institute (NHLBI) expert panel report (USA). Haemophilia. 2008;14(2):171–232.
18. Favaloro EJ. Clinical utility of the PFA-100. Semin Thromb Hemost. 2008;34(8):709–33.
19. Flood VH, Gill JC, Morateck PA, Christopherson PA, Friedman KD, Haberichter SL, et al. Common VWF exon 28 polymorphisms in African Americans affecting the VWF activity assay by ristocetin cofactor. Blood. 2010;116(2):280–6.
20. Patzke J, Budde U, Huber A, Mendez A, Muth H, Obser T, et al. Performance evaluation and multicentre study of a von Willebrand factor activity assay based on GPIb binding in the absence of ristocetin. Blood Coagul Fibrinolysis. 2014;25(8):860–70.
21. Graf L, Moffat KA, Carlino SA, Chan AK, Iorio A, Giulivi A, et al. Evaluation of an automated method for measuring von Willebrand factor activity in clinical samples without ristocetin. Int J Lab Hematol. 2014;36(3):341–51.
22. Favaloro EJ. Diagnosis and classification of von Willebrand disease: a review of the differential utility of various functional von Willebrand factor assays. Blood Coagul Fibrinolysis. 2011;22(7):553–64.
23. Riddell AF, Gomez K, Millar CM, Mellars G, Gill S, Brown SA, et al. Characterization of W1745C and S1783A: 2 novel mutations causing defective collagen binding in the A3 domain of von Willebrand factor. Blood. 2009;114(16):3489–96.
24. Flood VH, Schlauderaff AC, Haberichter SL, Slobodianuk TL, Jacobi PM, Bellissimo DB, et al. Crucial role for the VWF A1 domain in binding to type IV collagen. Blood. 2015;125(14):2297–304.
25. Flood VH, Christopherson PA, Gill JC, Friedman KD, Haberichter SL, Bellissimo DB, et al. Clinical and laboratory variability in a cohort of patients diagnosed with type 1 VWD in the United States. Blood. 2016;127(20):2481–8.
26. Sharma R, Flood VH. Advances in the diagnosis and treatment of Von Willebrand disease. Hematology Am Soc Hematol Educ Program. 2017;2017(1):379–84.
27. Doshi BS, Rogers RS, Whitworth HB, Stabnick EA, Britton J, Butler RB, et al. Utility of repeat testing in the evaluation for von Willebrand disease in pediatric patients. J Thromb Haemost. 2019.
28. Gill JC, Endres-Brooks J, Bauer PJ, Marks WJ Jr, Montgomery RR. The effect of ABO blood group on the diagnosis of von Willebrand disease. Blood. 1987;69(6):1691–5.
29. Laffan MA, Lester W, O'Donnell JS, Will A, Tait RC, Goodeve A, et al. The diagnosis and management of von Willebrand disease: a United Kingdom Haemophilia Centre Doctors Organization guideline approved by the British Committee for Standards in Haematology. Br J Haematol. 2014;167(4):453–65.
30. Dumont T, Allen L, Kives S. Can von Willebrand disease be investigated on combined hormonal contraceptives? J Pediatr Adolesc Gynecol. 2013;26(3):138–41.

31. Zia A, Callaghan MU, Callaghan JH, Sawni A, Bartlett H, Backos A, et al. Hypercoagulability in adolescent girls on oral contraceptives-global coagulation profile and estrogen receptor polymorphisms. Am J Hematol. 2015;90(8):725–31.

32. O'Brien SH. Evaluation and management of heavy menstrual bleeding in adolescents: the role of the hematologist. Blood. 2018;

33. Gresele P. Subcommittee on Platelet Physiology of the International Society on T, Hemostasis. Diagnosis of inherited platelet function disorders: guidance from the SSC of the ISTH. J Thromb Haemost. 2015;13(2):314–22.

34. Harrison P, Mackie I, Mumford A, Briggs C, Liesner R, Winter M, et al. Guidelines for the laboratory investigation of heritable disorders of platelet function. Br J Haematol. 2011;155(1):30–44.

35. Born GV. Aggregation of blood platelets by adenosine diphosphate and its reversal. Nature. 1962;194:927–9.

36. Hayward CPM, Moffat KA, Brunet J, Carlino SA, Plumhoff E, Meijer P, et al. Update on diagnostic testing for platelet function disorders: what is practical and useful? Int J Lab Hematol. 2019;41(Suppl 1):26–32.

37. Hayward CP, Moffat KA. Laboratory testing for bleeding disorders: strategic uses of high and low-yield tests. Int J Lab Hematol. 2013;35(3):322–33.

38. Sorokin V, Alkhoury R, Al-Rawabdeh S, Houston RH, Thornton D, Kerlin B, et al. Reference range of Platelet Delta granules in the pediatric age group: an ultrastructural study of platelet whole mount preparations from healthy volunteers. Pediatr Dev Pathol. 2016;19(6):498–501.

39. Bolton-Maggs PH, Patterson DA, Wensley RT, Tuddenham EG. Definition of the bleeding tendency in factor XI-deficient kindreds–a clinical and laboratory study. Thromb Haemost. 1995;73(2):194–202.

40. Sharief LA, Kadir RA. Congenital factor XIII deficiency in women: a systematic review of literature. Haemophilia. 2013;19(6):e349–57.

41. Quiroga T, Goycoolea M, Panes O, Aranda E, Martinez C, Belmont S, et al. High prevalence of bleeders of unknown cause among patients with inherited mucocutaneous bleeding. A prospective study of 280 patients and 299 controls. Haematologica. 2007;92(3):357–65.

42. van der Giessen LJ, Liekens D, Rutgers KJ, Hartman A, Mulder PG, Oranje AP. Validation of beighton score and prevalence of connective tissue signs in 773 Dutch children. J Rheumatol. 2001;28(12):2726–30.

43. Kendel NE, Haamid FW, Christian-Rancy M, O'Brien SH. Characterizing adolescents with heavy menstrual bleeding and generalized joint hypermobility. Pediatr Blood Cancer. 2019;66(6):e27675.

44. Hurst BS, Lange SS, Kullstam SM, Usadi RS, Matthews ML, Marshburn PB, et al. Obstetric and gynecologic challenges in women with Ehlers-Danlos syndrome. Obstet Gynecol. 2014;123(3):506–13.

45. Mast KJ, Nunes ME, Ruymann FB, Kerlin BA. Desmopressin responsiveness in children with Ehlers-Danlos syndrome associated bleeding symptoms. Br J Haematol. 2009;144(2):230–3.

46. De Paepe A, Malfait F. Bleeding and bruising in patients with Ehlers-Danlos syndrome and other collagen vascular disorders. Br J Haematol. 2004;127(5):491–500.

47. Apter D. Serum steroids and pituitary hormones in female puberty: a partly longitudinal study. Clin Endocrinol. 1980;12(2):107–20.

48. Pena AS, Doherty DA, Atkinson HC, Hickey M, Norman RJ, Hart R. The majority of irregular menstrual cycles in adolescence are ovulatory: results of a prospective study. Arch Dis Child. 2018;103(3):235–9.

49. Maslyanskaya S, Talib HJ, Northridge JL, Jacobs AM, Coble C, Coupey SM. Polycystic ovary syndrome: an under-recognized cause of abnormal uterine bleeding in adolescents admitted to a children's hospital. J Pediatr Adolesc Gynecol. 2017;30(3):349–55.

50. Bourne AW. Hyperthyroidism in functional menorrhagia. Proc R Soc Med. 1922;15(Obstet Gynaecol Sect):24–30.

51. Endrikat J, Muller U, Dusterberg B. A twelve-month comparative clinical investigation of two low-dose oral contraceptives containing 20 micrograms ethinylestradiol/75 micrograms gestodene and 30 micrograms ethinylestradiol/75 micrograms gestodene, with respect to efficacy, cycle control, and tolerance. Contraception. 1997;55(3):131–7.

52. Rosenberg MJ, Meyers A, Roy V. Efficacy, cycle control, and side effects of low- and lower-dose oral contraceptives: a randomized trial of 20 micrograms and 35 micrograms estrogen preparations. Contraception. 1999;60(6):321–9.

53. Salamonsen LA, Butt AR, Hammond FR, Garcia S, Zhang J. Production of endometrial matrix metalloproteinases, but not their tissue inhibitors, is modulated by progesterone withdrawal in an in vitro model for menstruation. J Clin Endocrinol Metab. 1997;82(5):1409–15.

54. Galant C, Berliere M, Dubois D, Verougstraete JC, Charles A, Lemoine P, et al. Focal expression and final activity of matrix metalloproteinases may explain irregular dysfunctional endometrial bleeding. Am J Pathol. 2004;165(1):83–94.

55. Pennesi CM, Kenney B, Thakkar R, Ching C, Hewitt G, McCracken K. Prolonged vaginal bleeding in an adolescent secondary to a foreign body: need for a comprehensive assessment and complex surgery. J Pediatr Adolesc Gynecol. 2018;31(6):640–3.

56. Deligeoroglou E, Karountzos V, Creatsas G. Abnormal uterine bleeding and dysfunctional uterine bleeding in pediatric and adolescent gynecology. Gynecol Endocrinol. 2013;29(1):74–8.

57. James AH. Heavy menstrual bleeding: work-up and management. Hematology Am Soc Hematol Educ Program. 2016;2016(1):236–42.

58. Arbel-DeRowe Y, Tepper R, Rosen DJ, Beyth Y. The contribution of pelvic ultrasonography to the diagnostic process in pediatric and adolescent gynecology. J Pediatr Adolesc Gynecol. 1997;10(1):3–12.

59. American College of O, Gynecologists. ACOG Technology Assessment in Obstetrics and Gynecology No. 5: sonohysterography. Obstet Gynecol. 2008;112(6):1467–9.

60. Farquhar C, Ekeroma A, Furness S, Arroll B. A systematic review of transvaginal ultrasonography, sonohysterography and hysteroscopy for the investigation of abnormal uterine bleeding in premenopausal women. Acta Obstet Gynecol Scand. 2003;82(6):493–504.

Screening Tools for Evaluating the Bleeding Adolescent

Kalinda Woods and Sue Kearney

Introduction

Bleeding has always been a distressing and obvious clinical symptom, a fact which is demonstrable through many eras in history and across cultures. Because bleeding is a common human experience, it can be challenging to differentiate normal versus pathologic bleeding. Historically, clinicians have relied heavily on a thorough assessment of the patient (including the interview and physical exam) to determine if further diagnostic testing is appropriate. However, when it comes to bleeding, approximately 1/3 of healthy individuals may report at least one hemorrhagic symptom by 30 years of age [1]. The significant overlap of lifetime cumulative bleeding incidence in normal and mild bleeding disorder patients highlights the challenges in discriminating between normal and abnormal hemostasis using an "individualized approach" to the bleeding history.

The adolescent population presents unique challenges when it comes to diagnosing abnormal bleeding. Adolescents have had less time to manifest bleeding symptoms, and as a group, they may have had less exposure to surgical and other hemostatic challenges. In addition, bruising and epistaxis are frequently reported at this age in the absence of a bleeding disorder [2] and may be erroneously attributed to their high level of activity. Finally, adolescents with heavy menstrual bleeding (HMB) are often loathe to seek medical attention. Estimates suggest that 5–44% of adolescents with HMB have an associated underlying and undiagnosed bleeding disorder [3].

Given these issues, investigators have sought to standardize the bleeding history in the form of bleeding assessment tools (BATs) in order to objectively quantify bleeding severity and increase diagnostic accuracy.

This chapter will:

(a) Review the bleeding assessment tools (BATs) used for both pediatric and adult populations with emphasis on those applicable to the adolescent.
(b) Review the application of these tools with reference to the published data on specific study populations and disease states.
(c) Review the opportunities and challenges of BATs.
(d) Discuss strategies for administration and data collection of future BATs.

K. Woods (✉)
Department of Gynecology and Obstetrics, Emory University School of Medicine, The Emory Clinic, Atlanta, GA, USA
e-mail: kalinda.d.woods@emory.edu

S. Kearney
Medical Director CHCMN Hemophilia and Thrombosis Center, Children's Hospital and Clinics of Minnesota, Minneapolis, MN, USA

© Springer Nature Switzerland AG 2020
L. V. Srivaths (ed.), *Hematology in the Adolescent Female*,
https://doi.org/10.1007/978-3-030-48446-0_2

The Bleeding Assessment Tool

Over many years, clinician-researchers have developed a variety of questionnaires to evaluate bleeding, which are collectively referred to as bleeding assessment tools or BATs. Bleeding assessment tools were designed and developed initially as research tools for the quantification of bleeding symptoms and the study of phenotype/genotype correlations. A BAT typically includes a specific set of questions to illicit the bleeding history and an interpretation grid to score the severity of each bleeding symptom [1]. The ideal BAT will provide a bleeding score (BS) based not only on incidence of bleeding but also on severity, frequency, and need for intervention. These tools have proven helpful not only for researchers but also for clinicians diagnosing and treating bleeding disorders. Clinicians can utilize these tools to establish an objective score or quantitative benchmark by which to determine the need for further diagnostic tests, to evaluate severity of bleeding symptoms, and to track patient response to therapy. Given the complexity and nuances of differentiating normal vs abnormal bleeding and the desire to reduce unnecessary testing, there has been a renewed interest in the use of BATs in recent years.

The Evolution of BAT

In the mid-1990s, the International Society on Thrombosis and Hemostasis (ISTH) Scientific and Standardization Committee (SSC) established a set of provisional criteria for the diagnosis of von Willebrand disease (vWD) type I which included thresholds for mucocutaneous bleeding symptoms to be considered significant [4]. The establishment of the ISTH vWD consensus criteria provided a platform for investigators to develop and validate BATs with the goal of an objective, quantitative assessment of bleeding and a standardized approach to diagnosis. Minimal criteria for significant bleeding were defined. See Table 2.1 [5].

Much of the initial work on the modern BAT was done by a group of investigators from

Table 2.1 Criteria for nontrivial bleeding

Epistaxis	Any nosebleed that causes interference or distress with daily or social activities. Significant features include bleeding greater than 10 minutes, a frequency of greater than five episodes/year, and no other identifiable cause
Cutaneous bleeding	Five or more bruises (>1 cm) in exposed areas; petechiae; hematomas without trauma
Minor cutaneous wound	Two or more bleeding episodes caused by superficial cuts lasting more than 10 minutes requiring frequent bandage changes
Oral cavity bleeding	Causes frankly bloody sputum or a swollen tongue or mouth and lasts greater than 10 minutes on more than one occasion
Hematemesis	Unexplained gastrointestinal bleeding
Hematuria	Unexplained macroscopic hematuria
Tooth extraction	Any unexpected bleeding requiring intervention by a dentist
Surgical bleeding	Any abnormal bleeding judged by the surgeon that causes a delay in discharge or that requires supportive treatment
Menorrhagia	Any bleeding that interferes with daily or social activities. Significant features include changing pads more than every 2 hours; lasting more than 7 days; large clots >1 cm combined with a history of flooding; or a PBAC score higher than 100
Postpartum bleeding	Bleeding lasting for more than 6 weeks that causes progressive anemia or is judged to be abnormal by the obstetrician
Muscle hematomas or hemarthrosis	Any spontaneous joint/muscle bleeding (not related to traumatic injuries) is considered significant
CNS bleeding	Any subdural or intracerebral hemorrhage requiring intervention
Other	Bleeding symptoms that occur during infancy

Adapted from Rodeghiero et al. [6]

Vicenza, Italy. Led by Rodegheiro, the "Vincenza BAT" has undergone several iterations [6]. The original Vincenza BAT queried bleeding symptoms including epistaxis, menstrual bleeding, and postsurgical bleeding. For each bleeding symptom, a score was given depending on the bleeding severity (0 for absent or trivial; 3 for those symptoms requiring medical intervention). The approximate time of administration of the original Vincenza BAT was 40 minutes. The Vincenza BAT was first studied in 42 obligatory carriers of type I vWD. The results of this study demonstrated that having at least three hemorrhagic symptoms or a BS of 3 in men and 5 in women was supportive of type I VWD (high specificity, moderate sensitivity) [7]. The Vincenza BAT was later revised in an attempt to improve the sensitivity. In this version, the scoring system reflected the absence of symptoms in the setting of significant hemostatic challenges (scoring −1), all the way up to a score of 4 if infusion of clotting fac-

tors or surgery were required. Version 2 of the Vincenza BAT was used to evaluate patients in the European Molecular and Clinical Markers for the Diagnosis and Management of Type 1 VWD Study (MCMDM-1 VWD), and the BS was strongly inversely correlated with vWF level [8]. A condensed version (version 3) of the MCMDM1-VWD Bleeding Questionnaire was subsequently developed, removing all details that did not directly affect the BS. This reduced the time of administration from 40 minutes to 5–10 minutes [9]. These tools have been studied in other bleeding disorders with good validity [10, 11]. See Table 2.2 for further details.

Table 2.2 Scoring comparison for BATs

Symptom	Score					
	−1	0[a]	1[a]	2	3	4
Epistaxis	–	No or trivial	Present	Packing, cauterization	Blood transfusion or replacement therapy	–
	–	No or trivial (≤5)	>5 or more than 10′	Consultation only	Packing or cauterization or antifibrinolytics	Blood transfusion or replacement therapy or desmopressin
	–	No or trivial	>5 or more than 10′	Consultation only	Packing or cauterization	Blood transfusion or replacement therapy
	–	No/trivial	> 5/y or more than 10′	Consultation only[b]	Packing or cauterization or antifibrinolytics	Blood transfusion or replacement therapy (use of hemostatic blood components and rFVlla) or desmopressin
Cutaneous	–	No or trivial	Petechiae or bruises	Hematomas	Consultation	–
	–	No or trivial (<1 cm)	>1 cm and no trauma	Consultation only	–	–
	–	No or trivial	> 1 cm and no trauma	Consultation only	–	–
	–	No/trivial	For bruises 5 or more (> 1 cm) in exposed areas	Consultation only[b]	Extensive	Spontaneous hematoma requiring blood transfusion
Minor wounds	–	No or trivial	Present (1–5 episodes/year)	Consultation	Surgical hemostasis	–
	–	No or trivial (<5)	>5 or more than 5′	Consultation only or Steri-Strips	Surgical hemostasis or antifibrinolytics	Blood transfusion or replacement therapy or desmopressin

(continued)

Table 2.2 (continued)

Symptom	Score					
	–	No or trivial	>5 or more than 5′	Consultation only	Surgical hemostasis	Blood transfusion or replacement therapy or desmopressin
	–	No/trivial	> 5/year or more than 10′	Consultation only[b]	Surgical hemostasis	Blood transfusion, replacement therapy, or desmopressin
Oral cavity	–	No or trivial	Present	Consultation only	Surgical hemostasis or blood transfusion	–
	–	No	Reported at least one	Consultation only	Surgical hemostasis or antifibrinolytics	Blood transfusion or replacement therapy or desmopressin
	–	No	Referred at least one	Consultation only	Surgical hemostasis or antifibrinolytics	Blood transfusion or replacement therapy or desmopressin
	–	No/trivial	Present	Consultation only[b]	Surgical hemostasis or antifibrinolytics	Blood transfusion, replacement therapy, or desmopressin
Gastrointestinal	–	No or trivial	Present	Consultation	Surgery or blood transfusion	–
	–	No	Identified cause	Consultation or spontaneous	Surgical hemostasis, antifibrinolytics, blood transfusion, replacement therapy, or desmopressin	–
	–	No	Associated with ulcer, portal hypertension, hemorrhoids, anglodysplasia	Spontaneous	Surgical hemostasis, antifibrinolytics, blood transfusion, replacement therapy, or desmopressin	–
	–	No or trivial	Present but not associated with ulcer, portal hypertension, hemorrhoids, anglodysplasia	Consultation only[b]	Surgical hemostasis, antifibrinolytic	Blood transfusion, replacement therapy, or desmopressin
Hematuria	–	–	–	–	–	–
	–	–	–	–	–	–
	–	–	–	–	–	–
	–	No or trivial	Present (macroscopic)	Consultation only[b]	Surgical hemostasis, antifibrinolytic	Blood transfusion, replacement therapy, or desmopressin
Tooth extraction	–	No or trivial	Present	Suturing or packing	Blood transfusion	–

Table 2.2 (continued)

Symptom	Score					
	No bleeding in at least 2 extractions	None done or no bleeding in 1 extraction	Reported, no consultation	Consultation only	Resuturing, repacking, antifibrinolytics	Blood transfusion, replacement therapy, or desmopressin
	No bleeding in at least 2 extractions	None done or no bleeding in 1 extraction	Reported, no consultation	Consultation only	Resuturing or packing	Blood transfusion, replacement therapy, or desmopressin
	–	No/trivial or none done	Reported in <25% of all procedures, no intervention[c]	Resuturing or packing	Blood transfusion, replacement therapy, or desmopressin	
Surgery	–	No or trivial	Present	Suturing or resurgery	Blood transfusion	–
	No bleeding in at least 2 surgeries	None done or no bleeding in 1 surgery	Reported, no consultation	Consultation only	Surgical hemostasis or antifibrinolytics	Blood transfusion, replacement therapy, or desmopressin
	No bleeding in at least 2 extractions	None done or no bleeding in 1 extraction	Reported, no consultation	Consultation only	Surgical hemostasis or antifibrinolytic	Blood transfusion, replacement therapy, or desmopressin
	–	No/trivial or none done	Reported in <25% of all procedures, no intervention[c]	Surgical hemostasis or antifibrinolytics	Blood transfusion, replacement therapy, or desmopressin	
Menorrhagia	–	No or trivial	Present	Consultation, pill use, iron therapy	Blood transfusion, hysterectomy, D&C	–
	–	No	Reported or consultation only	Antifibrinolytics or pill use	D&C, iron therapy	Blood transfusion or replacement therapy or desmopressin or hysterectomy
	–	No	Consultation only	Antifibrinolytics or pill use	D&C, iron therapy, endometrial ablation	Blood transfusion or replacement therapy or desmopressin or hysterectomy
	–	No/trivial	Consultation only[b] or changing pads more frequently than every 2 h or clot and flooding or PBAC score > 100[d]	Time off work/school >2/year or requiring antifibrinolytics, hormonal or iron therapy	Requiring combined treatment with antifibrinolytics and hormonal therapy or present since menarche and > 12 month	Acute menorrhagia requiring hospital admission and emergency treatment or requiring blood transfusion, replacement therapy, desmopressin, D&C, endometrial ablation, hysterectomy
Postpartum	–	No or trivial	Present, iron therapy	Blood transfusion, D&C, suturing	Hysterectomy	–

(continued)

Table 2.2 (continued)

Symptom	Score					
	No bleeding in at least two deliveries	None done or no bleeding in one delivery	Reported or consultation only	D&C, iron therapy, antifibrinol-ytics	Blood transfu-sion, replace-ment therapy, or desmopressin	Hysterectomy
	No bleeding in at least two deliveries	None done or no bleeding in one delivery	Consultation only	D&C, iron therapy, antifibrinol-ytics	Blood transfu-sion, replace-ment therapy, or desmopressin	Hysterectomy
	–	No/trivial or no deliveries	Consultation only[b] or use of Syntocinon or IV oxytocin >6 week	Iron therapy or antifibri-nolytics	Requiring blood transfusion, replacement therapy, desmopressin, or requiring examination under anesthesia and/or the use of uterine balloon/package to tamponade the uterus	Any procedure requiring critical care of surgical intervention (e.g., hysterectomy, internal iliac artery ligation, uterine artery emboliza-tion, uterine brace suture)
Hemar-throsis	–	No or trivial	Present	Consultation only	Blood transfu-sion, surgery	–
	–	Never	Posttrauma, no therapy	Spontane-ous, no therapy	Spontaneous or traumatic requir-ing desmopres-sin, or replacement therapy	Spontaneous or traumatic, requiring surgical intervention or blood transfusion
	–	Never	Posttrauma, no therapy	Spontane-ous, no therapy	Spontaneous or traumatic requir-ing desmopres-sin, or replacement therapy	Spontaneous or traumatic, requiring surgical intervention or blood transfusion
	–	Never	Posttrauma, no therapy	Spontane-ous, no therapy	Spontaneous or traumatic requir-ing desmopres-sin, or replacement therapy	Spontaneous or traumatic, requiring surgical intervention or blood transfusion
Central nervous system	–	–	–	–	–	–
	–	Never	–	–	Subdural, any intervention	Intracerebral, any intervention
	–	Never	–	–	Subdural, any intervention	Intracerebral, any intervention
	–	Never	–	–	Subdural, any intervention	Intracerebral, any intervention
Other bleeding[c]	–	–	–	–		

Table 2.2   (continued)

Symptom	Score					
	–	No	Reported	Consultation only	Surgical hemostasis, antifibrinolytics, iron therapy	Blood transfusion, replacement therapy, or desmopressin
	–	–	–	–	–	–
	–	No/trivial	Present	Consultation only[b]	Surgical hemostasis, antifibrinolytics	Blood transfusion, replacement therapy, or desmopressin

Notes: The white rows are the scoring system for the original Vicenza Bleeding Questionnaire,[5] the light gray rows for the EU MCMDM-1VWD Bleeding Questionnaire (the "Other" category is not scored) and Pediatric Bleeding Questionnaire,[18] the medium gray rows for the Condensed MCMDM–1VWD Bleeding Questionnaire,[7] and the dark gray rows are for the scoring used for both the ISTH-BAT[10] and Self-BAT[14]
[a]Distinction between 0 and 1 is of critical importance. Score 1 means that the symptom is judged as present in the patient's history by the interviewer but does not qualify for a score of 2 or more (as provided for ISTH-BAT scoring[10])
[b]Consultation only: the patient sought medical evaluation and was either referred to a specialist or offered detailed laboratory investigation (as provided for ISTH-BAT scoring[10])
[c]Example: 1 extraction/surgery resulting in bleeding (100%): the score to be assigned is 2; 2 extractions/surgeries, 1 resulting in bleeding (50%): the score to be assigned is 2; 3 extractions/surgeries, 1 resulting in bleeding (33%): the score to be assigned is 2; 4 extractions/surgeries, 1 resulting in bleeding (25%): the score to be assigned is 1
[d]If already available at the time of collection
[e]Includes umbilical stamp bleeding, cephalohematoma, cheek hematoma caused by sucking during breast/bottle feeding, conjunctival hemorrhage, or excessive bleeding following circumcision or venipuncture. Their presence in infancy requires detailed investigation independently from the overall score

In 2008, the ISTH/SSC Joint Working Group met to establish a consensus BAT. The group proposed a standardized bleeding questionnaire with a defined scoring system for calculating the overall bleeding for use in children and adults with inherited bleeding disorders [5]. Based heavily on the foundations of the Vincenza BAT, the ISTH-BAT was proposed as a consensus BAT and was recommended for universal adoption.

Modern Bleeding Assessment Tools

The ISTH-BAT

Launched in 2010, the ISTH-BAT was designed to achieve greater accuracy by considering not only the severity but also the frequency of bleeding episodes. The scoring system for this tool removed the −1 score for categories including dental extraction and surgery. Administration time for the ISTH-BAT is approximately 10–20 minutes. Normative values for adults and pediatrics were established by collating data from the prior Vincenza-based BAT studies including data from more than 1000 normal adults and 328 children. Abnormal bleeding is defined as a BS of > = 4 in adult males, > = 6 in adult females, and > =3 in children [12]. The ISTH-BAT has subsequently been coupled with an electronic repository, at the Rockefeller University Center for Clinical and Translational Science, with the goal of an expansive dataset on bleeding symptoms in different patient populations [5]. The ISTH-BAT can be found at https://www.isth.org/page/reference_tools [13], and its scoring system is depicted in Table 2.2.

The ISTH-BAT has not been extensively studied and validated in all populations or bleeding disorders, but research using this tool is ongoing. Using the ISTH-BAT, the resultant BS was able to discriminate between patients with vWD and those without a bleeding disorder [14], and higher BS [15] were inversely correlated with vW factor levels. The ISTH-BAT BS was also higher in patients with hemophilia A and B [16]. The BS correlation was mixed in patients with platelet dysfunction: a higher score was found in patients with a platelet function disorder in two studies [17, 18], but Lowe et al. reported that the ISTH-BAT score could not discriminate between patients with or without a platelet defect [19]. The ISTH-BAT BS has also been shown to correlate with the frequency and severity of bleeding symptoms in FXIII-deficient patients [20], thus supporting its future use to evaluate this patient population; however, this tool was not discriminatory in osteogenesis imperfecta [21]. The role of the ISTH-BAT in predicting future bleeding was evaluated, but unfortunately, the BS failed to predict risk of subsequent bleeding in a cohort of consecutive patients [22]. See Table 2.3 for further details on validity of the ISTH-BAT.

Table 2.3 Validity of the BATs in different clinical/research settings

Test (reference)	Age mean (range)	Dz	Study group	Subject number	Sensitivity	Specificity	PPV	NPV
Vincenza [6]	45 (N/A)	vWD	Referral	n = 257; 42 obligate carriers; 215 controls	69.1%	98.6%	33.0%	99.0%
MCMDM-1 VWD [7]	37 (1–91)	vWD	Referral	n = 712; 517 vWD family members; 195 controls	33.0%	88.0%	N/A	N/A
Condensed MCMDM-1 VWD [8]	40 (11–81)	vWD	Primary care	n = 259; 217 possible vWD, 42 known vWD	100.0%	87.0%	20.0%	100.0%
Condensed MCMDM-1 VWD [9]	20.2 (11–31)	MBD	Referral	n = 30	85.0%	90.0%	89.0%	86.0%
Condensed MCMDM-1 VWD [10]	(5–79)	MBD	Referral	n = 215	25–47%	81–98%	3.0%	78.0%
ISTH-BAT [19]	39(31–53)	Plt D/o	Referral	n = 100; 79 suspected plt d/o; 21 healthy	49.0%	53.0%	50.0%	54.0%
ISTH-BAT [18]	15.6 (1–63)	Plt D/o	Referral	n = 64; 48 with GT or BSS; 16 healthy controls	100.0%	76.2%	90.0%	100.0%
ISTH-BAT [17]	43.7	Plt D/o	Referral	n = 555 consecutive pts. with suspected plt d/o	76.9% (m); 52.1% (f)	62.4% (m); 86.1% (f)	N/A	N/A
Self-BAT [23]	43 (18–73)	vWD	Referral	n = 64	78.0%	27.0%	15.0%	88.0%
Self-BAT [23]	43(18–73)	vWD	Referral (females only)	n = 53	100.0%	21.0%	17.0%	100.0%

Table 2.3 (continued)

Test (reference)	Age mean (range)	Dz	Study group	Subject number	Sensitivity	Specificity	PPV	NPV
Self-BAT [24]	(18–72)	HC	Referral	n = 108; 97 HA carriers; 11 HB carriers	71.0%	51.0%	51.0%	71.0%
PBQ [25]	8.3(0.5–17)	vWD	Primary care	n = 151	83.0%	79.0%	14.0%	99.0%
PBQ (vs ISTH-BAT) [14]	5.7(1.1–16.9)	MBD	Referral	n = 100	47.7%	94.9%	87.5%	67.9%
PBQ (vs ISTH-BAT) [14]	5.7(1.1–16.9)	vWD	Referral	n = 100	65.2%	94.6%	83.3%	86.9%
PBQ [26]	<18	vWD	Referral	n = 1281 healthy; 35 with vWD	97.2%	97.1%	48.6%	99.9%
Self-PBQ [s]	9.6(0–18)	vWD	Referral	n = 155	78.0%	37.0%	18.0%	91.0%

The Self-BAT

It is important to note that heretofore all BATs were administered by an expert, a requirement which can have significant ramifications in terms of cost and resource utilization. Implementation of the ISTH-BAT may not be feasible in a busy clinical practice. As such, Deforest et al. sought to develop a self-administered BAT that could be completed without assistance. The development of this BAT required conversion of the ISTH-BAT to a grade 4 reading level. Normative values were re-established, and ultimately an optimized version of the "Self-BAT" was evaluated in first-time referrals to a hematology clinic. The Self-BAT is estimated to take 10 minutes to complete [23]. Refer to Table 2.3 for the scoring grid.

Similar to the ISTH-BAT, limited data on validity of the Self-BAT is available in various populations. In the seminal study of the Self-BAT, its use as a screening tool for VWD (particularly in females) was supported [23]. In hemophilia carriers, the Self-BAT BS inversely correlated with factor levels, and this correlation improved when only carriers with deficient factor levels (<0.5 IU/ml) were included, emphasizing that a good understanding of the study population is required in order to understand its usefulness as a tool [24]. See Table 2.3.

The Pediatric Bleeding Questionnaire

Given the unique challenges of clinical assessment in the pediatric population, a need was identified to tailor the BAT for the younger age group. Children and young adolescents may not have had exposure to hemostatic challenges (surgical, dental, menstrual, and postpartum bleeding), and thus it was felt that the criteria used for identification of bleeding disorders in adults may be overly stringent. In 2009, the Pediatric Bleeding Questionnaire (PBQ) was developed. It is also a derivation of the MCMDM-1 VWD Bleeding Questionnaire with the addition of pediatric-specific bleeding symptoms in an "Other" category. These symptoms include umbilical stump bleeding, cephalohematoma, post-circumcision bleeding, post-venipuncture bleeding, and macroscopic hematuria. Normative data have been obtained, and a bleeding score of <2 was determined to represent normal hemostasis [25]. Refer to Table 2.2 for the scoring grid.

The PBQ has been studied in children with vWD by several research groups and has been shown to be a useful tool to discriminate between affected and unaffected children [14, 25, 26]. Similarly to the ISTH-BAT, the PBQ has not been proven to be a good screening tool for future bleeding risk. In a study investigating 60 children with vWD, the PBQ was not able to predict operative bleeding in elective pediatric surgeries [27]. See Table 2.3.

The Self-PBQ

Of note, Casey et al. generated a Self-PBQ by combining features of the PBQ and the ISTH-BAT. As with the Self-BAT, the questionnaire was translated into a fourth grade reading level. This tool was then evaluated in a population of children referred to a hematologist for bleeding. A positive BS was > = 3. The Self-PBQ was felt to be a reasonable screening tool for the assessment of children with vWD; however it was noted that in cases where there is a significant family history, a normal BS should not preclude diagnostic testing [28]. See Table 2.3.

Menorrhagia-Specific BAT

The Pictorial Blood Assessment Chart

In the late 1980s, Highman et al. designed a chart and scoring system to assess menstrual blood loss. In this tool, termed the Pictorial Blood Assessment Chart (PBAC), the subject's description of the staining of pads or tampons was scored. A total score of greater than 100 per cycle was associated with menstrual blood loss >80 ml. When administered correctly, this tool was felt to improve diagnostic accuracy of HMB [29]. The median time to completion is 10 minutes. This has subsequently been extensively studied in a variety of populations and is felt to have a high level of sensitivity and specificity. Although the PBAC is considered a validated tool for diagnosis of HMB at a cutoff of 80 ml blood loss per cycle, it is unknown if it is a use-

ful tool to assess the effectiveness of HMB treatment, in either a research or a clinical setting [30]. See Fig. 2.1 [31].

The Philipp Screening Tool

In 2008, Philipp et al. developed a screening tool with the goal of helping gynecologists assess which women with menorrhagia to refer for a comprehensive hemostatic evaluation. A group of 146 adolescents with a physician diagnosis of menorrhagia underwent comprehensive hemostatic testing for the diagnosis of bleeding disorders, including von Willebrand disease, platelet dysfunction, and coagulation factor deficiencies. A questionnaire of bleeding symptoms was then administered. Bleeding symptoms with high predictive values for laboratory hemostatic abnormalities were then combined and used as single variables to calculate sensitivity, specificity, and positive and negative predictive values in order to develop a short screening tool to identify women for further evaluation [32]. The Philipp screening tool consists of eight questions in the following four categories: (1) duration of menses ≥7 days and "flooding" or impairment of daily activities with menses, (2) a history of treatment for anemia, (3) a family history of a diagnosed bleeding disorder, or (4) a history of excessive bleeding with tooth extraction, tonsillectomy, adenoidectomy, delivery, or miscarriage, or bleeding complications from surgery. Further refinements have included pairing the Phillip questionnaire with the PBAC, using a higher PBAC cutoff value of 185, and the addition of serum ferritin, all of which increased the sensitivity of the screening tool and further solidified that targeted questions could increase the discerning power of the clinical history [33].

The Warner Criteria

Many early clinical trials confirmed HMB by measurement of blood in sanitary products. Given that this approach is not feasible in clinical practice, Warner et al. sought to identify features

DAY	DAY 1	DAY 2	DAY 3	DAY 4	DAY 5	DAY 6	DAY 7	DAY 8	DAY 9	DAY 10	TOTAL TALLIES	MULTIPLYING FACTOR	ROW TOTAL
(pad – light stain)												×1	
(pad – moderate stain)												×5	
(pad – heavy stain)												×20	
(tampon – light stain)												×1	
(tampon – moderate stain)												×5	
(tampon – heavy stain)												×10	
Small blood clots (= Dime)												×1	
Large blood clots (≥ Quarter)												×5	
Menstrual accidents												×5	
Total Score (Sum of rows)													

How to use the Pictorial Blood Assessment Chart:

- Record the number of tampons and sanitary pads used each day during your period by placing a tally mark under the day next to the box representing the amount of bleeding noted each time you change your pads or tampon (see example at right)
- Record clots by indicating whether they are the size of a dime or a quarter coin in the small and in the large blood clot row under the relevant day.
- Record any incidences of flooding (accidents) by placing a tally mark in the menstrual accident row.

Scoring the Chart:
At the end of your period tabulate a "**Total Score**" by mutiplying the total number or tallies in each row by the "**Multiplying Factor**" at the end of the row. Then sum the "**Row Totals**" to obtain the final "**Total Score**"

Example:
Ms. Smith in the first day of her period, she used 7 pads (5 lightly stained, 1 moderately and 1 heavy stained). She also used 1 moderately stained tampon and had 3 blood clots 1 small and 2 large. She also had one incidence of flooding.

Days	D1	D2	D3	D4
(pad – light stain)	IIII			
(pad – moderate stain)	I			
(pad – heavy stain)	I			
(tampon – light stain)				
(tampon – moderate stain)	I			
Small blood clots (= Dime)	I			
Large blood clots (≥ Quarter)	II			
Menstrual accidents	I			
Total Score				

Fig. 2.1 Pictorial blood loss assessment. (With permission from Springer; El-Nashar, S.A., Shazly, S.A.M. & Famuyide, A.O. Gynecol Surg (2015) 12: 157.) chart

in the clinical history that could predict losses of >80 ml. In 2004, Warner et al. published their more objective symptom-based dataset which determined that the presence of large clots (>1 inch in diameter), low ferritin, and "flooding," defined as changing a pad or tampon hourly or more, were predictive of HMB (defined as >80 ml menstrual blood loss) [34].

Other Specialized BATs

Epistaxis

In 1988, Katsanis et al. published an epistaxis scoring system (ESS) that classified the severity of nosebleeds based on frequency, duration, amount, proportion of life with recurrent nosebleeds, and site. Children with "severe" epistaxis based on the ESS were more likely to have a personal history of bleeding at other sites, a personal history of nasal cautery, a positive family history

of bleeding, as well as laboratory findings of anemia, iron deficiency, and abnormal coagulation testing [35].

Immune Thrombocytopenia

In 2013, Rodegheiro et al. published a proposed consensus-based immune thrombocytopenia (ITP)-specific bleeding assessment tool which included definitions, terminology, and a scoring system for bleeding manifestations in three major domains: skin, visible mucosae, and organs [36]. Bleeding after hemostatic challenges or surgeries was also scored. Severity was graded from 0 to 3 or 4 (with grade 5 reserved for fatal bleeding).

Rare Bleeding Disorders

Given concern that patients with rare bleeding disorders (RBD) were not always captured using previously published BAT, in 2016, the European Network of Rare Bleeding Disorders (EN-RBD) group developed a new bleeding scoring system based on data from 492 patients enrolled in the EN-RBD database. RBD include fibrinogen, factor (F) II, FV, FV + FVIII, VVII, FX, FXI, and FXIII deficiencies. The RBD-BAT was designed to circumvent issues related to age, sex, and the timing of administration of the questionnaire. The RBD-BAT was able to differentiate patients with RBD from healthy individuals with a sensitivity of 67.1% and a specificity of 73.8%. There was a significant negative correlation between the bleeding score and a coagulant factor level especially for fibrinogen and factor XIII deficiencies. Based on symptom data from persons with RBD, the investigators also developed a formula to assess the probability of having a RBD [37].

Alternate Methods of Administering the BAT

As health care has become increasingly technology-forward, new methods of administration of BAT have been trialed. Jacobson et al. created a mobile application used to quantify severity of menstrual bleeding. This was compared with the PBAC in a randomized crossover study design and was found to be feasible as a research tool and the preferred method for recording bleeding in the adolescent population [38].

Reyen et al. capitalized on commonly used social media platforms to promote a website entitled "Let's Talk Period!" in order to increase awareness of undiagnosed bleeding disorders. The website was also a platform in which users could complete an online Self-BAT. This study demonstrated that this format is an effective strategy to reach target populations, but further work is needed to understand if this format will overcome current barriers to the identification and management of women with previously undiagnosed bleeding disorders. Unrestricted access to the Self-BAT can be found at http://letstalkperiod.ca [39].

Benefits and Challenges of the BAT

Benefits

In research, standardization of the BAT has the obvious advantage of facilitating comparison across studies.

In clinical use, the BAT has several possible roles:

(a) Screening: For the practicing clinician, the BAT can be used as a screening tool in both primary and tertiary care settings during the initial evaluation [15]. A structured and uniform approach to the diagnosis of common bleeding disorders may assist nonspecialists in knowing when to refer.

(b) Diagnostic evaluation: The greatest utility of the BAT may lie in the negative predictive value of the bleeding score. When used properly, a low score could highlight patients for whom further testing is not required. For example, in one study, a normal activated partial thromboplastin time and a normal bleeding score almost completely excluded the presence of a bleeding disorder in patients referred for hematologic evaluation [11].

(c) Evaluation of disease severity: Clinicians can also use the BAT to standardize the evaluation of disease severity in those who have already been diagnosed [6].

(d) Assist in disease management: One of the most imperative clinical needs is to predict the inherent bleeding risk such that physicians can intervene in a prophylactic way prior to major bleeding events. There is supporting data that a history of bleeding correlates with higher risk of future bleeding in vWD [8]; however this has not been the case in other studies [22, 27].

Challenges of the BAT

(a) Validity: When evaluating the clinical utility of the various bleeding assessment tools, it is crucial to bear in mind the specific goal and setting of use. One tool may not be generalizable to all situations. Aspects that may impact the validity of the BAT include:

- (i) The administration (Self vs Expert).
- (ii) The setting of the test (Primary vs Tertiary Care).
- (iii) The disease severity (Mild vs Severe).
- (iv) The age of the patient.
- (v) The disease.

(b) Sub-optimal sensitivity/specificity: Criticisms of some BATs note that the scoring is often based on the worst single bleeding episode and may not account for frequency of bleeding symptoms and a plateau effect. This was addressed within the scoring for the ISTH-BAT. In some studies, the sensitivity of the BAT can be enhanced with the combination of simple laboratory tests [40].

Conclusion

In conclusion, while a good clinical assessment remains the fundamental tool of the diagnostician, the development of standardized and validated bleeding assessment tools or BATs to assess for abnormal bleeding can greatly enhance the approach to the bleeding patient. The selective use of a BAT can also limit unnecessary testing and improve the management of the bleeding patient. This is of particular relevance to the adolescent patient in whom the absence of symptoms does not always reflect the hemostatic potential.

In adolescent girls, heavy menstrual bleeding can be associated with significant morbidity. HMB can adversely affect quality of life, academic achievements, interpersonal relationships, friendships, and peer bonding. The impact of an undiagnosed or misdiagnosed bleeding disorder resulting HMB cannot be understated. Therefore, assessment of HMB using simple and low-tech methods such as PBAC in combination with standardized questionnaires can be useful for early recognition and appropriate management of this group.

There exists great opportunity for further study of these tools in the information age. Utilization of smartphone applications and digital media to collect and transmit data on a more precise and measurable platform is the future of diagnostic medicine. The adolescent population in particular, having grown up with technology, are often more comfortable with electronic data and sharing information via mobile applications. Badawy et al. found that adolescents with chronic health conditions (CHC) can improve treatment adherence via use of texting and mobile phone apps [41]. The use of technology in screening, diagnosis, and management of bleeding disorders in adolescents is yet another frontier and presents a unique opportunity for the development of more efficient tools that can improve the quality of life for adolescents with bleeding disorders.

References

1. Tosetto A, et al. Bleeders, bleeding rates and bleeding score. J Thromb Haemost. 2013;11(Suppl. 1):142–50.
2. Nosek-Cenkowska B, Cheang MS, Pizzi NJ, Israels ED, Gerrard JM. Bleeding/bruising symptomatology in children with and without bleeding disorders. Thromb Haemost. 1991;65(3):237–41.
3. James AH. Bleeding disorders in adolescents. Obstet Gynecol Clin N Am. 2009;36(1):153–62.
4. Sadler JE, Rodrigheiro F. Provisional criteria for the diagnosis of VWD. J Thromb Haemost. 2005;3:775–7.
5. Rodegheiro F, Tosetto A, Abshire T, Arnold DM, Coller B, James P, ISTH/SSC joint VWF Perinatal/ Pediatric Hemostasis Subcommittees Working Group. ISTH/SSC bleeding assessment tool: a standardized questionnaire and a proposal for a new bleeding score for inherited bleeding disorders. J Thrombosis Haemost. 2010;8(9):2063–5.
6. Rydz N, James P. The evolution and value of bleeding assessment tools. J Thromb Haemost. 2012;10(11):2223–9.
7. Rodegheiro F, Castaman G, Tosetto A, Batlle J, Baudo F, Capelletti A, Cassana P, De Bosch N, Eikenboom JCJ, Federicia B, Lethagen S, Linari S, Srivastava A. The discriminant power of bleeding history for the diagnosis of type I von Willebrand disease: an international, multicenter study. J Thromb Haemost. 2005;3:2619–26.
8. Tosetto A, Rodegheiro F, Castaman G, et al. A quantitative analysis of bleeding symptoms in type 1 von Willebrand disease: results from a multicenter European study (MCMDM-1 vWD). J Thromb Haemost. 2006;4(4):766–73.
9. Bowman M, Mundell G, Grabell J, Hopman WM, Rapson D, Lillicrap D, James P. Generation and validation of the condensed MCMDM-1 VWD bleeding questionnaire for von Willebrand disease. J Thromb Haemost. 2006;4:766–73.

10. Azzam H, Goneim H, El-Saddik A, Azmy E, Hassan M, El-Sharawy S. The condensed MCMDM-1 VWD bleeding questionnaire as a predictor of bleeding disorders in women with unexplained menorrhagia. Blood Coagul Fibrinolysis. 2012;23:311–5.

11. Tosetto A, Castaman G, Plug I, Rodeghiero F, Eikenboom J. Prospective evaluation of the clinical utility of quantitative bleeding severity assessments in patients referred for hemostatic evaluation. J Thromb Haemost. 2011;9:1143–8.

12. Elbatarny M, Zimmerman Program Investigators, et al. Normal range of bleeding scores for the ISTH-BAT; adult and pediatric data from the merging project. Haemophilia. 2014;20(6):831–5.

13. Bowman M, James P. Bleeding scores for the diagnosis of von Willebrand disease. Semin Thromb Hemost. 2017;43:530–9.

14. Bidlingmaier C, Grote V, Budde U, Olivieri M, Kurnik K. Prospective evaluation of a pediatric bleeding questionnaire and the ISTH bleeding assessment tool in children and parents in routine clinical practice. J Thromb Haemost. 2012;10:1335–41.

15. Pathare A, Al Omrani S, Al Hajri F, Al Obaidani N, Al Balushi B, Al FK. Bleeding score in type 1 von Willebrand disease patients using the ISTH-BAT questionnaire. Int J Lab Hem. 2018;40:175–80.

16. Borhany M, Fatime N, Abid M, Shamsi T, Othman M. Application of the ISTH bleeding score in hemophilia. Transfus Apher Sci. 2018;57(4):556–60.

17. Adler M, Kaufmann J, Alberio L, Nagler M. Diagnostic utility of the ISTH bleeding assessment tool in patients with suspected platelet function disorders. J Thromb Haemost. 2019;17(7):1104–12.

18. Kaur H, Borhany M, Azzam H, Costa-Lima C, Ozelo M, Othman M. The utility of international society on thrombosis and Haemostasis-bleeding assessment tool and other bleeding questionnaires in assessing the bleeding phenotype in two platelet function defects. Blood Coagul Fibrinolysis. 2016;27(5):589–93.

19. Lowe GC, Lordkipanidze M, Watson SP, Group UGs. Utility of the ISTH bleeding assessment tool in predicting platelet defects in participants with suspected inherited platelet function disorders. J Thromb Haemost. 2013;11:1663–8.

20. Naderi M, Cohan N, Haghpanah S, Miri-Aliabad G, Shahramian I, Ahmadinejad M, Sadeghi S, Dorgalaleh A, Khazaei HA, Karimi M. Correlation of bleeding score with frequency and severity of bleeding symptoms in FXIII deficiency assessing by the ISTH bleeding assessment tool. Transfus Apher Sci. 2019;58(4):495.

21. Gooijer K, Rondeel JMM, von Dijk FS, Harsevoort AGJ, Janus GJM, Fanken AAM. Bleeding and bruising in Osteogenesis Imperfecta: International Society of Thrombosis and Haemostasis bleeding assessment tool and haemostasis laboratory assessment in 22 individuals. Br J Haemotol. 2019;187(4):509–17.

22. Fasulo MR, Biguzzi E, Abbattista M, Stufano F, Pagliari MT, Mancini I, Gorski MM, Cannavo A, Corgiolu M, Peyvandi F, Rosendaal FR. The ISHT bleeding assessment tool and the risk of future bleeding. J Thromb Haemost. 2018;16:125–30.

23. Deforest M, Grabell J, Albert S, et al. Generation and optimization of the self-administered bleeding assessment tool and its validation as a screening test for von Willebrand disease. Haemophilia. 2015;21(5):e384–8.

24. Young JE, Grabell J, Tuttle A, Bowman M, Hopman WM, Good D, Rydz N, Mahlangu JN, James PD. Evaluation of a self-administered bleeding assessment tool (Self-BAT) in haemophilia carriers and correlations with quality of life. Haemophilia. 2017;23(6):e536–8.

25. Bowman M, Riddel J, Rand ML, Tosetto A, Silva M, James PD. Evaluation of the diagnostic utility for von Willebrand disease of a pediatric bleeding questionnaire. J Thromb Haemost. 2009;7(8):1418–21.

26. Mittal N, Pederson R, James P, Shott S, Valentino L. Utility of a pediatric bleeding questionnaire as a screening tool for von Willebrand disease in apparently healthy children. Haemophilia. 2015;21(6):806–11.

27. Sim AY, Bowman M, Hopman W, Engen D, Silva M, James P. Predicting operative bleeding in elective pediatric surgeries using the pediatric bleeding questionnaire (PBQ). J Pediatr Hematol Oncol. 2014;36:e246–7.

28. Casey LJ, Tuttle A, Grabell J, Hopman W, Moorehead PC, Blanchette VS, Wu JK, Steele M, Klaasen RJ, Silva M, Rand M, James P. Generation and optimization of the self-administered pediatric bleeding questionnaire and its validation as a screening tool for von Willebrand disease. Pediatr Blood Cancer. 2017;21(5):e384–8.

29. Highman JM, O'Brien PM, Shaw RW. Assessment of menstrual blood loss using a pictorial chart. Br J Obstet Gynaecol. 1990;97(8):234–9.

30. Herman MC. Is the PBAC score associated with treatment outcome after endometrial ablation for HMB? Br J Obstet Gynaecol. 2017;1:277–88.

31. El-Nashar SA, Shazly SAM. Famuyide, Pictorial blood loss assessment chart for quantification of menstrual blood loss: a systematic review. A.O. Gynecol Surg. 2015;12:157.

32. Phillipp CS, Faiz A, Dowling NF, et al. Development of a screening tool for identifying women with menorrhagia for hemostatic evaluation. Am J Obstet Gynecol. 2008;198(2):163.e1–8.

33. Philipp CS, Faiz A, Heit JA, et al. Evaluation of a screening tool for bleeding disorders in a US multisite cohort of women with menorrhagia. Amer J Obstet Gynecol. 2011;204(3):e1–7.

34. Warner PE, Critchley HO, LUmsden MA, Campbell-Brown M, Douglas A, Murray GD. Menorrhagia I: measured blood loss, clinical features and outcome in women with heavy periods: a survey with follow-up data. Am J Obstet Gynecol. 2004;190(5):1216–23.

35. Katsanis E, Luke K, Hsu E, Li M, Lillicrap D. Prevalence and significance of mild bleeding disorders in children with recurrent epistaxis. J Pediatr. 1988;113:73–6.

36. Rodegheiro F, et al. Standardization of bleeding assessment in immune thrombocytopenia: report from the International Working Group. Blood. 2013;121(14):2596–606.
37. Palla R, Siboni S, Menegatti M, Musallam K, Peyvandi F, EN RBD Group. Establishment of a bleeding score as a diagnostic tool for patients with rare bleeding disorders. Thromb Res. 2016;148:128–34.
38. Jacobson AE, et al. Mobile application vs paper pictorial blood assessment chart to track menses in young women: a randomized cross-over design. J Pediatr Adolesc Gynecol. 2018;31:84–8.
39. Reynen E, et al. Let's talk period! Preliminary results of an online bleeding awareness knowledge translation project and bleeding assessment tool promoted on social media. Haemophilia. 2017:e282–6.
40. Alberto Tosetto MD. Bleeding assessment tools: limits and advantages for the diagnosis and prognosis of inherited bleeding disorders. Semin Thromb Hemost. 2016;42(5):463–70.
41. Badawy SM, et al. Text messaging and mobile phone apps as interventions to improve adherence in adolescents with chronic health conditions. JMIR Mhealth Uhealth 2017;5(5):e66.

von Willebrand Disease

Trinh Nguyen and Lakshmi V. Srivaths

Introduction

Erik von Willebrand described "hereditary pseudohemophilia" in 1926 after studying a family of bleeders from Åland [1, 2]. The factor responsible for this disease was later named von Willebrand factor (VWF) [1], and the *VWF* gene was subsequently cloned in 1985 [1, 3]. von Willebrand disease (VWD) is the most common inherited bleeding disorder [4–6]. The bleeding manifestations in VWD range from mild to severe; however due to the hemostatic challenges of menstruation and childbirth, bleeding is more commonly reported in post-menarchal females, including heavy menstrual bleeding (HMB), pregnancy and postpartum hemorrhage (PPH), and other gynecologic bleeding [4, 7]. This chapter reviews the epidemiology, pathophysiology, clinical manifestations, evaluation, and management of VWD with emphasis on female-specific bleeding details and challenges.

Epidemiology

VWD occurs in all ethnicities [8]. The estimated prevalence of VWD in the general population is 0.6–1.3% [4, 5] with a reported symptomatic

T. Nguyen · L. V. Srivaths (✉)
Department of Pediatrics, Section of Hematology, Baylor College of Medicine, Houston, TX, USA
e-mail: lvsrivat@texaschildrens.org

prevalence of 1 in 1000 individuals [9]. Although VWD is autosomally inherited [6, 7], there is a disproportionally higher frequency of females diagnosed with VWD due to their obstetric and gynecological hemostatic challenges [6, 7]. Among females with HMB, the estimated prevalence of VWD is 5–20% in adult women [10, 11] and 5–36% in adolescent females [4, 10, 12]. These prevalence data are likely an underestimation, as many females with bleeding symptoms may not seek medical attention [4, 5, 13], influenced by sociocultural factors [14]. Lack of provider awareness of bleeding disorder screening and assessment may also contribute to underdetection of VWD [13, 15, 16].

Pathophysiology

VWF is a large multimeric glycoprotein which binds collagen at sites of vascular injury, mediating platelet adhesion and aggregation, and stabilizing and transporting FVIII in circulation [17, 18], thereby having a dual role in primary and secondary hemostasis [18]. The *VWF* gene is located on the short arm of chromosome 12, spanning 178-kb consisting of 52 exons [17–19]. VWF is produced by vascular endothelial cells and megakaryocytes [20, 21]. A prepropolypeptide VWF transcript is synthesized in the endoplasmic reticulum (ER) [19, 21] which undergoes posttranslational modifications and dimerization of the VWF monomer to form

© Springer Nature Switzerland AG 2020
L. V. Srivaths (ed.), *Hematology in the Adolescent Female*,
https://doi.org/10.1007/978-3-030-48446-0_3

dimers and multimers of varying sizes from 500 to >20,000 kDa [19, 21]. The ultra-large molecular weight multimers (ULMWM) and the high molecular weight multimers (HMWM) are the most "biologically active" [21]. The VWF multimers are stored as ULMWM in the cigar-shaped Weibel-Palade bodies of the endothelial cells [20, 22] and released upon vascular damage. In circulation, they are rendered less thrombogenic with degradation by ADAMTS13 (a disintegrin and metalloprotease with a thrombospondin type 1 motif, member 13) [18, 22].

VWD is a spectrum of disorders characterized by quantitative or qualitative deficiencies of the VWF. Inheritance is autosomal dominant except in types 2 N and 3 VWD, which have autosomal recessive inheritance (Table 3.1) [17]. *VWF* gene variants have incomplete penetrance and variable expressivity. As a result, crossover of mild bleeding symptomatology also seen in the normal population makes definitive diagnosis of milder phenotypes difficult [9, 23].

Type 1 VWD is the most common, representing 60–80% of VWD cases reported [1, 3, 6, 14].

Table 3.1 Genetics of von Willebrand disease

Type of VWD	Mode of inheritance	Sites of mutations	Genetic defect
Type 1[c]	AD[a]	Spans *VWF* gene	Mostly missense mutations
Type 2A[c]	AD	A1 domain A2 domain D3 domain Cysteine knot D2 domain	Missense mutations
Type 2B	AD	A1 domain	Missense mutation[d]
Type 2 M	AD	A1 domain A3 domain	Missense mutations[e]
Type 2 N	AR[b]	D' domain Propeptide cleavage site D3 domain	Missense mutations
Type 3	AR	Spans *VWF* gene	Mostly null alleles

[a]Autosomal dominant
[b]Autosomal recessive
[c]Generally AD, but may be AR
[d]Resulting in gain of function
[e]Resulting in loss of function

Mutations causing type 1 VWD have been discovered in only 70% of the patients [1, 17]. Most are missense mutations spanning the entire gene [17], leading to defective pathophysiological mechanisms including aberrant storage, secretion, and accelerated clearance of VWF [17, 20]. This results in mild to moderate deficiencies of VWF antigen (VWF:Ag) and platelet binding function measured as VWF activity (VWF:Act). The VWF:Act/VWF:Ag ratio is >0.6 due to proportionately decreased protein and function. Multimer analysis will show a decrease in all multimer sizes.

Type 2A VWD is the second most common type, representing 20–25% of VWD cases [17, 21], and characterized by missense mutations that affect the assembly of the HMWM and/or allow for increased ADAMTS13-mediated proteolysis, resulting in loss of HMWM, low VWF:Ag, and an even lower VWF:Act. The VWF:Act/VWF:Ag ratio is typically <0.6 [24]. Multimer analysis will show loss of HMWM.

Type 2B VWD results from a gain-of-function missense mutation in the GPIbα-binding domain of the *VWF*, with increased affinity and binding to platelets [17, 20, 23], resulting in increased clearance of VWF and platelets, with development of thrombocytopenia [17, 20, 23]. VWF:Ag and VWF:Act are both low, with VWF:Act/VWF:Ag ratio < 0.6. Multimer analysis will show loss of HMWM and intermediate multimers.

Mutation of the GPIb gene (GPIBA) causes a platelet-type VWD (pseudo-VWD) due to a gain-of-function mutation increasing the binding affinity of platelets for VWF [17, 19, 24]. Clinical presentation and lab analysis are similar to type 2B VWD, but the mutation is not in the *VWF* gene [17].

Type 2 M VWD results from loss-of-function *VWF* missense mutations affecting GPIbα or collagen binding, resulting in decreased platelet-binding [17, 20, 23]. Mutations in GPIbα will result in decreased VWF:Act and VWF:Act/VWF:Ag ratio <0.6 due to decreased binding of VWF to GPIbα; however, VWF:Ag and multimer assays will be normal. In contrast, mutations affecting VWF binding to collagen will result in normal VW studies except VWF collagen binding assay [17, 20, 23].

Type 2 N VWD results from *VWF* missense mutations leading to decreased binding of VWF to FVIII and increased proteolysis and mild to moderate deficiency of FVIII with levels between 5% and 40% [17, 24]. In addition to autosomal recessive inheritance pattern, individuals with type 2 N VWD may inherit one type 2 N and one type 1 VWD allele [24]. This compound hetero-zygous inheritance pattern is associated with low VWF:Ag and VWF:Act [24].

Type 3 VWD is the least common and most severe type of VWD [5, 17]. Mutations span the *VWF* gene [17] including large deletions and null and missense mutations, resulting in essentially no production or secretion of VWF. VWF:Ag and VWF:Act are <5%, and consequently FVIII activity (FVIII:C) is <10% [17, 20, 23]. In addition to autosomal recessive inheritance pattern, inheritance of two mutant co-dominant alleles can occur when both parents have type 1 VWD [1, 17, 23].

Bleeding manifestations in types 2 N and 3 VWD include typical mucosal symptoms; how-ever, more severe bleeding such as gastrointesti-nal bleeding or even hemarthrosis, similar to persons with hemophilia, can occur [5, 17, 24].

Reports from the Zimmerman and the Low VWF in Ireland Cohort (LoViC) studies have shown that patients with low VWF levels have clinically significant bleeding history and ele-vated bleeding scores similar to patients with type 1 VWD [25, 58]. The interim report of a study on adolescents with low VWF reported gynecologic and other bleeding and associated complications [26]. Clinical guidelines from the National Heart, Lung, and Blood Institute, the European Group on VWD, and the UK Doctors' Haemophilia Organisation state that patients with decreased levels of VWF should be considered as two subsets: patients with significant reduction of VWF levels (<30 IU/dL) with significant bleed-ing manifestations and more likely to have iden-tifiable *VWF* gene mutations inherited in an autosomal dominant pattern be labeled as type 1 VWD [27]. In contrast, patients with milder reduction in VWF levels (30–50 IU/dL) and vari-able bleeding manifestations with less frequent VWF gene variations can be called as having "low VWF levels" [27]. Recent studies have shown both reduced synthesis and secretion from endothelial cells and enhanced clearance of VWF as potential causative mechanisms in patients with low VWF levels [28].

Acquired von Willebrand Syndrome (AVWS) is a rare bleeding disorder with similar clinical manifestations and laboratory results as inher-ited VWD [10, 22]. Typically there is no per-sonal or family history of bleeding prior to clinical presentation [10]. Etiologies causing AVWS include autoimmune disorders, malig-nancy, and congenital or acquired heart diseases, which result in increased clearance of normally produced VWF:Ag by antibodies, shear stress destruction and loss of HMWM, increased prote-olysis, and/or adsorption of VWF by malignant cells [10]. Therapy for AVWS includes hemo-static therapy as well as treating the underlying cause which usually causes resolution of AVWS [10, 21, 22].

Genetic and Physiologic Modifiers of VWD

Genetic modifiers outside of the *VWF* gene may be associated with lower VWF levels. One nota-ble genetic modifier is the ABO blood group, wherein blood type O has been shown to be asso-ciated with 25% lower VWF levels when com-pared to other blood types [1, 17, 20, 23]. Genome-wide association studies have identified several genetic loci that are associated with vari-able VWF levels in patients with VWD and healthy individuals [1, 9, 23]. Recent studies have documented the significance of increased clearance of VWF through various mechanisms with regard to the pathophysiology of type 1 VWD and also some types 2 and 3 VWD [28]. The interim report of a study on adolescents with low VWF documented the presence of VWF clearance receptor gene variants in post-menarchal adolescent females with HMB [26].

Physiologic and other modifiers of VWF lev-els include age, ethnicity, stress, anxiety, inflammation, thyroid abnormalities, estrogen use, timing of menstrual cycle, and pregnancy [2, 7, 14, 29]. Individuals of African or Korean ancestry have been demonstrated to have higher VWF:Ag [5, 20] levels than Caucasians. VWF rises by 1–2% per year [9] and sometimes normalizes, but what is unknown is whether the bleeding tendency is mitigated by higher VWF levels.

Presenting Features

Bleeding Manifestations and Complications

Signs and symptoms of VWD depend on the type and severity of the disease [12]. Bleeding manifestations include easy bruising, mucocutaneous bleeding including epistaxis, gingival bleeding, hematuria, and gastrointestinal bleeding, post-surgery and post-trauma bleeding, heavy menstrual and other gynecological bleeding, and bleeding with pregnancy and parturition [4, 12, 22, 30]. HMB is the most common presentation in females with VWD, with up to 75–93% of females with VWD reporting HMB [7, 31].

Heavy Menstrual Bleeding

HMB (previously termed menorrhagia) is the most common presentation of VWD in females of reproductive age by self-report and by objective confirmation [7, 13, 32], and HMB at menarche is often the first sign of VWD in affected individuals [15, 16, 33].

As only 40–50% of women with subjective HMB were found to have objective confirmation of HMB [34], objective criteria have been developed to standardize HMB evaluations which include the following:

- Bleeding lasting for ≥7 days.
- Loss of >80 mL blood per menstrual cycle.
- Soaking through pads/tampons every 1 hour.
- Soaking onto clothes, beddings, or linens.
- Passing clots.

- Pictorial blood assessment chart (PBAC) score of >100.
- Presence of anemia.
- Presence of low ferritin.

Other Gynecologkical Bleeding

Females with VWD are at risk of bleeding during gynecologic procedures and more likely to require transfusion support [6, 31]. Incidence of fibroids [1, 4, 31, 34] and endometriosis [1, 4, 31, 34] in females with VWD is reported to be higher than in controls, though the data is limited. Bleeding into corpus luteal cysts at ovulation leading to mid-cycle pain termed mittelschmerz [7, 12] and hemorrhagic ovarian cysts (HOC) have been reported with increased frequency in females with VWD (52% in VWD vs. 22% in controls) [35]. Ruptured corpus luteal or HOC as a rare complication may lead to hemoperitoneum, need for transfusion support, and acute surgical intervention [6]. Rarely, hemoperitoneum has preceded the diagnosis of VWD [6].

Bleeding During Pregnancy and Postpartum

VWF levels increase 2–3-fold during pregnancy [1, 21, 36]; however, median levels remain lower in females with than those without VWD [10]. The rise in VWF:Ag is not sufficient enough in type 3 VWD and does not alleviate the bleeding predisposition in type 2 VWD as the qualitative defect persists [1, 36]. Moreover, a corresponding rise in VWF:Ag may exacerbate the thrombocytopenia in women with type 2B VWD [36]. A retrospective study by James and Jamison reported a tenfold risk of antepartum bleeding in females with VWD [37].

Both primary (within the first 24 hours) and secondary PPH (after the first 24 hours) occur at higher frequency in females with VWD than in the general population [36–38] with bleeding risk persisting up to 6 weeks postpartum [36, 37, 39]. James et al. reported a rapid decline in VWF and

FVIII levels by 1 week post- delivery, reaching baseline levels by 3 weeks postpartum in females with VWD [40]. In addition, females with VWD treated with products to raise VWF levels at delivery and postpartum did not achieve levels as seen in females without VWD, suggesting they still remain at risk for PPH [40].

Diagnosis

Diagnosis of VWD is based on a combination of personal and family history of bleeding as well as laboratory assays of VWF:Ag, VWF:Act, and FVIII:C [5, 20, 23, 57]. Menstrual and bleeding assessment scores have been developed to help screen patients with bleeding manifestations for VWD testing.

Bleeding Assessment

The Pictorial Blood Assessment Chart (PBAC) score is a useful clinical tool to quantify menstrual bleeding, with a score of >100 associated with the diagnosis of HMB [41]. A single center study in adolescents suggested score of >165 as indicating HMB in the adolescent population [42]. The American College of Obstetricians and Gynecologists (ACOG) 2019 guidelines recommend using the PBAC score with the bleeding questionnaire developed by Philipp et al. as a screening tool for bleeding evaluation in adolescents presenting with HMB [33, 43]. Whereas the questionnaire was only 62% sensitive for bleeding disorders in adolescents, the sensitivity improved to 95% when used with a PBAC score of >100 [43].

Various bleeding assessment tools (BATs) have been devised to standardize bleeding evaluation and for comparison of bleeding phenotypes [44]. In 2010, ISTH published the ISTH-BAT, with a positive/abnormal bleeding score (BS) of ≥4 in adult males, ≥6 in adult females, and ≥ 3 in children [44]. The Self-BAT, which is a modified ISTH-BAT, was validated as a screening tool with sensitivity of 78% for diagnosis of VWD in adults only [44]. The pediatric bleeding questionnaire

(PBQ) was developed from the MCMDM-1 VWD bleeding questionnaire with the addition of pediatric-specific bleeding symptoms such as umbilical stump bleeding, cephalohematoma, and post-circumcision bleeding and had a sensitivity of 83% and specificity of 79% for the diagnosis of VWD in children with BS ≥2 [44]. A Self-PBQ, modified from the PBQ and ISTH-BAT, was recently shown to have sensitivity of 78% and specificity of 37% for the diagnosis of VWD in children with BS ≥3 [45]. Limitations of BATs include lack of specificity and being age-dependent and time-consuming [1, 5, 10, 20].

Laboratory Evaluation (Fig. 3.1)

Initial evaluation for an individual presenting with a possible bleeding disorder should include a complete blood count to look for anemia and thrombocytopenia and coagulation studies including prothrombin time, activated partial thromboplastin time, and serum fibrinogen level to assess for other coagulation disorders (Table 3.2) [4, 15, 20, 36].

The platelet function analyzer (PFA-100® Dade-Behring Inc., Miami, FL, USA) was demonstrated to be an appropriate screening tool for VWD in adult women with HMB with sensitivity of 80–100% [46]. PFA-100®may miss milder forms of VWD, however [10]. For adolescents presenting with HMB, Naik et.al reported that the PFA-100® had no diagnostic utility in screening for VWD, with sensitivity of only 52% [47].

Diagnostic Assays for VWD

Testing for VWD should include VWF:Ag, VWF:Act (such as the VWF:RCo assay and VWF:Gp1b assay), and FVIII:C (Table 3.3) [1, 5, 17, 24].

The VWF:RCo assay is insensitive at VWF levels <10–20% and has a high coefficient of variation [5, 17]. In recent years, newer VWF functional assays using recombinant GPIb fragments with higher sensitivity and precision have replaced the VWF:RCo assay in some laboratories [1, 5, 9,

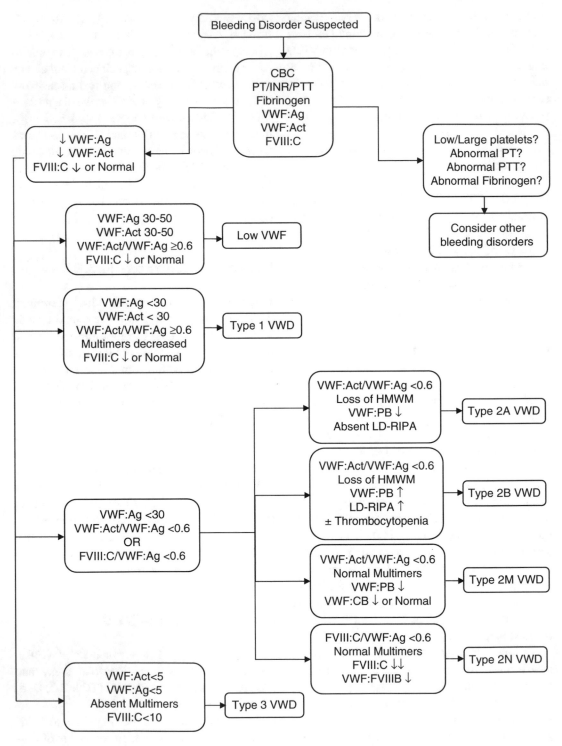

Fig. 3.1 Flow diagram for evaluation for von Willebrand disease

Table 3.2 Screening tests for suspected bleeding disorders

Test	Function
Complete blood count	Screening for anemia and thrombocytopenia
Prothrombin time Activated partial thromboplastin time Fibrinogen	Screening for coagulation factor deficiencies
VWF:Ag assay VWF:Act assay 1. Ristocetin-dependent functional assays (VWF:RCo and VWF-GPIbR). 2. Ristocetin-independent functional assays (VWF:GP1bM).	Screening for von Willebrand disease
FVIII:C assay	Screening for FVIII deficiency and von Willebrand disease

20]. The VWF-GPIbR binding assay continues to use ristocetin to trigger VWF-GPIb binding and therefore has similar limitations as the VWF:RCo assay. The VWF:GPIbM utilizes the spontaneous binding of VWF with a recombinant mutant gain-of-function GPIb fragment independent of ristocetin [5, 9, 20] and has higher sensitivity, lower limit of detection of 2 IU/dL, and greater precision [5]. As plasma levels of VWF can vary significantly over time due to many factors, guidelines recommend repeat testing to ensure consistency in levels prior to assigning diagnosis.

A low VWF:Act/VWF:Ag ratio <0.6 is associated with type 2 VWD diagnosis (type 2A, 2B, 2 M), while type 1 VWD and type 2 N have a higher ratio of ≥0.6 [10, 17, 24]. Analysis of VWF multimers will show normal or mild reduction of all multimer sizes in type 1 VWD and low

Table 3.3 Diagnosis of von Willebrand disease

VWD type	VWF/FVIII assays (IU/dL)	VWF:Act/VWF:Ag Ratio	Multimers	Other diagnostic tests
Low VWF	VWF:Act[a] 30–50 VWF:Ag[b] 30–50 FVIII:C[c]↓ or normal	≥0.6	Normal	
Type 1	VWF:Act[a]<30 VWF:Ag[b] < 30 FVIII:C[c]↓ or normal	≥0.6	Normal or decreased in all multimer sizes	
Type 2A	VWF:Act[a]<30 VWF:Ag[b] < 30–200 FVIII:C[c] ↓ or normal	<0.6	Loss of HMWM	VWF:PB[d]↓ LD-RIPA[e] – Absent
Type 2B	VWF:Act[a]<30 VWF:Ag[b] < 30–200 FVIII:C[c]↓ or normal	<0.6	Loss of HMWM and intermediate multimers	VWF:PB[d]↑ LD-RIPA[e]↑ ± thrombocytopenia
Type 2 M	VWF:Act[a]<30 VWF:Ag[b] < 30–200 FVIII:C[c]↓ or normal	<0.6	Normal	VWF:PB[d]↓ VWF:CB[f]↓ or normal
Type 2 N	VWF:Act[a] 30–200 VWF:Ag[b] 30–200 FVIII:C[c]↓↓ (5–40%)	>0.6	Normal	FVIII:C/VWF:Ag <0.6 VWF:FVIIIB[g] ↓
Type 3[h]	VWF:Act[a]<5 VWF:Ag[b] < 5 FVIII:C[c] < 10	N/A	Absent	

[a]VWF:Act IU/dL
[b]VWF:Ag IU/dL
[c]FVIII:C IU/dL
[d]VWF:PB = von Willebrand factor – platelet binding
[e]LD-RIPA = low dose Ristocetin-induced platelet aggregation
[f]VWF:CB = von Willebrand factor – collagen binding
[g]VWF:FVIIIB = von Willebrand factor – FVIII binding
[h]Consider genetic testing for types 3, 2A, 2B, 2M and 2N when diagnosis is not clear

VWF activity, essentially no multimers present in type 3 VWD, and loss of HMWM in types 2A and 2B VWD [10, 17, 24].

Factor VIII activity will be normal or slightly reduced in type 1 VWD, low VWF, and types 2A, 2B, and 2 M VWD, low in type 2 N VWD, and very low in type 3 VWD [1, 10, 17, 24]. The FVIII:C/VWF:Ag ratio is <0.6 in type 2 N [3, 20]. The binding affinity of patient's VWF for FVIII (VWF:FVIIIB) is decreased in type 2 N VWD, helping to differentiate it from hemophilia [10, 17, 19, 24].

In the absence of thrombocytopenia, it may be challenging to differentiate type 2A from type 2B VWD. The VWF-platelet binding assay (VWF:PB) assesses the ability of patient plasma to bind to commercial platelets, which is increased in type 2B VWD [24]. The response to low-dose ristocetin-induced platelet aggregation (LD-RIPA) is increased in type 2B VWD, as spontaneous aggregation occurs even at low doses ($\leq$0.6 mg/mL) of ristocetin [24]. Similarly, type 2B VWD may be differentiated from platelet-type VWD by normal VWF:PB utilizing the patient's plasma, in the latter [24].

Type 2 M VWD may have normal VWF:Ag, VWF:Act, FVIII:C, and multimers, when the defect is in the binding of collagen. The VWF collagen binding assay is low in these subtypes; however, there are multiple types of collagen, each requiring specific testing [10, 14, 24]. This diagnosis may be missed if genetic testing is not completed. Reduced collagen binding may also be seen in type 1 and type 3 VWD due to low VWF:Ag and type 2A and type 2B VWD due to decreased HMWM [19].

Measurement of the VWF propeptide (VWFpp) and the elevated VWFpp/VWF:Ag ratio may be helpful to identify accelerated clearance defects including type 1C VWD, some type 2 VWD variants, and AVWS [10, 23, 24].

Genetic Analysis

Gene sequencing of *VWF* is not routinely performed but may be warranted in type 3 and some type 2 VWD variants, particularly type 2A, 2B, 2M and 2N when diagnosis is not clear [1, 10, 17, 24]. Genetic analysis may be warranted for prenatal diagnosis and counseling and for differentiation between type 2 N VWD and hemophilia A as management is different in these disorders [23]. Traditional mutation analysis utilized PCR and Sanger sequencing [24]; however new developments including next-generation sequencing allow for more than one gene to be analyzed simultaneously and detection of deletions/duplications that cause VWD [23].

Most of the mutations for VWD Type 2A cluster in A1 and A2 domains, encoded by exon 28 [48]. The D3 domain (exons 22 and 25–27) is the site of >25% of 2A mutations, and rarer mutations are found in the cysteine knot (CK, exon 52) and D2 domains (exons 11–17) with occasional mutations elsewhere in the gene [48]. Type 2B VWD mutations have a restricted location within the A1 domain encoded by the 5′ end of exon 28 [48]. Type 2 M mutations are located in the A1 domain (exon 28) or A3 domain (exons 28–32) [48]. Type 2 N mutations lie predominantly in the D′ domain (exons 18–20), and few may lie close to the propeptide cleavage site (exon 17) and in the D3 domain (exons 24–25) [48]. Targeted analysis of exon 28 is a starting point for type 2 VWD genetic analysis [48], and if this does not detect a causative genetic variant, then an extended exon analysis of the *VWF* gene may be undertaken.

Exon 28 polymorphism p.D1472H has been associated with lower in vitro VWF:RCo/VWF:Ag ratio without increased bleeding phenotype [49]. The presence of this mutation has led to mis-labeling patients as having VWD with resultant unnecessary therapy [49]. To date, over 750 mutations have been identified in the *VWF* gene with only ~220 proven to cause disease in vitro or in vivo [3]. Recent studies have shown mutations of clearance receptors and glycosylation enzymes as causing low VWF levels due to increased clearance [26, 28], which may in part explain the pathophysiology in some patients lacking *VWF* gene variations. Other genetic modifiers such as ABO blood type, through increased clearance and/or other unidentified mechanisms, have also been associated with low VWF levels. A study to compare genetic variations with bleeding manifestations, response to medications, and outcome in adolescent females with HMB and low VWF is currently underway [26] (clinicaltrials.gov, #NCT02933411).

Time of Testing, Sample Collection, Processing, and Handling

As VWF levels have been shown to vary due to various physiologic factors, testing is best done in post-menarchal females during menstrual cycles and when they are not taking estrogen therapy. Sidonio et al. demonstrated the cost-effectiveness of testing for VWD in adolescents with HMB prior to initiation of oral contraception (OC) [32]. Pregnancy, acute inflammation, exercise, stress, and anxiety of venipuncture can lead to falsely elevated levels. Traumatic blood draws, agitation of blood samples, delay in transport, and processing can also lead to erroneous values.

Management

General Management

Management of bleeding manifestations in adolescent females with VWD includes both VWD-specific hemostatic therapy to increase VWF levels and supportive therapy with antifibrinolytics and hormonal therapy for HMB (Table 3.4). Females with VWD should be advised to avoid nonsteroidal anti-inflammatory drugs or other agents affecting platelet function and increasing bleeding risk [21, 33, 36, 39].

Factor-Based Therapy

DDAVP (1-deamino-8-D-arginine vasopressin), a synthetic analog of desmopressin, acts by stimulating release of VWF and FVIII from endothelial Weibel-Palade bodies [2, 4, 6, 50]. DDAVP is approved for use via intravenous (IV) or intra-

Table 3.4 von Willebrand disease therapy

Therapeutic category	Options
VWD-specific hemostatic therapy	DDAVP[a] Plasma-derived VWF/FVIII concentrate Recombinant VWF
General hemostatic therapy	Antifibrinolytics Tranexamic acid Aminocaproic acid
Hormonal therapy[b]	Estrogen Progesterone Combination
Surgical/procedural therapy	Surgical Foley balloon tamponade Uterine artery embolization Uterine packing[c] Endometrial ablation[c] Dilation and curcttage[c] Hysterectomy[c]
Other factors	Recombinant factor VII for VWD type 3 with inhibitor
Treatment for anemia	Oral or intravenous iron PRBC transfusion

VWD = von Willebrand Disease
[a]Need to assess patient response to DDAVP prior to use
[b]Various formulations including oral pills, patches, injections, implants, intrauterine device
[c]If no longer desire fertility

nasal (IN) routes in the USA. The subcutaneous (SQ) route is not approved in the USA. Assessment of response to therapy with challenge test (dose of 0.3 microgram/kg IV given with timed analysis of VWF:Ag, VWF:Act, and FVIII:C, at 0 hour, 1 hour, and 4 hours) is necessary to avoid unwarranted use in nonresponders [5, 17, 36]. Response to IN route is required even if there is a response to IV DDAVP dose [21]. Stimate (CSL Behring LLC, Kiel, Germany) (1.5 mg/mL solution) is administered as 150 microgram per puff per nostril (<50 kg:1 puff in one nostril; ≥50 kg:1 puff each in both nostrils) [17, 51], and a 2–4-fold rise in levels [1] denotes response. Adverse effects include headaches, facial flushing, hypertension, hypotension, hyponatremia, and rarely seizures [4, 5, 21]. Desmopressin is effective in ~80% of type 1 VWD patients [5] and ~13% in type 2 patients [52]. The response may be short-lived in type 2 N VWD [52]. Desmopressin is relatively contraindicated in type 2B VWD as it may exacerbate the thrombocytopenia [17, 21] and is not effective in type 3 VWD [21].

Plasma-derived VWF/FVIII (pd-VWF/FVIII) concentrates are available for treatment of patients with VWD who do not respond to or unable to tolerate DDAVP and type 1 VWD and low VWF level patients with severe or prolonged bleeding and type 2 and 3 VWD [12, 17, 21]. Many pd-VWF/FVIII concentrates are commercially available with varying concentrations of VWF:Act and FVIII (Humate-P®, Alphanate®, Wilate®) [1]. Dosing recommendations are generally based on the desired goal of VWF:Act and/or FVIII:C.

A recombinant VWF (rVWF), vonicog alfa (Vonvendi®, Baxalta, Bannockburn, IL, USA) was FDA approved in 2015 and 2018 for adults ≥18 years for on-demand management of bleeding [52, 53] and perioperative management of bleeding, respectively. Manufactured from genetically engineered CHO cell line co-expressing the VWF and FVIII genes and devoid of human or animal proteins, the risks of pathogen transmission and allergic reaction are essentially eliminated [18, 52]. This rVWF contains the ULMWM and HMWM and has greater activity than its pd-VWF/FVIII counterpart [18, 22, 52]. Initial dose of 40–50 IU/kg is recommended for minor bleeds and 50–80 IU/kg for major bleeds [18, 53] with subsequent doses and frequency dependent on location and extent of bleeding [53]. For patients with baseline FVIII:C < 40% or unknown levels, it is recommended to infuse an approved rFVIII product with the first dose rVWF [53]. Currently an uncontrolled, open-label, phase 3a, multicenter study on the long-term safety and efficacy of rVWF including pediatric patients aged 12–18 with severe VWD is underway (www.clinicaltrials.govIdentifier# NCT03879135).

Patients with type 3 VWD especially with large deletions are at risk of developing antibodies to VWF [19]. Pd-VWF/FVIII concentrates are contraindicated in these individuals with life-threatening anaphylactic reactions [52], and rVWF and recombinant factor VII may be utilized as treatment options.

Non-factor Therapy

Antifibrinolytics prevent the conversion of plasminogen to plasmin, thereby inhibiting fibrinolysis and stabilizing the clot [6, 21]. Tranexamic acid (TA; Lysteda®) (given as PO at 1300 mg three times a day for 5 days for HMB, FDA approved for use in adult women >18 years of age, IV dose of 10–15 mg/kg every 8 hours, or as a mouthwash) and epsilon-aminocaproic acid (EACA; Amicar®, Xanodyne Pharmaceuticals, Inc. Newport, KY, USA) (given PO at 50–100 mg/kg/dose every 6 hours or IV every 6–8 hours) can be administered for up to 7 days in the setting of mucosal or menstrual bleeding [21].

Hormonal therapy (estrogen, progesterone, or combination of both) available in various formulations (oral pills, patches, injections, implants, and intrauterine devices) has been used for HMB control in females with VWD [2, 5, 54]. The levonorgestrel-releasing intra-uterine system (LNG-IUD) (Mirena; Schering Oy, Turku, Finland) has been shown to be effective in both adolescents and adult women with VWD [4, 59]. Successful and sustained placement may require hemostatic prophylaxis to minimize bleeding complications [34, 59].

In patients with low VWF levels, general hemostatic therapy such as antifibrinolytics and hormonal therapy are offered upfront for mild to moderate bleeding, with factor-based therapy reserved for patients with severe bleeding complications.

Management of Heavy Menstrual Bleeding

Treatment options for HMB include hormonal therapy, DDAVP, and factor concentrates for severe bleeding and DDAVP non-responders [1, 5, 54]. TA and/or EACA can be used as primary or adjunctive therapies. There are few data available on long-term VWF replacement to reduce HMB. A survey on HTCs by Ragni et al. showed 13 women receiving VWF infusions as third-line treatment, at 50 IU/kg/dose for up to 5 days per cycle with 100% reported reduction in all [54]. A new study comparing rVWF to TA for HMB in type 1 VWD is underway (VWDMin trial) (ClinicalTrials.gov Identifier NCT02606045).

Surgical options including endometrial ablation, dilation and curettage, and hysterectomy may be options for woman who no longer desire fertility; however, these are not typically offered to adolescents in order to preserve fertility [4, 12, 51]. Other methods including Foley balloon tamponade of the endometrial cavity, uterine artery embolization, and uterine packing remain options for females with HMB and VWD [4].

Management of Bleeding During Pregnancy and Postpartum

Pregnant females with VWD should be managed by a multidisciplinary team [33, 36, 39], with delivery planned at a center with lab and blood bank support [36, 39]. Females with VWD are at a high risk for spinal or epidural hematoma [33]. Females with VWF and FVIII levels >50 IU/dL may be candidates for epidural anesthesia as well as vaginal delivery [21, 40]. Assistive devices such as forceps or vacuum suctioning should be avoided to prevent trauma [36, 39]. Close monitoring of blood counts and coagulation labs are recommended during pregnancy and postpartum [36, 39]. Hemostatic therapy includes antifibrinolytics, DDAVP, and VWF [36]. Desmopressin (after cord clamping) [21] and factor concentrates in the third trimester have been recommended to achieve VWF:Act and FVIII:C goal >100 IU/dL [1] and >50 IU/dL, respectively, for 3 days after vaginal delivery and 5 days following caesarean section [36]. James et al. reported that even when treated with VWF, females with VWD appear to be at risk of PPH [40].

Hormonal therapy, DDAVP, factor concentrates, antifibrinolytics, and surgical and procedural methods form the armamentarium for management of other gynecological bleeding complications.

Management of Anemia and Iron Deficiency

Iron deficiency anemia due to chronic blood loss can be managed by IV or oral iron supplementation. When severe, red cell transfusions may be required. Correction of the underlying problem remains the mainstay of therapy for iron deficiency anemia from chronic HMB.

Complications

Gynecologic Complications

Bleeding during pregnancy and PPH [7] increase maternal and fetal morbidity and mortality, hospitalization, and transfusion requirement [37, 55]. The rate of hysterectomy in females with VWD is doubled when compared to controls [1], and vulvar and perineal hematomas occur with higher frequency [32, 37]. HOC can rupture causing intraperitoneal bleeding or retroperitoneal hematoma, and endometriosis can lead to increased morbidity and infertility [31].

Hematologic Complications

Females with HMB, bleeding during pregnancy, and PPH and males and females with recurrent and prolonged mucocutaneous bleeding may develop iron deficiency and anemia from chronic blood loss. Females with VWD have reported higher incidence of anemia [4, 6, 7]. Iron deficiency can cause fatigue and impaired learning and negatively impact concentration, verbal learning, and memory.

Angiodysplasia is a rare vascular malformation [22, 56], reported in patients lacking HMWM as seen in type 2A, type 2B, type 3 VWD, and AVWS [22]. Lesions typically occur in the cecum and ascending colon and are associated with severe, life-threatening, and recurrent gastrointestinal bleeding [22, 56]. Plasma-derived concentrates may not be effective, whereas rVWF with ULM may be beneficial [22]. Surgical resection, embolization [22], and use of anti-angiogenics such as atorvastatin [22, 51], thalidomide [22, 51], and octreotide [5, 51] have been reported to be successful.

Quality of Life Issues

Bleeding and the associated pain and discomfort in patients with VWD can affect day-to-day activities and negatively impact their family life, travel, sports participation, school attendance, work life, social functioning, and overall physical, emotional, and psychological well-being, leading to decreased health-related quality of life scores [7, 54].

Summary

A cross-sectional study of the Female Universal Data Collection data by Srivaths et al. [13] showed significant delay in diagnosis of bleeding disorder in adults compared to adolescents (median delay of 10 years in pre-menopausal adult women vs. 4 years in post-menarchal adolescents) with adults having more bleeding complications, anemia and gynecological procedures/surgeries, thereby stressing the importance of early recognition of symptoms and diagnosis of bleeding disorder [13]. Prior studies have also demonstrated delay in diagnosis from the time of bleeding symptom to presentation by 4–14 years in women with VWD [15]. Despite long-standing recommendation from the ACOG and guidelines from the American Academy of Pediatrics advising the screening of adolescents with HMB for bleeding disorders particularly VWD, studies have shown that <25% of post-pubertal girls and adolescents with HMB are screened for VWD [15, 16, 33]. Ongoing global efforts to increase patient and provider awareness and improve provider adherence to guidelines for comprehensive evaluation and optimal management of VWD especially in females with HMB and gynecologic/obstetric bleeding complications will pave way for prompt diagnosis and appropriate therapy and thereby avoid complications and improve overall quality of life of these patients.

References

1. Leebeek FW, Eikenboom JC. Von Willebrand's disease. N Engl J Med. 2016;375(21):2067–80.
2. Lee CA, Abdul-Kadir R. von Willebrand disease and women's health. Semin Hematol. 2005;42:42–8.
3. de Jong A, Eikenboom J. Von Willebrand disease mutation spectrum and associated mutation mechanisms. Thromb Res. 2017;159:65–75.
4. James AH. Bleeding disorders in adolescents. Obstet Gynecol Clin N Am. 2009;36:153–62.
5. Sharma R, Flood VH. Advances in the diagnosis and treatment of Von Willebrand disease. Blood. 2017;130:2386–91.
6. Kujovich JL. von Willebrand's disease and menorrhagia: prevalence, diagnosis, and management. Am J Hematol. 2005;79:220–8.
7. Kouides PA. Obstetric and gynaecological aspects of von Willebrand disease. Best Pract Res Clin Haematol. 2001;14:381–99.
8. Srivastava A, Rodeghiero F. Epidemiology of von Willebrand disease in developing countries. Semin Thromb Hemost. 2005;31:569–76.
9. Bowman ML, James PD. Controversies in the diagnosis of type 1 von Willebrand disease. Int J Lab Hematol. 2017;39(Suppl 1):61–8.
10. James AH, Eikenboom J, Federici AB. State of the art: von Willebrand disease. Haemophilia. 2016;22(Suppl 5):54–9.
11. James A, Matchar DB, Myers ER. Testing for von Willebrand disease in women with menorrhagia: a systematic review. Obstet Gynecol. 2004;104:381–8.
12. James AH, Kouides PA, Abdul-Kadir R, Edlund M, Federici AB, Halimeh S, Kamphuisen PW, Konkle BA, Martínez-Perez O, McLintock C, Peyvandi F, Winikoff R. Von Willebrand disease and other bleeding disorders in women: consensus on diagnosis and management from an international expert panel. Am J Obstet Gynecol. 2009;201:12.e1–8.
13. Srivaths LV, Zhang QC, Byams VR, Dietrich JE, James AH, Kouides PA, Kulkarni R, Hemophilia Treatment Centers Network Investigators. Differences in bleeding phenotype and provider interventions in postmenarchal adolescents when compared to adult women with bleeding disorders and heavy menstrual bleeding. Haemophilia. 2018;24:63–9.
14. Shankar M, Lee CA, Sabin CA, Economides DL, Kadir RA. von Willebrand disease in women with menorrhagia: a systematic review. BJOG. 2004;111:734–40.
15. Khamees D, Klima J, O'Brien SH. Population screening for von Willebrand disease in adolescents with heavy menstrual bleeding. J Pediatr. 2015;166:195–7.
16. Jacobson AE, Vesely SK, Koch T, Campbell J, O'Brien SH. Pattern of von Willebrand disease screening in girls and adolescents with heavy menstrual bleeding. Obstet Gynecol. 2018;131:1121–9.
17. Lillicrap D. von Willebrand disease: advances in pathogenetic understanding, diagnosis, and therapy. Blood. 2013;122:3735–40.

18. Gill JC, Castaman G, Windyga J, Kouides P, Ragni M, Leebeek FW, Obermann-Slupetzky O, Chapman M, Fritsch S, Pavlova BG, Presch I, Ewenstein B. Hemostatic efficacy, safety, and pharmacokinetics of a recombinant von Willebrand factor in severe von Willebrand disease. Blood. 2015;126:2038–46.

19. Baronciani L, Goodeve A, Peyvandi F. Molecular diagnosis of von Willebrand disease. Haemophilia. 2017;23:188–97.

20. de Jong A, Eikenboom J. Developments in the diagnostic procedures for von Willebrand disease. J Thromb Haemost. 2016;14:449–60.

21. Curnow J, Pasalic L, Favaloro EJ. Treatment of von Willebrand disease. Semin Thromb Hemost. 2016;42:133–46.

22. Selvam S, James P. Angiodysplasia in von Willebrand disease: understanding the clinical and basic science. Semin Thromb Hemost. 2017;43(6):572–80.

23. Goodeve A. Diagnosing von Willebrand disease: genetic analysis. Hematology Am Soc Hematol Educ Program. 2016;2016:678–82.

24. Roberts JC, Flood VH. Laboratory diagnosis of von Willebrand disease. Int J Lab Hematol. 2015;37(Suppl 1):11–7.

25. Lavin M, Aguila S, Schneppenhcim S, Dalton N, Jones KL, O'Sullivan JM, O'Connell NM, Ryan K, White B, Byrne M, Rafferty M, Doyle MM, Nolan M, Preston RJS, Budde U, James P, Di Paola J, O'Donnell JS. Novel insights into the clinical phenotype and pathophysiology underlying low VWF levels. Blood. 2017;130:2344–53.

26. Srivaths L, Di Paola J, Minard CG et al. Genotypic and phenotypic analysis of adolescents with heavy menstrual bleeding and low Von Willebrand activity – interim report of a multi-center study. Oral presentation, American Society of Hematology Annual Meeting, 2019.

27. Lavin M, O'Donnell JS. How I treat low von Willebrand factor levels. Blood. 2019;133(8):795–804. Epub 2018 Dec 21.

28. O'Sullivan JM, Ward S, Lavin M, O'Donnell JS. von Willebrand factor clearance – biological mechanisms and clinical significance. Br J Haematol. 2018;183(2):185–95.

29. Dumont T, Allen L, Kives S. Can von Willebrand disease be investigated on combined hormonal contraceptives? J Pediatr Adolesc Gynecol. 2013;26:138–41.

30. Chen YC, Chao TY, Cheng SN, Hu SH, Liu JY. Prevalence of von Willebrand disease in women with iron deficiency anaemia and menorrhagia in Taiwan. Haemophilia. 2008;14:768–74.

31. James AH. More than menorrhagia: a review of the obstetric and gynaecological manifestations of von Willebrand disease. Thromb Res. 2007;120(Suppl 1):S17–20.

32. Sidonio RF Jr, Smith KJ, Ragni MV. Cost-utility analysis of von Willebrand disease screening in adolescents with menorrhagia. J Pediatr. 2010;157:456–60, 460.e1.

33. Committee Opinion No.785: Screening and management of bleeding disorders in adolescents with heavy menstrual bleeding. Obstet Gynecol. 2019;134:e71–e83.

34. Kadir RA, Chi C. Women and von Willebrand disease: controversies in diagnosis and management. Semin Thromb Hemost. 2006;32(6):605–15.

35. James AH. Von Willebrand disease. Obstet Gynecol Surv. 2006;61:136–45.

36. Reynen E, James P. Von Willebrand disease and pregnancy: a review of evidence and expert opinion. Semin Thromb Hemost. 2016;42:717–23.

37. James AH, Jamison MG. Bleeding events and other complications during pregnancy and childbirth in women with von Willebrand disease. J Thromb Haemost. 2007;5:1165–9.

38. Malec LM, Moore CG, Yabes J, Li J, Ragni MV. Postpartum haemorrhage in women with von Willebrand disease: an observational study of the Pennsylvania Health Care Cost Containment Council (PHC4) database. Haemophilia. 2015;21:e442–5.

39. Roth CK, Syed LJ. von Willebrand disease in pregnancy. Nurs Womens Health. 2016;20:501–5.

40. James AH, Konkle BA, Kouides P, Ragni MV, Thames B, Gupta S, Sood S, Fletcher SK, Philipp CS. Postpartum von Willebrand factor levels in women with and without von Willebrand disease and implications for prophylaxis. Haemophilia. 2015;21:81–7.

41. Higham JM, O'Brien PM, Shaw RW. Assessment of menstrual blood loss using a pictorial chart. Br J Obstet Gynaecol. 1990;97:734–9.

42. Sanchez J, Andrabi S, Bercaw JL, Dietrich JE. Quantifying the PBAC in a pediatric and adolescent gynecology population. Pediatr Hematol Oncol. 2012;29(5):479–84.

43. Phillip CS, Faiz A, Dowling NF, Beckman M, Owens S, Ayers C, Bachmann G. Development of a screening tool for identifying women with menorrhagia for hemostatic evaluation. Am J Obstet Gynecol. 2008;198:163.e1–163.38.

44. Bowman ML, James PD. Bleeding scores for the diagnosis of von Willebrand disease. Semin Thromb Hemost. 2017;43:530–9.

45. Casey LJ, Tuttle A, Grabell J, Hopman W, Moorehead PC, Blanchette VS, Wu JK, Steele M, Klaassen RJ, Silva M, Rand ML, James PD. Generation and optimization of the self-administered pediatric bleeding questionnaire and its validation as a screening tool for von Willebrand disease. Pediatr Blood Cancer. 2017;64:e.26588.

46. James AH, Lukes AS, Brancazio LR, Thames E, Ortel TL. Use of a new platelet function analyzer to detect von Willebrand disease in women with menorrhagia. Am J Obstet Gynecol. 2004;191:449–55.

47. Naik S, Teruya J, Dietrich JE, Jariwala P, Soundar E, Venkateswaran L. Utility of platelet function analyzer as a screening tool for the diagnosis of von Willebrand disease in adolescents with menorrhagia. Pediatr Blood Cancer. 2013;60:1184–7.

48. Castaman G, Hillarp A, Goodeve A. Laboratory aspects of von Willebrand disease: test repertoire and options for activity assays and genetic analysis. Haemophilia. 2014;20(Suppl 4):65–70.

49. Francis JC, Hui SK, Mahoney D Jr, Dietrich JE, Friedman KD, Soundar E, Srivaths LV. Diagnostic challenges in patients with bleeding phenotype and von Willebrand exon 28 polymorphism p.D1472H. Haemophilia. 2014;20:e211–4.

50. James AH, Kouides PA, Abdul-Kadir R, Dietrich JE, Edlund M, Federici AB, Halimeh S, Kamphuisen PW, Lee CA, Martínez-Perez O, McLintock C, Peyvandi F, Philipp C, Wilkinson J, Winikoff R. Evaluation and management of acute menorrhagia in women with and without underlying bleeding disorders: consensus from an international expert panel. Eur J Obstet Gynecol Reprod Biol. 2011;158:124–34.

51. Saccullo G, Makris M. Prophylaxis in von Willebrand disease: coming of age? Semin Thromb Hemost. 2016;42:498–506.

52. Franchini M, Mannucci PM. Von Willebrand factor (Vonvendi®): the first recombinant product licensed for the treatment of von Willebrand disease. Expert Rev Hematol. 2016;9:825–30.

53. Vonvendi® [Package insert]. Lexington: Baxalta US Inc; 2018.

54. Ragni MV, Machin N, Malec LM, James AH, Kessler CM, Konkle BA, Kouides PA, Neff AT, Philipp CS, Brambilla DJ. Von Willebrand factor for menorrhagia: a survey and literature review. Haemophilia. 2016;22:397–402.

55. Ragni MV, Machin N, James AH, Seaman CD, Malec LM, Kessler CM, Konkle BA, Kouides PA, Neff AT, Philipp CS, Brooks MM. Feasibility of the Von Willebrand disease PREVENT trial. Thromb Res. 2017;156:8–13.

56. Ramsay DM, Buist TAS, Macleod DA, Heading RC. Persistent gastrointestinal bleeding due to angiodysplasia of the gut in von Willebrand's disease. Lancet. 1976;2:275–8.

57. Sadler JE, Rodeghiero F, ISTH SSC Subcommittee on von Willebrand Factor. Provisional criteria for the diagnosis of VWD type 1. J Thromb Haemost. 2005;3:775–7.

58. Flood VH, Christopherson PA, Gill JC, Friedman KD, Haberichter SL, Bellissimo DB, Udani RA, Dasgupta M, Hoffman RG, Ragni MV, Shapiro AD, Lusher JM, Lentz SR, Abshire TC, Leissinger C, Hoots WK, Manco-Johnson MJ, Gruppo RA, Boggio LN, Montgomery KT, Goodeve AC, James PD, Lillicrap D, Peake IR, Montgomery RR. Clinical and laboratory variability in a cohort of patients diagnosed with type 1 VWD in the United States. Blood. 2016;127(20):2481–8.

59. Adeyemi-Fowode OA, Santos XM, Dietrich JE, Srivaths L. Levonorgestrel-releasing intrauterine device use in female adolescents with heavy menstrual bleeding and bleeding disorders: single institution review. J Pediatr Adolesc Gynecol. 2017;30(4):479–83.

Hemophilia Carriers

4

Allison P. Wheeler and Robert F. Sidonio

For many years it has been recognized that the hemorrhagic disorder now known as hemophilia is a hereditary disease of males transmitted to them only through females. From both the sociologic and medical points of view it would be important to detect those females who are conductors of the genetic defect responsible for this disease [1].

Hemophilia Background and History

The earliest references to bleeding consistent with hemophilia date back as far as the second century AD with specific warnings regarding circumcision bleeding in the Talmud. As early as 1820, there was an understanding of both the clinical manifestations and inheritance pattern of the disease [2]. Hemophilia further became intertwined with history through the royal families of Europe and Russia, beginning with Queen Victoria and her children, Leopold who was affected with hemophilia B and Alice and Beatrice who were both carriers [2]. Understanding of the pathophysiology of hemophilia began in the early twentieth

A. P. Wheeler (✉)
Vanderbilt University Medical Center, Department of Pathology, Microbiology & Immunology, Nashville, TN, USA
e-mail: Allison.P.Wheeler@VUMC.org

R. F. Sidonio
Aflac Cancer and Blood Disorders, Emory University, Department of Pediatrics, Atlanta, GA, USA

century after it was clearly defined by a prolonged clotting time. The discrepancy between factor VIII (hemophilia A) and IX (hemophilia B) deficiency was finally determined in the 1950s, along with the X-linked recessive inheritance pattern. Both deficiencies are defined by residual factor activity, and due to the inheritance pattern, the majority of affected persons are males. Females are typically heterozygous for the mutations and thus referred to as carriers of the disease.

Historically females were considered to be asymptomatic, their carrier state defined by mutation testing or family history, the latter being the only viable option until the latter part of the twentieth century. The term carrier in classical genetics conveys that the person will thus lack symptoms from the variant likely contributing to this long-held belief. An obligate hemophilia carrier was historically defined by pedigree analysis, receiving the designation if one of the following were identified: (1) daughter of a father with hemophilia; (2) mother of one son with hemophilia, plus another family member with hemophilia or who is a known carrier of the hemophilia gene; and (3) mothers of two sons with hemophilia. Additional methods of carrier detection were investigated, but because of their cumbersome nature, these were not incorporated into modern clinical practice [3]. Genetic testing can now be incorporated into identification of carriers; however there have always been ethical questions surrounding the genetic testing of minors for asymptomatic conditions [4]. This par-

© Springer Nature Switzerland AG 2020
L. V. Srivaths (ed.), *Hematology in the Adolescent Female*,
https://doi.org/10.1007/978-3-030-48446-0_4

adigm has been challenged recently as accumulating data suggests hemophilia carriers are at risk for bleeding regardless of their factor level. Merskey [5] first described hemophilia A carriers with normal factor VIII activity and a bleeding phenotype, and subsequent landmark papers by Mauser Bunschoten [6] and Plug [7] further demonstrated clinically significant bleeding symptoms in up to 40–60% of hemophilia carriers. Over the last 70 years, the hemophilia carrier has been studied with a focus on laboratory testing and a bleeding phenotype worth clinical consideration and potential treatment.

Factor Activity in Hemophilia Carriers

The testing of factor activity can provide insight into the hemophilia carrier status and her potential bleeding tendency, although imperfectly in an individual. Based on the Lyon hypothesis, female carriers of hemophilia should expect to have random inactivation of one X chromosome in each cell, resulting in a factor activity of approximately 50% [8]. However, this has imperfectly explained the bleeding tendency and does not explain the large number of extreme lyonization leading to levels in the moderate and severe hemophilia range. Multiple variables have historically been suggested to influence factor activity, including maternal versus paternal inheritance [9, 10], age and blood type [11] in factor VIII activity in carriers, as well as blood type, von Willebrand factor, body mass index, and C-reactive protein in non-factor VIII carriers. However, in a case control designed study with genetic confirmation, only von Willebrand factor antigen and activity were noted to significantly modify factor VIII activity [12]. Overall, the majority of carriers demonstrate factor activities within the lower end of the normal range, but there is noted variation due to the acute phase reactant nature of FVIII (Table 4.1) [3, 6, 7, 10–15]. While statistically these levels are different than non-carriers (Table 4.1), they are neither able to provide diagnostic benefit nor explain the bleeding phenotype reported by these women given that most of the reported activities

Table 4.1 Factor VIII and factor IX activity measurements in hemophilia carriers +/− controls

	Factor VIII/IX Activity (U/dL) – carriers, mean (range)	Factor VIII/IX activity (U/dL) – Controls, mean (range)
Chediak 1980 [9]	56 (14–128) [n = 62]	104 (50–195) [n = 53]
Wahlberg 1982[a] [10]	62 (15–120) [n = 38]	76 (27–159) [n = 40]
Graham 1986 [11] and Green 1986 [3]	54 [n = 332]	106 [n = 136]
Mauser-Bunschoten 1988[b] [6]	84 (60–177) [n = 17]	99 (60–160) [n = 25]
Plug 2006[a] [7]	60 (5–219) [n = 225]	102 (45–328) [n = 143]
Ay 2010[c] [12]	74 (51–103) [n = 42]	142 (109–169) [n = 42]
Meisbach 2011 [13]	55 (4–114) [n = 46]	
Paroskie 2015 [14]	83 (37–195) [n = 34]	134 (68–242) [n = 29]
Boban 2017 [15]	61 (5–153) [n = 126] {FVIII} 59 (1–149) [n = 48] {FIX}	

[a]Median (range)
[b]Combines factor VIII and IX activity subjects
[c]Median (interquartile range)

would be considered adequate for hemostasis. Additionally, there is a paucity of data on the possible discrepancy between one-stage and chromogenic assays. This discrepancy is well described in males with mild hemophilia A and thus could explain the increased bleeding phenotype of those carriers with mild FVIII/FIX deficiency.

Bleeding Symptoms in Hemophilia Carriers

Bleeding symptoms in carriers were initially described excluding menstrual bleeding and focused on bleeding after injury and surgical procedures [5]. While the later observations have persisted, the importance of reproductive tract bleeding has been demonstrated in multiple studies.

Table 4.2 Percentage of hemophilia carriers who report the following bleeding symptoms (approximations provided when necessary)

	Range (%)	Merskey 1951 [5]	Mauser Bunschoten 1988[a] [6]	Plug 2006 [7]	Olsson 2014[a] [16]	Paroskie 2015 [14]
Cutaneous bleeding	16–70	53	37, 24	19	18, 16	70
Oral bleeding	11–50	47		27	12, 11	50
Post-surgical	11–45	11	30, 11	28	32, 36	45
Postpartum	0–47		22, 0		20, 47	30
Hematomas	21–35				25, 21	35
Hemarthrosis	3–20			8	3, 5	20
Heavy menstrual bleeding	10–65		31, 10	48	36, 47	65
Epistaxis	8–43		8, 12	43	22, 37	40
Minor wounds	0–37	16	20, 0	21	30, 37	25
Gastrointestinal bleeding	4–11				4, 11	10

[a]Hemophilia A carriers, hemophilia B carriers

The majority of studies investigating the bleeding tendency in hemophilia carriers have been based on self-reported bleeding, as opposed to direct, prospective, or retrospective observation [5–7, 14, 16]. Reported symptoms included epistaxis, easy bruising, heavy menstrual bleeding (HMB), and post-procedural bleeding with the frequency of each symptom varying significantly between studies (Table 4.2). In a number of studies, carriers were compared with non-carriers, demonstrating both increased bleeding and decreased factor VIII or IX activity [6, 10]. One study compared bleeding symptoms and factor VIII activity among carriers and demonstrated that in females with factor VIII activity <0.40 IU/mL, there was increased bleeding, specifically from small "wounds" and following surgical procedures or dental extraction [7]. Contrarily, an increased bleeding tendency was independent of the factor VIII activity with many women demonstrating increased bleeding despite normal factor VIII activity in more recent studies [13, 14, 17]. This increase in bleeding tendency, despite normal, or near normal, factor VIII activity begs the question what other unknown modifiers predict the bleeding phenotype. Interestingly, FVIII mutation and severity of hemophilia in affected males predicted carrier bleeding symptoms in one small study [13]; however confirmatory studies in larger populations have failed to demonstrate this genetic modifier (personal communication).

Joint bleeding, the pathognomonic hemophilia bleeding symptom, has been self-reported in carriers [7, 17] and confirmed by physical examination characteristics and focused imaging. The Normal Joint study provided standardization of range of motion (ROM) evaluation and joint examination in healthy individuals of varying age and BMI [18]. Further, a reduction in joint range of motion, a surrogate for hemarthrosis, in males with hemophilia occurs over time and in a manner related to hemophilia severity [19]. Using the Centers for Disease Control and Prevention (CDC) Universal Data Collection (UDC) dataset, bleeding disorder data collected from 136 federally funded Hemophilia Treatment Centers (HTCs), joint range of motion of female carriers of hemophilia was compared to historical normal controls. Joint range of motion was reduced overall in hemophilia carriers, and FVIII/FIX deficiency severity (mild, moderate, and severe deficiency, as well as normal levels) was associated with increasing joint injury [20]. In a single institutional study ($n = 9$), female carriers with greater than 10% asymmetry in their joint exams or reduced joint ROM compared to age and BMI matched controls were asked to undergo imaging of the affected as well as the contralateral joint. MRIs (T2* sequence) demonstrated hemophilic joint changes suggestive of previous joint bleeding, including hemosiderin deposition most commonly found in affected ankles [21]. These studies support the notion that female carriers of hemophilia with mildly reduced or normal FVIII/FIX are experiencing mild clinical and subclinical joint bleeding in their first three decades of life.

HMB has always been difficult to evaluate and quantify given that it is common and occurs in up to 40% of adolescents [22]. While HMB has been clinically defined as bleeding or greater than 7 days or blood loss of greater than 80 mL per menses, quantification has been performed with the pictorial bleeding assessment chart (PBAC). The PBAC provides a visual assessment technique that quantifies the volume of blood in used pads and tampons to assess for light, normal, or heavy menses [23]. As expected, and seen with other bleeding disorders, hemophilia carriers frequently report HMB. In self-reported studies, 35 to 94% of carriers reported HMB [16, 17], and up to 20% of carriers report the need for a hysterectomy secondary to excessive blood loss [7]. While prospective evaluation of the PBAC has not been conducted in hemophilia carriers, PBAC scores were significantly higher in carriers compared to non-carrier women (423 versus 182.5, $P = 0.018$) when asked to recall their recent cycles. Additionally, there is an increased failure rate of combined oral contraceptive pills in efforts to control this HMB [14]. Overall, future studies need to be conducted to understand the menstrual bleeding phenotype and to investigate the optimal treatment modalities.

Quality of Life in Hemophilia Carriers

As expected, the bleeding symptoms in hemophilia patients have been associated with a decreased quality of life and recently demonstrated in hemophilia carriers. A Swedish study compared hemophilia carriers, stratifying them by bleeding score to controls, and demonstrated that overall carriers had a comparable quality of life to normal control females. However, those carriers with increased bleeding tendency demonstrated reduced quality of life in certain health domains: in mental health (presence of depressive feelings or nervousness), general health (perception of poorer personal health and expectation of deteriorating), and social function (limitations

of social activities) [24]. A second cross-sectional study compared hemophilia carriers to controls demonstrated reduced quality of life in the health domains of pain and general health [25]. To further complicate our understanding, in another study, there was no correlation between increased bleeding scores and decreased quality of life [26]. Taken together, these studies demonstrate that hemophilia carriers do exhibit some reduction in quality of life; however the etiology is not entirely clear based on the current literature. Additionally, the various studies relied on mostly non-disease-specific patient-reported outcome instruments that may not fully capture the effect of bleeding on a woman's quality of life. There is clearly a need for additional research to improve our understanding of this group of women.

Bleeding Scores in Hemophilia Carriers

Given the general acceptance of an increased bleeding phenotype in female carriers of hemophilia, identification and an objective approach to bleeding assessment is warranted. Bleeding assessment tools (BATs), originally designed to investigate whether a patient with bleeding symptoms should be evaluated for von Willebrand Disease, have given providers an objective means of assessing bleeding symptoms and to compare across bleeding disorders. In an effort to evaluate the utility of the ISTH-BAT, 168 hemophilia carriers were characterized in a cross-sectional study and compared with historical controls diagnosed with type 1 von Willebrand disease and type 3 von Willebrand disease heterozygotes. The ISTH-BAT scores of the hemophilia carriers fell in between the two von Willebrand disease groups in terms of bleeding tendency; carriers with either reduced or normal factor VIII activity demonstrated positive bleeding scores [27]. Further investigation into the predictability of BATs of 108 hemophilia A and B carriers using both the ISTH-BAT (expert administered) and self-BAT bleeding scores demonstrated good correlation. In this study, a self-BAT score of ≥ 6 demonstrated a positive predictive value of 0.51 and negative predictive value of 0.71 for the identification of low factor VIII or IX [26]. Taken together, one can assess that there is utility for BATs in bleeding assessment of hemophilia carriers. This is particularly important in this population as there is a lack of correlation of factor level to bleeding score.

The assessment and quantification of HMB as with normal women and those with bleeding disorders has largely relied on the semi-quantitative measurement with the PBAC. PBAC scores consistent with a clinical definition of HMB (> 100) have been reported in 57% of carriers of hemophilia, compared with 74% of women with von Willebrand disease, 59% of women with factor XI deficiency, and 29% of controls [28]. While additional studies have used the PBAC to quantify HMB in hemophilia carriers, as well as monitor response to therapy in women with HMB with or without bleeding disorders, there have not been any attempts to systematically validate the score in the hemophilia carrier population or compare PBAC scores to factor VIII or IX activities. At this time, it is reasonable to consider the PBAC as a means of menstrual bleeding assessment and to utilize it in response to menstrual reduction strategies.

Treatment Options for Hemophilia Carriers

The treatment of bleeding in carriers of hemophilia requires a multifaceted approach, considering the patient's bleeding history, including specific bleeding symptoms and historical response to treatment. Additionally, one needs to consider the baseline FVIII or FIX level when choosing an appropriate hemostatic medication. To that end, in hemophilia A and B carriers with levels ≥50% and no significant personal bleeding history, it is reasonable to consider the liberal use of antifibrinolytics, with only rare use of factor concentrates. In carriers with lower factor activity and/or a more severe bleeding phenotype, one can use similar guidelines for males with hemophilia, focusing on the baseline factor activity and dosing per the relevant hemophilia severity range. Hematologic medications available to aid in cessation or prevention of bleeding include

recombinant or plasma-derived factor concentrates and antifibrinolytic medications in both hemophilia A and B carriers, as well as 1-desamino-8-D-arginine vasopressin (DDAVP) in hemophilia A carriers (Table 4.3). Additionally, topical hemostatic agents can be considered, such

Table 4.3 Treatment recommendations regarding medical management of hemophilia A and B carriers[b]

	Hemophilia A carriers	Hemophilia B carriers
Heavy menstrual bleeding	Antifibrinolytics[c] Hormonal management [a] Goal FVIII >50%, DDAVP if applicable[d]	Antifibrinolytics[c] Hormonal management [a] Goal FIX >50%
Delivery	Goal FVIII >50%	Goal FIX >50%
Bleeding postpartum	Antifibrinolytics[c] Goal FVIII >50%	Antifibrinolytics[c] Goal FIX >50%
Surgery	Goal FVIII 50–80%	Goal FIX 60–80%
Dental extraction	Antifibrinolytics[c] Goal FVIII >50%, DDAVP if applicable[d]	Antifibrinolytics[c] Goal FIX >50%
Medical intervention (scope, puncture, biopsy)	Goal FVIII >50%, DDAVP if applicable[d]	Goal FIX >50%
Severe trauma	Goal FVIII 80–100%	Goal FIX 60–80%
Bleeding	Goal FVIII >50%, DDAVP if applicable[d]	Goal FIX >50%
Severe bleeding	Goal FVIII 80–100%	Goal FIX 60–80%

[a]Hormonal management should be adjusted based on patient response to therapy and additional considerations (e.g., presence of hormonally influenced headaches); options include combined estrogen and progesterone therapy versus progesterone only therapy
[b]Duration of therapy, including factor replacement, should be determined based on severity and anticipated duration of bleeding symptoms
[c]Tranexamic acid or aminocaproic acid dosing for menstrual bleeding should continue for 5 days; alternative symptoms frequently require that treatment continue up to 2–3 days beyond the resolution of bleeding
[d]Therapy with DDAVP should only occur if the patient has demonstrated response to this medication as discussed in the text. Further, consideration into fluid management should be made, and concentrated/recombinant factor replacement should be considered in the setting of increased IV fluid needs and/or breastfeeding given the paucity of data regarding the transmission of DDAVP via breast milk

as intranasal preparations of antifibrinolytics or various topical hemostatic agents available for small wounds. Additionally, one can consider non-hemostatic hormonal therapies such as combined oral contraceptives, progestins, or long-acting reversible contraception to address reproductive tract bleeding.

DDAVP, a synthetic analog of vasopressin, in high doses increases both factor VIII and von Willebrand factor through release of these clotting proteins from endothelial cell storage sites [29]. This medication has demonstrated hemostatic efficacy in persons with mild hemophilia A, von Willebrand disease, low VWF, and mild qualitative platelet function disorders (typically delta storage pool deficiency) and hemophilia A carriers. The response of hemophilia A carriers has been investigated by two groups. An early study investigating the response of hemophilia A carriers ($n = 20$) and subjects with von Willebrand disease ($n = 10$) demonstrated a more significant increase in von Willebrand factor compared to factor VIII in carriers, as evidenced by a decrease in the factor VIII/von Willebrand factor ratio after administration of DDAVP [30]. A more recent manuscript studied the response of 17 hemophilia A carriers and nine normal control female patients to DDAVP. Following high-dose DDAVP, the factor VIII did not increase as effectively as von Willebrand factor in carriers when compared to controls. Interestingly measurements of global coagulation (thromboelastography and thrombin generation) were similar between the two groups; the only measurement that differed between the two groups was median peak thrombin at 4 hours, which was decreased in hemophilia A carriers [31]. This specific study which sought to characterize the pharmacologic stress response on VWF and FVIII than demonstrate hemostatic efficacy illustrated the limitations of high-dose DDAVP in hemophilia A carriers. Although the guidelines are not clearly defined, it is reasonable to consider high-dose DDAVP in hemophilia A carriers with mild and moderate FVIII deficiency. The goal of DDAVP administration should be a demonstrated response, defined

loosely as a 1–two-fold response of elevation of FVIII above baseline, reaching at least 50–60% activity at 1–3 hours.

In hemophilia B carriers or hemophilia A carriers without verified response or anticipated lack of response, it is reasonable to consider the use of plasma-derived or recombinant FVIII/FIX products utilizing the same severity-based guidelines in place for males with hemophilia and consider similar goals for procedures and activity.

Antifibrinolytic mediations, specifically tranexamic acid and aminocaproic acid, promote clot stability. Both medications are lysine derivatives that bind to the lysine-bindings sites within the plasminogen/plasmin molecule effectively inhibiting fibrinolysis. Tranexamic acid has been FDA approved for the treatment of HMB (https://www.accessdata.fda.gov/drugsatfda_docs/anda/2014/202286Orig1s000.pdf), and aminocaproic acid has been FDA approved for the treatment of acute bleeding due to increased fibrinolysis. (https://www.accessdata.fda.gov/drugsatfda_docs/label/2004/15197scm036,scf037,scp038,scm039_amicar_lbl.pdf). Both medications are most commonly used in combination with other hemostatic therapies such as high-dose DDAVP or factor concentrates for surgical or dental prophylaxis or to aid in menstrual control [32].

Control of HMB provides an additional set of challenges for the hemophilia carrier; however there are numerous hormonal methods of menstrual regulation to consider. Generally, 40% of adolescent women experience HMB [33], and 20% of those women ultimately will be diagnosed with a congenital bleeding disorder, including 8–9% with clotting factor deficiencies [34]. Reduction of menstrual bleeding among adolescent girls with a congenital bleeding disorder and HMB has been achieved through a variety of means as would be utilized in those teenagers without a bleeding disorder. These commonly employed strategies which include progesterone-only therapy (depot medroxyprogesterone acetate, levonorgestrel-releasing intrauterine system) and combined estrogen and progesterone therapy (combined oral contraceptive pills, transdermal patch) were variably effective with menstrual bleeding control achieved in 42–89% [35]. There is a significant data gap and limited investigation into effective strategies in this population with some studies ongoing (ATHENA 1). While there have not been studies comparing various menstrual reduction strategies in hemophilia carriers compared to other bleeding disorders, these are all reasonable options to aid in menstrual control as monotherapy or in conjunction with hematologic medications as discussed above.

Conclusion

Hemophilia carriers over the past 50–75 years have demonstrated that some of these women do bleed more than the general population, negating the notion of the asymptomatic carrier state. We believe that female carriers of hemophilia have been accepted as persons with a bleeding disorder requiring monitoring and treatment management. However, there is still significant work that needs to be done to improve our understanding of this population. Overall, the bleeding phenotype of these women and the explanation as to why some women will exhibit a more severe bleeding phenotype independent of factor activity remain unclear and warrant further investigation to improve our clinical and pathological understanding of this population. Considering the adolescent population, there are a number of aspects of future research to consider. First, further investigation into reduction of menstrual bleeding is truly warranted, including, but not limited to, combination medications. Currently there is a black box warning on tranexamic acid for concurrent use with combined estrogen and progesterone hormonal medications (https://www.accessdata.fda.gov/drugsatfda_docs/anda/2014/202286Orig1s000.pdf); however one might question if this safety concern persists for persons with bleeding disorders. Second, the use of prophylactic factor replacement has never been investigated in this patient population, either for primary or secondary prevention of bleeding. Further one might question the need for situational prophylactic therapy in the setting of athletics in these females, especially considering the reports outlining subclinical and clinical joint bleeding. Considering older female hemophilia carriers, there are a number of questions to ask to optimize care of women during pregnancy. Factor VIII levels rise during pregnancy [36], but factor IX does not, leading to the potential for increased bleeding, and postpartum hemorrhage affects both groups of women leading to questions about optimal therapy for efficacy and safety of both the mother and fetus/child. Additionally, there is significant variability seen in bleeding with menopause, and determining the best approach for treatment in these women has not been studied to our knowledge. Overall, despite significant advances in our understanding of hemophilia carriers, there is still significant work to be done to provide complete lifelong care to this patient population.

References

1. Margoulis A and Ratnoff OD. A laboratory study of the carrier state in classic hemophilia. J Clin Invest. 1956;35(11):1316–23.
2. Ingram GIC. The history of haemophilia. J clin path. 1976;29:469–79.
3. Green, et al. Carrier detection in hemophilia A: a cooperative international study. 2. The efficacy of a universal discriminant. Blood. 1986;67:1560–67.
4. Miller R. Genetic Counselling for Hemophilia. Treatment of Hemophilia. 2002;25:1–15.
5. Merskey C and Mcfarlane RG. The Female Carriers of Haemophilia A Clinical and Laboratory Study. Lancet. 1951;1(6653):487–90.
6. Mauser-Bunschoten, et al. Bleeding Symptoms in Carriers of Hemophilia. Thrombosis and Haemostasis. 1988;59(3):349–52.
7. Plug, et al. Bleeding in carriers of hemophilia. Blood. 2006;108:52–6.
8. Lyon MF. Sex Chromatin and Gene Action in the Mammalian X-Chromosome.
9. Chediak, et al. Lower factor VIII coagulant in daughters of subjects with hemophilia A compared to other obligate carriers. Blood. 1980;55:552–8.
10. Wahlberg T, Blomback M and Brodin U. Carriers and Noncarriers of Haemophilia A: 1. Multivariate Analysis of Pedigree Data, Screen Blood Coagulation Tests and Factor VIII Variables. Thrombosis Research. 1982;25:401–14.
11. Graham, et al. Carrier detection in hemophilia A: a cooperative international study. 1. The carrier phenotype. Blood. 1986;67:1554–9.

12. Ay C, et al. Determinants of factor VIII plasma levels in carriers of haemophilia A and in control women. Haemophilia. 2010;16:111–7.
13. Miesbach, et al. Associated between phenotype and genotype in carriers of haemophilia A. Haemophilia. 2011;17:246–51.
14. Paroskie, et al. A cross-sectional study of bleeding phenotype in haemophilia A carriers. British Journal of Haematology. 2015;170:223–8.
15. Boban et al. Comparative study of the prevalence of clotting factor deficiency in carriers of haemophilia A and haemophilia B. Haemophilia. 2017;23(5):e471–3.
16. Olsson, et al. Clotting factor level is not a good predictor of bleeding in carriers of haemophilia A and B. Blood coagulation and Fibrinolysis. 2014;25:471–5.
17. Paroskie, et al. Both Hemophilia Health Care Providers and Hemophilia A Carriers Report that Carriers have Excessive Bleeding. J Pediatr Hematol Oncol. 2014;36(4):e224-e230.
18. Soucie, et al. Range of motion measurements: reference values and a database for comparison studies. Haemophila. 2011;17:500–7.
19. Soucie, et al. Joint range-of-motion limitations among young males with hemophilia: prevalence and risk factors. Blood. 2004;103:2467–73.
20. Sidonio, et al. Females with FVIII and FIX deficiency have reduced joint range of motion. Am J Hematol. 2014;89(8):831–6.
21. Gilbert, et al. Haemophilia A Carriers Demonstrate Pathological and Radiological Evidence of Structural Joint Changes. Haemophilia. 2014;20(6);e426-e429.
22. Haamid, et al. Heavy Menstrual Bleeding in Adolescents. J Pediatr Adolesc Gynecol. 2017;30:335–40.
23. Janssen, et al. A Simple Visual Assessment Technique to Discriminate Between Menorrhagia and Normal Menstrual Blood Loss. Obstet Gynecol. 1995;85:977–82.
24. Olsson, et al. Association between bleeding tendency and health-related quality of life in carriers of moderate and severe hameophilia. Haemophilia 2015;21:742–6.
25. Gilbert, et al. Hameophilia A Carriers Experience Reduced Health-Related Quality of Life. Haemophilia. 2015;21(6):761–5.
26. Young, et al. Evaluation of the self-administered bleeding assessment tool (Self-BAT) in haemophliia carriers and correlations with quality of life. Haemophilia. 2017;23(6):e536-e538.
27. James, et al. Evaluation of the utility of the ISTH-BAT in haemophilia carriers: a multinational study. Haemophilia. 2016;22:912–8.
28. Kadir, et al. Assessment of menstrual blood loss and gynaecological problems in patients with inherited bleeding disorders. Haemophilia. 1999;5:40–8.
29. Mannucci, et al. 1-Deamino-8-d-arginine vasopressin: a new pharmacological approach to the management of haemophilia and von Willebrands' disease. Lancet. 1977;1(8017):869–72.
30. Casonato et al. DDAVP infusion in haemophilia A carriers: different behavior of plasma factor VIII and von Willebrand factor. Blood Coagulation and Fibrinolysis. 1996;7:549–53.
31. Candy, et al. A decreased and less sustained desmopressin response in hemophilia A carriers contributes to bleeding. Blood Advances. 2018;2(20):2629–36.
32. Mauser-Bunschoten EP. Symptomatic Carriers of Hemophilia. Treatment of Hemophilia. 2008;46:1–11.
33. Friebert, et al. Bleeding disorders among young women: A population-based prevalence study. Acta Obstericia et Gynecologica. 2006;85:200–6.
34. Ahuja SP and Hertweck SP. Overview of Bleeding Disorders in Adolescent Females with Menorrhagia. J Pediatr Adolesc Gynecol. 2010;23:S15–21.
35. Alaqzam, et al. Treatment Modalities in Adolescents Who Present with Heavy Menstrual Bleeding. J Pediatr Adolesc Gynecol. 2018;31:451–8.
36. Drury-Stewart, et al. Complex changes in von Willebrand factor-associated parameters are acquired during uncomplicated pregnancy. PLoS One. 2014;9(11):e112935.

Rare Coagulation Factor Deficiencies

5

Shilpa Jain and Suchitra S. Acharya

Introduction

Rare coagulation factor deficiencies (RCFDs) comprise inherited quantitative and/or qualitative deficiencies of coagulation factors (F), viz., fibrinogen (FI), prothrombin (FII), FV, FVII, FX, FXI, and FXIII, and combined factor deficiencies such as FV+FVIII and FII, FVII, FIX, and FX (vitamin K-dependent coagulation factor deficiency [VKCFD]) [1]. The clinical manifestations can be widely heterogeneous ranging from a mild bleeding phenotype to more severe symptoms and life-threatening bleeds. The hemostatic challenges of the female reproductive life make them more likely to be symptomatic even with the heterozygous state, presenting with excessive bleeding during menstruation, pregnancy, miscarriage, or childbirth [2]. Heavy menstrual bleeding (HMB) can lead to significant pain, anemia, and limitation in daily activities, with an adverse impact on quality of life, family/social interactions, and increased absenteeism from school/work [2, 3]. Pregnancy and childbirth are associated with increased maternal and fetal/neonatal bleeding complications [2]. However, the identification of these disorders in the adolescent age group is challenged by the overlap with normal physiological symptoms secondary to anovulation, paucity of accurate diagnostic assays, and a frequent lack of family history to suggest an inherited bleeding disorder. This chapter will review the impact of RCFDs in adolescent girls including clinical presentations, diagnosis, and management dilemmas.

Epidemiology and Clinical Presentation

The worldwide prevalence of RCFDs has been estimated to be between 3% and 5% of all inherited coagulation disorders with recent reports of 8% prevalence rate derived from the World Federation of Hemophilia (WFH) survey (http://wfh.org) in 2016 and the Rare Bleeding Disorders Database (RBDD) (www.rbdd.org) in 2012 [1, 4–6]. Increased prevalence of RCFDs is particularly noted in countries with a high rate of consanguinity and endogamous marriages, such as the Middle East, Arabian Peninsula, North Africa, and India [7–11], and historically in outports of Newfoundland and Labrador, the easternmost provinces of Canada [12].

The prevalence of 1 symptomatic person per 500,000 population (homozygous or compound

S. Jain
Division of Pediatric Hematology-Oncology, Women and Children's Hospital of Buffalo and Hemophilia Center of Western New York, Buffalo, NY, USA

S. S. Acharya (✉)
Hemostasis and Thrombosis Center, Northwell Health Bleeding Disorders and Thrombosis Program Cohen Children's Medical Center, Northwell Health Zucker School of Medicine at Hofstra/Northwell, Hempstead, NY, USA
e-mail: Sacharya@northwell.edu

© Springer Nature Switzerland AG 2020
L. V. Srivaths (ed.), *Hematology in the Adolescent Female*,
https://doi.org/10.1007/978-3-030-48446-0_5

heterozygous) for FVII deficiency, constituting 28–36% of all RCFDs, makes this the most common deficiency [1], closely followed by FXI deficiency which accounts for 23–32% of all RCFDs. Less prevalent are deficiencies of FI, FV, and FX (7–10% each), FXIII (~6%), and FV+FVIII deficiency (~2–3%) [5, 12, 13]. The rarest of the RCFDs are FII deficiency with a prevalence of ~1 per 2 million (2%) [1, 12] and less than 50 families worldwide with VKCFD that have been reported [14, 15].

There is no inherent predilection for race- or ethnicity-based RCFDs, with the exception of FXI deficiency, which is prevalent among Ashkenazi Jews; 1 out of every 450 individuals is affected [16–18]. In addition, the North American Registry of Rare Bleeding Disorders reported FII deficiency disproportionately affecting Latinos [4].

Inheritance

Most RCFDs are autosomal recessive (AR) in inheritance equally affecting males and females. Some FXI deficiency and dysfibrinogenemia may also have an autosomal dominant transmission [1]. Heterozygous individuals can have variable corresponding factor levels that render an unpredictable bleeding phenotype. Combined FV+FVIII deficiency and VKCFD are caused by mutations in genes outside those encoding the coagulation factors themselves and are true AR disorders in that heterozygosity may confers low normal factor levels making them asymptomatic.

Clinical Manifestations of RCFDs

Classification of RCFDs

The RCFDs are characterized by a wide range of clinical phenotypes and bleeding sites [13]. There is great variability in bleeding patterns in individuals with the same RCFD and between clinical bleeding symptoms and residual clotting factor levels among the different RCFDs posing a barrier to a uniform classification. Data from the European Network of Rare Bleeding Disorders (EN-RBD) indicated a strong association of clinical bleeding severity with factor activity levels for FI, FII, FX, and FXIII, a weak correlation with FV and FVII levels, and no association with FXI activity [19]. This implies that a single classification of clinical severity for all types of RCFDs may not be appropriate, unlike hemophilia A or B, as the factor activity levels to ensure absence of clinical symptoms are dissimilar between individual RCFDs [13, 19]. Based on the EN-RBD data, it is proposed that the classification of RCFDs be based on location, bleeding trigger, and potential clinical impact, as *severe*, associated with risk of spontaneous major bleeding; *moderate,* with spontaneous mild bleeding events; and *mild*, with bleeding occurring only after trauma and otherwise asymptomatic [13, 19]. This classification has some practical utility for most of the RCFDs except for FXI deficiency.

Clinical Bleeding Symptoms and Assessment

The hallmark of RCFDs across all ages and genotypes is mucocutaneous bleeding (oral, nasal, gastrointestinal, genitourinary, and menstrual) and that associated with surgery including dental procedures [20], although the absence of bleeding episodes especially after surgical challenges does not necessarily exclude a RCFD [21, 22]. Soft tissue and joint bleeding have been reported with all RCFDs but are more common in severe FI, FII, FX, and FXIII deficiencies [1, 19, 21, 23, 24]. Gastrointestinal bleeding is a common manifestation with severe FX deficiency and occasionally with FV+FVIII deficiency but less frequently reported with all other RCFDs [1, 19]. Umbilical cord and CNS bleeding are prevalent with severe FI, FII, FX, and FXIII deficiencies and rarely with severe FVII deficiency [1, 13, 19, 21, 25]. FXI deficiency rarely presents with spontaneous bleeding even at moderately reduced levels (<15–20%) but may present after trauma and surgery in tissues with abundant fibrinolytic activity such as the nasopharynx and urogenital tract [1, 18, 19, 26, 27]. Combined

FV+FVIII deficiency is also associated with a mild bleeding phenotype and commonly presents with mucocutaneous, HMB, post-partum, or post-surgical bleeds [28]. In contrast, those affected with VKCFD often present in infancy or early childhood with CNS or umbilical stump bleeding [15, 29].

Various non-coagulation-related phenotypic manifestations (dysmorphic features resembling warfarin embryopathy, developmental delay, and skeletal defects) have been reported to be associated with certain RCFDs, especially FX and VKCFD [15, 30]. There have also been reports of arterial and venous thromboembolic events in FI and FVII deficiency and after FXI concentrate infusions [19, 31–32].

The optimal assessment of the presence and severity of bleeding symptoms in a patient referred for evaluation of a bleeding disorder is vital for further workup and management. Using the data from the EN-RBD database, a bleeding assessment tool (BAT) has been specifically designed for RBDs, given the phenotypic heterogeneity of these disorders in order to avoid subjective interpretation of symptoms by patients specifically in mild cases [33]. A bleeding score (BS) of 1.5 using the BAT was found to be able to discriminate between patients with and without a RCFD with a sensitivity of ~67% and specificity of 74%, and a negative correlation was observed between BS and factor activity level [33]. However, the validity and reliability of the BAT in RCFDs need to be further explored.

Gynecological and Obstetric Bleeding Manifestations

In addition to the systemic bleeding symptoms manifested by RCFDs, women are disproportionately affected as compared to men because of the unique challenges during their reproductive years, even in the heterozygous state. The specific hemorrhagic manifestations experienced by adolescent girls can be HMB, ovarian bleeding cysts and hemoperitoneum, post-partum hemorrhage, and gynecological disorders such as uterine fibroids, endometrial hyperplasia and polyps,

and bleeding after procedures. These can be associated with significant morbidity, chronic iron deficiency anemia and pain, and impaired quality of life due to limitation in social activities, work, and education [3].

Heavy menstrual bleeding is the most common bleeding symptom reported in up to 70% of women with RCFDs irrespective of the type of bleeding disorder and factor level [34, 35]. Girls with RCFDs may experience even heavier menstrual bleeding during anovulatory cycles which are more likely to occur starting with menarche and adolescence. The prevalence of RCFDs in adolescents presenting with HMB is reported to be 13–20% although the exact prevalence in each disorder is difficult to ascertain [3].

A higher risk of gynecological conditions associated with bleeding such as hemorrhagic ovarian cysts, endometriosis, and structural lesions (e.g., fibroids, endometrial hyperplasia, and polyps) has been reported [34, 35]. Of these, hemorrhagic ovarian cysts resulting in hemoperitoneum are highly suggestive of a bleeding disorder. Furthermore, adolescents with RCFDs may also be vulnerable to obstetric complications including post-partum hemorrhage (secondary or delayed) [36] and recurrent miscarriages given the roles of FXIII and FI in placental implantation and pregnancy maintenance [23, 36–38]. Yet another frequently missed complication in teens with RCFDs is vaginal or vulvar hematomas which should trigger a bleeding workup. The rate of bleeding complications may require these girls/women to undergo unnecessary interventions such as hysterectomy, endometrial ablation, dilatation, and curettage to decrease menstrual flow which can worsen the bleeding [2]. Paradoxically, thrombotic episodes have been reported with FI and FVII deficiencies in the post-partum and post-surgical settings [38, 39]. Accurate and timely diagnosis of a bleeding disorder can help reduce the severity of menstrual and post-partum bleeding through non-surgical means and prevent some of these grave complications.

Given this heterogeneity of the bleeding phenotype, the role of contributing factors such as the fibrinolytic potential of the site of injury, activation of the thrombin-activatable fibrinolysis inhibitor (TAFI) with FXI deficiency, coexistence of inherited thrombophilia, additional source of functional FV from platelets, and reduced levels of tissue factor pathway inhibitor (TFPI) associated with FV deficiency needs to be explored.

Inhibitor Development

Although there is a better understanding of inhibitor development in hemophilia A and B, there is a paucity of data pertaining to inhibitors in persons with RCFDs given their rarity. The management of bleeding after inhibitor development in RCFDs becomes even more challenging for providers with scant available data. Alloantibodies complicating replacement for FV, VII, XI, and FXIII deficiencies are more commonly encountered. These antibodies are of the IgG subclass but have not been well characterized. There have only been anecdotal reports in the literature which describe their development after replacement with plasma and plasma-derived concentrates [40–43].

Diagnostic Evaluation and Considerations

Laboratory Diagnosis

The initial laboratory evaluation for diagnosis of RCFDs requires screening coagulation studies (prothrombin time [PT], activated partial thromboplastin time [aPTT]). Prolongation of these tests requires characterizing factor activity levels for the diagnosis (Fig. 5.1). The thrombin and reptilase times are required to accurately diagnose FI deficiency. Quantitative or qualitative deficiency can be diagnosed based on the concordance/discordance of factor antigen and activity levels particularly important in FI and FII deficiencies. Normal antigen levels with decreased activity signify a dysfunctional protein which in these RCFDs can increase thrombotic risk with coexisting prothrombotic risk factors [13, 47].

A lack of standardization of currently available factor assays can cause a discrepancy in factor levels hindering an accurate classification. The RBD Working Group has proposed using the

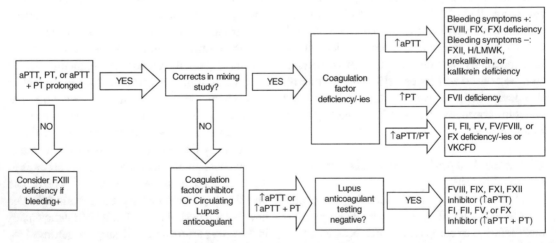

Fig. 5.1 Schematic depicting basic process for evaluating coagulation profile abnormalities. If readily available, initial testing should consist of a mixing study to determine whether the coagulation study abnormality is due to a coagulation factor deficiency or inhibitor. The possible factors involved may then be narrowed down based on which coagulation studies (aPTT only, PT only, aPTT, and PT) are abnormal. Note: PT and aPTT are normal in

FXIII deficiency because fibrin generation is not impaired. aPTT activated partial thromboplastin time, FI fibrinogen, FII factor II, FIX factor IX, FV factor V, FVII factor VII, FVIII factor VIII, FX factor X, FXI factor XI, FXII factor XII, FXIII factor XIII, H/LMWK high-/low-molecular-weight kininogen, PT prothrombin time, VKCFD vitamin K-dependent clotting factor deficiency

Clauss method for measuring FI level and recombinant thromboplastin reagents for FVII activity assays for accuracy [19, 44].

A resurgence in interest in using global assays of thrombin generation (TG) and viscoelastic testing (TEG/ROTEM) may provide an overall view of hemostasis in an individual along with individual factor activity levels. These viscoelastic assays enable assessment of clot kinetics, fibrinolysis, and individual hemostatic capacity which may correlate better with symptom severity to predict bleeding risk and determine treatment effectiveness [45–49] with ongoing efforts toward their standardization [23, 26, 50–52].

Molecular Diagnosis

The molecular diagnosis of most RCFDs can be established by identification of the causative mutation in the genes encoding the corresponding coagulation factors with two exceptions: (1) combined FV+FVIII deficiency which results from a common molecular defect affecting intracellular processing of both proteins (MCFD2 and LMAN1) [60] and (2) VKCFD which has two subtypes based on the mutated enzyme involved in vitamin K metabolism, namely, GGCX and VKORC1 [15, 29].

The most prevalent mutations found among RCFDs are missense mutations reported in 52–57% of patients followed by small insertions/deletions in 20–30% mostly in FI and FV deficiencies. Splicing and nonsense mutations are uncommon, reported in <15% of patients [53].

Prenatal diagnosis for known familial mutations can be offered by obtaining fetal DNA via amniocentesis or chorionic villus sampling [54] along with linkage and sequence analyses against the proband and parents in a fetus suspected to have a RCFD if conceived from consanguinity by heterozygous parents. Early diagnosis may allow for decisions regarding termination vs continuation of pregnancy with appropriate plans for delivery as indicated. Furthermore, in vitro fertilization can enable selection of healthy embryos using pre-implantation genetic determination (PGD) as previously attempted in hemophilia [54, 55].

Harmonizing data from national and international databases on gene mutations would be extremely valuable to determine common and recurrent mutations for each disorder in specific regions of the world enabling their use for quick and convenient genotyping. Currently, the data on phenotype and genetic variants of RCFDs can be found in the following databases: (1) RBDD project (http://eu.rbdd.org); (2) the International Society on Thrombosis and Haemostasis (ISTH) website (http://www.isth.org/?MutationsRareBleeding); and (3) the European Association for Haemophilia and Allied Disorders Coagulation Factor Variant Databases (http://www.eahad-db.org/citations.html.php). Recent projects in the UK ThromboGenomics (https://haemgen.haem.cam.ac.uk/) and USA ATHN 10 (https://athn.org) have been undertaken to offer comprehensive genetic testing using next-generation sequencing. Detection of novel polymorphisms and relation to a specific RCFD would be important to establish by obtaining data on allele frequency in this population. The continuous characterization of novel molecular defects combined with functional studies will provide a better understanding of the complexity of these disorders and implications on phenotype.

Management

Adolescent girls with RCFDs face bleeding challenges during their menses as well as during pregnancy and delivery. This necessitates care at specialized centers through a multidisciplinary clinic where hematologists and gynecologists/adolescent medicine physicians collaborate under one roof to offer comprehensive care, regular follow-ups, and anticipatory guidance for bleeds and surgeries through their reproductive life and beyond. The goals of treatment for acute HMB are to appropriately treat and prevent life-threatening hemorrhage, restore and maintain iron levels, improve quality of life, and monitor ongoing maintenance therapy to reduce morbidity.

Recommendations regarding the management of other bleeding episodes and surgeries are mainly based on existing literature and expert consensus [17].

In general, the need for hemostatic therapy is based on severity, residual factor activity, personal or family history of bleeding or thrombosis, and site of bleeding (areas with abundant fibrinolysis).

The management for RCFDs here will focus on clotting factor replacement therapies only as use of hormonal measures for HMB management is described elsewhere.

Replacement Products

Specific factor replacement products are available in the USA to treat or prevent bleeding with deficiencies of FI, FVII, FX, and FXIII, and a concentrate is available in Europe for FXI deficiency. Single factor concentrates are not available for FII and FV deficiencies. Most of the factor products are plasma-derived (PD) with recombinant options available for FVII and FXIII deficiency. Dosing with specific products requires knowledge with respect to half-life of the product and hemostatic levels (Table 5.1).

In situations of non-availability of specific factor concentrate, alternate sources of factor include fresh frozen plasma (FFP) and cryoprecipitate. Prothrombin complex concentrates (PCCs) are highly purified concentrates of specific coagulation factors obtained from pooled normal plasma,

Table 5.1 Factor replacement products for treatment or prevention of bleeding in RCFDs

Replacement product	Content	Viral Inactivation	Therapeutic options	
			First-line	Second-line
Single-factor concentrates				
RiaSTAP (CSL Behring)	pd-fibrinogen	Yes	Fibrinogen (FI) deficiency	Cryoprecipitate, FFP
Fibryga (Octapharma)	pd-fibrinogen	Yes	Fibrinogen (FI) deficiency	Cryoprecipitate, FFP
FibCLOT(LFB, Les Ulis)[a]	pd-fibrinogen	Yes	Fibrinogen (FI) deficiency	Cryoprecipitate, FFP
NovoSeven (NovoNordisk)	rFVIIa	N/A	FVII deficiency	PCC, FFP
Coagadex (Bio Products Laboratory)	pd- FX	Yes	FX deficiency	PCC, FFP
Hemoleven (LFB) (unlicensed)[a]	pd-FXI	Yes	FXI deficiency	FFP
	pd-FXIII	Yes	FXIII deficiency	FFP, Cryoprecipitate
Corifact (CSL Behring)	rFXIII-A	N/A	FXIII A-subunit deficiency	FFP, Cryoprecipitate
Tretten (NovoNordisk)	rFVIII or pd-FVIII	N/A (rFVIII)	FVIII deficiency (FV+FVIII)	FFP
FVIII (numerous options)			FV (See below)	
PCCs				
3-factor PCCs				
Profilnine (Grifols)	FII > FIX = FX > FVII	Yes	FII deficiency	FX deficiency, VKCFD
Bebulin (Shire)	FX > FII > FIX> FVII	Yes	FX deficiency	FII deficiency, VKCFD
4-factor PCCs				
Kcentra (CSL Behring)	FX > FII > FIX > FVII	Yes	VKCFD	FII and FX deficiencies
Octaplex (Octapharma)[a]	FII > FX > FIX > FVII	Yes	FII deficiency	FX deficiency, VKCFD
Beriplex (CSL Behring)[a]	FX > FII > FIX > FVII	Yes	VKCFD	FII and FX deficiencies
FFP				
SD-Fresh Frozen Plasma (Octaplas, Octapharma)	All coagulation factors	No	FV deficiency FXI deficiency	All RBDs VKCFD
Cryoprecipitate	FVIII, fibrinogen, VWF, and FXIII	No		Fibrinogen deficiency FXIII deficiency

N/A Not Applicable
[a]Not available in USA

namely, FII, FIX, FX, and FVII, in varying amounts depending on the product [56]. For FII deficiency, PCCs are the preferred replacement product of choice [56], whereas FFP is the mainstay of treatment for FV deficiency. In the USA, FFP or solvent detergent-treated FFP is used for FXI deficiency when hemostasis is required during trauma, surgery, and delivery [56]. The risk of developing thrombosis with FI and FXI deficiency should be considered during bleed prevention and management and should be tailored to the bleeding/thrombosis phenotype in the individual and family. Cryoprecipitate is a by-product of FFP which is obtained after thawing a single donor volume of FFP at 4 °C and is rich in von Willebrand factor, FVIII, FXIII, and FI. It can be used for replacement of FI and FXIII, when the specific purified plasma-derived and recombinant factor products are not available (Table 5.1) [56–59].

For combined FV+FVIII deficiency, hemostasis for major bleeds/surgeries is achieved by administering FFP to replace FV along with a FVIII concentrate to replace FVIII [60]. For minor bleeding episodes/surgeries, desmopressin (DDAVP) can be used to increase FVIII levels [60–61]. FFP or PCCs are recommended for treatment of bleeding or for surgical coverage in VKCFD, in addition to maintenance oral vitamin K [29].

Although FFP and cryoprecipitate are widely available and relatively inexpensive, they have several disadvantages compared with single-factor concentrates and PCCs. Variable factor levels make accurate dosing a challenge requiring large volumes to be infused with the risk for fluid overload and transfusion-associated acute lung injury (TRALI). Inability to virally inactivate them with potential risk of pathogen transmission and requirement of blood group matching prior to the transfusion and thawing process for cryoprecipitate delaying administration are other challenges.

Ancillary Therapies

Adjunctive agents to factor replacement products include systemic antifibrinolytics (i.e., tranexamic acid and ε-aminocaproic acid) and topical hemostatic agents (e.g., fibrin glue, collagen). Antifibrinolytics may be used alone for less severe forms of mucosal tract bleeding, minor (e.g., dental) procedures, or HMB; however, caution needs to be exercised in the presence of upper urinary tract bleeding when intrarenal obstruction from glomerular capillary thrombosis or clots in the renal pelvis and ureters can occur.

Prophylactic Replacement Therapy

Prophylactic hemostatic therapy in RCFDs, primary or secondary, may be valuable in girls with RCFDs for management of HMB, at the time of childbirth and preventing PPH. Currently, prophylactic fibrinogen replacement is recommended during pregnancy to maintain trough levels of >1 g/L and >1.5 g/L soon after implantation and during labor to prevent adverse outcomes [17]. However, the indications for prophylaxis in RCFDs are not well-studied because of their rarity. The only RCFD for which routine prophylaxis is recommended from the time of diagnosis is severe FXIII deficiency because of the risk for serious, even life-threatening, bleeding events such as ICH even later in life [62]. Secondary prophylaxis may be considered after musculoskeletal bleeding or life-threatening hemorrhage, particularly in deficiencies of FXIII, FX, and FVII and in severe cases of FI and FV deficiencies [1, 57, 63, 64]. Parenteral administration of high-dose VK is effective in complete or partial correction of the coagulation factor defects associated with inherited VKCFD.

Novel Treatments

Recent development of non-factor replacement therapies that promote hemostasis by alternate mechanisms may have a promising role in the treatment of patients affected with RCFDs. One such novel hemostatic drug is a bispecific recombinant antibody, Hemlibra (emicizumab-kxwh), which was recently approved by FDA (November 2017) for use in hemophilia A patients which leads to effective thrombin generation by binding to FIXa and FX, thus mimicking the cofactor activity of FVIII [65]. Other approaches to increase thrombin generation which may be revolutionary in the treatment of RCFDs include downregulation or inhibition of activity of natural anticoagulants such as anti-TFPI monoclonal antibody (Concizumab) and RNA interference molecule (ALN-AT3/Fitusiran) targeting anti-thrombin III [66–68]. Other targets that have been explored are activated protein C and an engineered factor Va mutant which have shown improved thrombin generation and hemostasis in hemophilia mice models [69, 70].

These alternative therapeutic agents have demonstrated favorable safety profile after either weekly or monthly subcutaneous injections and have been effective in hemophilia. Their role needs to be explored in RCFDs especially with FVII/FXI/FX deficiency but might not be useful for other RBDs such as dysfibrinogenemia or FXIII deficiency.

Future Directions

There is a dilemma in predicting bleeding risk in adolescents presenting with HMB as the sole symptom of an underlying RCFD, especially in the heterozygous state, and in the absence of previous hemostatic challenges. Management of RCFDs is still based on expert opinion and on provider's personal experiences. A multidisciplinary approach to patient care with a tiered approach toward diagnosis and management is ideal. Development of guidelines for management of women-specific bleeding manifestations for each type of RCFD would require detailed evaluation of each factor deficiency to determine the hemostatic level of individual factors and formulate an algorithm for the use of replacement products, along with a combination of hormonal and antifibrinolytic therapy. Harmonization of data can be achieved by developing accurate data collection tools through international registries using common definitions, standardizing factor assay methodology, evaluating thrombin generation through TG assays and clot characteristics through viscoelastic testing, and studying disease modifiers that may contribute to the phenotypic heterogeneity of these disorders. Finally, conducting in vitro expression studies of each gene mutation is important to establish the mechanistic link between gene mutations and observed disease phenotypes.

References

1. Peyvandi F, Palla R, Menegatti M, Mannucci PM. Introduction. Rare Bleeding Disorders: general aspects of clinical features, diagnosis, and management. Semin Thromb Hemost. 2009;35(4):349–55.
2. Peyvandi F, Garagiola I, Menegatti M. Gynecological and obstetrical manifestations of inherited bleeding disorders in women. J Thromb Haemost. 2011;9(Suppl 1):236–45.
3. Kulkarni R. Improving care and treatment options for women and girls with bleeding disorders. Eur J Haematol. 2015;95(Suppl 81):2–10.
4. Acharya SS, Coughlin A, Dimichele DM. and the North American Rare Bleeding Disorder Study Group. Rare Bleeding Disorder Registry: deficiencies of factors II, V, VII, X, XIII, fibrinogen and dysfibrinogenemias. J Thromb Haemost. 2004;2(2):248–56.
5. Hemophilia WFo. World Federation of Hemophilia Report on the Annual Global Survey 20162017 12/12/2017. Available from: http://www1.wfh.org/publications/files/pdf-1690.pdf.
6. Peyvandi F, Palla R, Menegatti M, Siboni SM, Halimeh S, Faeser B, et al. Coagulation factor activity and clinical bleeding severity in rare bleeding disorders: results from the European Network of Rare Bleeding Disorders. J Thromb Haemost. 2012;10(4):615–21.
7. Borhany M, Pahore Z, Ul Qadr Z, Rehan M, Naz A, Khan A, et al. Bleeding disorders in the tribe: result of consanguineous inbreeding. Orphanet J Rare Dis. 2010;5:23.
8. Peretz H, Mulai A, Usher S, Zivelin A, Segal A, Weisman Z, et al. The two common mutations causing factor XI deficiency in Jews stem from distinct founders: one of ancient Middle Eastern origin and another of more recent European origin. Blood. 1997;90(7):2654–9.
9. Saadat M, Ansari-Lari M, Farhud DD. Consanguineous marriage in Iran. Ann Hum Biol. 2004;31(2):263–9.
10. Tonbary YA, Elashry R, Zaki MS. Descriptive epidemiology of hemophilia and other coagulation disorders in Mansoura, Egypt: retrospective analysis. Mediterr J Hematol Infect Dis. 2010;2(3):e2010025.
11. Viswabandya A, Baidya S, Nair SC, Abraham A, George B, Mathews V, et al. Correlating clinical manifestations with factor levels in rare bleeding disorders: a report from Southern India. Haemophilia. 2012;18(3):e195–200.
12. Scully MF, Stoffman J, Boyd S. The unusual pattern of hereditary bleeding disorders in the province of Newfoundland and Labrador-Canada's most Eastern Province. Transfus Apher Sci. 2018;57(6):713–6.
13. Peyvandi F, Menegatti M, Palla R. Rare Bleeding Disorders: worldwide efforts for classification, diagnosis, and management. Semin Thromb Hemost. 2013;39(6):579–84.
14. Castaman G, Linari S. Diagnosis and treatment of von Willebrand disease and Rare Bleeding Disorders. J Clin Med. 2017;6(4).

15. Weston BW, Monahan PE. Familial deficiency of vitamin K-dependent clotting factors. Haemophilia. 2008;14(6):1209–13.
16. Asakai R, Chung DW, Davie EW, Seligsohn U. Factor XI deficiency in Ashkenazi Jews in Israel. N Engl J Med. 1991;325(3):153–8.
17. Mumford AD, Ackroyd S, Alikhan R, Bowles L, Chowdary P, Grainger J, et al. Guideline for the diagnosis and management of the rare coagulation disorders: a United Kingdom Haemophilia Centre Doctors' Organization guideline on behalf of the British Committee for Standards in Haematology. Br J Haematol. 2014;167(3):304–26.
18. Seligsohn U. Factor XI deficiency in humans. J Thromb Haemost. 2009;7(Suppl 1):84–7.
19. Peyvandi F, Di Michele D, Bolton-Maggs PH, Lee CA, Tripodi A, Srivastava A, et al. Classification of rare bleeding disorders (RBDs) based on the association between coagulant factor activity and clinical bleeding severity. J Thromb Haemost. 2012;10(9):1938–43.
20. Byams VR, Kouides PA, Kulkarni R, Baker JR, Brown DL, Gill JC, et al. Surveillance of female patients with inherited bleeding disorders in United States. Haemophilia Treatment Centres. Haemophilia. 2011;17(Suppl 1):6–13.
21. Mannucci PM, Duga S, Peyvandi F. Recessively inherited coagulation disorders. Blood. 2004;104(5):1243–52.
22. Peyvandi F, Spreafico M. National and international registries of rare bleeding disorders. Blood Transfus. 2008;6(Suppl 2):s45–8.
23. Acharya SS, Dimichele DM. Rare inherited disorders of fibrinogen. Haemophilia. 2008;14(6):1151–8.
24. Ejaz MS, Latif N, Memon A. Hereditary prothrombin deficiency. J Pak Med Assoc. 2009;59(9):637–9.
25. Lapecorella M, Mariani G. International Registry on congenital factor VII deficiency: defining the clinical picture and optimizing therapeutic options. Haemophilia. 2008;14(6):1170–5.
26. Bolton-Maggs PH. Factor XI deficiency--resolving the enigma? Hematology Am Soc Hematol Educ Program. 2009;97–105.
27. Palla R, Peyvandi F, Shapiro AD. Rare bleeding disorders: diagnosis and treatment. Blood. 2015;125(13):2052–61.
28. Peyvandi F, Tuddenham EG, Akhtari AM, Lak M, Mannucci PM. Bleeding symptoms in 27 Iranian patients with the combined deficiency of factor V and factor VIII. Br J Haematol. 1998;100(4):773–6.
29. Napolitano M, Mariani G, Lapecorella M. Hereditary combined deficiency of the vitamin K-dependent clotting factors. Orphanet J Rare Dis. 2010;5:21.
30. Girolami A, Ruzzon E, Tezza F, Scandellari R, Scapin M, Scarparo P. Congenital FX deficiency combined with other clotting defects or with other abnormalities: a critical evaluation of the literature. Haemophilia. 2008;14(2):323–8.
31. Meijers JC, Tekelenburg WL, Bouma BN, Bertina RM, Rosendaal FR. High levels of coagulation factor XI as a risk factor for venous thrombosis. N Engl J Med. 2000;342(10):696–701.
32. Salomon O, Steinberg DM, Dardik R, Rosenberg N, Zivelin A, Tamarin I, et al. Inherited factor XI deficiency confers no protection against acute myocardial infarction. J Thromb Haemost. 2003;1(4):658–61.
33. Palla R, Siboni SM, Menegatti M, Musallam KM, Peyvandi F. European Network of Rare Bleeding Disorders. Establishment of a bleeding score as a diagnostic tool for patients with rare bleeding disorders. Thromb Res. 2016;148:128–34.
34. James AH. Women and bleeding disorders. Haemophilia. 2010;16(Suppl 5):160–7.
35. Lee CA, Chi C, Pavord SR, Bolton-Maggs PH, Pollard D, Hinchcliffe-Wood A, et al. The obstetric and gynaecological management of women with inherited bleeding disorders--review with guidelines produced by a taskforce of UK Haemophilia Centre Doctors' Organization. Haemophilia. 2006;12(4):301–36.
36. Pike GN, Bolton-Maggs PH. Factor deficiencies in pregnancy. Hematol Oncol Clin North Am. 2011;25(2):359–78, viii-ix.
37. Inbal A, Muszbek L. Coagulation factor deficiencies and pregnancy loss. Semin Thromb Hemost. 2003;29(2):171–4.
38. Lak M, Keihani M, Elahi F, Peyvandi F, Mannucci PM. Bleeding and thrombosis in 55 patients with inherited afibrinogenaemia. Br J Haematol. 1999;107(1):204–6.
39. Girolami A, Peroni E, Girolami B, Ferrari S, Lombardi AM. Congenital FXI and FVII deficiency asume an apparent opposite protection against arterial or venous thrombosis: an intriguing observation. Hematology. 2016;21(8):486–9.
40. Perez Botero J, Burns D, Thompson CA, Pruthi RK. Successful treatment with thalidomide of a patient with congenital factor V deficiency and factor V inhibitor with recurrent gastrointestinal bleeding from small bowel arteriovenous malformations. Haemophilia. 2013;19:e59–61.
41. Batorova A, Mariani G, Kavakli K, de Saez AR, Caliskan U, Karimi M, et al. Inhibitors to factor VII in congenital factor VII deficiency. Haemophilia. 2014;20:e188–91.
42. Livnat T, Tamarin I, Mor Y, Winckler H, Horowitz Z, Korianski Y, et al. Recombinant activated factor VII and tranexamic acid are haemostatically effective during major surgery in factor XI-deficient patients with inhibitor antibodies. Thromb Haemost. 2009;102:487–92.
43. Muszbek L, Penzes K, Katona E. Auto- and allo-antibodies against factor XIII: laboratory diagnosis and clinical consequences. J Thromb Haemost. 2018;16:822.
44. Monagle P, Barnes C, Ignjatovic V, Furmedge J, Newall F, Chan A, et al. Developmental haemostasis. Impact for clinical haemostasis laboratories. Thromb Haemost. 2006;95(2):362–72.
45. Livnat T, Shenkman B, Martinowitz U, Zivelin A, Dardik R, Tamarin I, et al. The impact of thrombin generation and rotation thromboelastometry on assessment of severity of factor XI deficiency. Thromb Res. 2015;136(2):465–73.

46. Rugeri L, Quelin F, Chatard B, De Mazancourt P, Negrier C, Dargaud Y. Thrombin generation in patients with factor XI deficiency and clinical bleeding risk. Haemophilia. 2010;16(5):771–7.

47. Spiezia L, Radu C, Campello E, Bulato C, Bertini D, Barillari G, et al. Whole blood rotation thromboelastometry (ROTEM) in nine severe factor V deficient patients and evaluation of the role of intraplatelet factor V. Haemophilia. 2012;18(3):463–8.

48. Zekavat OR, Haghpanah S, Dehghani J, Afrasiabi A, Peyvandi F, Karimi M. Comparison of thrombin generation assays with conventional coagulation tests in evaluation of bleeding risk in patients with rare bleeding disorders. Clin Appl Thromb Hemost. 2014;20(6):637–44.

49. Zia AN, Chitlur M, Rajpurkar M, Ozgonenel B, Lusher J, Callaghan JH, et al. Thromboelastography identifies children with rare bleeding disorders and predicts bleeding phenotype. Haemophilia. 2015;21(1):124–32.

50. de Moerloose P, Neerman-Arbez M. Congenital fibrinogen disorders. Semin Thromb Hemost. 2009;35(4):356–66.

51. Riddell A, Abdul-Kadir R, Pollard D, Tuddenham E, Gomez K. Monitoring low dose recombinant factor VIIa therapy in patients with severe factor XI deficiency undergoing surgery. Thromb Haemost. 2011;106(3):521–7.

52. van Veen JJ, Hampton KK, Maclean R, Fairlie F, Makris M. Blood product support for delivery in severe factor X deficiency: the use of thrombin generation to guide therapy. Blood Transfus. 2007;5(4):204–9.

53. Peyvandi F, Kunicki T, Lillicrap D. Genetic sequence analysis of inherited bleeding diseases. Blood. 2013;122(20):3423–31.

54. Peyvandi F, Garagiola I, Mortarino M. Prenatal diagnosis and preimplantation genetic diagnosis: novel technologies and state of the art of PGD in different regions of the world. Haemophilia. 2011;17(Suppl 1):14–7.

55. Chen J, Wang J, Lin XY, Xu YW, He ZH, Li HY, et al. Genetic diagnosis in Hemophilia A from southern China: five novel mutations and one preimplantation genetic analysis. Int J Lab Hematol. 2017;39(2):191–201.

56. MASAC Recommendations concerning products licensed for the treatment of hemophilia and other bleeding disorders.: National Hemophilia Foundation; Revised August 2017 [Available from: https://www.hemophilia.org/Researchers-Healthcare-Providers/Medical-and-Scientific-Advisory-Council-MASAC/MASAC-Recommendations.

57. Ashley C, Chang E, Davis J, Mangione A, Frame V, Nugent DJ. Efficacy and safety of prophylactic treatment with plasma-derived factor XIII concentrate (human) in patients with congenital factor XIII deficiency. Haemophilia. 2015;21(1):102–8.

58. Carcao M, Fukutake K, Inbal A, Kerlin B, Lassila R, Oldenburg J, et al. Developing the first recombinant factor XIII for congenital factor XIII deficiency: clinical challenges and successes. Semin Thromb Hemost. 2017;43(1):59–68.

59. Nugent DJ, Ashley C, Garcia-Talavera J, Lo LC, Mehdi AS, Mangione A. Pharmacokinetics and safety of plasma-derived factor XIII concentrate (human) in patients with congenital factor XIII deficiency. Haemophilia. 2015;21(1):95–101.

60. Zheng C, Zhang B. Combined deficiency of coagulation factors V and VIII: an update. Semin Thromb Hemost. 2013;39(6):613–20.

61. Mansouritorghabeh H, Shirdel A. Desmopressin acetate as a haemostatic elevator in individuals with combined deficiency of factors V and VIII: a clinical trial. J Thromb Haemost. 2016;14(2):336–9.

62. Todd T, Perry DJ. A review of long-term prophylaxis in the rare inherited coagulation factor deficiencies. Haemophilia. 2010;16(4):569–83.

63. Kuperman AA, Barg AA, Fruchtman Y, Shaoul E, Rosenberg N, Kenet G, et al. Primary prophylaxis for children with severe congenital factor VII deficiency - clinical and laboratory assessment. Blood Cells Mol Dis. 2017;67:86–90.

64. Napolitano M, Giansily-Blaizot M, Dolce A, Schved JF, Auerswald G, Ingerslev J, et al. Prophylaxis in congenital factor VII deficiency: indications, efficacy and safety. Results from the Seven Treatment Evaluation Registry (STER). Haematologica. 2013;98(4):538–44.

65. Oldenburg J, Mahlangu JN, Kim B, Schmitt C, Callaghan MU, Young G, et al. Emicizumab prophylaxis in Hemophilia A with inhibitors. N Engl J Med. 2017;377:809–18.

66. Pasi KJ, Rangarajan S, Georgiev P, Mant T, Creagh MD, Lissitchkov T, et al. Targeting of Antithrombin in Hemophilia A or B with RNAi therapy. N Engl J Med. 2017;377:819–28.

67. Sehgal A, Barros S, Ivanciu L, Cooley B, Qin J, Racie T, et al. An RNAi therapeutic targeting antithrombin to rebalance the coagulation system and promote hemostasis in hemophilia. Nat Med. 2015;21:492–7.

68. Chowdary P, Lethagen S, Friedrich U, Brand B, Hay C, Abdul Karim F, et al. Safety and pharmacokinetics of anti-TFPI antibody (concizumab) in healthy volunteers and patients with hemophilia: a randomized first human dose trial. J Thromb Haemost. 2015;13:743–54.

69. Polderdijk SG, Adams TE, Ivanciu L, Camire RM, Baglin TP, Huntington JA. Design and characterization of an APC-specific serpin for the treatment of hemophilia. Blood. 2017;129:105–13.

70. von Drygalski A, Cramer TJ, Bhat V, Griffin JH, Gale AJ, Mosnier LO. Improved hemostasis in hemophilia mice by means of an engineered factor Va mutant. J Thromb Haemost. 2014;12:363–72.

Platelet Disorders in the Adolescent Female

Deepti Warad, Meera Chitlur, and Claire Philipp

Introduction

Platelets play an essential role in primary hemostasis where they adhere to the site of vascular injury and result in the formation of a platelet plug. The activated platelet then provides a negatively charged phospholipid surface where the coagulation factors are assembled to facilitate cell-based thrombin generation. Congenital or acquired platelet disorders associated with a decrease/abnormality in platelet number or function can therefore result in a bleeding diathesis. Bleeding manifestations in patients with platelet disorders typically involve skin and mucous membranes, with heavy menstrual bleeding (HMB) being a common complaint in adolescent females with platelet disorders [1, 2]. Management of HMB in the adolescent female with a platelet disorder is often challenging and requires a multidisciplinary approach with a hematologist being an essential part of the team along with adolescent medicine and/or gynecol-

D. Warad (✉)
Mayo Clinic, Rochester, MN, USA
e-mail: warad.deepti@mayo.edu

M. Chitlur
Wayne State University, Children's Hospital of Michigan, Detroit, MI, USA

C. Philipp
Rutgers Robert Wood Johnson Medical School, New Brunswick, NJ, USA

ogy physician. Here we discuss the clinical manifestations, evaluation, approach to diagnosis, and management of platelet disorders in adolescents.

Platelet Disorders

A systematic classification is essential for a stepwise approach toward diagnosis of platelet disorders. Platelet abnormalities may be classified as quantitative or qualitative, although there is much overlap, and then further classified as congenital (inherited) or acquired (Fig. 6.1).

Disorders of Platelet Number

Acquired Thrombocytopenia

Immune thrombocytopenia (ITP) is an acquired autoimmune disorder characterized by low circulating platelet count <100,000/mm^3, which may occur in the absence (primary ITP) or presence (secondary ITP) of an underlying disease, as a result of both destruction of platelets and impaired megakaryopoiesis. In most cases, primary ITP is mediated by IgG autoantibodies against GPIIb/IIIa antigen on the platelets [3]. Primary ITP is most commonly seen in children between 1 and 6 years of age, while secondary forms predominate in the adolescent and adult age groups. Although ITP is thought to be pri-

© Springer Nature Switzerland AG 2020
L. V. Srivaths (ed.), *Hematology in the Adolescent Female*,
https://doi.org/10.1007/978-3-030-48446-0_6

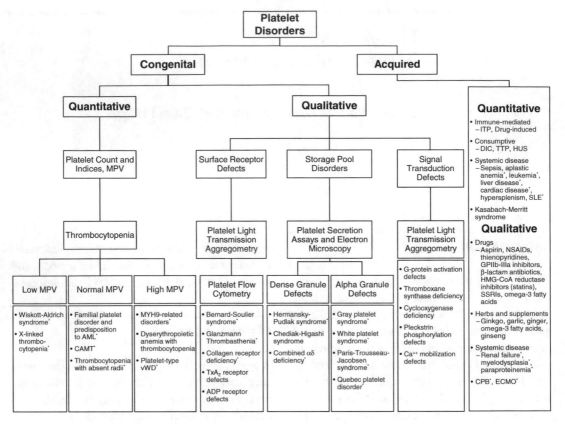

Fig. 6.1 Algorithmic approach for classification and diagnosis of platelet disorders. *Disorders that may present with impaired platelet function in addition to thrombocytopenia. ADP adenosine diphosphate, AML acute myeloid leukemia, CAMT congenital amegakaryocytic thrombocytopenia, CPB cardiopulmonary bypass, DIC disseminated intravascular coagulation, ECMO extracor-poreal membrane oxygenation, HUS hemolytic uremic syndrome, ITP immune thrombocytopenic purpura, MPV mean platelet volume, NSAIDs nonsteroidal anti-inflammatory drugs, SLE systemic lupus erythematosus, SSRIs selective serotonin reuptake inhibitors, TTP thrombotic thrombocytopenic purpura

marily a disorder of platelet number, there is evidence to indicate that function may be significantly affected [4].

Thrombocytopenia may also accompany other systemic and immune-mediated disorders as well as consumptive coagulopathy (Fig. 6.1).

Congenital Thrombocytopenia

Congenital (inherited) thrombocytopenia presents most often as a part of genetic syndromes. In addition to a mild to moderate decrease in platelet count, these platelets may have impaired function [5]. Individuals may display other phenotypic abnormalities such as sensorineural hearing loss, skeletal deformities, oculocutaneous albinism, renal abnormalities, immunodeficiency, skin changes such as eczema, or pancreatic insufficiency providing clues to the underlying diagnosis [6, 7].

Disorders of Platelet Function

Inherited Platelet Function Disorders

Surface Receptor Defects

Autosomal recessive disorders such as Glanzmann thrombasthenia (GT) and Bernard-Soulier syndrome (BSS) are rare bleeding disorders characterized by inherited deficiencies of platelet

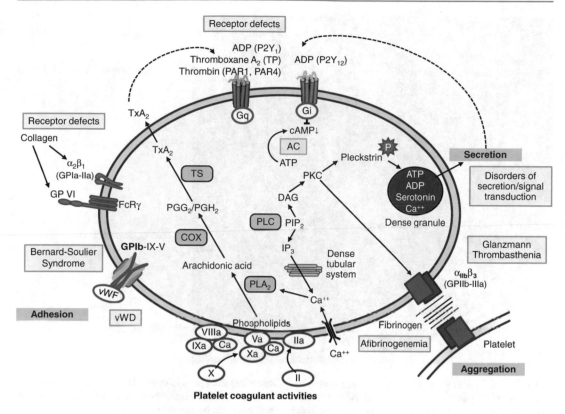

Fig. 6.2 Overview of congenital platelet function disorders. A brief overview of the cell surface membrane receptors and intracellular pathways associated with platelet signaling, adhesion, activation, secretion, and aggregation. AC adenylyl cyclase, ADP adenosine diphosphate, ATP adenosine triphosphate, cAMP cyclic adenosine monophosphate, COX cyclooxygenase, DAG diacylglycerol, FcRγ Fc receptor-γ, GP glycoprotein, P phosphorylation, PGG$_2$/PGH$_2$ prostaglandins G$_2$ and H$_2$, PIP$_2$ phosphatidylinositol 4,5-bisphosphate, PLA$_2$ phospholipase A$_2$, PLC phospholipase C, PKC protein kinase C, IP$_3$ inositol-1,4,5-trisphosphate, TS thromboxane synthase, TxA$_2$ thromboxane A$_2$, vWD von Willebrand disease, vWF von Willebrand factor

glycoprotein (GP) IIb/IIIa (fibrinogen receptor) [8] and GP1b/IX (von Willebrand Factor (vWF) receptor) [9], respectively. Collagen receptor GPVI deficiency has also been described [10] (Fig. 6.2).

Platelet-type von Willebrand disease (PT-vWD) occurs due to gain-of-function mutation in the GP1BA gene encoding for surface glycoprotein Ibα (GPIbα) resulting in enhanced affinity for vWF. Increased clearance of platelets from circulation leads to mild thrombocytopenia as well as loss of high molecular weight vWF multimers. Platelet flow cytometry and gene mutation analyses help differentiating from type 2B vWD.

Soluble agonist receptor deficiencies are rarer. Deficiencies of thromboxane A2 (TXA2) recep-

tor, alpha 2 (α2) adrenergic receptor, and P$_2$Y$_{12}$ receptor have been described [11] (Fig. 6.2).

Signal Transduction Deficiency
Signal transduction pathway defects are a heterogeneous group of bleeding disorders caused by adenosine diphosphate (ADP) or epinephrine receptor deficiencies or abnormalities in the signal transduction that involve G-protein activation, phospholipase C activation, calcium mobilization, protein (pleckstrin) phosphorylation, and tyrosine phosphorylation [11] (Fig. 6.2). Defects in TXA2 pathway resemble aspirin effects on platelet aggregation studies due to impaired dense granule secretion [11–13]. Response to agonists such as arachidonate is obtunded, and no secondary wave is observed

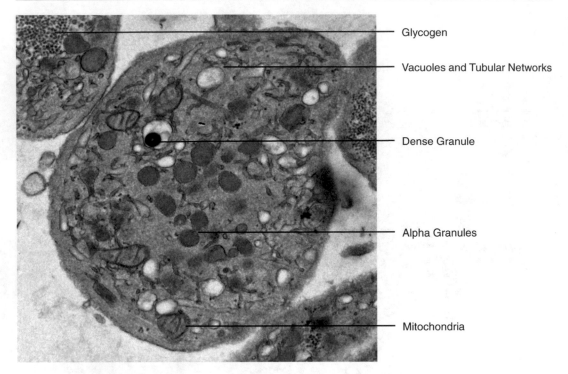

Glycogen

Vacuoles and Tubular Networks

Dense Granule

Alpha Granules

Mitochondria

Fig. 6.3 Platelet ultrastructure by thin-section light transmission electron microscopy. Platelet morphology including size, shape, and state of activation, subcellular organelles such as alpha granules, canalicular systems, Golgi complex, mitochondria, and presence of aberrant inclusions can be assessed

with addition of epinephrine. Decrease in serum and urine thromboxane B2 may be noted.

Storage Pool Deficiency

Platelet storage pool deficiencies are characterized by abnormal dense (δ) and/or alpha (α) granules (Fig. 6.3). The prototypic disease of α granule deficiency is gray platelet syndrome (GPS) due to the characteristic pale and agranular appearance of platelets on peripheral smear examination. Platelet light transmission electron microscopy can be confirmatory with absent or markedly decreased α granules in thin-section preparations [14, 15]. Dense (δ) granule deficiency is seen in rare syndromes such as Hermansky-Pudlak (HPS) and Chediak-Higashi syndromes (CHS). Decreased platelet ATP release and/or confirmation of absent or markedly decreased dense granules by whole mount transmission electron microscopy are helpful diagnostically [16–19]. Platelet function tests such as PFA-100® and platelet aggregation lack sufficient sensitivity and may be normal in storage pool disorders.

Acquired Disorders of Platelet Function

A number of medications, including commonly used drugs such as aspirin, nonsteroidal anti-inflammatory drugs (NSAIDs), P_2Y_{12} inhibitors such as thienopyridines (ticlopidine, prasugrel, and clopidogrel) and ticagrelor, and GPIIb/IIIa receptor inhibitors such as abciximab, eptifibatide, and tirofiban, cause acquired platelet dysfunction [20–22]. Platelet dysfunction may also accompany systemic disorders such as uremia, myelodysplasia and myeloproliferative disorders, systemic lupus erythematosus, and liver cirrhosis (Fig. 6.1).

Clinical Features of Platelet Disorders

Bleeding Phenotype in Adolescents with Platelet Disorders

Mucocutaneous bleeding symptoms such as bruising, epistaxis, bleeding post trauma, surgery, or tooth extraction and HMB (defined as uterine bleeding that is abnormal in duration and volume) are common manifestations of inherited or acquired platelet disorders and may be secondary to platelet disorders of number and/or function [1, 2, 23]. The most frequent bleeding symptom is HMB occurring in % of female adolescent with platelet function disorders [1]. It is important to note that HMB may be the presenting symptom in adolescents with thrombocytopenia as well as mild platelet function disorders, although platelets are not thought to play a major role in endometrial hemostasis [24]. Epistaxis and easy bruisability also occur frequently in adolescents with platelet function disorders. Gingival and/or oral mucosal bleeding is far less common, occurring in 4–5% [1]. Muscle, joint, gastrointestinal, or genitourinary tract bleeding can also be seen in disorders of platelet function [2]. The risk of excessive bleeding with surgery in individuals with inherited platelet function disorders in one study was reported to be 24.8% with a 13.4% incidence of bleeding in inherited disorders of platelet number [25]. Similar types of bleeding symptoms are reported in adolescents with more severe inherited platelet function disorders including BSS, GT, and GPS, although bleeding manifestations are variable and can sometimes be severe requiring blood transfusions and be associated with significant anemia [8, 26–30]. Intracranial hemorrhage (ICH) and gastrointestinal (GI) hemorrhage have been reported to occur in some of these patients as well [8, 29]. HMB is frequently reported in females with GT and bleeding can be very severe at menarche [30].

The extent of bleeding symptoms in adolescents with inherited platelet disorders can be demonstrated using standardized bleeding questionnaires [31–33]. Quantification of bleeding symptoms in a national registry of children including adolescents with inherited platelet disorders using a pediatric bleeding questionnaire demonstrated elevated bleeding scores in 71.4% of inherited platelet function disorders with or without thrombocytopenia compared to 41.4% of children followed for congenital isolated thrombocytopenia [31]. In another study using a quantitative pediatric bleeding questionnaire in children and adolescents with various inherited platelet disorders, 96% had an abnormal score. GT patients and patients with nonspecific platelet function disorders had the highest bleeding scores, while patients with MHY9 macrothrombocytopenia had the lowest [32]. Patients with BSS and GT had higher bleeding scores using the International Society of Hemostasis and Thrombosis Bleeding Assessment Tool (ISTH-BAT) than controls [33].

In adolescents with severe ITP, ecchymosis is the most common bleeding symptom occurring in the majority of cases, with epistaxis, oral bleeds, GI bleeding, and hematuria occurring less frequently and ICH rarely [34]. Significant bleeding is rarely reported in primary ITP with platelet counts >30,000/cu mm and occurs most often when platelet counts are <10,000/cu mm [35]. "Wet" bleeding, indicating the presence of mucous membrane bleeding, has been considered a risk factor for ICH in ITP and has been used as an indication for treatment to prevent major bleeding including ICH [4, 36]. In addition, ICH is also noted to occur more frequently in patients over 10 years of age, and age is therefore often considered an indication for treatment [35]. In a retrospective gender-related analysis of ITP patients, HMB was found in 18% of young women with ITP [37]. The overall incidence of HMB in adolescents with thrombocytopenia is reported to be 13–20% [38, 39] . Patients with ITP bleed less than those with aplastic anemia or chemotherapy-induced thrombocytopenia at equivalent platelet counts [36]. The bleeding phenotype in ITP depends on the platelet number, function of the platelets, the presence of additional bleeding disorders, and concurrent use of drugs or presence of infections which may interfere with coagulation [4].

Platelet Disorders in Adolescents Presenting with Bleeding Symptoms

Heavy Menstrual Bleeding
HMB is estimated to occur in approximately 20–37% of the female adolescent population [40–42]. Although HMB in adolescents can most frequently be attributed to anovulation and immaturity of the hypothalamic-pituitary-ovarian-uterine axis, bleeding disorders have been identified as a common cause of HMB in adolescents [39, 41, 43–47]. Among bleeding disorders, platelet function disorders have been reported in 5–44% of adolescents presenting with HMB [41, 43, 44, 47–51]. A number of studies have found platelet function disorders to be the most common bleeding disorder in this population [43, 44, 50, 52]. The frequency with which platelet function disorders are observed in this population varies based on whether platelet aggregation testing is performed as part of a comprehensive hemostatic evaluation in all patients, whether platelet ATP release is included in the testing, and how abnormal platelet function is assessed and defined [46]. Thrombocytopenia has also been observed in adolescents with HMB [47]. The most common quantitative platelet disorder associated with HMB in adolescents is ITP.

Epistaxis
Between 2% and 6% of children under 19 years of age referred for epistaxis have been reported to have an underlying platelet function defect [53, 54]. More than 90% of children with epistaxis found to have a bleeding disorder also have other bleeding symptoms, compared to 34% of children with epistaxis and no underlying bleeding disorder. Features of epistaxis significantly more common in patients with platelet function disorders include epistaxis requiring medical attention, >5 episodes/year, duration >10 min, bleeding occurring from both nostrils, and lack of seasonal correlation [55].

Evaluation

A complete history including bleeding symptoms, menstrual history, family history of bleeding symptoms and diagnosed bleeding disorders, medication history, and surgical and dental procedures and whether associated with excessive bleeding should be performed in adolescents presenting for evaluation [39]. CBC and iron studies should also be obtained in female adolescents with associated HMB as approximately 50–65% of adolescents with HMB have been found to have iron deficiency and/or anemia [47, 56].

Bleeding Assessment and Screening Tools

Standardized bleeding questionnaires and bleeding scores have been developed to determine the extent of bleeding symptoms in adolescents with bleeding disorders, including platelet function disorders [32, 33, 57–59]. A bleeding assessment tool has also been developed for ITP [60, 61].

Organ-specific short screening tools for both HMB (e.g., Philipp Screening Tool) and epistaxis have been developed applicable to adolescents presenting with these symptoms [55, 56, 62]. These screening tools may be useful in assisting clinicians in primary care settings to determine which adolescents should undergo comprehensive hemostatic laboratory testing for bleeding disorders, including platelet function disorders [55, 56, 62, 63].

Laboratory Testing

Platelet Number and Morphology

Automated Platelet Count
Platelet count derived using automated hematology analyzers is a rapid and convenient initial screen to assess quantitative abnormalities.

Automated analyzers primarily operate based on two principal mechanisms, impedance method or light scatter method. Platelets are distinguished from other cells in the impedance method based on their size as measured by change in electric potential that is proportional to the size of the cell passing through the counter aperture. This method can fail to identify platelets accurately when interference from other blood components such as microcytic red blood cells (RBCs) or fragments of RBCs or white blood cells is present causing overlap in platelet size distribution. Light or fluorescence scatter method provides better differentiation of platelets as cells are measured from multiple angles by a laser beam to identify cells based on size and cytoplasmic complexity [64].

Other useful platelet indices can be obtained by automated methods such as mean platelet volume (MPV) and can help in narrowing the diagnosis. Normal MPV ranges between 5 and 11 fl in most laboratories. Small platelet size (MPV <5 fl) are characteristic of certain disorders such as Wiskott-Aldrich syndrome (WAS), whereas large platelets (MPV >11 fl) can been seen in disorders such as ITP and BSS (Table 6.1).

Either method can be affected by pre-analytical factors such as specimen clotting due to insufficient mixing and platelet clumping due to platelet activation during sample collection. EDTA-dependent in vitro platelet clumping may result in pseudothrombocytopenia that can be avoided by utilizing sodium citrate or acid-citrate-dextrose (ACD) tubes for testing [65].

Light Microscopy and Manual Platelet Count

The importance of manual review of peripheral blood morphology cannot be overemphasized. The presence of macro- and microthrombocytes can be assessed by light microscopy. Many automated analyzers may not be able to detect platelets accurately based on their size if they are excessively large or small, as can occur in BSS or WAS, respectively. Visualization of platelet clumps suggests pseudothrombocytopenia, while pale agranular-appearing platelets are indicative

of GPS. The presence of intracytoplasmic inclusions, such as Döhle bodies in neutrophils, is diagnostic of MYH9-related disorders. Fragmented red blood cells are representative of microangiopathic hemolysis as seen in hemolytic uremic syndrome or thrombotic thrombocytopenic purpura (HUS/TTP) or disseminated intravascular coagulation (DIC). Increased reticulated platelets or young platelets with higher RNA content are indicative of increased platelet turnover as seen in ITP or any peripheral destructive process.

Manual platelet count by hemocytometer can be used to verify platelet count when automated counts are abnormal and unable to quantify platelet count accurately [66].

Electron Microscopy

Platelet light transmission electron microscopy (PTEM) is the preferred method for diagnosis of storage pool disorders affecting α and δ granules as most of these disorders may have completely normal or marginally abnormal platelet function results. Platelet ultrastructure is visualized by two methods, whole mount and thin-section preparation. In addition, leucocyte morphology can also be assessed by buffy coat preparations. Dense granules are primarily evaluated by whole mount preparation and appear as dark opaque inclusions due to their high calcium content. Alpha granules, other cellular organelles such as mitochondria, inclusions, and leucocytes are visualized by thin-section preparation (Fig. 6.3). Disorders associated with dense granule deficiency include HPS, CHS, WAS, and thrombocytopenia with absent radii syndrome (TAR), whereas α granule deficiency is seen classically in GPS and in other rare disorders such as white platelet syndrome, X-linked GATA1 macrothrombocytopenia, and York platelet syndrome. Combined deficiency is observed in α-δ platelet storage pool deficiency, while giant α granules characterize Paris-Trousseau-Jacobsen syndrome. Abnormal cytoplasmic inclusions in leucocytes are seen in CHS (Table 6.1).

Table 6.1 Laboratory diagnosis of inherited platelet disorders

	Inheritance	Platelet count	Peripheral blood smear	Platelet aggregation	Platelet ATP secretion	Flow cytometry	Diagnostic EM features	Gene mutation
Congenital thrombocytopenias								
Wiskott-Aldrich syndrome	X-R	Severe ↓	Small platelets	AA ↓ ADP ↓ Epi ↓ Col ↓ Risto ↓	↓ ↓ ↓ ↓ ↓	↓ GPIIb ↓ GPIIIa ↓ P-selectin ↓ PAC-1 ↓ CD63 on ADP stimulation	Small size, variable and distorted shape with numerous microvillosities, degranulated cytoplasm (scarce granules or lysosomes, rare mitochondria), and the distension of the canalicular system	*WAS*
MYH9-related disorders	AD	Mild to mod. ↓	Large platelets, leukocyte inclusions	NL	NL	NL	Inclusions in white cells NL platelet ultrastructure	*MYH9*
Familial platelet disorder and predisposition to AML	AD	Mild to mod. ↓	NL	AA ↓ ADP ↓ Epi ↓ Col ↓ Risto NL/↓	↓ ↓ ↓	↓ p-selectin on stimulation ↓ PAC-1 and fibrinogen binding	↓ Alpha, or dense granules, or both	*RUNX1*
Congenital amegakaryocytic thrombocytopenia	AR	Severe ↓	NL	NL	NL	↓ c-Mpl expression	NL	*MPL*
X-linked thrombocytopenia with dyserythropoiesis	X-R	Severe ↓	Large platelets	NL	NL	↓ p-selectin on stimulation	Large in size Hypogranular platelets Gray platelets with ↑DTS	*GATA-1*
Surface receptor defects								
Glanzmann thrombasthenia	AR	Mild to mod. ↓	Large platelets	AA ↓ ADP ↓ Epi ↓ Col ↓ Risto NL	NL NL NL NL NL	Absent GPIIb, GPIIIa	Large size	*ITGA2B, ITGB3*
Bernard-Soulier syndrome	AR	Mod. to severe ↓	Giant platelets	AA NL ADP NL Epi NL Col NL Risto ↓	NL NL NL NL NL	Absent GPIbα, GPIX	Giant platelets Megakaryocytes with abnormal membrane system	*GP1BA, GP1BB, GP9*

Disorder	Inheritance		Morphology	Aggregation		Activation	EM/Smear	Gene
Collagen receptor GPVI deficiency	AR	Mild ↓ or NL	NL	AA NL ADP NL Epi NL Col ↓ Risto NL	NL NL NL → NL	↓ GPVI ↓ P-selectin	NL	*GP6*
ADP receptor defect	AR	NL	NL	AA ↓ 2nd W ADP ↓ Epi ↓ 2nd W Col NL Risto NL	→ → → NL NL	↓ P-selectin ↓ PAC-1 On ADP ↓ ASP activity	NL	*P2RY12*
Thromboxane A2 receptor deficiency	AR	NL	NL	AA ↓ or delayed ADP NL Epi No 2nd wave Col NL Risto NL U46619 ↓	→ NL NL↓	No specific assay NL	NL	*TBXA2R*
Storage pool disorders								
Gray platelet syndrome	AD or AR	Mild ↓	Large and pale platelets	AA NL/↓ ADP NL/↓ Epi NL/↓ Col NL/↓ Risto NL/↓	NL/↓ NL/↓ NL/↓ NL/↓ NL/↓	↓ P-selectin upon sTRAP, ADP or convulxin stimulation	Large Lack alpha granules Few (<10%) platelets have visible granules DTS↑ Rare Golgi (<30% of platelets)	*NBEAL2, GFI1B*
White platelet syndrome	AD	Mild ↓	Large platelets	AA ↓ ADP ↓ Epi ↓ Col ↓ Risto ↓/NL	→ → → ↓/NL	↓ P-selectin upon sTRAP, ADP or convulxin stimulation	Large Lack alpha granules Few (30%) platelets are hypogranular DTS↑ Frequent Golgi (>30% of platelets)	Unknown
Paris-Trousseau Jacobsen syndrome	AD	Mod. to severe ↓	NL or large platelets	NL	NL	N/A	Large hypogranular platelets Giant α-granules	Del11q23 (*FLI1*)

(continued)

Table 6.1 (continued)

	Inheritance	Platelet count	Peripheral blood smear	Platelet aggregation	Platelet ATP secretion	Flow cytometry	Diagnostic EM features	Gene mutation
Quebec platelet disorder	AD	Mild ↓ or NL	NL	AA NL ADP NL/↓ Epi ↓ Col NL/↓ Risto NL	NL NL No 2nd W NL NL	↓ p-selectin ↓ Annexin V binding	NL	Elevated u-PA
Hermansky-Pudlak syndrome	AD or AR	NL	NL	AA NL ADP NL Epi ↓ 2nd W Col NL Risto NL	↓ ↓ ↓ ↓	↓ Serotonin	Absent dense body by whole mount	HPS1-7 AP3B1, AP3D1 DTNBP1, BLOC1S3, BLOC1S6 PLDN
Chediak-Higashi syndrome	AR	NL	Leukocyte inclusions	AA NL ADP ↓ Epi ↓ 2nd W Col NL Risto NL	NL/↓ NL/↓ NL/↓ NL/↓ NL/↓	↓ Dense granule mepacrine uptake and release	Leukocyte lysosomal inclusions ↓ Dense body	LYST
Combined αδ granule deficiency	AR/AD	NL	NL	AA NL/↓ ADP NL/↓ Epi NL/↓ Col NL/↓ Risto NL/↓	↓ ↓ ↓ ↓ ↓	↓ P-selectin ↓ serotonin	↓ Alpha and dense granules	Unknown
Signal transduction defects								
G-protein activation defect	AD	NL	NL	AA NL/↓ ADP ↓ Epi ↓ Col ↓ Risto NL/↓	NL/↓ ↓ ↓ NL/↓	↓ Activation with PAC-1	NL	GNAS

Disorder	Inheritance			Platelet aggregation		Assay		Gene
Thromboxane synthase deficiency	AD	NL	NL	AA absent ADP ↓ 2nd W Epi ↓ Col ↓ Risto NL	→ → → NL/↓	No specific assay NL	NL	TBXAS1
Cyclooxygenase deficiency	AD	NL	NL	AA absent ADP ↓ 2nd W Epi ↓ Col ↓ Risto NL	→ → → NL	No specific assay NL	NL	PTGS1
Pleckstrin phosphorylation defects	Unknown	NL	NL	AA NL ADP ↓ Epi ↓ Col NL U44069 ↓	NL → NL/↓	↓ Serotonin	NL	Unknown
Calcium mobilization defects	Unknown	NL	NL	AA NL ADP ↓ Epi ↓ Col NL/↓ U44069 ↓	NL → NL/↓	↓ Serotonin	NL	Unknown

Large platelet: more than half the size of red cells, Giant platelet: as big as red cells

↓ decreased, *2nd W* secondary wave, *AA* arachidonic acid, *AD* autosomal dominant, *ADP* adenosine diphosphate, *AML* acute myeloid leukemia, *AR* autosomal recessive, *Col* collagen, *DTS* dense tubular system, *Epi* epinephrine, *NL* normal, *PAC-1* procaspase-activating compound 1, *Risto* ristocetin, *sTRAP* soluble thrombin receptor agonist peptide, *u-PA* urokinase-type plasminogen activator, *VASP* vasodilator-stimulated phosphoprotein, *X-R* X-linked recessive

Platelet Function Analysis

Platelet Function Analyzer (PFA-100®) and Other Point-of-Care Tests

Platelet function analysis by PFA-100® (Siemens, Tarrytown, NY) is a widely available in vitro test for global platelet function designed as a replacement for the bleeding time which is now universally considered obsolete. Citrated whole blood is passed at high shear rate through an aperture in membranes coated with either collagen/epinephrine or collagen/adenosine diphosphate (ADP) as agonists. PFA-100 measures the aperture closure times (CTs) mimicking in vivo changes during primary hemostasis [67]. Therefore, PFA-100 may be useful as a screening test for vWD, particularly types 2A, 2B, and 3. In females, including adolescents, presenting with HMB, 80% sensitivity for vWD has been observed, with an inverse correlation between the closure time and VWF ristocetin cofactor [68]. This test is useful in screening severe platelet function disorders such as GT; however, the sensitivity is poor for the mild platelet function disorders, e.g., platelet storage pool disorders, often found in adolescents presenting with HMB [68]. Antiplatelet therapy with aspirin may also be predictably measured with PFA-100. Due to lack of sensitivity to P_2Y_{12} receptor antagonists, the INNOVANCE® PFA-200 has been developed for detecting platelet function inhibition by this class of drugs and may also be abnormal in inherited P_2Y_{12} defects [67]. Results may be compromised by preanalytical variables related to sample handling as well as thrombocytopenia and low hematocrit. Platelet reactivity can also be measured by the VerifyNow® P_2Y_{12} assay (Instrumentation Laboratory, Bedford, MA) which measures ADP-induced platelet activation in whole blood and by the MultiPlate analyzer® (Roche Diagnostics, Rotkreuz, Switzerland) which measures changes in electrical impedance by multiple electrode aggregometry.

Platelet Aggregation and Secretion

In vitro platelet aggregation assays allow evaluation of platelet function, primarily reflecting activation and aggregation, in a more specific fashion due to the use of different agonists at various concentrations that target specific receptors on the cell membrane surface. Commonly used agonists include collagen (activates receptors GPVI and GPIa/IIa), ADP (activates receptors P_2Y_1 and P_2Y_{12}), epinephrine (activates the $\alpha2$ receptor), arachidonic acid (activates the cyclooxygenase pathway), ristocetin (activates VWF binding to GPIb/V/IX), and thrombin receptor activation peptide (TRAP, activates the thrombin receptors PAR_1 and PAR_4).

The two methods usually employed in most laboratories are light transmission aggregometry (LTA) and whole blood aggregometry (WBA) [23]. LTA is considered the gold standard of platelet function testing that measures change in light transmission optically when agonists are stirred in patient's platelet-rich plasma (PRP) causing activation and aggregation. The increase in light transmission is recorded as a function of time on a graph. The resultant patterns, i.e., primary and secondary waves as well as deaggregation, are unique to each agonist that facilitate qualitative interpretation of abnormalities, if present. Percent aggregation, maximum amplitude, and rate of aggregation are also important parameters to be considered for quantitative interpretation. The WBA is based on similar principles measuring platelet aggregation by electrical impedance resulting in time-dependent curves. The advantages of WBA include smaller blood volume requirement, increased sensitivity to most agonists, and platelet function testing in the presence of other blood components that more closely mimics the in vivo setting. Classic examples of platelet aggregation abnormalities include absence of aggregation to all agonists except ristocetin in GT as platelets are deficient in GPIIb/IIIa receptors, while in BSS, platelets fail to aggregate with ristocetin only, due to lack of GP1b receptors. These assays, however, are not predictably sensitive to storage pool and secretion defects (Table 6.1).

The most commonly available secretion assay is the platelet adenosine triphosphate (ATP) release as an alternative to the gold standard radioactive ^{14}C-labelled serotonin release assay. Platelet ATP release is a marker for dense granule function and can be measured simultaneously with aggregation using specialized instruments.

The secretion of ATP from dense granules is quantified by lumiaggregometry measuring luminescence generated by ATP-dependent cleavage of luciferin by the firefly enzyme luciferase. Evaluation of α-granule secretion may be performed by flow cytometric measurement of surface P-selectin expression or, alternatively, by quantification of soluble α-granule contents in sample supernatants [69, 70] .

Platelet Surface Receptors and Activation

Platelet flow cytometric analysis is a reliable method to assess hereditary platelet disorders due to quantitative surface GP deficiencies and is a useful adjunctive test for platelet function evaluation. Surface expression levels can be measured by using fluorescent-conjugated GP-specific antibodies, and their fluorescence intensities can be compared to normal ranges of various GPs. Platelet activation causes conformational change and surface expression of activation markers such as P-selectin and annexin V that are markers of platelet granular secretion. Markedly decreased GPIIb and GPIIIa expression levels are diagnostic for GT, while BSS is characterized by markedly decreased GPIX and GPIbα expression. Identification of decreased GPVI or GPIa expression suggests collagen receptor deficiency (Table 6.1).

Gene Analysis

With expanding knowledge of inherited platelet disorders, genetic analyses can aid as a confirmatory test and facilitate genotype-phenotype correlation. Molecular diagnosis allows accurate diagnosis, especially for patients with subtle and nonspecific abnormalities, tailoring therapy, as well as individual and kindred counseling. For example, NBEAL2 gene mutation is associated with GPS, PLAU mutation in Quebec platelet syndrome, HPS mutations in Hermansky-Pudlak syndrome, MYH9 in MYH9-related disorders, MPL mutation in congenital amegakaryocytic thrombocytopenia (CAMT), and WAS mutation in Wiskott-Aldrich syndrome (Table 6.1). The International Society on Thrombosis and Haemostasis (ISTH) Genomics in Thrombosis

and Hemostasis Subcommittee has published guidelines for genetic testing in inherited platelet disorders with a curated list of 61 disease-causing defects related to platelet function and thrombopoietic disorders [71, 72]. Single gene tests as well as platelet disorder gene panels based on technologies such as whole exome sequencing and next-generation sequencing are available commercially for testing.

Management

General principles Since bleeding in patients with platelet disorders is typically mild except in a few inherited disorders of platelet function such as GT, and most bleeding manifestations involve skin and mucous membrane, intervention is often not required. Local measures like ice and application of pressure may be sufficient to manage minor bleeding.

Antifibrinolytic agents If intervention is warranted, antifibrinolytic (AF) agents are the mainstay of management of skin and mucous membrane bleeding. The two agents commonly used include epsilon aminocaproic acid (Amicar®) and tranexamic acid (Lysteda®). These agents are lysine analogues which prevent plasminogen from binding to fibrin and thereby prevent plasminogen activation and fibrinolysis. Tranexamic acid has been shown to significantly reduce menstrual blood flow in females with HMB and platelet function disorders [73]. Although data on the efficacy, dosing, and timing of antifibrinolytics in patients with bleeding disorders and other bleeding symptoms is extremely limited, these agents remain the standard of care for the management of mucosal bleeding and the prevention of bleeding with minor surgery, especially those involving mucous membranes [74]. Antifibrinolytic agents may be used orally or intravenously. The dose for tranexamic acid is 25 mg/kg body weight given every 8 hours, in patients with normal renal function, while reduced dosing at 15–20 mg/kg is recommended with renal impairment. Amicar is dosed at 50–75 mg/kg body weight every 6 hours for continued bleeding. The duration of therapy is approximately 3–5 days for minor bleeding or surgery and 5–7 days for major bleeding or surgery.

Recombinant FVIIa The mechanism of action of rFVIIa is hypothesized to be increased thrombin generation by tissue factor-independent processes along with increased adhesion of platelets to the extracellular matrix and enhanced platelet aggregation [75, 76]. In the international GT registry, the dose of rFVIIa found to be effective for the management of spontaneous bleeding and for the prevention of bleeding with surgery is 90–140 μg/kg every ≤2.5 hours [76]. The risk of excessive thrombin generation resulting in thrombosis must be recognized and has been infrequently reported [75, 77].

DDAVP The utility of DDAVP in patients with mild hemophilia and vWD has been well established, as the drug increases plasma concentrations of VWF and FVIII by releasing stored VWF and FVIII from the endothelial lining. In platelet disorders the effect of DDAVP is secondary to increased adhesion of platelets to the subendothelial matrix and increased aggregation at high shear with a resulting decrease in the bleeding time [75]. DDAVP has been shown to be effective in storage pool disorders, platelet signal transduction abnormalities, TXA receptor deficiency, and May-Hegglin anomaly in small case series. The dose most commonly used is 0.3 μg/kg as a single intravenous dose in pre-procedural settings [78]. Intranasal DDAVP has been shown to be effective in managing HMB in patients with platelet dysfunction [73].

Platelet transfusions Although platelet transfusions intuitively would "fix" the problem, they are often deferred and used only as a last resort for several reasons including the need for hospitalization (even short term) for infusion, the potential risks associated with exposure to blood products such as allergic reactions/anaphylaxis, febrile reactions, transfusion-associated lung injury, and the development of alloantibodies. HLA-matched, single-donor leucocyte-depleted platelet concentrates should be considered in order to decrease the risk of development of anti-HLA antibodies.

Hormonal therapy Patients with severe platelet disorders like GT and BSS can present with severe bleeding at the time of menarche, often requiring blood transfusions. HMB may also be a recurring issue in these patients requiring the continuous use of hormonal therapy. Progesterone-only agents, combined oral contraceptives (COC), or IV estrogen may be required, depending on the severity of bleeding. Intrauterine devices like the Mirena® IUD have been shown to be effective in decreasing the bleeding and improving the QoL in patients with bleeding disorders and associated HMB [79]. Milder platelet disorders may not be associated with severe HMB but may still require outpatient intervention with hormonal therapies and/or antifibrinolytics.

Thrombopoietin (TPO) mimetics TPO mimetics are typically utilized to raise the platelet count in both acute and chronic ITP. The two agents currently available include Romiplostim (N-Plate®) and Elthrombopag (Promacta®). These agents stimulate the TPO receptor and result in enhanced megakaryopoiesis and platelet production. They have been shown to be effective in both improving the platelet count and in the management of bleeding in patients with MYH9-related platelet disorders [80].

Hematopoietic stem cell transplant (HSCT) and gene therapy HSCT is a consideration for patients with recurrent severe bleeding and/or platelet alloantibodies and resultant platelet refractoriness. As of 2015, 19 cases of GT had undergone HSCT. Cord blood, HLA identical siblings, HLA-matched unrelated donors, and matched family donors have been utilized. Both reduced and conventional conditioning regimens have been reported to have been used successfully with sustained engraftment [81]. Gene therapy is also still in the experimental stage for GT. Transplanting autologous hematopoietic stem cells transduced with genes encoding for normal GPIIb/IIIa could result in de novo synthesis of the normal integrin within the mega-karyocyte and resultant normal expression of the receptor on the platelet surface. This has been shown to be successful in a dog gene therapy model followed for up to 5 years, but it remains to be seen if this is a feasible option in humans [82].

Major bleeding Management of major or life-threatening bleeding includes acute intervention to assist in hemostasis and also the management of acute and chronic anemia. AF in this situation are used as adjunctive agents, with platelet transfusions being the mainstay of therapy to restore hemostasis in both thrombocytopenia and platelet dysfunction. Platelet transfusions are extremely effective in stopping bleeding except in situations associated with immune-mediated destruction of platelets or development of alloantibodies resulting in refractoriness to platelet transfusions. Recombinant activated FVII has been shown to be effective in managing bleeding especially in GT [77].

Major bleeding in ITP The intent of treatment is to raise the platelet count acutely to stop the bleeding. The established first-line therapy for bleeding in ITP includes intravenous immune globulin (IVIG), oral prednisone/IV steroids, and anti-D (in those who are RhD positive). In acute situations it is often necessary to utilize multiple modalities simultaneously to expeditiously raise the platelet count. The modalities that are commonly used together are IVIG and steroids, as this combination has been shown to increase the platelet count in as few as 24 hours. In addition, the use of AF agents and hormonal therapies (COC or IV estrogen) is essential to control uterine bleeding [83]. Platelet transfusions are usually reserved for major bleeding events such as ICH, as they may only elevate the counts for a very short duration or may not be effective at all. In the event of life-threatening HMB, all the above modalities in addition to platelet and red cell transfusions may become necessary [83]. Once the acute bleeding is controlled, secondary treatment options such as TPO receptor agonists or other immunosuppressive agents like ritux-imab and continuous hormonal therapies may be necessary to maintain adequate platelet counts and prevent recurrence of HMB or other major bleeding [4]. Data from the Intercontinental Cooperative ITP study group looking at bleeding manifestations and management in chronic ITP reported no ICH in 343 patients enrolled on study with complete data available. Platelet transfusions were used uncommonly, with 54% of platelet transfusions being used in patients with bleeding from more than two sites. Splenectomy may also be considered for management of both acute and chronic thrombocytopenia associated with bleeding, but is rarely considered in the acute setting [84].

Supportive management In addition to the management of acute bleeding, it is imperative that issues such as anemia and QoL be addressed appropriately. Chronic anemia is associated with significant deterioration of the QoL secondary to fatigue, which is often ignored as a clinical symptom. Appropriate multidisciplinary care with a hematologist in the loop may be beneficial. Lack of compliance with oral iron supplementation secondary to GI side effects of iron therapy is very common and requires close follow-up and frequent monitoring [85]. In view of the increased likelihood of exposure to blood and blood products in patients with platelet disorders, it is also important to ensure that patients are vaccinated against hepatitis B. Preventive measures such as adequate dental hygiene (to prevent gingival bleeding) and avoidance of aspirin and NSAIDs must be emphasized [75].

Conclusion

HMB and other mucocutaneous bleeding symptoms such as epistaxis are common bleeding symptoms in adolescent females. While severe platelet disorders often present earlier in childhood, mild platelet disorders are an important cause of bleeding symptoms, especially HMB, in adolescent females. A systematic and stepwise approach using standardized questionnaires and bleeding scores and meticulous correlation of clinical history, physical examination, and laboratory findings can facilitate accurate diagnosis. Multidisciplinary team involvement is essential to ensure optimum treatment and to maintain high quality of life.

References

1. Amesse LS, Pfaff-Amesse T, Gunning WT, Duffy N, French JA 2nd. Clinical and laboratory characteristics of adolescents with platelet function disorders and heavy menstrual bleeding. Exp Hematol Oncol. 2013;2(1):3.
2. Philipp CS. Platelet disorders in adolescents. J Pediatr Adolesc Gynecol. 2010;23(6 Suppl):S11–4.
3. Neunert CE. Current management of immune thrombocytopenia. Hematology Am Soc Hematol Educ Program. 2013;2013:276–82.
4. Kuhne T. Diagnosis and management of immune thrombocytopenia in childhood. Hamostaseologie. 2017;37(1):36–44.
5. Bolton-Maggs PH, Chalmers EA, Collins PW, Harrison P, Kitchen S, Liesner RJ, et al. A review of inherited platelet disorders with guidelines for their management on behalf of the UKHCDO. Br J Haematol. 2006;135(5):603–33.
6. Nurden P, Nurden AT. Congenital disorders associated with platelet dysfunctions. Thromb Haemost. 2008;99(2):253–63.
7. Wei AH, Schoenwaelder SM, Andrews RK, Jackson SP. New insights into the haemostatic function of platelets. Br J Haematol. 2009;147(4):415–30.
8. George JN, Caen JP, Nurden AT. Glanzmann's thrombasthenia: the spectrum of clinical disease. Blood. 1990;75(7):1383–95.
9. Jenkins CS, Phillips DR, Clemetson KJ, Meyer D, Larrieu MJ, Luscher EF. Platelet membrane glycoproteins implicated in ristocetin-induced aggregation. Studies of the proteins on platelets from patients with Bernard-Soulier syndrome and von Willebrand's disease. J Clin Invest. 1976;57(1):112–24.
10. Arthur JF, Dunkley S, Andrews RK. Platelet glycoprotein VI-related clinical defects. Br J Haematol. 2007;139(3):363–72.
11. Rao AK, Gabbeta J. Congenital disorders of platelet signal transduction. Arterioscler Thromb Vasc Biol. 2000;20(2):285–9.
12. Fuse I, Hattori A, Mito M, Higuchi W, Yahata K, Shibata A, et al. Pathogenetic analysis of five cases with a platelet disorder characterized by the absence of thromboxane A2 (TXA2)-induced platelet aggregation in spite of normal TXA2 binding activity. Thromb Haemost. 1996;76(6):1080–5.
13. Fuse I, Higuchi W, Aizawa Y. Pathogenesis of a bleeding disorder characterized by platelet unresponsiveness to thromboxane A2. Semin Thromb Hemost. 2000;26(1):43–5.
14. Raccuglia G. Gray platelet syndrome. A variety of qualitative platelet disorder. Am J Med. 1971;51(6):818–28.
15. White JG. Ultrastructural studies of the gray platelet syndrome. Am J Pathol. 1979;95(2):445–62.
16. Holmsen H, Weiss HJ. Secretable storage pools in platelets. Annu Rev Med. 1979;30:119–34.
17. Meyers KM, Holmsen H, Seachord CL, Hopkins GE, Borchard RE, Padgett GA. Storage pool deficiency in platelets from Chediak-Higashi cattle. Am J Phys. 1979;237(3):R239–48.
18. White JG. Platelet granule disorders. Crit Rev Oncol Hematol. 1986;4(4):337–77.
19. Witkop CJ, Krumwiede M, Sedano H, White JG. Reliability of absent platelet dense bodies as a diagnostic criterion for Hermansky-Pudlak syndrome. Am J Hematol. 1987;26(4):305–11.
20. Goldenberg NA, Jacobson L, Manco-Johnson MJ. Brief communication: duration of platelet dysfunction after a 7-day course of Ibuprofen. Ann Intern Med. 2005;142(7):506–9.
21. Kottke-Marchant K, Powers JB, Brooks L, Kundu S, Christie DJ. The effect of antiplatelet drugs, heparin, and preanalytical variables on platelet function detected by the platelet function analyzer (PFA-100). Clin Appl Thromb Hemost. 1999;5(2):122–30.
22. Madan M, Berkowitz SD, Christie DJ, Jennings LK, Smit AC, Sigmon KN, et al. Rapid assessment of glycoprotein IIb/IIIa blockade with the platelet function analyzer (PFA-100) during percutaneous coronary intervention. Am Heart J. 2001;141(2):226–33.
23. Podda G, Femia EA, Cattaneo M. Current and emerging approaches for evaluating platelet disorders. Int J Lab Hematol. 2016;38(Suppl 1):50–8.
24. Deligeoroglou E, Karountzos V. Abnormal Uterine Bleeding including coagulopathies and other menstrual disorders. Best Pract Res Clin Obstet Gynaecol. 2018;48:51–61.
25. Orsini S, Noris P, Bury L, Heller PG, Santoro C, Kadir RA, et al. Bleeding risk of surgery and its prevention in patients with inherited platelet disorders. Haematologica. 2017;102(7):1192–203.
26. Gunay-Aygun M, Zivony-Elboum Y, Gumruk F, Geiger D, Cetin M, Khayat M, et al. Gray platelet syndrome: natural history of a large patient cohort and locus assignment to chromosome 3p. Blood. 2010;116(23):4990–5001.
27. Kongalappa S, Reddy JM, Durugappa T, D'Souza F, Subramanian S, Prakash A. Glanzmann Thrombasthenia in children: experience from a Tertiary Care Center in Southern India. J Pediatr Hematol Oncol. 2019;41(2):e68–71.
28. Markovitch O, Ellis M, Holzinger M, Goldberger S, Beyth Y. Severe juvenile vaginal bleeding due to Glanzmann's thrombasthenia: case report and review of the literature. Am J Hematol. 1998;57(3):225–7.
29. Savoia A, Pastore A, De Rocco D, Civaschi E, Di Stazio M, Bottega R, et al. Clinical and genetic aspects of Bernard-Soulier syndrome: searching for

genotype/phenotype correlations. Haematologica. 2011;96(3):417–23.

30. Rajpurkar M, O'Brien SH, Haamid FW, Cooper DL, Gunawardena S, Chitlur M. Heavy menstrual bleeding as a common presenting symptom of rare platelet disorders: illustrative case examples. J Pediatr Adolesc Gynecol. 2016;29(6):537–41.

31. Revel-Vilk S, Richter C, Ben-Ami T, Yacobovich J, Aviner S, Ben-Barak A, et al. Quantitation of bleeding symptoms in a national registry of patients with inherited platelet disorders. Blood Cells Mol Dis. 2017;67:59–62.

32. Biss TT, Blanchette VS, Clark DS, Wakefield CD, James PD, Rand ML. Use of a quantitative pediatric bleeding questionnaire to assess mucocutaneous bleeding symptoms in children with a platelet function disorder. J Thromb Haemost. 2010;8(6):1416–9.

33. Kaur H, Borhany M, Azzam H, Costa-Lima C, Ozelo M, Othman M. The utility of International Society on thrombosis and haemostasis-bleeding assessment tool and other bleeding questionnaires in assessing the bleeding phenotype in two platelet function defects. Blood Coagul Fibrinol Int J Haemost Thromb. 2016;27(5):589–93.

34. Chandra J, Ravi R, Singh V, Narayan S, Sharma S, Dutta AK. Bleeding manifestations in severely thrombocytopenic children with immune thrombocytopenic purpura. Hematology (Amsterdam, Netherlands). 2006;11(2):131–3.

35. Arnold DM. Bleeding complications in immune thrombocytopenia. Hematology Am Soc Hematol Educ Program. 2015;2015:237–42.

36. Provan D, Newland AC. Current Management of Primary Immune Thrombocytopenia. Adv Ther. 2015;32(10):875–87.

37. Andres E, Mecili M, Fothergill H, Zimmer J, Vogel T, Maloisel F. Gender-related analysis of the clinical presentation, treatment response and outcome in patients with immune thrombocytopenia. Presse Med. 2012;41(9 Pt 1):e426–31.

38. Ahuja SP, Hertweck SP. Overview of bleeding disorders in adolescent females with menorrhagia. J Pediatr Adolesc Gynecol. 2010;23(6 Suppl):S15–21.

39. Haamid F, Sass AE, Dietrich JE. Heavy menstrual bleeding in adolescents. J Pediatr Adolesc Gynecol. 2017;30(3):335–40.

40. Gray SH, Emans SJ. Abnormal vaginal bleeding in adolescents. Pediatr Rev. 2007;28(5):175–82.

41. Gursel T, Biri A, Kaya Z, Sivaslioglu S, Albayrak M. The frequency of menorrhagia and bleeding disorders in university students. Pediatr Hematol Oncol. 2014;31(5):467–74.

42. Friberg B, Orno AK, Lindgren A, Lethagen S. Bleeding disorders among young women: a population-based prevalence study. Acta Obstet Gynecol Scand. 2006;85(2):200–6.

43. Philipp CS, Faiz A, Dowling N, Dilley A, Michaels LA, Ayers C, et al. Age and the prevalence of bleeding disorders in women with menorrhagia. Obstet Gynecol. 2005;105(1):61–6.

44. Vo KT, Grooms L, Klima J, Holland-Hall C, O'Brien SH. Menstrual bleeding patterns and prevalence of bleeding disorders in a multidisciplinary adolescent haematology clinic. Haemophilia. 2013;19(1):71–5.

45. Bevan JA, Maloney KW, Hillery CA, Gill JC, Montgomery RR, Scott JP. Bleeding disorders: a common cause of menorrhagia in adolescents. J Pediatr. 2001;138(6):856–61.

46. Zia A, Rajpurkar M. Challenges of diagnosing and managing the adolescent with heavy menstrual bleeding. Thromb Res. 2016;143:91–100.

47. O'Brien B, Mason J, Kimble R. Bleeding disorders in adolescents with heavy menstrual bleeding: the Queensland Statewide Paediatric and Adolescent Gynaecology Service. J Pediatr Adolesc Gynecol. 2019;32(2):122–7.

48. Mikhail S, Varadarajan R, Kouides P. The prevalence of disorders of haemostasis in adolescents with menorrhagia referred to a haemophilia treatment centre. Haemophilia. 2007;13(5):627–32.

49. Mills HL, Abdel-Baki MS, Teruya J, Dietrich JE, Shah MD, Mahoney D Jr, et al. Platelet function defects in adolescents with heavy menstrual bleeding. Haemophilia. 2014;20(2):249–54.

50. Seravalli V, Linari S, Peruzzi E, Dei M, Paladino E, Bruni V. Prevalence of hemostatic disorders in adolescents with abnormal uterine bleeding. J Pediatr Adolesc Gynecol. 2013;26(5):285–9.

51. Jayasinghe Y, Moore P, Donath S, Campbell J, Monagle P, Grover S. Bleeding disorders in teenagers presenting with menorrhagia. Aust N Z J Obstet Gynaecol. 2005;45(5):439–43.

52. Philipp CS, Dilley A, Miller CH, Evatt B, Baranwal A, Schwartz R, et al. Platelet functional defects in women with unexplained menorrhagia. J Thromb Haemost. 2003;1(3):477–84.

53. Elden L, Reinders M, Witmer C. Predictors of bleeding disorders in children with epistaxis: value of preoperative tests and clinical screening. Int J Pediatr Otorhinolaryngol. 2012;76(6):767–71.

54. Sandoval C, Dong S, Visintainer P, Ozkaynak MF, Jayabose S. Clinical and laboratory features of 178 children with recurrent epistaxis. J Pediatr Hematol Oncol. 2002;24(1):47–9.

55. Stokhuijzen E, Segbefia CI, Biss TT, Clark DS, James PD, Riddel J, et al. Severity and features of epistaxis in children with a mucocutaneous bleeding disorder. J Pediatr. 2018;193:183-9.e2.

56. Philipp CS, Faiz A, Heit JA, Kouides PA, Lukes A, Stein SF, et al. Evaluation of a screening tool for bleeding disorders in a US multisite cohort of women with menorrhagia. Am J Obstet Gynecol. 2011;204(3):209 e1–7.

57. Rodeghiero F, Tosetto A, Abshire T, Arnold DM, Coller B, James P, et al. ISTH/SSC bleeding assessment tool: a standardized questionnaire and a proposal for a new bleeding score for inherited bleeding disorders. J Thromb Haemost. 2010;8(9):2063–5.

58. Bidlingmaier C, Grote V, Budde U, Olivieri M, Kurnik K. Prospective evaluation of a pediatric bleed-

ing questionnaire and the ISTH bleeding assessment tool in children and parents in routine clinical practice. J Thromb Haemost. 2012;10(7):1335–41.

59. Elbatarny M, Mollah S, Grabell J, Bae S, Deforest M, Tuttle A, et al. Normal range of bleeding scores for the ISTH-BAT: adult and pediatric data from the merging project. Haemophilia. 2014;20(6):831–5.

60. Page LK, Psaila B, Provan D, Michael Hamilton J, Jenkins JM, Elish AS, et al. The immune thrombocytopenic purpura (ITP) bleeding score: assessment of bleeding in patients with ITP. Br J Haematol. 2007;138(2):245–8.

61. Kumar M, Dutta S, Bhattyacharyya M. Application of ITP-BAT bleeding score in clinical practice. Int J Hematol. 2015;101(2):207–8.

62. Philipp CS, Faiz A, Dowling NF, Beckman M, Owens S, Ayers C, et al. Development of a screening tool for identifying women with menorrhagia for hemostatic evaluation. Am J Obstet Gynecol. 2008;198(2):163. e1–8.

63. Zia A, Stanek J, Christian-Rancy M, Ahuja SP, Savelli S, O'Brien SH. Utility of a screening tool for haemostatic defects in a multicentre cohort of adolescents with heavy menstrual bleeding. Haemophilia. 2018;24(6):957–63.

64. Briggs C, Harrison P, Machin SJ. Continuing developments with the automated platelet count. Int J Lab Hematol. 2007;29(2):77–91.

65. Kunz D. Possibilities and limitations of automated platelet counting procedures in the thrombocytopenic range. Semin Thromb Hemost. 2001;27(3):229–35.

66. Sutor AH, Grohmann A, Kaufmehl K, Wundisch T. Problems with platelet counting in thrombocytopenia. A rapid manual method to measure low platelet counts. Semin Thromb Hemost. 2001;27(3):237–43.

67. Rand ML, Reddy EC, Israels SJ. Laboratory diagnosis of inherited platelet function disorders. Transfus Apher Sci. 2018;57(4):485–93.

68. Philipp CS, Miller CH, Faiz A, Dilley A, Michaels LA, Ayers C, et al. Screening women with menorrhagia for underlying bleeding disorders: the utility of the platelet function analyser and bleeding time. Haemophilia. 2005;11(5):497–503.

69. Mumford AD, Frelinger AL 3rd, Gachet C, Gresele P, Noris P, Harrison P, et al. A review of platelet secretion assays for the diagnosis of inherited platelet secretion disorders. Thromb Haemost. 2015;114(1):14–25.

70. Gresele P. Subcommittee on Platelet Physiology of the International Society on T, Hemostasis. Diagnosis of inherited platelet function disorders: guidance from the SSC of the ISTH. J Thromb Haemost. 2015;13(2):314–22.

71. Gresele P, Bury L, Falcinelli E. Inherited platelet function disorders: algorithms for phenotypic and genetic investigation. Semin Thromb Hemost. 2016;42(3):292–305.

72. Megy K, Downes K, Simeoni I, Bury L, Morales J, Mapeta R, et al. Curated disease-causing genes for bleeding, thrombotic, and platelet disorders: communication from the SSC of the ISTH. J Thromb Haemost. 2019;17(8):1253–60.

73. Kouides PA, Byams VR, Philipp CS, Stein SF, Heit JA, Lukes AS, et al. Multisite management study of menorrhagia with abnormal laboratory haemostasis: a prospective crossover study of intranasal desmopressin and oral tranexamic acid. Br J Haematol. 2009;145(2):212–20.

74. O'Brien SH. Common management issues in pediatric patients with mild bleeding disorders. Semin Thromb Hemost. 2012;38(7):720–6.

75. Nurden AT, Freson K, Seligsohn U. Inherited platelet disorders. Haemophilia. 2012;18(Suppl 4):154–60.

76. Lee A, Poon MC. Inherited platelet functional disorders: general principles and practical aspects of management. Transfus Apher Sci. 2018;57(4):494–501.

77. Recht M, Rajpurkar M, Chitlur M, d'Oiron R, Zotz R, Di Minno G, et al. Independent adjudicator assessments of platelet refractoriness and rFVIIa efficacy in bleeding episodes and surgeries from the multinational Glanzmann's thrombasthenia registry. Am J Hematol. 2017;92(7):646–52.

78. Desborough MJ, Oakland KA, Landoni G, Crivellari M, Doree C, Estcourt LJ, et al. Desmopressin for treatment of platelet dysfunction and reversal of antiplatelet agents: a systematic review and meta-analysis of randomized controlled trials. J Thromb Haemost. 2017;15(2):263–72.

79. Kingman CE, Kadir RA, Lee CA, Economides DL. The use of levonorgestrel-releasing intrauterine system for treatment of menorrhagia in women with inherited bleeding disorders. Br J Obstet Gynecol. 2004;111(12):1425–8.

80. Zaninetti C, Barozzi S, Bozzi V, Gresele P, Balduini CL, Pecci A. Eltrombopag in preparation for surgery in patients with severe MYH9-related thrombocytopenia. Am J Hematol. 2019;94(8):E199–201.

81. Solh T, Botsford A, Solh M. Glanzmann's thrombasthenia: pathogenesis, diagnosis, and current and emerging treatment options. J Blood Med. 2015;6:219–27.

82. Poon MC, Di Minno G, d'Oiron R, Zotz R. New insights into the treatment of Glanzmann Thrombasthenia. Transfus Med Rev. 2016;30(2):92–9.

83. James AH, Kouides PA, Abdul-Kadir R, Dietrich JE, Edlund M, Federici AB, et al. Evaluation and management of acute menorrhagia in women with and without underlying bleeding disorders: consensus from an international expert panel. Eur J Obstet Gynecol Reprod Biol. 2011;158(2):124–34.

84. Neunert CE, Buchanan GR, Imbach P, Bolton-Maggs PH, Bennett CM, Neufeld E, et al. Bleeding manifestations and management of children with persistent and chronic immune thrombocytopenia: data from the Intercontinental Cooperative ITP Study Group (ICIS). Blood. 2013;121(22):4457–62.

85. Cooke AG, McCavit TL, Buchanan GR, Powers JM. Iron deficiency anemia in adolescents who present with heavy menstrual bleeding. J Pediatr Adolesc Gynecol. 2017;30(2):247–50.

Fibrinolytic Pathway Disorders

7

Shveta Gupta and Sweta Gupta

Fibrinolytic Pathway Overview and Regulation

The three main components of blood coagulation include primary hemostasis, secondary hemostasis, and the fibrinolytic system. The coagulation and fibrinolytic systems are highly regulated and inter-related through mechanisms that ensure balanced hemostasis. The typical physiologic response to vessel injury is initial adherence of platelets to sub-endothelial sites followed by platelet activation and platelet plug formation. The activated platelets facilitate the assembly of activated coagulation factors leading to production of thrombin, which catalyzes the conversion of fibrinogen to insoluble fibrin. Fibrin plays an essential role in hemostasis as both the primary product of the coagulation cascade and the substrate for fibrinolysis [1]. Fibrin formed as a result of action of thrombin on fibrinogen triggers the conversion of circulating pro-enzyme plasminogen to plasmin. Plasmin is generated from the zymogen plasminogen on the surface of the fibrin clot, or on cell surfaces, by either tissue

plasminogen activator (tPA) or urokinase-type plasminogen activator (uPA) [2]. tPA is synthesized and released by endothelial cells. tPA is a weak activator of plasminogen; however, fibrin greatly enhances its catalytic potential. uPA is produced by monocytes, macrophages, and urinary epithelium and can effectively activate plasminogen both in presence and absence of fibrin but has much lower affinity for fibrin as compared with tPA [3]. Once formed plasmin is the main fibrinolytic enzyme that proteolyzes fibrin into fibrin degradation products (FDP). Plasmin increases the efficiency of the plasminogen activators, hence exerting positive feedback on its own activation. Both tPA and uPA are cleared by the liver after forming complexes with a low-density lipoprotein (LDL)-receptor-like protein; however, in addition, inhibitors are also essential for effective fibrinolytic homeostasis [4]. Excessive circulating plasmin and plasminogen activators are most commonly neutralized by serine protease inhibitors, or serpins which include plasminogen activator inhibitor-1 (PAI-1), plasminogen activator inhibitor-2 (PAI-2), and α2-antiplasmin (A2AP). Other non-serpin inhibitors which play minor roles in plasmin inhibition include thrombin-activatable fibrinolysis inhibitor (TAFI), α2-macroglobulin, C1-esterase inhibitor, and members of the contact pathway of the coagulation cascade [5]. The plasminogen activators tPA and uPA are rapidly inhibited by PAI-1, which is released into the circulation from

S. Gupta (✉)
Arnold Palmer Hospital for Children, Orlando, FL, USA
e-mail: shveta.gupta@orlandohealth.com

S. Gupta
Indiana Hemophilia and Thrombosis Center, Indianapolis, IN, USA

© Springer Nature Switzerland AG 2020
L. V. Srivaths (ed.), *Hematology in the Adolescent Female*,
https://doi.org/10.1007/978-3-030-48446-0_7

Fig. 7.1 Pathway of
fibrinolysis. Dotted lines
indicate inhibition.
Black arrows indicate
stimulation. A2AP
α2-antiplasmin; PAI-1
plasminogen activator
inhibitor-1; tPA
tissue-type plasminogen
activator; uPA
urokinase-type
plasminogen activator;
FDP fibrin degradation
products; TAFI
thrombin-activatable
fibrinolysis inhibitor

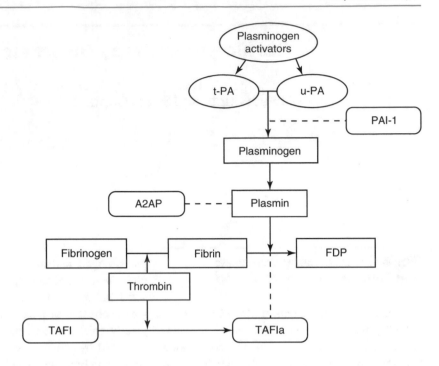

endothelial cells, platelets, and other cells. In pregnancy, PAI-2 is additionally a major tPA and uPA inhibitor. The main physiological plasmin inhibitor is A2AP. Fibrin-bound plasmin is protected from A2AP inhibition allowing for fibrinolysis to effectively proceed. Activated TAFI is a carboxypeptidase that removes C-terminal lysine residues on fibrin, thereby decreasing plasmin generation and stabilization of fibrin-containing thrombi [6] (Fig. 7.1).

Hyperfibrinolysis can result in bleeding, whereas hypofibrinolytic states with decreased activation of fibrinolysis can result in impaired clot dissolution and are a recognized acquired cause of thrombosis in multiple disease states [5].

Congenital Hyperfibrinolytic Disorders

Hemorrhagic diathesis secondary to hyperfibrinolysis is characterized by normal primary hemostasis but delayed bleeding because of premature dissolution of the hemostatic plug and may be reminiscent of the bleeding that occurs with FXIII deficiency. Bleeding disorders occur when the fibrinolytic process is accelerated, as a

result of either (1) decreased fibrinolytic inhibition due to deficiency of main inhibitors, PAI-1 or A2AP, or (2) increased fibrinolytic activation as a result of excess uPA or tPA. Key characteristic features of the fibrinolytic disorders are summarized in Table 7.1.

Deficiency of Fibrinolytic Inhibitors

Alpha 2 Antiplasmin Deficiency (Excessive Plasmin Activity)

Background A2AP is the major physiologic plasmin inhibitor. It is a member of serpin family of enzyme inhibitors and is synthesized in the liver with a half-life of 2–6 days. Other functions of A2AP include increased resistance of fibrin to plasmin by promoting competitive inhibition of plasminogen binding to fibrin and crosslinking of the alpha chains of fibrin along with activated FXIII [5]. The first case of A2AP deficiency was reported in 1978 and was named Miyasoto disease after the patient's surname who presented with recurrent bleeding [7]. The disorder is inherited in an autosomal recessive manner and is very rare, although the exact prevalence is unknown.

Table 7.1 Characteristic features of congenital fibrinolytic disorders

Defect	Genetic mutation	Inheritance	Key bleeding Symptoms	Diagnosis	Treatment
A2AP deficiency	*SERPINE 2*	AR	Mucocutaenous bleeding, intramedullary hemorrhage, umbilical bleeding, reproductive tract bleeding	Reduced antiplasmin activity	Antifibrinolytics Agents and/or Fresh frozen plasma for severe bleeding
PAI-1 deficiency	*SERPINE 1*	AR	Mucocutaenous bleeding, delayed Bleeding post-surgery and trauma, reproductive tract bleeding, delayed wound healing	Absent PAI-1 activity with absent to low/ normal antigen	
Quebec platelet disorder	*PLAU*	AD	Mucocutaenous bleeding, muscle and joint bleeds, spontaneous hematuria		Antifibrinolytic agents

A2AP α2-antiplasmin, *PAI-1* Plasminogen activator inhibitor-1, *AR* autosomal recessive, *AD* autosomal dominant

Clinical Manifestations Homozygous A2AP deficiency results in moderate to severe bleeding symptoms often presenting in childhood. Umbilical bleeding may be the first manifestation of the disease. Other symptoms range from easy bruising, mucosal bleeding, soft tissue hematomas, hemarthroses, bleeding following dental or surgical procedures, and trauma [8]. Interestingly multiple patients with an unusual clinical manifestation of spontaneous or post-traumatic diaphyseal intramedullary hemorrhage of the long bones have been described [9, 10]. Heterozygous individuals, in contrast, may have milder bleeding or may be asymptomatic. The most common bleeding symptoms described are commonly either post-surgical or post-traumatic; however, severe bleeding manifestation like gastrointestinal bleeding or umbilical stump bleeding has also been reported [11]. Elderly patients with heterozygous A2AP deficiency may manifest increased bleeding symptoms due to fall in plasma levels with increasing age [12].

Implications in Young Women Symptoms of heavy menstrual bleeding (HMB) and postpartum bleeding and obstetric complications such as preterm delivery and miscarriages have been reported in both homozygous and heterozygous states [6, 13]. Although it appears to be a relevant issue, the true prevalence of female-specific bleeding issues in A2AP deficiency states is challenging to estimate given the low prevalence of this disorder [14].

PAI-1 Deficiency (Excessive Plasminogen Activation)

Background Complete quantitative deficiency and qualitative defects in *PAI-1 result in a moderate to severe bleeding phenotype in humans* [15–25]. *PAI-1 deficiency is an autosomal recessive disorder. Due to its rarity, its prevalence is unknown, although cases have been reported worldwide. Heterozygotes of PAI-1 deficiency do not manifest with bleeding symptoms. Fay et al. reported the* first genetic defect *SERPINE1* (c.699_700dupTA) in a young Amish homozygous PAI-1-deficient female in 1992 with undetectable PAI-1 levels, who presented with bleeding post-trauma and surgery [16]. Since then, several extended family members have been diagnosed to carry the same mutation.

Clinical Manifestations Individuals with PAI-1 deficiency manifest with bruising, epistaxis, oral bleeds, muscle hematomas after injury or trauma, hemarthrosis, prolonged wound healing, and post-traumatic, post-surgical bleeding, and women can present with HMB, hemorrhagic rupture of ovarian cysts, antenatal bleeding, and postpartum hemorrhage. Other genetic defects leading to compound heterozygous and homozygous states with variable bleeding phenotypes have been described in the literature [15–26]. In a recent NIH-funded research study, it was discovered that complete deficiency of PAI-1 is associated with varying degrees of cardiac fibrosis resulting in poor ejection fraction, as seen in the Amish population in Berne, Indiana [27].

Implications in Young Women PAI-1 deficiency has major implications in the reproductive years manifesting mainly as HMB and pregnancy-related hemorrhage. Per published reports, the severity of menorrhagia can be variable resulting in anemia warranting iron supplements to packed red cell transfusions due to massive hemorrhage, as described in a 15-year-old Japanese girl with her first menstrual cycle [24, 26, 28, 29]. Pregnancies can be complicated with miscarriage, antepartum and postpartum hemorrhage, severe enough to require fresh frozen plasma (FFP) and blood transfusions. Preterm labor is also common in these individuals [25, 29]. In populations where consanguinity is common or there is a founder effect as seen in the Berne Amish in Indiana, male partners should be investigated for carrier status, as this can have implications for the neonate. Reported pregnancies have had good outcomes except for complications of prematurity. Other gynecological implications include rupture of hemorrhagic ovarian cysts and rare cases of hemoperitoneum [29]. In the light of the recent discovery of PAI-1 deficiency and its link to cardiac fibrosis, pregnant women should be closely monitored if they have poor ejection fraction, and their care should be coordinated by a cardiologist, hematologist, high-risk obstetrician, and maternal-fetal medicine specialist [13, 26, 27].

Increased Fibrinolytic Stimulants

Quebec Platelet Disorder (Excessive Plasminogen Activation)

Background Quebec platelet disorder (QPD) is an autosomal dominant gain-of-function defect as a result of tandem duplication of a 78-kb genomic segment involving the PLAU gene that leads to increase intra-platelet expression of uPA, hence hyperfibrinolysis [30]. It was first described in 1984 with most known cases traced to a single family of French ancestry in Quebec, Canada. Although the worldwide distribution of QPD is

unknown, the prevalence in Quebec is estimated to be 1:220,000 [31].

Clinical Manifestations Delayed bleeding after dental procedures, surgery, or trauma is frequently reported in the setting of disordered fibrinolysis in QPD [32]. Other bleeding symptoms, mostly trauma related, include easy bruising, prolonged bleeding from cuts, and joint bleeds. Spontaneous episodes of hematuria have been reported in approximately 50% of affected individuals with majority being mild and self-resolving. Impaired wound healing in the setting of associated thrombocytopenia has been reported [33].

Implications in Young Women Although HMB has been described in some women, no unfavorable obstetric outcomes including miscarriages or infertility have been reported. However, two women requiring postpartum red cell transfusion have been described in the literature [6].

Diagnosis for Disorders of Congenital Hyperfibrinolysis

General Diagnostic Considerations

Fibrinolysis is difficult to measure directly, and assays remain poorly predictive of bleeding. Therefore, developing a reliable test of fibrinolysis for clinical use has been difficult, and this may lead to underestimation of fibrinolytic disorders. The routine laboratory coagulation screening tests including platelet count, prothrombin time, activated partial thromboplastin time, fibrinogen, thrombin time, and PFA-100 are usually normal in patient with A2AP or PAI-1 deficiencies and QPD [5]. With a high index of clinical suspicion, further evaluation of fibrinolytic system may be performed which can include measurement of individual components or global evaluation of fibrinolytic activity, although due to the complexity of the system, the design of a "gold standard" assay has remained an elusive goal. The global measurement of fibrinolytic activity encompasses different assays which either utilize (1) whole blood thromboelastography and global fibrinolytic capacity (GFC) in whole blood; (2) plasma turbidity assays, simultaneous thrombin and plasmin generation assays, and GFC in plasma; and (3) euglobulin fraction of plasma-euglobulin clot lysis time (ECLT) and its various modifications [34]. ECLT is not infrequently utilized to screen for hyperfibrinolysis. If the time taken to clot dissolution (usually 60–120 minutes) is shortened, it's indicative of increased fibrinolysis; however, normal ECLT does not rule out hyperfibrinolysis. The lack of global validation for ECLT and poor sensitivity has led to fibrinolysis-specific assays to substitute ECLT in many instances [35]. Thromboelastography (TEG) or rotation thromboelastometry (ROTEM) measures the viscoelastic changes of the coagulation and fibrinolytic components of hemostasis using citrated whole blood after re-calcification and addition of coagulation activators. They provide insight into the extent of fibrinolysis present by measuring the difference between maximum viscosity (referred to as MA using TEG, maximal clot firmness (MCF) using ROTEM) achieved after the clot formation and the clot viscosity at 30 and 60 minutes thereafter (clot lysis). Several parameters may be incorporated to reflect endogenous fibrinolytic activity, and modifications have been proposed to more accurately assess fibrinolysis including APTEM test for ROTEM [36]. At present, thromboelastometry is limited by the fact that it can be performed only at specialty centers by trained personnel, by its variable reproducibility, and by the requirement for fresh samples of blood. In clinical practice, the use of thromboelastography for assessment of the fibrinolytic system has been demonstrated for massive hyperfibrinolysis especially in the setting of trauma and limited use in detecting subtle defects [34].

Specific Diagnostic Considerations

A2AP Deficiency   In the event A2AP deficiency is suspected based on either clinical history or shortened ECLT, specific A2AP activity and antigen assays should be performed. A deficiency can be either (1) quantitative (type 1), a decrease in both antigen and activity, or (2) qualitative (type 2), a decrease in activity with normal or low normal antigen levels [8]. Patients with homozygous or compound heterozygous deficiency typically have A2AP activity levels below 10%, whereas the heterozygotes have levels ranging from 35 to 70% of normal [14]. Clinically significant hyperfibrinolysis is predicted to occur with A2AP activity levels of less than 60% [37].

PAI-1 Deficiency   A short ECLT or thromboelastogram detecting hyperfibrinolysis may indicate PAI-1 deficiency, but a definitive test involves measurement of antigenic [enzyme-linked immunosorbent assay (ELISA)] and functional (chromogenic test) PAI-1. Oftentimes, an activity level of zero is reported to be within the *normal* limits of assay detection [28]. PAI-1 also has diurnal variation with higher values observed in the morning and nadir values in the afternoon [38]. Dysfunctional PAI-1 is extremely difficult to detect as normal antigen with low activity might be found in normal individuals also. Iwaki et al. have recently reported a sophisticated method of PAI-1 assay using AlphaLISA® technology (PerkinElmer Japan, Yokohama, Japan) for a case with dysfunctional PAI-1 [23]. Diagnosis is based on high index of clinical suspicion, ruling out common mucocutaneous bleeding disorders including von Willebrand disease and platelet function defects and absent to low PAI-1 activity and antigen levels substantiated with genetic testing, if feasible. Recently, the use of Nijmegen Hemostasis Assay (NHA) was reported to simultaneously measure thrombin and plasmin generation in ten patients with complete PAI-1 deficiency. Low thrombin generation parameters with increased plasmin peak and plasmin potential were noted as expected [39].

QPD   Positive family history in the setting of bleeding symptoms often raises clinical suspicion for QPD given the autosomal dominant inheritance and high penetrance. Although the platelet morphology is normal in patients with QPD, platelet aggregation analysis may reveal a characteristic pattern of absent aggregation with ADP and collagen. Mild thrombocytopenia and mild factor V deficiency may be present [40]. Plasma tests including plasminogen, uPA, and other assays for systemic fibrinolysis are normal in QPD. Due to the isolated intra-platelet excess of uPA, the urinary levels of uPA are also normal [41]. The definitive diagnosis should be made by performing a PCR assay for *PLAU* duplication mutation testing [42].

Treatment for Disorders of Congenital Hyperfibrinolysis

The treatment for acute bleeding or for peri-procedural prophylaxis in patients with congenital hyperfibrinolytic disorders consists of antifibrinolytic agents, tranexamic acid (TA) or epsilon aminocaproic acid (EACA). These are lysine analogues that decrease plasminogen activation by inhibiting plasminogen binding to fibrin and clot stabilization. Intravenous and oral routes have been used for EACA and TA. Dosing of EACA includes 50–100 mg/kg/dose orally or intravenously every 6 hours with a maximum dose of 3 grams/dose; dosing of TA includes 25 mg/kg three times a day or 1300 mg three times a day orally or 10 mg/kg/dose intravenously every 6–8 hrs. For pregnant women with complete PAI-1 deficiency, the use of antifibrinolytic agents in standard dosing is recommended for intermittent bleeding in the first and second trimester, continuous prophylactic use from 26 weeks' gestation through delivery, and for at least 2 weeks postpartum. There are no studies regarding the safety of EACA or TA during breastfeeding although, anecdotally, no adverse effects on the pregnancy or neonate have been reported [29]. EACA has been classified as category C and TA as category B by the United States Food and Drug Administration (FDA). Amish PAI-1-deficient women have routinely utilized an herbal over-the-counter progesterone-containing cream, Progesta-Care (*Life-Flo*, www.life-flo. com) during menses either alone or in addition to oral EACA/TA which results in an improvement of their reported menstrual blood flow. The cream contains 20 mg of progesterone per pump with the patient using one pump daily applied to the abdomen and thighs [29].

Additionally, for A2AP and PAI-1 deficiencies, although the use of fresh frozen plasma (FFP) has been described, it is however not recommended due to variable A2AP or PAI activities and risks of dilutional coagulopathy [8]. There are no purified or recombinant PAI-1 or A2AP replacement concentrates currently available. Desmopressin (DDVAP) should be avoided in treatment of hyperfibrinolytic disorders as it can induce secretion of plasminogen activator [6]. Antifibrinolytic therapy is the mainstay of treatment for Quebec platelet disorder and not DDAVP or platelet transfusions as used in other platelet function disorders [32, 43]. The administration of platelets in patients with QPD has failed to demonstrate reduction in bleeding symptoms [31].

Acquired Fibrinolytic Disorders

Hyperfibrinolysis results in bleeding complications and is seen in chronic liver disease which causes decreased synthesis of A2AP [44], nephrotic syndrome resulting in urinary loss of A2AP [45], and disseminated intravascular coagulation (DIC) that results in bleeding due to consumption of circulating fibrinogen. Other conditions associated with excessive fibrinolysis due to varying mechanisms include heat stroke, extensive trauma, amyloidosis, malignancies like acute promyelocytic leukemia [46], gastric cancer, adenocarcinoma, prostatic cancer, and medical interventions like cardiopulmonary bypass and thrombolysis [5, 46–48].

Hypofibrinolysis results in an acquired tendency to thrombosis; these conditions include antiphospholipid antibody syndrome, hypothyroidism, alcoholic liver disease, and multiple myeloma. Supportive care and treatment of the underlying cause is recommended to abate the risk of bleeding or clotting [5, 49–52] .

Fibrinolytic Pathway Disorders in Bleeding of Unknown Cause

There are a significant number of patients with bleeding tendencies along with positive family history where no diagnosis can be established despite thorough investigation of hemostatic parameters [53]. Although hyperfibrinolysis has been discussed as a possible cause for mild-moderate bleeding symptoms of unknown cause (BUC), fibrinolysis testing is not a part of the routine coagulation work-up. Gebhart et al. [54] investigated components of the fibrinolytic pathway in 270 adult patients (median age 44 years), with BUC who showed lower levels of tPA-PAI-1 complexes and PAI-1 and higher levels of TAFI and A2AP. Szczepaniak et al. [55] also demonstrated that the fibrinolytic system can play an etiological role in patients with BUC in women with HMB with no underlying hemorrhagic diathesis identified. Analysis of the clot characteristics in 52 women aged less than 50 years with HMB showed increased clot permeability with looser plasma fibrin clots and higher susceptibility to clot lysis. Alternatively, Agren et al. [56] showed low PAI-1 activity levels are common in normal population, and no statistically significant difference was noted when levels were compared between healthy donors and those with bleeding tendency.

Summary

Disorders of fibrinolysis result in bleeding of varying severity with no pathognomonic features distinguishing one disorder from the other. Additionally, these hyperfibrinolytic states are rare and challenging to diagnose due to lack of standardized, reproducible assays which are not widely available. It is likely that the cases reported in the medical literature to date are just the tip of the iceberg, emphasizing the need for further research in these rare bleeding disorders. A hematologist should have a high index of suspicion for fibrinolytic disorders if there is delayed bleeding after surgery or trauma and/or reproductive tract bleeding wherein tier-one evaluation for common bleeding disorders has not yielded conclusive results. Global assays may prove useful in these rare scenarios [36, 39]. Identification of the genetic mutation resulting in the defective protein should be attempted, which would help identify carriers in the family and aid genetic counselling for future generations. Treatment relies on the use of antifibrinolytic therapy and as needed FFP for severe bleeding presentations. The Registry for Bleeding Disorders Surveillance is a component of the Community Counts, a CDC public health surveillance project, which is collecting detailed information from HTCs regarding all bleeding disorders, including the rare fibrinolytic disorders which will eventually serve as a rich database for research and hypothesis generation [57]. However due to the rarity of these conditions, multinational registries for each of the individual disorders should be created to formulate standard care guidelines where none exist.

References

1. Stump DC, Taylor FB, Nesheim ME, Giles AR, Dzik WH, Bovill EG. Pathologic fibrinolysis as a cause of clinical bleeding. Semin Thromb Hemost. 1990;16:260–73.
2. Lijnen HR. Elements of the fibrinolytic system. Ann N Y Acad Sci. 2001;936:226–36.
3. Cesarman-Maus G, Hajjar KA. Molecular mechanisms of fibrinolysis. Br J Haematol. 2005;129:307–21.
4. Rijken DC, Lijnen HR. New insights into the molecular mechanisms of the fibrinolytic system. J Thromb Haemost. 2009;7:4–13.
5. Chapin JC, Hajjar KA. Fibrinolysis and the control of blood coagulation. Blood Rev. 2015;29:17–24.
6. Saes JL, Schols SEM, van Heerde WL, Nijziel MR. Hemorrhagic disorders of fibrinolysis: a clinical review. J Thromb Haemost. 2018;16:1498–509.
7. Koie K, Kamiya T, Ogata K, Takamatsu J. Alpha2-plasmin-inhibitor deficiency (Miyasato disease). Lancet. 1978;2:1334–6.
8. Carpenter SL, Mathew P. Alpha2-antiplasmin and its deficiency: fibrinolysis out of balance. Haemophilia. 2008;14:1250–4.
9. Devaussuzenet VM, Ducou-le-Pointe HA, Doco AM, Mary PM, Montagne JR, Favier R. A case of intramedullary haematoma associated with congenital alpha2-plasmin inhibitor deficiency. Pediatr Radiol. 1998;28:978–80.
10. Takahashi Y, Tanaka T, Nakajima N, Yoshioka A, Fukui H, Miyauchi Y, et al. Intramedullary multiple hematomas in siblings with congenital alpha-2-plasmin inhibitor deficiency: orthopedic surgery with protection by tranexamic acid. Haemostasis. 1991;21:321–7.
11. Kordich L, Feldman L, Porterie P, Lago O. Severe hemorrhagic tendency in heterozygous alpha 2-antiplasmin deficiency. Thromb Res. 1985;40:645–51.

12. Ikematsu S, Fukutake K, Aoki N. Heterozygote for plasmin inhibitor deficiency developing hemorrhagic tendency with advancing age. Thromb Res. 1996;82:129–16.

13. Dawley B, Alpha II. Antiplasmin deficiency complicating pregnancy: a case report. Obstet Gynecol Int. 2011;2011:698648.

14. Jain S, Acharya SS. Inherited disorders of the fibrinolytic pathway. Transfus Apher Sci. 2019; https://doi.org/10.1016/j.transci.2019.08.007.

15. Schleef RR, Higgins DL, Pillemer E, Levitt LJ. Bleeding diathesis due to decreased functional activity of type 1 plasminogen activator inhibitor. J Clin Invest. 1989;83:1747–52.

16. Fay WP, Shapiro AD, Shih JL, Schleef RR, Ginsburg D. Brief report: complete deficiency of plasminogen-activator inhibitor type 1 due to a frame-shift mutation. N Engl J Med. 1992;327:1729–33.

17. Fay WP, Parker AC, Condrey LR, Shapiro AD. Human plasminogen activator inhibitor-1 (PAI-1) deficiency: characterization of a large kindred with a null mutation in the PAI-1 gene. Blood. 1997;90:204–8.

18. Kuhli C, Lüchtenberg M, Scharrer I, Hattenbach L-O. Massive subhyaloidal hemorrhage associated with severe PAI-1 deficiency. Graefes Arch Clin Exp Ophthalmol. 2005;243:963–6.

19. Minowa H, Takahashi Y, Tanaka T, Naganuma K, Ida S, Maki I, et al. Four cases of bleeding diathesis in children due to congenital plasminogen activator inhibitor-1 deficiency. Haemostasis. 1999;29:286–91.

20. Morimoto Y, Yoshioka A, Imai Y, Takahashi Y, Minowa H, Kirita T. Haemostatic management of intraoral bleeding in patients with congenital deficiency of alpha2-plasmin inhibitor or plasminogen activator inhibitor-1. Haemophilia. 2004;10:669–74.

21. Takahashi Y, Tanaka T, Minowa H, Ookubo Y, Sugimoto M, Nakajima M, et al. Hereditary partial deficiency of plasminogen activator inhibitor-1 associated with a lifelong bleeding tendency. Int J Hematol. 1996;64:61–8.

22. Diéval J, Nguyen G, Gross S, Delobel J, Kruithof EK. A lifelong bleeding disorder associated with a deficiency of plasminogen activator inhibitor type 1. Blood. 1991;77:528–32.

23. Iwaki T, Nagahashi K, Takano K, Suzuki-Inoue K, Kanayama N, Umemura K, et al. Mutation in a highly conserved glycine residue in strand 5B of plasminogen activator inhibitor 1 causes polymerisation. Thromb Haemost. 2017;117:860–9.

24. Iwaki T, Tanaka A, Miyawaki Y, Suzuki A, Kobayashi T, Takamatsu J, et al. Life-threatening hemorrhage and prolonged wound healing are remarkable phenotypes manifested by complete plasminogen activator inhibitor-1 deficiency in humans. J Thromb Haemost. 2011;9:1200–6.

25. Iwaki T, Nagahashi K, Kobayashi T, Umemura K, Terao T, Kanayama N. The first report of uncontrollable subchorionic and retroplacental haemorrhage inducing preterm labour in complete PAI-1 deficiency in a human. Thromb Res. 2012;129:e161–3.

26. Heiman M, Gupta S, Khan SS, Vaughan DE, Shapiro AD. Complete plasminogen activator inhibitor 1 deficiency. In: Adam MP, Ardinger HH, Pagon RA, Wallace SE, Bean LJ, Stephens K, et al., editors. GeneReviews®. Seattle: University of Washington, Seattle; 1993. http://www.ncbi.nlm.nih.gov/books/NBK447152/. Accessed 22 Sep 2019.

27. Flevaris P, Khan SS, Eren M, Schuldt AJT, Shah SJ, Lee DC, et al. Plasminogen activator inhibitor type I controls cardiomyocyte transforming growth factor-β and cardiac fibrosis. Circulation. 2017;136:664–79.

28. Mehta R, Shapiro AD. Plasminogen activator inhibitor type 1 deficiency. Haemophilia. 2008;14:1255–60.

29. Heiman M, Gupta S, Shapiro AD. The obstetric, gynaecological and fertility implications of homozygous PAI-1 deficiency: single-centre experience. Haemophilia. 2014;20:407–12.

30. Diamandis M, Veljkovic DK, Maurer-Spurej E, Rivard GE, Hayward CPM. Quebec platelet disorder: features, pathogenesis and treatment. Blood Coagul Fibrinolysis. 2008;19:109–19.

31. Blavignac J, Bunimov N, Rivard GE, Hayward CPM. Quebec platelet disorder: update on pathogenesis, diagnosis, and treatment. Semin Thromb Hemost. 2011;37:713–20.

32. McKay H, Derome F, Haq MA, Whittaker S, Arnold E, Adam F, et al. Bleeding risks associated with inheritance of the Quebec platelet disorder. Blood. 2004;104:159–65.

33. Hayward CPM, Rivard GE. Quebec platelet disorder. Expert Rev Hematol. 2011;4:137–41.

34. Ilich A, Bokarev I, Key NS. Global assays of fibrinolysis. Int J Lab Hematol. 2017;39:441–7.

35. Longstaff C. Measuring fibrinolysis: from research to routine diagnostic assays. J Thromb Haemost. 2018;16:652–62.

36. van Geffen M, van Heerde WL. Global haemostasis assays, from bench to bedside. Thromb Res. 2012;129:681–7.

37. Okajima K, Kohno I, Soe G, Okabe H, Takatsuki K, Binder BR. Direct evidence for systemic fibrinogenolysis in patients with acquired alpha 2-plasmin inhibitor deficiency. Am J Hematol. 1994;45:16–24.

38. Angleton P, Chandler WL, Schmer G. Diurnal variation of tissue-type plasminogen activator and its rapid inhibitor (PAI-1). Circulation. 1989;79:101–6.

39. Saes JL, Schols SEM, Betbadal KF, van Geffen M, Verbeek-Knobbe K, Gupta S, et al. Thrombin and plasmin generation in patients with plasminogen or plasminogen activator inhibitor type 1 deficiency. Haemophilia. 2019; https://doi.org/10.1111/hae.13842.

40. Janeway CM, Rivard GE, Tracy PB, Mann KG. Factor V Quebec revisited. Blood. 1996;87:3571–8.

41. Kahr WH, Zheng S, Sheth PM, Pai M, Cowie A, Bouchard M, et al. Platelets from patients with the Quebec platelet disorder contain and secrete abnormal amounts of urokinase-type plasminogen activator. Blood. 2001;98:257–65.

42. Diamandis M, Paterson AD, Rommens JM, Veljkovic DK, Blavignac J, Bulman DE, et al. Quebec platelet disorder is linked to the urokinase plasminogen activator gene (PLAU) and increases expression of the linked allele in megakaryocytes. Blood. 2009;113:1543–6.

43. Hayward CPM, Rao AK, Cattaneo M. Congenital platelet disorders: overview of their mechanisms, diagnostic evaluation and treatment. Haemophilia. 2006;12(Suppl 3):128–36.

44. Tripodi A, Mannucci PM. The coagulopathy of chronic liver disease. N Engl J Med. 2011;365:147–56.

45. Malyszko J, Malyszko JS, Mysliwiec M. Markers of endothelial cell injury and thrombin activatable fibrinolysis inhibitor in nephrotic syndrome. Blood Coagul Fibrinolysis. 2002;13:615–21.

46. Sallah S, Gagnon GA. Reversion of primary hyperfibrinogenolysis in patients with hormone-refractory prostate cancer using docetaxel. Cancer Investig. 2000;18:191–6.

47. Edmunds LH. Managing fibrinolysis without aprotinin. Ann Thorac Surg. 2010;89:324–31.

48. Hess JR, Brohi K, Dutton RP, Hauser CJ, Holcomb JB, Kluger Y, et al. The coagulopathy of trauma: a review of mechanisms. J Trauma. 2008;65:748–54.

49. Cesarman-Maus G, Ríos-Luna NP, Deora AB, Huang B, Villa R, Cravioto Mdel C, et al. Autoantibodies against the fibrinolytic receptor, annexin 2, in antiphospholipid syndrome. Blood. 2006;107:4375–82.

50. Krone KA, Allen KL, McCrae KR. Impaired fibrinolysis in the antiphospholipid syndrome. Curr Rheumatol Rep. 2010;12:53–7.

51. Mazur P, Sokołowski G, Hubalewska-Dydejczyk A, Płaczkiewicz-Jankowska E, Undas A. Prothrombotic alterations in plasma fibrin clot properties in thyroid disorders and their post-treatment modifications. Thromb Res. 2014;134:510–7.

52. van Marion AMW, Auwerda JJA, Minnema MC, van Oosterom R, Adelmeijer J, de Groot PG, et al. Hypofibrinolysis during induction treatment of multiple myeloma may increase the risk of venous thrombosis. Thromb Haemost. 2005;94:1341–3.

53. Quiroga T, Mezzano D. Is my patient a bleeder? A diagnostic framework for mild bleeding disorders. Hematol Am Soc Hematol Educ Program. 2012;2012:466–74.

54. Gebhart J, Kepa S, Hofer S, Koder S, Kaider A, Wolberg AS, et al. Fibrinolysis in patients with a mild-to-moderate bleeding tendency of unknown cause. Ann Hematol. 2017;96:489–95.

55. Szczepaniak P, Zabczyk M, Undas A. Increased plasma clot permeability and susceptibility to lysis are associated with heavy menstrual bleeding of unknown cause: a case-control study. PLoS One. 2015;10:e0125069.

56. Agren A, Wiman B, Stiller V, Lindmarker P, Sten-Linder M, Carlsson A, et al. Evaluation of low PAI-1 activity as a risk factor for hemorrhagic diathesis. J Thromb Haemost. 2006;4:201–8.

57. Gupta S, Acharya S, Roberson C, Lail A, Soucie JM, Shapiro A. Potential of the community counts registry to characterize rare bleeding disorders. Haemophilia. 2019; https://doi.org/10.1111/hae.13847.

Hypermobility Syndromes in Heavy Menstrual Bleeding

8

Genevieve Moyer, Patricia Huguelet, and Pamela Trapane

Overview of Joint Hypermobility

Introduction

Joint hypermobility (JH) is a term used to describe an increase in range of motion across one or more joints. Joint hypermobility is a common feature of inherited connective tissue disorders (CTD), most notably, Ehlers-Danlos Syndrome (EDS), including the hypermobile subtype (hEDS). EDS comprises a clinically heterogeneous group of diseases characterized by abnormalities in one of several types of the extracellular matrix protein, collagen. The classification of EDS has evolved from the Berlin nosology in 1988 and the Villefranche nosology in 1998 to the newest classification system created in 2017 by the

International EDS Consortium which recognizes 13 EDS subtypes (Table 8.1) [2–4]. These EDS subtypes are distinguished from other CTD syndromes that can be associated with JH as well as "hypermobility spectrum disorders" which includes all other individuals with symptomatic joint hypermobility that do not fit into the hypermobile EDS criteria (Table 8.2) [4, 5]. Other connective tissue diseases that have been associated with JH include Marfan syndrome, Loeys-Dietz syndrome, pseudoxanthoma elasticum, hyperhomocysteinemia, Beals syndrome, arterial tortuosity syndrome, lateral meningocele syndrome, hereditary cutis laxa syndromes, skeletal dysplasias, hereditary myopathies, and other chromosomal and congenital anomaly/intellectual disability disorders [5].

In addition to generalized joint hypermobility (GJH), other clinical features associated with EDS can include varying degrees of skin fragility and hyperextensibility, poor wound healing, atrophic scarring, and, rarely, vascular and hollow viscus rupture [7]. Disease manifestations that are shared between EDS and other CTD associated with GJH include chronic pain, autonomic dysfunction, gastrointestinal disorders, genitourinary dysfunction, and psychologic impairment [5]. Many GJH disorders are also associated with an increased risk of bleeding manifested by easy bruising, surgical bleeding, and heavy menstrual bleeding (HMB). Despite a growing body of research, GJH disorders continue to be associated

G. Moyer (✉)
University of Colorado Anschutz Medical Campus, Aurora, CO, USA

Children's Hospital Colorado, Aurora, CO, USA

University of Colorado Anschutz Medical Campus Hemophilia and Thrombosis Center, Aurora, CO, USA
e-mail: genevieve.moyer@cuanschutz.edu

P. Huguelet
University of Colorado Anschutz Medical Campus, Aurora, CO, USA

Children's Hospital Colorado, Aurora, CO, USA

P. Trapane
University of Florida Health, Gainesville, FL, USA

© Springer Nature Switzerland AG 2020
L. V. Srivaths (ed.), *Hematology in the Adolescent Female*,
https://doi.org/10.1007/978-3-030-48446-0_8

Table 8.1 2017 international EDS consortium EDS nosology [4]

EDS subtype	Disease manifestations	Genetic basis	Inheritance
Classical	Hyperextensible skin, atrophic scars	COL5A1, COL5A2, COL1A1	AD
Classical-like	Hyperextensible skin	TNXB	AR
Cardiac-valvular	Cardiac valve involvement, hyperextensible skin	COL1A2	AR
Vascular	Extensive bruising, vascular rupture	COL3A1, COL1A1	AD
Hypermobile	Joint hypermobility, musculoskeletal pain	None confirmed	AD
Arthrochalasia	Joint hypermobility	COL1A1, COL1A2	AD
Dermatosparaxis	Hyperextensible and extremely fragile skin	ADAMTS2	AR
Kyphoscoliotic	Congenital hypotonia and progressive scoliosis	PLOD1, FKBP14	AR
Brittle cornea syndrome	Thin cornea and early-onset keratoconus/globus	ZNF469, PRDM5	AR
Spondylodysplastic	Congenital hypotonia and short stature	B4GALT7, B3GALT6, SLC39A13	AR
Musculocontractural	Hyperextensible skin, facial dysmorphia, and joint contractures	CHST13, DSE	AR
Myopathic	Congenital hypotonia, proximal contractures	COL12A1	AD or AR
Periodontal	Severe, early-onset periodontitis	C1R, C1S	AD

Table 8.2 Joint hypermobility classification [5]

Hypermobile type	Subtype	Criteria
Asymptomatic, non-syndromic JH	Limited joint hypermobility (LJH)	Involvement of JH at usually less than 5 joints without other syndromic features
	Peripheral joint hypermobility (PJH)	JH at hands and/or feet, sparing large and axial joint involvement without other syndromic features
	Generalized joint hypermobility (GJH)	Involvement of JH at usually 8 or more joints without other syndromic features
Hypermobile Ehlers-Danlos syndrome (hEDS)/ syndromic joint hypermobility		GJH plus involvement of two or more of: (i) Musculoskeletal involvement[a] (ii) Systemic involvement[b] (iii) Positive family history in first degree relative.
Hypermobility spectrum disorders (HSD)	Generalized HSD (G-HSD)	Individuals with symptomatic GJH that do not meet criteria for hEDS but do have one or more additional musculoskeletal abnormalities[c]
	Peripheral HSD (P-HSD)	Individuals with symptomatic PJH and one or more additional musculoskeletal abnormalities[c]
	Localized HSD (L-HSD)	Individuals with symptomatic LJH and one or more additional musculoskeletal abnormalities[c]
	Historical HSD (H-HSD)	Self-reported history of GJH without current objective GJH and one or more additional musculoskeletal abnormalities[c]

[a]Musculoskeletal involvement includes one of the following: daily musculoskeletal pain in two limbs for at least 2 months, chronic widespread pain for at least 3 months, and recurrent joint dislocations

[b]Systemic involvement includes five or more of the following: velvety skin, hyperextensible skin (2 cm at volar aspect of hands), unexplained striae, bilateral piezogenic papules of the heels, recurrent abdominal hernias, two or more atrophic scars, prolapse of the pelvic, uterine or rectal floor, dental crowding and high/narrow palate, arachnodactyly, mitral valve prolapse, aortic root dilation, and arm span to height ratio ≥ 1.05

[c]Musculoskeletal abnormalities can include musculoskeletal pain, dislocations, physical traits such as scoliosis or flat foot, degenerative joint and bone disease, and neurodevelopmental abnormalities including hypotonia and motor delay [6]

with challenges in diagnosis and treatment due to the heterogeneity of clinical presentation even within a given diagnosis, an evolving nosology, and disease rarity.

Epidemiology

Symptomatic GJH has been estimated to be present in up to 20 per 1,000 individuals with most of these cases attributed to some form of EDS which has an estimated overall prevalence of about 1 in 1,500 individuals worldwide. The most common EDS subtype, hEDS, has an estimated prevalence of 1 out of 10,000 individuals [8, 9]. Although hEDS is thought to be inherited in an autosomal dominant fashion, the lack of one clear genetic etiology means that other modes of inheritance may also exist. Hypermobile EDS tends to be more common in females with a female to male ratio as high as 9:1, which may in part be caused by a bias related to the lifetime impact of male testosterone on joint mobility and attenuation of pain perception [10–12].

Pathophysiology

In many conditions associated with GJH, specific molecular markers have been causally linked to defects in extracellular matrix protein elements which lead to consistent syndromic features. Most EDS subtypes are associated with genetic defects in the synthesis of or post-translational modification of types I, III, V, and pro-collagen. While many forms of EDS have been linked to specific molecular aberrations, hEDS has no clearly established genetic marker. While some cases of hEDS have been associated with haploinsufficiency of tenascin XB (TNXB), a statistically significant relationship has not been established to implicate this as a singular cause [11, 13, 14]. What is shared among conditions that lead to GJH is that these inherited defects lead to an alteration

in the structure or function of the extracellular matrix that provides support to the musculoskeletal system. In addition to the genetic basis of disease, the clinical manifestation of symptoms related to hEDS and other GJH conditions is also heavily dependent on a variety of life experiences and environmental exposures, such that it is believed that many at-risk individuals may lead asymptomatic lives or never present for medical evaluation of GJH [11]. The accumulation of trauma, suboptimal musculoskeletal mechanics, defects in proprioception, and the presence of underlying bone or joint disease can all impact the degree of GJH acquisition and associated symptoms across the lifespan of a susceptible individual. Inflammatory joint and tissue diseases, hypothyroidism, and nutritional deficiencies can lead to acquired forms of GJH even in the absence of an underlying genetic predisposition [5].

Disease Manifestations

Non-bleeding Co-morbidities

The extra-articular symptoms that are experienced by those with GJH are diverse and vary across disorders. As mentioned above, many individuals with GJH experience symptoms related to alterations in underlying connective tissues including tissue laxity and fragility, skin hyperextensibility, atrophic scarring, obstetric and gynecologic complaints, acute and chronic pain, fatigue, anxiety, postural orthostatic hypotension (POTS) and dysautonomia, osteoporosis and osteoarthritis, gastrointestinal disorders, pelvic/urinary disorders, and mast cell activation disorders [5, 14–16].

Hemostasis-Related Co-morbidities

Bleeding is a common finding across several disorders associated with GJH as well as across the EDS subtypes. To date, no unifying hemostatic defect has been clearly described, and even in the case of clinically overt bleeding, laboratory testing is often normal. Dysfunctional collagen/VWF interaction and the fragility of capillaries and perivascular connective tissues have been blamed as the likely culprits behind the increased bleeding symptoms seen in patients with connective tissue disorders and hEDS [17, 18]. GJH is also thought to exacerbate the symptoms of other inherited bleeding disorders such as von Willebrand disease [19, 20]. While factor deficiencies and platelet function and storage pool defects have been described in individuals with GJH, these cases are exceptions. In one cohort study of patients with EDS, 83% of subjects had abnormal platelet function, with abnormalities in response to adenosine triphosphate (ADP) being the most common aggregation defect. Subjects with abnormalities in platelet aggregation testing were more likely to have abnormal bleeding as measured by the International Society on Thrombosis and Hemostasis-Scientific and Standardization Committee Bleeding Assessment Tool (ISTH-SCC BAT), and 90% of patients with a score > 5 had at least one platelet function abnormality. The authors of this study explained their results by hypothesizing that abnormalities in collagen biosynthesis may lead to increased activation and exhaustion of platelets which decreases their ability to react to other agonists [21].

Bleeding symptoms can range from mild bruising and mucosal bleeding to life-threatening hemorrhage secondary to surgical intervention or vascular rupture, with the latter most commonly seen in vascular subtype EDS and in Loeys-Dietz syndrome [17, 21, 22]. In the case of pseudoxanthoma elasticum, hemorrhage most commonly affects the gastrointestinal tract though abnormal uterine and intra-articular bleeding have also been reported [23].

To date, there is very little published research dedicated to the gynecologic symptoms of females with GJH, and this is an area in need of further investigation. However, available data does suggest abnormal uterine bleeding, and other gynecologic symptoms are common manifestations of these disorders. In one report, up to 76% of 386 women with hypermobile EDS reported a history of HMB at some point in their life [24]. The only analysis to date that has specifically assessed menstrual symptoms of adolescent girls with EDS evaluated 30 subjects and found that 73% of girls had menses that lasted at least 7 days or longer and 80% of girls reported menstrual flow as "heavy" or "very heavy" by the Menstrual Impact Questionnaire (MIQ). In this same study, HMB was severe enough to lead to a negative impact on school and extracurricular activities in as many as 60% of subjects [25]. Dysmenorrhea is also common and has been reported by as many as 93.6% of women with hEDS [26]. One notable case report describes a 16-year-old female with EDS who presented with brisk vaginal bleeding after she developed a tear in her vaginal wall and posterior fourchette during her sexual debut [27]. It has been noted that young girls may note a worsening of extragynecologic symptoms related to the GJH complex with onset of puberty [24]. As is too often the case for all women with bleeding disorders, individuals with GJH often experience a significant delay in the evaluation and management of AUB by either hematology or gynecology specialists [25].

Although not commonly encountered in the adolescent population, it is worth noting that compared to the general population, obstetric complications are also much more common in individuals with EDS. EDS is associated with more than double the rate of preterm birth, spontaneous abortion, and postpartum hemorrhage [26, 28, 29]. Maternal death has been reported in up to 5% of cases pregnancy in women with vascular type EDS [30]. Obstetric complications are also common among women with Loeys-Dietz, pseudoxanthoma elasticum, and Marfan syndrome [31–35]. Unique obstetric complications that may occur with these syndromes include an increased risk of gastrointestinal hemorrhage in those with pseudoxanthoma elasticum, aortic dissection in patients with Marfan syndrome, and postpartum hemorrhage in both Loeys-Dietz and Marfan syndrome [31, 32, 36, 37]. Because young girls with GJH may present first with HMB, it is important to assess for these underly-

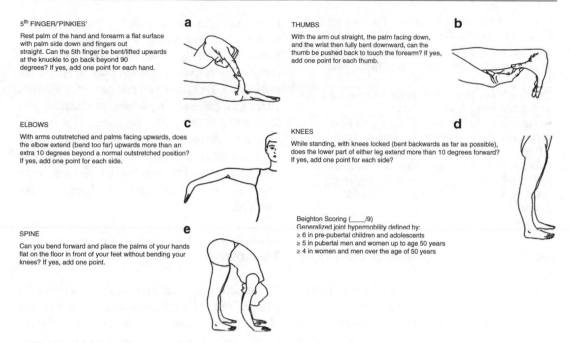

5th FINGER/'PINKIES'

Rest palm of the hand and forearm a flat surface with palm side down and fingers out straight. Can the 5th finger be bent/lifted upwards at the knuckle to go back beyond 90 degrees? If yes, add one point for each hand.

a

THUMBS

With the arm out straight, the palm facing down, and the wrist then fully bent downward, can the thumb be pushed back to touch the forearm? If yes, add one point for each thumb.

b

ELBOWS

With arms outstretched and palms facing upwards, does the elbow extend (bend too far) upwards more than an extra 10 degrees beyond a normal outstretched position? If yes, add one point for each side.

c

KNEES

While standing, with knees locked (bent backwards as far as possible), does the lower part of either leg extend more than 10 degrees forward? If yes, add one point for each side?

d

Beighton Scoring (_____/9)
Generalized joint hypermobility defined by:
≥ 6 in pre-pubertal children and adolescents
≥ 5 in pubertal men and women up to age 50 years
≥ 4 in women and men over the age of 50 years

SPINE

Can you bend forward and place the palms of your hands flat on the floor in front of your feet without bending your knees? If yes, add one point.

e

Fig. 8.1 The Beighton scoring system for assessing joint hypermobility. (**a**) 5th finger/pinkies, (**b**) Thumbs, (**c**) Elbows, (**d**) Knees, (**e**) Spine [1]

ing disorders before these patients become pregnant so that pre-conception counseling and directed screening can be offered when appropriate.

In addition to abnormal bleeding and obstetric complications, other gynecologic disorders that can be seen in both women and girls with GJH include dyspareunia and sexual dysfunction, pelvic pain, uterine prolapse, and cystocele. It is believed that these conditions may be related to the joint laxity and supportive tissue fragility seen across CTDs [26, 38].

Screening and Diagnosis

The process of diagnosing a GJH syndrome can be lengthy and challenging and is often associated with numerous subspecialty consultations [28]. Part of the diagnostic challenge in this group is related to the heterogeneity seen both across and within GJH conditions. Clinical tools that can aid in the screening, diagnosis, and management of patients with GJH range from clinic-based assessments to imaging and genetic testing.

The most commonly used clinical tool for the diagnosis of GJH is the Beighton score which assesses range of motion in the first and fifth fingers, elbows, knees, and spine (Fig. 8.1). Because generalized mobility decreases across the lifespan, the scoring system accounts for differences in age [39]. In addition to the physical observations provided by the Beighton score, the five-point questionnaire allows for detection of historical GJH in individuals whose joint disease may have led to restrictive arthropathy that may mask the presence of previously hypermobile joints (Table 8.3). In this five-point questionnaire, answering "yes" to two or more questions predicts joint hypermobility with 80–85% sensitivity and 80–90% specificity [40]. Although infrequently used, the tourniquet test for capillary fragility is worth noting for its historical significance. This test, which may also be known as the Rumpel-Leede or Hess test, is performed by inflating a blood pressure cuff to a point between the patients' systolic and diastolic blood pressure for 10 minutes. A circle with a 5 cm diameter is drawn in the area where the cuff is applied and the number of petechiae are counted with more

Table 8.3 Five-point questionnaire for assessing generalized joint hypermobility [1]

Question 1: Can you now (or could you ever) place your hands flat on the floor without bending your knees?
Question 2: Can you now (or could you ever) bend your thumb to touch your forearm?
Question 3: As a child, did you amuse your friends by contorting your body into strange shapes or could you do the splits?
Question 4: As a child or teenager, did your shoulder or kneecap dislocate on more than one occasion?
Question 5: Do you consider yourself "double jointed"?

than 15 indicating the presence of capillary fragility [41, 42].

Because cardiovascular complications including aortic root dilation, mitral valve prolapse, and other congenital disorders are common manifestations of many GJH conditions, appropriate disease classification is important so that cardiac screening can be instituted in appropriate cases. The GJH conditions most commonly associated with cardiovascular complications include classical EDS, cardiac-valvular and vascular EDS, as well as Marfan syndrome; however, abnormalities have also been reported in other EDS subtypes including the kyphoscoliotic type due to LYSYL hydroxylase-1 deficiency, spondylodysplastic type, and musculocontractural type [43]. Because the adolescent female with these syndromes may first present for management of a bleeding diathesis, it is important for the subspecialties involved in the management of hemostatic disorders and HMB to be aware of the need for echocardiographic screening in such individuals so that timely referrals are made. Screening echocardiogram should be performed in all individuals with GJH in whom these high-risk syndromes cannot be definitively ruled out. In most of these conditions, echocardiographic screening should include measurement of aortic root size and valve evaluation and should be performed at diagnosis or by 5 years of age and repeated yearly [43].

Because hEDS has no known genetic cause, the diagnosis can be made by any clinician through analysis of the diagnostic criteria.

However, referral to a medical geneticist is often an important component of the evaluation of an individual with GJH. Genetic testing can help to confirm the diagnosis of many rare types of EDS and other GJH syndromes and can offer families additional guidance regarding inheritance patterns and screening considerations. If a specific alternative diagnosis is suspected, genetic testing for that grouping of disorders (e.g., Loeys-Dietz syndrome) should be sent, but delaying a diagnosis until the time of genetic evaluation is not required.

Treatment

Multidisciplinary management is essential for the optimal care of individuals with GJH. Because of the heterogeneity of disorders and disease manifestations associated with GJH, management should be individualized for each patient. Subspecialty consultation by orthopedics and physical therapy should be pursued at a minimum. For patients who are undergoing surgery, patients should be evaluated by cardiology, hematology, and anesthesiology. Other subspecialties that often play an important role in the management of these patients include obstetrics and gynecology, neurology, and psychology.

For all individuals with GJH, a healthy lifestyle including appropriate physical activities and a well-balanced diet including at least the recommended daily amount of ascorbic acid intake are encouraged. Early evaluation and anticipatory guidance by physical therapy may lead to improvement in joint stability, proprioception, muscle strength, and balance [44]. Water-based exercise may be uniquely well suited for individuals with GJH as it leads to minimal strain on affected joints; however, no specific physical therapy interventions have proven more beneficial than another, and this is another area where additional research is required. It is also important for all patients with GJH to be counseled on the importance of pacing, physical activity modification, and use of protective equipment to reduce the risk of injury, accelerated joint disease, and exacerbation of chronic pain and fatigue.

Because chronic pain is a common feature of GJH, patients should establish care with a medical provider who can support long-term management of such symptoms. Options for pain management may include topical analgesics, muscle relaxants, and short-term benzodiazepines. Tricyclic antidepressants, SSRIs, and antiepileptics may be helpful for the treatment of neuropathic pain [14, 45]. Opioids and tramadol should be reserved for cases where other first and second line agents are no longer efficacious and for severe, acute pain.

Management of Bleeding

Individuals with GJH who experience abnormal bruising or bleeding as well as those who are undergoing surgical intervention should be counseled on avoiding drugs that interfere with hemostasis such as antiplatelet agents and fish oil supplementation. For the management of bruising, supplementation of up to 4gm per day of ascorbic acid has been recommended by some investigators, though controlled studies regarding its efficacy are lacking [46]. For more severe bleeding in individuals with hEDS and other GJH syndromes, Table 8.4 provides a summary of available treatment options.

DDAVP has been the most thoroughly studied intervention with good results in most studies, particularly in those with abnormal platelet function defects [47, 48]. In the case of hEDS, in addition to increasing circulating factor VIII, DDAVP is also believed to increase circulating ultra-large von Willebrand factor multimers which may have the ability to overcome the underlying impairment in binding defective collagen to VWF and platelets [47–49]. Several case reports across multiple subtypes of EDS have demonstrated the ability of DDAVP administration to improve clinically relevant hemostasis [47, 48, 50, 51]. In one cohort of 19 children with EDS, DDAVP was found to reduce the mean bleeding time on average from 11.26 minutes to 5.95 minutes [48].

Other hemostatic agents may also have an important role in the management of excess

Table 8.4 Hemostatic medications for abnormal bleeding in individuals with GJH

General bleeding		
Medication name	Class of drug	Dosing
Tranexamic acid (Lysteda)	Antifibrinolytic	1300 mg PO TID or 1000 mg IV Q8hours
Aminocaproic acid (Amicar)	Antifibrinolytic	50–100 mg/kg PO Q4hours
DDAVP (Stimate)	Vasopressin analog	150mcg per actuation. 1 actuation in each nostril Qday up to 3 consecutive days
DDAVP (desmopressin)	Vasopressin analog	0.3mcg/kg IV × Qday up to 3 consecutive days
NovoSeven RT	Recombinant coagulation factor VIIa	10–30 mcg/kg IV Q2–3 hours

PO oral, *IV* intravenous, *Q* every, *TID* three times daily, *kg* kilogram, *mcg* microgram

bleeding in those with GJH disorders, though less data is available to definitively support their use. Antifibrinolytics such as tranexamic acid are associated with a low risk of adverse events and may be helpful in patients with GJH-associated bleeding, particularly in conjunction with DDAVP [49]. The use of NovoSeven has been reported for intraoperative management in those with hypermobile and vascular type EDS, though it should be reserved for significant bleeding and in cases when more conservative interventions have failed as it is associated with an increased risk of thrombosis [49, 52].

Because GJH may exacerbate other inherited or acquired bleeding diatheses, it is important for individuals who are afflicted by severe bleeding symptoms or who are planning to undergo surgical intervention to be evaluated by a hematologist and screened for common disorders of hemostasis. If specific factor deficiencies, von Willebrand disease, or platelet function defects are discovered, management of these conditions should be approached with additional caution in those with GJH.

Treatment of Abnormal Uterine Bleeding

When available, early referral of adolescent females to both a gynecologist and hematologist is recommended, ideally prior to onset of menarche. Although there is limited published data regarding optimal management strategies for HMB, several treatment options exist that may improve HMB symptoms. Early initiation of these interventions may reduce school absenteeism, emotional distress associated with HMB, and the development of iron deficiency and anemia.

In one observational study, 63% of adolescent females with GJH and HMB were adequately managed with long-term oral hormonal contraceptive therapy, either combination pills or progestin-only therapy [25]. The levonorgestrel intrauterine device (LNG-IUD) is an alternative option that has proven to be very effective at controlling HMB in young women with bleeding disorders; however, extreme caution should be used in patients with vascular EDS given a lack of evidence supporting its use in this population and a theoretical risk of spontaneous uterine rupture in these patients. Antifibrinolytics and DDAVP have demonstrated adjunctive benefit in the treatment of HMB [25, 50, 53]. Scheduled non-opioid analgesics including acetaminophen, nonsteroidal anti-inflammatory agents (NSAIDs), or cyclooxygenase-2 inhibitors may be useful, although NSAID use should be used judiciously in those with more prominent bleeding symptoms or who are at high risk for cardiovascular disease.

The impact of iron deficiency on cognitive function of adolescent females is well established, and studies using iron supplementation in iron-deficient girls with HMB have been associated with improved memory and learning ability [54, 55]. All women who are evaluated for abnormal uterine bleeding should undergo screening with a CBC and ferritin to identify cases of iron deficiency and anemia, and appropriate replacement therapy should be provided.

References

1. Society TE-D. Assessing joint hypermobility: the Ehlers-Danlos Society; 2019. Available from: https://www.ehlers-danlos.com/assessing-joint-hypermobility/.
2. Beighton P, de Paepe A, Danks D, Finidori G, Gedde-Dahl T, Goodman R, et al. International nosology of heritable disorders of connective tissue, Berlin, 1986. Am J Med Genet. 1988;29(3):581–94.
3. Beighton P, De Paepe A, Steinmann B, Tsipouras P, Wenstrup RJ. Ehlers-Danlos syndromes: revised nosology, Villefranche, 1997. Ehlers-Danlos National Foundation (USA) and Ehlers-Danlos Support Group (UK). Am J Med Genet. 1998;77(1):31–7.
4. Malfait F, Francomano C, Byers P, Belmont J, Berglund B, Black J, et al. The 2017 international classification of the Ehlers-Danlos syndromes. Am J Med Genet C Semin Med Genet. 2017;175(1):8–26.
5. Castori M, Tinkle B, Levy H, Grahame R, Malfait F, Hakim A. A framework for the classification of joint hypermobility and related conditions. Am J Med Genet C Semin Med Genet. 2017;175(1):148–57.
6. Castori M, Hakim A. Contemporary approach to joint hypermobility and related disorders. Curr Opin Pediatr. 2017;29(6):640–9.
7. De Paepe A, Malfait F. Bleeding and bruising in patients with Ehlers-Danlos syndrome and other collagen vascular disorders. Br J Haematol. 2004;127(5):491–500.
8. Hakim AJ, Sahota A. Joint hypermobility and skin elasticity: the hereditary disorders of connective tissue. Clin Dermatol. 2006;24(6):521–33.
9. Steinmann B, Royce PM, Superti-Furga A. In: Royce PM, Steinmann B, editors. Connective tissue and its heritable disorders. 2nd ed. New York: Wiley-Liss; 2002. p. 431–524.
10. Castori M, Sperduti I, Celletti C, Camerota F, Grammatico P. Symptom and joint mobility progression in the joint hypermobility syndrome (Ehlers-Danlos syndrome, hypermobility type). Clin Exp Rheumatol. 2011;29(6):998–1005.
11. Martin A. An acquired or heritable connective tissue disorder? A review of hypermobile Ehlers Danlos syndrome. Eur J Med Genet. 2019;62(7):103672.
12. Castori M, Dordoni C, Valiante M, Sperduti I, Ritelli M, Morlino S, et al. Nosology and inheritance pattern(s) of joint hypermobility syndrome and Ehlers-Danlos syndrome, hypermobility type: a study of intrafamilial and interfamilial variability in 23 Italian pedigrees. Am J Med Genet A. 2014;164A(12):3010–20.
13. Petersen JW, Douglas JY. Tenascin-X, collagen, and Ehlers-Danlos syndrome: tenascin-X gene defects can protect against adverse cardiovascular events. Med Hypotheses. 2013;81(3):443–7.
14. Tinkle B, Castori M, Berglund B, Cohen H, Grahame R, Kazkaz H, et al. Hypermobile Ehlers-Danlos syndrome (a.k.a. Ehlers-Danlos syndrome Type III and

Ehlers-Danlos syndrome hypermobility type): clinical description and natural history. Am J Med Genet C Semin Med Genet. 2017;175(1):48–69.

15. Mulvey MR, Macfarlane GJ, Beasley M, Symmons DP, Lovell K, Keeley P, et al. Modest association of joint hypermobility with disabling and limiting musculoskeletal pain: results from a large-scale general population-based survey. Arthritis Care Res (Hoboken). 2013;65(8):1325–33.

16. Morris SL, O'Sullivan PB, Murray KJ, Bear N, Hands B, Smith AJ. Hypermobility and musculoskeletal pain in adolescents. J Pediatr. 2017;181:213–21.e1.

17. Key NS, DE Paepe A, Malfait F, Shovlin CL. Vascular haemostasis. Haemophilia. 2010;16(Suppl 5):146–51.

18. Cunniff C, Williamson-Kruse L. Ehlers-Danlos syndrome, type VIII presenting with periodontitis and prolonged bleeding time. Clin Dysmorphol. 1995;4(2):145–9.

19. Hall SA, Meier ER, Gupta S, Nakar C, Rampersad A, Bakeer N, et al. Clinical features of children, adolescents, and adults with coexisting hypermobility syndromes and von Willebrand disease. Pediatr Blood Cancer. 2018;65(12):e27370.

20. Ott HW, Perkhofer S, Coucke PJ, de Paepe A, Spannagl M. Identification of von Willebrand disease type 1 in a patient with Ehlers-Danlos syndrome classic type. Haemophilia. 2016;22(4):e309–11.

21. Artoni A, Bassotti A, Abbattista M, Marinelli B, Lecchi A, Gianniello F, et al. Hemostatic abnormalities in patients with Ehlers-Danlos syndrome. J Thromb Haemost. 2018;16(12):2425–31.

22. Anstey A, Mayne K, Winter M, Van de Pette J, Pope FM. Platelet and coagulation studies in Ehlers-Danlos syndrome. Br J Dermatol. 1991;125(2):155–63.

23. Bick R. Vascular thrombohemorrhagic disorders: hereditary and acquired. Clin Appl Thromb Hemost. 2001;7(3):178–94.

24. Hugon-Rodin J, Lebegue G, Becourt S, Hamonet C, Gompel A. Gynecologic symptoms and the influence on reproductive life in 386 women with hypermobility type Ehlers-Danlos syndrome: a cohort study. Orphanet J Rare Dis. 2016;11(1):124.

25. Kendel NE, Haamid FW, Christian-Rancy M, O'Brien SH. Characterizing adolescents with heavy menstrual bleeding and generalized joint hypermobility. Pediatr Blood Cancer. 2019;66(6):e27675.

26. Hurst BS, Lange SS, Kullstam SM, Usadi RS, Matthews ML, Marshburn PB, et al. Obstetric and gynecologic challenges in women with Ehlers-Danlos syndrome. Obstet Gynecol. 2014;123(3):506–13.

27. Howard JM, Diaz MC, Soler ME. Hemorrhagic shock resulting from post-coital vaginal bleeding in an adolescent with Ehlers-Danlos type IV. Pediatr Emerg Care. 2009;25(6):397–8.

28. Castori M, Morlino S, Dordoni C, Celletti C, Camerota F, Ritelli M, et al. Gynecologic and obstetric implications of the joint hypermobility syndrome (a.k.a. Ehlers-Danlos syndrome hypermobility type) in 82 Italian patients. Am J Med Genet A. 2012;158A(9):2176–82.

29. Lind J, Wallenburg HC. Pregnancy and the Ehlers-Danlos syndrome: a retrospective study in a Dutch population. Acta Obstet Gynecol Scand. 2002;81(4):293–300.

30. Murray ML, Pepin M, Peterson S, Byers PH. Pregnancy-related deaths and complications in women with vascular Ehlers-Danlos syndrome. Genet Med. 2014;16(12):874–80.

31. Cauldwell M, Steer PJ, Curtis S, Mohan AR, Dockree S, Mackillop L, et al. Maternal and fetal outcomes in pregnancies complicated by the inherited aortopathy Loeys-Dietz syndrome. BJOG. 2019;126(8):1025–31.

32. Curry RA, Gelson E, Swan L, Dob D, Babu-Narayan SV, Gatzoulis MA, et al. Marfan syndrome and pregnancy: maternal and neonatal outcomes. BJOG. 2014;121(5):610–7.

33. Rahman J, Rahman FZ, Rahman W, al-Suleiman SA, Rahman MS. Obstetric and gynecologic complications in women with Marfan syndrome. J Reprod Med. 2003;48(9):723–8.

34. Paternoster DM, Santarossa C, Vettore N, Dalla Pria S, Grella P. Obstetric complications in Marfan syndrome pregnancy. Minerva Ginecol. 1998;50(10):441–3.

35. Viljoen DL, Beatty S, Beighton P. The obstetric and gynaecological implications of pseudoxanthoma elasticum. Br J Obstet Gynaecol. 1987;94(9):884–8.

36. Camacho M, Rengel C, Lopez-Herrero E, Carrillo JL, Eslava AJ, Valdivielso P. Approach to the management of pregnancy in patients with pseudoxanthoma elasticum: a review. J Obstet Gynaecol. 2016;36(8):1061–6.

37. Irons DW, Pollard KP. Post partum haemorrhage secondary to Marfan disease of the uterine vasculature. Br J Obstet Gynaecol. 1993;100(3):279–81.

38. Sorokin Y, Johnson MP, Rogowski N, Richardson DA, Evans MI. Obstetric and gynecologic dysfunction in the Ehlers-Danlos syndrome. J Reprod Med. 1994;39(4):281–4.

39. Beighton P, Solomon L, Soskolne CL. Articular mobility in an African population. Ann Rheum Dis. 1973;32(5):413–8.

40. Hakim AJ, Grahame R. A simple questionnaire to detect hypermobility: an adjunct to the assessment of patients with diffuse musculoskeletal pain. Int J Clin Pract. 2003;57(3):163–6.

41. Stevens DJ. Vascular hemostasis: a review. Am J Med Technol. 1973;39(6):252–7.

42. Uden A. Collagen and bleeding diathesis in Ehlers-Danlos syndrome. Scand J Haematol. 1982;28(5):425–30.

43. Brady AF, Demirdas S, Fournel-Gigleux S, Ghali N, Giunta C, Kapferer-Seebacher I, et al. The Ehlers-Danlos syndromes, rare types. Am J Med Genet C Semin Med Genet. 2017;175(1):70–115.

44. Engelbert RH, Juul-Kristensen B, Pacey V, de Wandele I, Smeenk S, Woinarosky N, et al. The evidence-based rationale for physical therapy treatment of children, adolescents, and adults diagnosed with joint hypermobility syndrome/hypermobile Ehlers Danlos syndrome. Am J Med Genet C Semin Med Genet. 2017;175(1):158–67.

45. Chopra P, Tinkle B, Hamonet C, Brock I, Gompel A, Bulbena A, Francomano C. Pain management in the Ehlers-Danlos syndromes. Am J Med Genet C Semin Med Genet. 2017;175(1):212–9.

46. Bolton-Maggs PH, Perry DJ, Chalmers EA, Parapia LA, Wilde JT, Williams MD, et al. The rare coagulation disorders--review with guidelines for management from the United Kingdom Haemophilia Centre Doctors' Organisation. Haemophilia. 2004;10(5):593–628.

47. Stine KC, Becton DL. DDAVP therapy controls bleeding in Ehlers-Danlos syndrome. J Pediatr Hematol Oncol. 1997;19(2):156–8.

48. Mast KJ, Nunes ME, Ruymann FB, Kerlin BA. Desmopressin responsiveness in children with Ehlers-Danlos syndrome associated bleeding symptoms. Br J Haematol. 2009;144(2):230–3.

49. Lindsay H, Lee-Kim YJ, Srivaths LV. Perioperative hemostatic Management in Ehlers-Danlos syndrome: a report of 2 cases and literature review. J Pediatr Hematol Oncol. 2016;38(2):158–60.

50. Rochelson B, Caruso R, Davenport D, Kaelber A. The use of prophylactic desmopressin (DDAVP) in labor to prevent hemorrhage in a patient with Ehlers-Danlos syndrome. N Y State J Med. 1991;91(6):268–9.

51. Yasui H, Adachi Y, Minami T, Ishida T, Kato Y, Imai K. Combination therapy of DDAVP and conjugated estrogens for a recurrent large subcutaneous hematoma in Ehlers-Danlos syndrome. Am J Hematol. 2003;72(1):71–2.

52. Faber P, Craig WL, Duncan JL, Holliday K. The successful use of recombinant factor VIIa in a patient with vascular-type Ehlers-Danlos syndrome. Acta Anaesthesiol Scand. 2007;51(9):1277–9.

53. Adeyemi-Fowode O, Santos XM, Dietrich JE, Srivaths L. Levonorgestrel-releasing intrauterine device use in female adolescents with heavy menstrual bleeding and bleeding disorders: single institution review. J Pediatr Adolesc Gynecol. 2017;30:479–83.

54. Bruner AB, Joffe A, Duggan AK, Casella JF, Brandt J. Randomised study of cognitive effects of iron supplementation in non-anaemic iron-deficient adolescent girls. Lancet. 1996;348(9033):992–6.

55. Nelson M. Anaemia in adolescent girls: effects on cognitive function and activity. Proc Nutr Soc. 1996;55(1B):359–67.

Complications of Heavy Menstrual Bleeding in Adolescents

9

Irmel A. Ayala and Enitan Adegite

Abbreviations

CHC   Combined hormonal contraceptives
HMB   Heavy menstrual bleeding
HRQOL   Health-related quality of life

Introduction

Menarche usually occurs between 12 and 13 years of age [1]. The average blood loss during a normal menstrual cycle is 30–40 ml. Heavy menstrual bleeding (HMB), defined as bleeding lasting over 7 days or blood loss above 80 ml per menses or excessive menstrual loss that interferes with a woman's physical, social, or emotional quality of life, is a very common complaint, affecting up to 37% of adolescent females [2]. In clinical practice, measurement of HMB is difficult and thus the diagnosis is typically based on perception and description of menstrual loss. HMB can occur due to a number of etiologies such as anatomic pathology, hormonal imbalances, or underlying medical conditions. Ovulatory dysfunction and anovulation are the most common etiologies of HMB in adolescents [3]. Hemostatic defects are identified in up to 50% of all adolescents with HMB [4–6]. Excessive monthly menstrual iron losses without adequate iron supplementation in the diet gradually reduces iron stores eventually leading to iron deficiency. Initially, isolated iron deficiency will be detected by decreased serum ferritin levels; however, once iron stores are eventually depleted, the hemoglobin production will be affected and iron deficiency anemia will develop.

Iron Deficiency and Anemia

The most common complication of HMB is iron deficiency, with or without anemia. It is estimated that the prevalence of iron deficiency in the general adolescent female population in the USA is between 9% and 16% [7]. In contrast, iron deficiency is diagnosed in up to 50% of adolescent females with HMB. Menstrual blood loss is the most common cause of iron deficiency in the adolescent female, but other factors, including inadequate iron intake, also play a role in the development of iron deficiency.

In spite of all the advances that have been made in regard to the proper identification and

I. A. Ayala (✉)
Hemophilia and Bleeding Disorders Treatment Center, Johns Hopkins All Children's Hospital, Cancer and Blood Disorders Institute, St. Petersburg, FL, USA
e-mail: iayala1@jhmi.edu

E. Adegite
Section of Adolescent Medicine, St Christopher's Hospital for Children, Drexel University, Philadelphia, PA, USA

© Springer Nature Switzerland AG 2020
L. V. Srivaths (ed.), *Hematology in the Adolescent Female*,
https://doi.org/10.1007/978-3-030-48446-0_9

management of HMB, many of these patients do not undergo the necessary evaluation to rule out the presence of iron deficiency [8–10].

Iron deficiency anemia was the leading cause of years lived with disability among children and adolescents in the world [11]. In the general population, iron deficiency has been associated with symptoms including fatigue, irritability, decreased productivity, pica, restless legs syndrome, headaches, and cognitive impairment. In the setting of fatigue, it is believed that iron deficiency results in derangements of the muscle metabolism, possibly secondary to modifications at the level of glucose utilization as an energy source. These metabolic derangements lead to increased lactate accumulation and increased muscle fatigue, which manifests as diminished endurance [12]. Iron supplementation improves fatigue resistance that results from decreased lactate accumulation. When compared with healthy controls, fatigue scores are higher in patients with HMB.

The relationship between iron deficiency and impaired cognitive function in infants and young children is well established. Studies have demonstrated that iron deficiency in children affects concentration, attention, and memory. Importantly, longitudinal studies have shown that adolescents with a history of iron deficiency anemia as infants continued to have decreased scores in spatial memory and attention relative to peers with adequate iron status in infancy. Although the mechanism that explains how iron deficiency affects the brain is not yet well understood, possible explanations may include alterations in brain metabolism and neurotransmitter metabolism, among others [13].

In the adolescent population, scholastic performance, attention, concentration, verbal memory, recognition, speed, and intelligence scores were seen to be decreased in the presence of iron deficiency with or without anemia [14]. In limited studies it was seen that iron replacement improves attention scores, concentration, and intelligence quotient [15, 16].

Rare Complications of HMB

Hemorrhagic shock is a rare medical complication of HMB. Among rare complications of hypovolemic shock in the setting of HMB, non-arteritic ischemic anterior neuropathy may result in visual loss, secondary to the interruption of oxygen supply to the optic nerve head, anterior to the lamina cribosa [17]. Other rare complications of HMB include cerebral sinovenous thrombosis (CSVT) in the setting of severe anemia [18]. Indeed, although the relationship between cerebral sinovenous thrombosis and iron deficiency anemia has been reported in the pediatric population for about three decades, most recent literature has also shown a relationship in the adult population. In the pediatric population, the etiology of iron deficiency is most commonly secondary to a nutritional deficiency. In the adolescent and adult population, however, the most common etiology of iron deficiency anemia is heavy menstrual bleeding. Potential explanations for the relationship between the development of CSVT and anemia include the frequently observed iron deficiency-related thrombocytosis along with decreased red cell deformability, increased viscosity, hemodynamic changes, and endothelial injury.

Health-Related Quality of Life

In addition to the physical complications, HMB also leads to other complications including decreased health-related quality of life (HRQOL). HRQOL is a multifaceted concept that includes aspects related to the physical, mental, emotional, social functioning, and well-being. HRQOL focuses on the impact that health status exerts on quality of life [19]. Menstrual problems are worse in adolescents and women with bleeding disorders, given the increased prevalence of HMB among these individuals. The excessive blood loss can be debilitating and often interferes with daily activities, socialization, sports, and school participation. Studies in adult women with bleeding disorders have shown that HMB significantly affects HRQOL. Among women with bleeding disorders, HRQOL score mean was lower in patients with HMB than in patients without this complication. In fact, the mean HRQOL of females with bleeding disorders and HMB was similar to that of HIV-positive severe hemophilia patients [20–23].

Adolescent females with inherited bleeding disorders have a higher risk of menstrual complications given the immaturity of the hypothalamic pituitary axis at this stage of life. This frequently leads to anovulatory cycles with subsequent heavy, prolonged, and irregular menstrual periods. Although literature specific to the HRQOL in the adolescent population that experiences HMB is limited, studies have demonstrated that adolescents with HMB in the setting of bleeding disorders experience lower HRQOL than healthy peers. More importantly, compared with teenage boys with congenital bleeding disorders, young females reported worse HRQOL scores. Although studies have shown a relationship between menstrual problems in general and decreased HRQOL, few studies have also shown that HMB affected physical functioning, emotional health, and school functioning. Studies have also shown that up to 52% of adolescents with HMB missed school compared with 20% of adolescents with normal periods [24–26].

In addition to the decreased HRQOL attributed to the direct short-term effects of HMB alone, the complications of anemia and iron deficiency that result as a consequence of HMB also affect HRQOL. In the adolescent population, fatigue severity scores and HMB severity scores were significantly higher in young women with HMB as compared to healthy controls [27]. Intravenous iron therapy improved fatigue scores in patients with proven iron deficiency, with and without anemia [28].

Despite the high prevalence of iron deficiency with and without anemia, the condition continues to remain underdiagnosed, leading to multiple complications. Prompt recognition, accurate diagnosis, and appropriate intervention without delay in these young females will improve not only their quality of life but their overall health as well. Increased awareness and distinction between normal and abnormal menstruation among the primary care providers and specialists is of utmost importance given the relatively high prevalence of HMB in the adolescent population.

Complications of Medical Therapy

The management of HMB in the adolescents predominantly involves medications and treatment regimens and may range from observation with serial blood checks, to the use of NSAIDS, hormonal contraceptives, blood products, and anti-fibrinolytic agents. The utilization of the different treatment alternatives available for HMB depends in part on concurrent morbidities and choice of patient/family.

Complications of Combined Hormonal Contraceptive Methods

The most frequently used medical treatment for HMB involves the use of combined hormonal contraceptive (CHC) medications. The estrogenic side effects are often dose dependent. The most common side effects including headaches, nausea, vomiting, and breakthrough bleeding tend to resolve with time. Nausea and vomiting may resolve with the use of an antiemetic when combined hormonal contraceptives are used at high doses to manage HMB. In patients that develop headaches as a side effect of using CHC, the clinician should consider switching to a different pill with a lower dose of estrogen that has a less estrogenic progestin or using extended cycling medications, where the patient has fewer intervals of taking placebo pills.

Breakthrough bleeding in adolescents tends to be related to adherence, and a CHC with a different route of administration or with less frequent dosing intervals should be considered. In these situations, additional options include using a weekly CHC patch or monthly NuvaRing rather than taking pills by mouth daily. The use of aids such as reminders, alerts, or alarms on mobile devices and apps can support better adherence to the treatment.

Weight changes as a result of using CHC, one of the most commonly articulated concerns by adolescent patients, occur in less than 3% of that population [29]. It is important to note and discuss with the patients that weight gain especially in early adolescence in females is developmentally appropriate and should be expected, irrespective of CHC use.

The more severe side effects are related to thromboembolism, but this is fortunately a rare complication in the adolescent population. Older age (>35 years) and having other risks such as genetic thrombophilia or prolonged immobilization are the major factors related to thromboembolism [30].

Complications of Progestin-Only Methods

Depot Medroxyprogesterone Acetate

Amenorrhea occurs at a rate of about 55% in 12 months and 68% in 24 months secondary to the use of depot medroxyprogesterone acetate [31].

In a patient with HMB, this may be desired, but some adolescents and their parents experience discomfort with the thought of not having menses monthly as they feel it may be unnatural or anxiety provoking because they were reassured of not being pregnant by their monthly menses.

Other side effects include unscheduled vaginal bleeding and diminished bone density. Diminished bone density has been reported with prolonged use and is reversible if the patient is off this medication for at least 6 months [32].

Intrauterine System (IUS)

The levonogestrel intrauterine system (IUS) has been shown to be very efficacious in the management of HMB. It is gaining popularity in use in the adolescent population. Adolescents with HMB most often are nulliparous, and nulliparity is associated with increased pain at the time of insertion. 4% lidocaine gel and intramuscular ketorolac have been used with varying some success for analgesia prior to IUS insertion [33]. Patients who are not sexually active may elect to have the insertion done under general anesthesia or conscious sedation to ease pain and anxiety and ensure adequate positioning for the LNG IUS insertion [34].

Systemic progesterone side effects such as migraine, acne, weight gain, mastalgia, nausea, and mood disorders are minimal, and the main concern is an irregular menstrual pattern limited to the first 3–6 months following LNG-IUS insertion [35].

Procedure-related complications, such as pelvic pain, perforation, upper genital infection, and expulsion, are also relatively rare [36].

No perforations were reported in a review of 2036 adolescents using LNG IUS [35]. The hormonal methods have the added benefit of providing contraception and management of premenstrual symptoms, menstrual cramps, and acne.

NSAIDs

Nonsteroidal anti-inflammatory drugs such as mefenamic acid (MFA), naproxen, ibuprofen, flurbiprofen, meclofenamic acid, diclofenac, indomethacin, and acetylsalicylic acid are efficacious in management of HMB and have been shown to reduce HMB by over 25% in three quarters of women with HMB [37]. NSAIDS also have the added benefit of analgesia for cramps. The side effects were described as not severe and were gastrointestinal such as abdominal pain, constipation, nausea, and heartburn [38].

Complications of Hemostatic Medications

Desmopressin

Desmopressin is typically utilized in patients with von Willebrand disease, low factor VIII, and certain inherited platelet disorders. Common short-term side effects include hypertension, facial flushing, and headaches. The major risk of desmopressin is the development of dilutional hyponatremia which tends to occur more frequently with IV administration compared with the nasal administration and for which the intake of liquid is typically limited for 24 hours after its administration [39].

Tranexamic Acid

TA is a competitive plasminogen inhibitor approved for use in women 18 years and older. A competitive plasminogen inhibitor medication has been increasingly used in adolescent patients despite the lack of significant safety and efficacy data in that population until recently [40]. Tranexamic acid is often preferred by parents who do not want their daughters on hormonal contraceptive methods because of their perceived daughter's young age, beliefs about birth control, or preference for as needed medication rather than continuous medication for management of HMB (Table 9.1).

Transfusion-Related Complications

Unfortunately, some adolescents with HMB will ultimately need to receive transfusion with red cells as part of their treatment. Transfusion therapy is associated with infectious and noninfectious complications. Viruses, bacteria, and parasites can all be transmitted via transfusions. The risk of a viral infectious disease transmitted by transfused red cells is low in developed countries with an estimated risk of less than 1 in two mil-

Table 9.1 Adverse effects of tranexamic acid

% Reporting	Adverse effects of tranexamic acid
>10%	Central nervous system: Headaches- 50% Respiratory: URI-like symptoms- 25% Musculoskeletal: Back pain 21% Musculoskeletal pain 11% Gastrointestinal: Abdominal pain −20% Reported mostly with oral formulation
1–10%	Central nervous system: Fatigue 5% Hematology and oncology: Anemia 6% Musculoskeletal: Arthralgia Muscle cramps $\leq 7\%$ Muscle spasms $\leq 7\%$
<1%	Allergic dermatitis, allergic skin reaction, anaphylactic shock, anaphylactoid reaction, anaphylaxis, cerebral thrombosis, chromatopsia, conjunctivitis (ligneous), deep vein thrombosis, diarrhea, dizziness, hypersensitivity reaction, hypotension (with rapid IV injection), nausea, pulmonary embolism, renal cortical necrosis, retinal artery occlusion, retinal vein occlusion, seizure, ureteral obstruction, visual disturbance, vomiting [41, 42]

lion transfusions for the most concerning pathogens including the human immunodeficiency virus and hepatitis C virus. The administration of donor questionnaires and advanced testing methodologies has significantly reduced the risk of many viral infections. The possibility of emerging pathogens always needs to be considered. Transfusion therapy is also associated with bacterial contamination which is in fact more common than viral infection. Multiple steps have been implemented to decrease the possibility of bacterial contamination and related sepsis.

In spite of risk mitigation, it is estimated that noninfectious transfusion reactions occur with a rate of 2.4 reactions per 1000 units transfused. Non-hemolytic transfusion reactions, which include allergic and febrile non-hemolytic reactions, are the most common reported transfusion-related reactions [43]. Additional transfusion-related complications include hemolytic reactions, both acute (within 24 hrs of transfusion) and delayed. Acute hemolytic transfusion reactions are a very significant complication and account for approximately 25% of transfusion-related mortalities [43]. Other significant transfusion-related complications include TRALI or transfusion-associated acute lung injury and TACO, transfusion-associated circulatory overload. Rare complications of transfusions include post transfusion purpura and transfusion-related graft versus host disease [43].

Complications of Iron Therapy

First line treatment for iron deficiency involves the administration of oral iron supplementation. The most commonly reported side effects of oral iron supplementation include constipation, nausea, abdominal pain, diarrhea, and dark stools [44]. In addition to these well-known side effects of iron supplementation, recent studies suggest that oral iron supplementation also disrupts the colonic microbiota which could potentially promote the presence of potentially pathogenic bacteria. Gastrointestinal symptoms attributed to oral iron supplementation result in nonadherence and treatment failure. Intravenous iron therapy is used when oral iron is not tolerated, ineffective, or inappropriate. Although IV iron administration is considered safe, it carries the risk of severe hypersensitivity reactions which happens to a very small subset of patients. In addition, treatment with IV iron is expensive, compared with oral iron supplements [45].

Complications of Surgical Procedures

Surgical procedures are fortunately very rarely necessary in the management of HMB in adolescents as most cases will resolve with medical management.

Endometrial Ablation

The major complications of endometrial ablation include perforation, endometritis, myometritis, cervical laceration/tear or stenosis, pelvic sepsis, pelvic abscess, pelvic inflammatory disease, hematometra, uterine tamponade, blood transfusion, glycine toxicity, fluid overload, fluid deficit, bowel obstruction, and urinary incontinence. Minor complications include skin rash and burning sensation, headache, nausea, vomiting or severe pelvic pain, weakness or fatigue during the first 24 hours, backache during the first 24 hours, bradycardia, fever, chills, bloating, abdominal tenderness, dysuria, urinary tract infection, hydrosalpinx, spotting during the first 24 hours, vaginal bleeding, abdominal cramping, infection (leucorrhoea), and first-degree burn [46].

A prospective national audit of hysteroscopic endometrial ablation and resection (10,686 cases) in England and Wales between 1993 and 1994 assessed the incidence of complications and reported a total complication rate of 4.4% [47]. These rates have improved to about 1% with second-generation procedures [48, 49].

Hysterectomy

This surgical procedure provides definitive treatment for HMB and is typically reserved for women that are past childbearing years, so it is very rarely used in adolescents unless HMB is life-threatening and no other fertility sparing treatments are available.

In a Cochrane review by Majoribanks et al., hysterectomy complication rates vary depending on route which could be abdominal, laparoscopic, vaginal, and laparoscopically assisted vaginal. Some short-term complications include hemorrhage (serious blood loss), infection, and wound healing problems and may require a lengthy postoperative recovery period [50].

Fertility Concerns

Contraceptives: Return to Fertility

The reported 12-month conception rates in former cyclic OC users range from 72% to 94% and are similar to those observed in women discontinuing intrauterine devices (71–92%) and progestin-only contraceptives (70–95%) [50]. According to this review, 83.1% (95% CI = 78.2–88%) of women who discontinued contraception became pregnant within the first 12 months. Return of fertility at the first year was not significantly different for hormonal methods and IUD users [51].

Fertility after discontinuing using contraception is not affected by the use of contraception, type of contraception, duration of use, or type of progesterone, a concern a lot of parents of adolescents often have [52].

The long-term side effect of surgical methods such as endometrial ablation and hysterectomy is infertility.

Other Associated Gynecologic Conditions

These conditions are associated with increased morbidity in females with bleeding disorders and not necessarily a complication of heavy menstrual bleeding.

Anovulation

Physiologic immaturity of the reproductive axis, under the control of the hypothalamic–pituitary–adrenal and ovarian axis results in irregular menstrual cycles. This is predominant in the first few years after menarche. Menses often times do not occur monthly and may have periods of prolonged absence followed by periods of excessive bleeding that may last several days to weeks as a result of a hypertrophied endometrium that is unstable and sloughs off from lack of progestin. This unpredictability makes it important for females especially those with bleeding disorders to have easy access to menstrual hygiene products and early evaluation and management of prolonged menses.

Mittelschmerz: Ovulation Pain

This occurs mid cycle with the rupture and release of the dominant ovarian follicle and may be associated with bleeding into the peritoneum. This blood in the peritoneum is often irritating, and patients will present with moderate to severe abdominal and pelvic pain. A survey by Kouides et al. reports a 49% rate of ovulation pain in women with VWD type 1 [53].

Hemorrhagic Ovarian Cysts

Failure of the corpus luteum to regress but rather, it continuing to grow and increase in size, may result in bleeding, into the cyst and it's rupture may result in significant pelvic pain and discomfort. A review by James in 2005 lists multiple case reports when this was reported in females with bleeding disorders [54]. Supportive care with analgesics is the main mode of treatment, and some cases may require surgical treatment. Future cysts can be prevented by suppressing ovulation using contraceptives, the most frequently used method being the combined hormonal contraceptive pill.

Obstetric and Pregnancy-Related Complications

Increased factor levels in pregnancy contribute to it being a protective hypercoagulable state in females with bleeding disorders [54]. A review of 182 females with severe VWD did not show an increase in miscarriage rate [55]; however, a CDC survey by Kirtava et al. of 102 females with Von Willebrand disease reports that 1.3% experienced heavy bleeding that resulted in a loss of pregnancy as compared to a rate of 0.3% in controls [56]. Uterine atony is the predominant cause of postpartum hemorrhage (PPH) [57]. The CDC survey of these 102 females listed above reports PPH rates of 59% as compared to controls at 21% [56]. A study by Srivaths et al. of 269 females with heavy menstrual bleeding reports that 100% of the adolescents less than 18 years that were pregnant reported having bleeding complications during their pregnancy or in the postpartum period versus 53% of adult women [58]. It is important for the clinician providing care for these pregnant adolescents with bleeding disorders to be aware of the potential for complications and collaborate early with colleagues in obstetrics.

Financial Impact

HMB is associated with high healthcare costs. These costs are as a result of often multiple visits to medical offices, emergency rooms, referrals to specialists, prescription drug coverage, hospitalizations, admission to the ICU, and transfusion therapy. The costs related to the care of heavy menstrual bleeding in the USA is estimated at over 1 billion dollars annually [59, 60].

Annual estimates of direct costs excluding workup and investigations in the treatment of HMB inclusive of two clinician office visits per method were estimated to be $612 for a 1-year supply of oral contraceptive pills, $763 for the LNG IUS, $1938 for endometrial ablation, and $4782 for hysterectomy [61]. The annual estimate of lost wages secondary to HMB by women was $1692 in an evaluation done by Cote in 2000 [62, 63]. These estimates are modest as they do not include the financial costs of associated therapy and the fact that patients with HMB may need to be on medications and utilize additional treatment modalities for varied duration, ranging from a few years to several decades, depending on the cause of the heavy menstrual bleeding, which could range from immaturity of the hypothalamic-pituitary axis to a bleeding disorder.

References

1. Committee Opinion No. 651 Summary. Obstet Gynecol. 2015;126(6):1328.
2. Friberg B, Kristin Örnö A, Lindgren A, Lethagen S. Bleeding disorders among young women: a population-based prevalence study. Acta Obstet Gynecol Scand. 2006;85(2):200–6.
3. Munro MG, Critchley HOD, Broder MS, Fraser IS. FIGO classification system (PALM-COEIN) for causes of abnormal uterine bleeding in nongravid women of reproductive age. Int J Gynecol Obstet. 2011;113(1):3–13.
4. O'Brien B, Mason J, Kimble R. Bleeding disorders in adolescents with heavy menstrual bleeding: the Queensland Statewide Paediatric and adolescent Gynaecology Service. J Pediatr Adolesc Gynecol. 2019;32(2):122–7.
5. Díaz R, Dietrich JE, Mahoney D, Yee DL, Srivaths LV. Hemostatic abnormalities in young females with heavy menstrual bleeding. J Pediatr Adolesc Gynecol. 2014;27(6):324–9.
6. Mikhail S, Varadarajan R, Kouides P. The prevalence of disorders of haemostasis in adolescents with menorrhagia referred to a haemophilia treatment centre. Haemophilia. 2007;13(5):627–32.
7. Iron deficiency–United States, 1999–2000. MMWR Morb Mortal Wkly Rep. 2002;51(40):897–9.
8. Cooke AG, McCavit TL, Buchanan GR, Powers JM. Iron deficiency anemia in adolescents who present with heavy menstrual bleeding. J Pediatr Adolesc Gynecol. 2017;30(2):247–50.
9. Revel-Vilk S, Paltiel O, Lipschuetz M, et al. Underdiagnosed menorrhagia in adolescents is associated with underdiagnosed anemia. J Pediatr. 2012;160(3):468–72.
10. Johnson S, Lang A, Sturm M, O'Brien SH. Iron deficiency without anemia: a common yet underrecognized diagnosis in young women with heavy menstrual bleeding. J Pediatr Adolesc Gynecol. 2016;29(6):628–31.
11. Global Burden of Disease Pediatrics C, Kyu HH, Pinho C, et al. Global and national burden of diseases and injuries among children and adolescents between 1990 and 2013: findings from the global burden of disease 2013 study. JAMA Pediatr. 2016;170(3):267–87.
12. Boccio JR, Iyengar V. Iron deficiency: causes, consequences, and strategies to overcome this nutritional problem. Biol Trace Elem Res. 2003;94(1):1–32.
13. Jáuregui-Lobera I. Iron deficiency and cognitive functions. Neuropsychiatr Dis Treat. 2014;10:2087–95.
14. More S, Shivkumar VB, Gangane N, Shende S. Effects of iron deficiency on cognitive function in school going adolescent females in rural area of Central India. Anemia. 2013;2013:–819136.
15. Rezaeian A, Ghayour-Mobarhan M, Mazloum SR, Yavari M, Jafari S-A. Effects of iron supplementation twice a week on attention score and haematologic measures in female high school students. Singap Med J. 2014;55(11):587–92.
16. Murray-Kolb LE, Beard JL. Iron treatment normalizes cognitive functioning in young women. Am J Clin Nutr. 2007;85(3):778–87.
17. Koh K-L, Sonny Teo KS, Chong M-F, Wan Hitam W-H. Non-arteritic anterior ischaemic optic neuropathy secondary to menorrhagia in a young healthy woman. BMJ Case Rep. 2018;2018:bcr2018225113.
18. Corrales-Medina FF, Grant L, Egas-Bejar D, Valdivia-Ascuna Z, Rodriguez N, Mancias P. Cerebral Sinovenous thrombosis associated with Iron deficiency anemia secondary to severe menorrhagia. J Child Neurol. 2013;29(9):NP62–4.
19. Healthy People 2020. Foundation Health Measure Report. Health-Related Quality of Life and Well-Being. US Department of Health and Human Services, Office of Disease Prevention and Health Promotion;November 2010.
20. Shankar M, Chi C, Kadir RA. Review of quality of life: menorrhagia in women with or with-

out inherited bleeding disorders. Haemophilia. 2007;14(1):071027033511001.

21. Kadir RA, Edlund M, Von Mackensen S. The impact of menstrual disorders on quality of life in women with inherited bleeding disorders. Haemophilia. 2010;16(5):832–9.

22. Peuranpää P, Heliövaara-Peippo S, Fraser I, Paavonen J, Hurskainen R. Effects of anemia and iron deficiency on quality of life in women with heavy menstrual bleeding. Acta Obstet Gynecol Scand. 2014;93(7):654–60.

23. Rae C, Furlong W, Horsman J, et al. Bleeding disorders, menorrhagia and iron deficiency: impacts on health-related quality of life. Haemophilia. 2013;19(3):385–91.

24. Nur Azurah AG, Sanci L, Moore E, Grover S. The quality of life of adolescents with menstrual problems. J Pediatr Adolesc Gynecol. 2013;26(2):102–8.

25. Pawar A, Krishnan R, Davis K, Bosma K, Kulkarni R. Perceptions about quality of life in a school-based population of adolescents with menorrhagia: implications for adolescents with bleeding disorders. Haemophilia. 2008;14(3):579–83.

26. Limperg PF, Joosten MMH, Fijnvandraat K, Peters M, Grootenhuis MA, Haverman L. Male gender, school attendance and sports participation are positively associated with health-related quality of life in children and adolescents with congenital bleeding disorders. Haemophilia. 2018;24(3):395–404.

27. Wang W, Bourgeois T, Klima J, Berlan ED, Fischer AN, O'Brien SH. Iron deficiency and fatigue in adolescent females with heavy menstrual bleeding. Haemophilia. 2012;19(2):225–30.

28. Sharma R, Stanek JR, Koch TL, Grooms L, O'Brien SH. Intravenous iron therapy in non-anemic iron-deficient menstruating adolescent females with fatigue. Am J Hematol. 2016;91(10):973–7.

29. Lethaby A, Wise MR, Weterings MA, Bofill Rodriguez M, Brown J. Combined hormonal contraceptives for heavy menstrual bleeding. Cochrane Database Syst Rev. 2019;2(2):–CD000154.

30. Curtis KM, Tepper NK, Jatlaoui TC, et al. U.S. medical eligibility criteria for contraceptive use, 2016. MMWR Recomm Rep. 2016;65(3):1–103.

31. Schwallie PC, Assenzo JR. Contraceptive use—efficacy study utilizing medroxyprogesterone acetate* administered as an intramuscular injection once every 90 days*Depo-Provera, Upjohn; sterile aqueous suspension of medroxyprogesterone acetate. Fertil Steril. 1973;24(5):331–9.

32. Gai L, Zhang J, Zhang H, Gai P, Zhou L, Liu Y. The effect of depot medroxyprogesterone acetate (DMPA) on bone mineral density (BMD) and evaluating changes in BMD after discontinuation of DMPA in Chinese women of reproductive age. Contraception. 2011;83(3):218–22.

33. Lohr PA, Lyus R, Prager S. Use of intrauterine devices in nulliparous women. Contraception. 2017;95(6):529–37.

34. Adams Hillard PJ. Menstrual suppression with the Levonorgestrel intrauterine system in girls with developmental delay. J Pediatr Adolesc Gynecol. 2012;25(5):308–13.

35. Patseadou M, Michala L. Usage of the levonorgestrel-releasing intrauterine system (LNG-IUS) in adolescence: what is the evidence so far? Arch Gynecol Obstet. 2016;295(3):529–41.

36. Luukkainen T, Lähteenmäki P, Toivonen J. Levonorgestrel-releasing intrauterine device. Ann Med. 1990;22(2):85–90.

37. Roy SN, Bhattacharya S. Benefits and risks of pharmacological agents used for the treatment of menorrhagia. Drug Saf. 2004;27(2):75–90.

38. Bofill Rodriguez M, Lethaby A, Farquhar C. Nonsteroidal anti-inflammatory drugs for heavy menstrual bleeding. Cochrane Database Syst Rev. 2019;9(9):–CD000400.

39. Ozgönenel B, Rajpurkar M, Lusher JM. How do you treat bleeding disorders with desmopressin? Postgrad Med J. 2007;83(977):159–63.

40. O'Brien SH, Saini S, Ziegler H, et al. An open-label, single-arm, efficacy study of tranexamic acid in adolescents with heavy menstrual bleeding. J Pediatr Adolesc Gynecol. 2019;32(3):305–11.

41. Lukes AS, Moore KA, Muse KN, et al. Tranexamic acid treatment for heavy menstrual bleeding. Obstet Gynecol. 2010;116(4):865–75.

42. Muse K, Lukes AS, Gersten J, Waldbaum A, Mabey RG, Trott E. Long-term evaluation of safety and health-related quality of life in women with heavy menstrual bleeding treated with oral tranexamic acid. Womens Health. 2011;7(6):699–707.

43. Carson JL, Triulzi DJ, Ness PM. Indications for and adverse effects of red-cell transfusion. N Engl J Med. 2017;377(13):1261–72.

44. Tolkien Z, Stecher L, Mander AP, Pereira DIA, Powell JJ. Ferrous sulfate supplementation causes significant gastrointestinal side-effects in adults: a systematic review and meta-analysis. PLoS One. 2015;10(2):–e0117383.

45. Szebeni J, Fishbane S, Hedenus M, et al. Hypersensitivity to intravenous iron: classification, terminology, mechanisms and management. Br J Pharmacol. 2015;172(21):5025–36.

46. Bofill Rodriguez M, Lethaby A, Grigore M, Brown J, Hickey M, Farquhar C. Endometrial resection and ablation techniques for heavy menstrual bleeding. Cochrane Database Syst Rev. 2019;1:CD001501.

47. Overton C, Hargreaves J, Maresh M. A national survey of the complications of endometrial destruction for menstrual disorders: the MISTLETOE study. BJOG. 1997;104(12):1351–9.

48. Athanatos D, Pados G, Venetis CA, et al. Novasure impedance control system versus microwave endometrial ablation for the treatment of dysfunctional uterine bleeding: a double-blind, randomized controlled trial. Clin Exp Obstet Gynecol. 2015;42(3):347–51.

49. Laberge PY, Garza-Leal J, Fortin C, et al. A randomized, controlled, multi-center trial of the safety and

efficacy of the minerva endometrial ablation system. one-year follow-up results. J Minim Invasive Gynecol. 2016;23(7):S44.

50. Marjoribanks J, Lethaby A, Farquhar C. Surgery versus medical therapy for heavy menstrual bleeding. Cochrane Database Syst Rev. 2016;

51. Barnhart KT, Schreiber CA. Return to fertility following discontinuation of oral contraceptives. Fertil Steril. 2009;91(3):659–63.

52. Girum T, Wasie A. Return of fertility after discontinuation of contraception: a systematic review and meta-analysis. Contracept Reprod Med. 2018;3:9–9.

53. Kouides PA, Phatak PD, Burkart P, et al. Gynaecological and obstetrical morbidity in women with type I von Willebrand disease: results of a patient survey. Haemophilia. 2000;6(6):643–8.

54. James AH. More than menorrhagia: a review of the obstetric and gynaecological manifestations of bleeding disorders. Haemophilia. 2005;11(4):295–307.

55. Lak M, Peyvandi F, Mannucci PM. Clinical manifestations and complications of childbirth and replacement therapy in 385 Iranian patients with type 3 von Willebrand disease. Br J Haematol. 2000;111(4):1236–9.

56. Kirtava A, Drews C, Lally C, Dilley A, Evatt B. Medical, reproductive and psychosocial experiences of women diagnosed with von Willebrand's disease receiving care in haemophilia treatment centres: a case-control study. Haemophilia. 2003;9(3):292–7.

57. Gabbe SG, Niebyl JR, Simpson JL. Obstetrics : normal and problem pregnancies. New York: Churchill Livingstone; 2002.

58. Srivaths LV, Zhang QC, Byams VR, et al. Differences in bleeding phenotype and provider interventions in postmenarchal adolescents when compared to adult women with bleeding disorders and heavy menstrual bleeding. Haemophilia. 2018;24(1):63–9.

59. Liu Z, Doan QV, Blumenthal P, Dubois RW. A systematic review evaluating health-related quality of life, work impairment, and health-care costs and utilization in abnormal uterine bleeding. Value Health. 2007;10(3):183–94.

60. Miller JD, Lenhart GM, Bonafede MM, Basinski CM, Lukes AS, Troeger KA. Cost effectiveness of endometrial ablation with the NovaSure(®) system versus other global ablation modalities and hysterectomy for treatment of abnormal uterine bleeding: US commercial and Medicaid payer perspectives. Int J Women's Health. 2015;7:59–73.

61. Blumenthal PD, Trussell J, Singh RH, et al. Cost-effectiveness of treatments for dysfunctional uterine bleeding in women who need contraception. Contraception. 2006;74(3):249–58.

62. Côté I, Jacobs P, Cumming D. Work loss associated with increased menstrual loss in the United States. Obstet Gynecol. 2002;100(4):683–7.

63. Côté I, Jacobs P, Cumming DC. Use of health services associated with increased menstrual loss in the United States. Am J Obstet Gynecol. 2003;188(2):343–8.

Hormonal Therapy for Heavy Menstrual Bleeding

10

Maureen K. Baldwin and Jennifer L. Bercaw-Pratt

Introduction

The goals of treatment of heavy menstrual bleeding are to reduce morbidity, restore and maintain normal blood volumes, prevent life-threatening hemorrhage, and improve quality of life [1, 2]. Hormonal therapies are safe and effective and are the mainstay of the treatment of heavy menstrual bleeding in adolescent females [3]. The treatment of heavy menstrual bleeding can be divided into the treatment of acute bleeding followed by maintenance of the chronic problem. Typically, hormonal therapies used to treat acute heavy menstrual bleeding include intravenous conjugated equine estrogen, combined oral estrogen-progestin pills, and oral progestins [3]. Once the acute bleeding has been controlled, multiple hormonal therapy options exist for long-term maintenance of heavy menstrual bleeding. These hormonal therapies include the levonorgestrel intrauterine system (LNG-IUS), combined hormonal options, and oral/injectable/subdermal progestins [3].

Estrogen and Progesterone in the Normal Menstrual Cycle

Understanding the normal menstrual cycle is imperative to understand how hormonal therapies are effective in treating heavy menstrual bleeding. The menstrual cycle occurs due to interaction with the hypothalamus/pituitary gland, ovary, and uterus to control the production of estrogen and progesterone. During the follicular phase of the menstrual cycle, follicle-stimulating hormone (FSH) stimulates the ovarian follicle to produce estrogen, which then has negative feedback on FSH and promotes luteinizing hormone (LH) secretion and ovulation. The resulting corpus luteum subsequently produces progesterone, which then suppresses LH. After approximately 2 weeks, production of progesterone gradually declines, leading to the signal cascade for the initiation of menstrual shedding and endometrial repair mechanisms.

Normal and induced menstrual cycles occur as a result of estrogen-stimulated endometrial proliferation, followed by a secretory transformation induced by the progestogen. Synchronous shedding of the endometrial lining occurs in response to the decline or withdrawal of the progestogen. Progestogen withdrawal induces a number of events, including production of tissue remodeling enzymes, prostaglandins, and cytokines. These lead to tissue breakdown and bleeding. Events that lead to the cessation of bleeding include

M. K. Baldwin
Department of Obstetrics and Gynecology, Oregon Health & Science University, Portland, OR, USA

J. L. Bercaw-Pratt (✉)
Department of Obstetrics and Gynecology, Baylor College of Medicine, Houston, TX, USA
e-mail: jbercaw@bcm.edu

© Springer Nature Switzerland AG 2020
L. V. Srivaths (ed.), *Hematology in the Adolescent Female*,
https://doi.org/10.1007/978-3-030-48446-0_10

collapse of the spiral arteries, platelet plugging, fibrin formation, and estrogen-induced proliferation [4].

The same mechanisms that play a role in normal endometrial cycling are present during the use of exogenous hormone therapies, though are subject to pharmacokinetics and dosing regimens. The cyclic fashion of many contraceptive hormone therapies is designed to mimic the natural menstrual cycle. With continuous administration of combined contraceptive hormone therapies, the endometrium remains inactive, and ovulation is suppressed, though breakthrough bleeding can occur. Usually breakthrough bleeding occurs in the setting of a proliferative endometrium, vessel fragility, or progestogen withdrawal and can occur more frequently in those with heavier baseline bleeding [5]. With continuous administration of progestin-only therapies, there is a dose-dependent inhibition of ovulation and typically an inactive endometrium, depending on endogenous follicular activity and estrogen production.

Estrogen Therapies

High-dose estrogen such as intravenous conjugated equine estrogen is used in the treatment of acute heavy menstrual bleeding [6]. The mechanism of action is by promoting platelet aggregation; increasing fibrinogen, factor V, and VI levels; and increasing production of both estrogen and progesterone receptors [6, 7]. In a randomized, double-blind, placebo-controlled trial, acute bleeding had ceased by 6 hours in 72% of participants receiving 25 mg intravenous estrogen every 4 hours versus 38% who received placebo ($p = 0.02$). The onset of action is too rapid to be attributed to induction of a trophic effect, and it is effective for both secretory and proliferative endometria [6]. Once the acute heavy menstrual bleeding has resolved, the patient is transitioned to any of the multiple hormonal therapies that exist for maintenance. Long-term unopposed estrogen treatment should not be used in the treatment of heavy menstrual bleeding due to risk of the development of endometrial cancer [2].

Combined Therapies

Combined therapies were developed primarily as contraceptives and thus block follicle development (an estrogen effect) and follicle rupture (a progestogen effect). The effect of combined methods on the endometrium depends on whether they are used cyclically or continuously. With cyclic use, initially there is early proliferation and then secretory transformation, followed by cyclic bleeding during the hormone-free interval. With continuous use, most patients experience an inactive endometrium, though breakthrough bleeding is a common problem.

The estrogen most commonly used in contraceptive formulations, such as the pill, patch, and vaginal ring, is ethinyl estradiol (EE); but mestranol and estradiol valerate (E2V) are also available in combination with progestins. Mestranol is metabolized to ethinyl estradiol with an equivalence of 50 mcg of mestranol to 30 mcg of EE [8]. Estradiol valerate is an estrogen formulation available since 2010 as a contraceptive in combination with dienogest [9]. E2V is quickly metabolized to the physiologic estradiol, 17β-estradiol, and valeric acid, so is considered much less potent than EE.

The amount of estrogen used in traditional oral contraceptive pills has been steadily decreasing since the early formulation of the pill. The first oral contraceptive pill approved by the US Food and Drug Administration was Enovid 10 which contained 150 mcg of mestranol and norethynodrel [10]. In contrast, contemporary oral contraceptive pills have between 10 and 50 mcg of EE. The bioactivity of the estrogen in traditional combined oral contraceptives exceeds the physiologic levels of the reproductive years [10]. This amount of circulating estrogen underscores the potential risk of thromboembolic events when using hormonal therapies containing EE [10]. The dominant hormone in the combined regimens is the progestin, which is dosed for ovulatory suppression and maintains a thin, inactive endometrium when used continuously. The progestin formulations used in combined hormonal therapies are numerous [11]. Progestins are classified by either their chemical structures or the time of their introduction to the market. A unique progestin used is drospirenone, which is the only available derivative of spironolactone, so it retains some of spironolactone's inherent anti-mineralocorticoid and anti-androgenic activity [10].

Estrogen provides endometrial stabilization and is generally associated with a predictable bleeding pattern when administered cyclically. As stated earlier, combined oral contraceptive pills thin endometrium and inhibit ovulation with resulting decreased menstrual blood loss of 43% [12]. However, at higher doses, EE is associated with endometrial proliferation and a thickened endometrial lining. Higher-dose regimens or "pill tapers" are frequently prescribed, particularly in the acute setting. The superior effectiveness of this strategy, while described in many textbooks and supported anecdotally, is unsubstantiated by clinical research. There is no evidence that higher doses are more effective for suppression of acute bleeding. Since the hormonal effects of exogenously administered gonadal steroids require receptor binding, activation, and then downstream effects, all therapies require patience.

Estradiol valerate (E2V) with dienogest (DNG) has been evaluated and FDA-approved for treatment of heavy menstrual bleeding with average reduction in measured menstrual blood loss (MBL) of approximately 68% versus placebo [13]. Patients should be advised that the phasic pill package should be used in the correct order and as prescribed and that there are only two hormone-free pills. The package uses an estrogen step-down and progestin step-up approach. A randomized trial of adults aged 18 or older compared MBL after E2V/DNG (n = 220) versus placebo (n = 135) for seven treatment cycles. Successful treatment with mean 50% reduction in MBL from baseline and less than 80 mL MBL was achieved by 63.6% of those receiving E2V/DNG and 11.9% of placebo.

Oral combined hormone pills are commercially available in cyclic and extended regimens but are frequently used off-label in continuous fashion. Packaging includes 24/4, 21/7, and 84/7 day hormone versus hormone-free pills. Patients frequently attempt complete menstrual suppression with continuous regimens by skipping the hormone-free interval. Continuous and extended regimens are subject to breakthrough bleeding, particularly for those with baseline heavy menstrual bleeding, a thickened endometrial lining, or poor adherence. To achieve a thin endometrial lining without bothersome bleeding, some providers recommend a few cycles of cyclic regimen followed by continuous cycling.

Breakthrough bleeding during continuous and extended cycling can be self-managed using a flexibly timed short hormone-free interval of about 4 days [14]. This is frequently described to patients as the "rule of 3s," which involves inducing a withdrawal bleed by stopping pills/ring if [1] bleeding or spotting has occurred for 3 days; [2] the combined regimen has been used for the last 3 weeks; and [3] the method is restarted in 3 days even if bleeding/spotting has persisted [15, 16]. This method maintains contraception while inducing a self-limited breakthrough bleeding episode. Patients who desire continuous suppression may find it useful to determine the optimal interval and timing for management of their withdrawal bleeding, including timing bleeding to avoid vacations or other special events [9, 11].

Progestin Therapies

Some patients have a contraindication to estrogen and are only candidates for progestogen agents, which can be administered by oral, intramuscular, subdermal, or intrauterine routes [17]. The mechanisms of action for the progestogen agents include stabilizing the endometrial lining, inhibiting the growth of the endometrium, inhibiting angiogenesis, and stimulating the conversion of estrogen to the less active estrone. Continuous progestin administration results in dose-dependent suppression of ovulation and down-regulation of estrogen and progestin receptors, leading to an unresponsive endometrium and subsequent amenorrhea in many women [18].

The wide variation in dose and type of progestin in current therapies has varying effects on bleeding pattern, which is particularly dependent on the pharmacokinetics of delivery. Evidence supports effective menstrual suppression with both progestin-only and combined medications; however, comparative data is lacking, particularly in adolescents. What is clear is that the historically recommended secretory or luteal phase cyclic oral progestin regimens, such as days 19 to 26, are less effective than dosing during days 5–26, so is no longer recommended for management [19]. The oral progestin options that are currently available in the US market are norethindrone (norethisterone), norethindrone acetate, micronized progesterone, and medroxyprogesterone acetate. A cyclic 4 mg drospirenone-only pill has also recently become available in the USA and is approved for contraception. It does provide ovulatory suppression and a predictable bleeding pattern with 24/4 cyclic administration. Additional delivery systems include the etonogestrel contraceptive implant, levonorgestrel intrauterine system, and depot medroxyprogesterone acetate. None of these have been studied for acute HMB.

Norethindrone (NET; 0.35 mg) and norethindrone acetate (NETA; 5 mg) are the most frequently utilized progestin-only oral options for heavy menstrual bleeding [20, 21]. NET is a derivative of the precursor NETA, which is rapidly hydrolyzed during first-pass metabolism [22]. Milligram for milligram, they can be considered to have equivalent bioactivity, despite the magnitude of difference between their commercially available doses. The dose required of each for inhibition of ovulation not in combination with estrogen is 0.4 mg for NET and 0.5 mg for NETA (Table 10.1) [23]. No intermediate dose is available; thus many providers use higher-dose regimens of NET to achieve endometrial suppression. Approximately 0.35% of NET is aromatized to ethinyl estradiol, equivalent to approximately 30–60 mcg EE after 5–10 mg NETA [23].

Oral medroxyprogesterone acetate (MPA) is one of the more commonly researched medication regimens for acute heavy menstrual bleeding but is not frequently used due to poor patient tolerance due to side effects such as bloating and fatigue. In the acute setting, use has been described as 60–120 mg on the first day, followed by 20 mg daily for 10 days, with over 50% of

Table 10.1 Dose-dependent effects by progestogens on endometrium, ovulation, and receptor binding affinity [23]

Progestin	TFD (mg/cycle)	OID (mg/day)	PR (%)	AR (%)	ER (%)
Medroxyprogesterone acetate	50		115	5	0
Norethisterone acetate	50	0.5			
Norethisterone	120	0.4	75	15	0
Levonorgestrel	5	0.06	150	45	0
Norgestimate	7	0.2	15	0	0
Etonogestrel	2	0.06	150	20	0
Drospirenone	50	2.0	35	65	0

TFD transformation dose in adult female (typical PR-mediated progestogenic effect on the endometrium), *OID* ovulation-inhibiting dose (without additional estrogen), *PR* progesterone receptor, *AR* androgen receptor, *ER* estrogen receptor

adolescent subjects experiencing bleeding cessation by 2 days and all subjects by 4 days [24]. For chronic HMB, typically MPA is used with cyclic dosing in non-contraceptive regimens such as 5–20 mg daily for cycle days 5 through 26 [19].

Some providers prefer oral micronized progesterone, but it has not been evaluated for management of heavy menstrual bleeding. One study compared management of anovulatory bleeding in older patients (ages 35–60) with natural micronized progesterone (NMP) 100 mg TID versus NET 5 mg TID administered cycle days 15–24 for 6 months. Side effect profiles and satisfaction were similar, but a proliferative endometrium and breakthrough bleeding was experienced more frequently by the NMP group [25].

Providing a loading dose of progestin or a step-down "taper" approach to dosing is common in the setting of acute heavy menstrual bleeding for progestin-only as well as combined therapies [20]. Dosing regimens range from 0.7 mg NET daily for 3–7 days to 10–15 mg NETA daily (5 mg BID to TID), prior to decreasing doses in a step-down fashion, attempting to avoid the bleeding episode that would occur after progestin withdrawal [26].

Breakthrough bleeding during use of progestin-only therapies is a commonly cited reason for discontinuation but does not affect all patients [20]. Various therapies and interventions, such as non-steroidal anti-inflammatory medications, matrix metalloproteinase inhibitors (doxycycline), estrogen receptor modulators, and low-dose estrogens, have been studied for their temporary or long-term effect on improvement of unscheduled bleeding [27].

Comparative Effectiveness of Hormonal Therapies

There have not been comparative studies for heavy menstrual bleeding outcomes between various types of oral combined therapies based on dose or type of progestin. Therefore, gynecologists prescribe the lowest dose, least expensive, and best tolerated medication that the patient will continue using. Typically, the non-phasic medication on formulary is both successful and well tolerated. We recommend prescribing a 12-month supply with typically 3 months dispensed per pharmacy visit, depending on state pharmacy regulations. Several states now allow pharmacist prescribing after appropriate training.

Oral combined pills and the vaginal ring are equally effective in reducing menstrual blood loss [28]. Fifty women ages 25–40 with heavy menstrual bleeding based on a pictorial bleeding assessment chart (PBAC) score >100 underwent six treatment cycles, including 3 weeks of combined vaginal ring or 30 mcg EE/150 mcg LNG oral pill, followed by 1 hormone-free week. Both resulted in approximately 70% reduction in PBAC scores. Bleeding pattern and compliance (88% versus 75%) were better with the vaginal ring. The combined ring can also be used continuously for up to 4 weeks of active medication and is well tolerated by teens who have already used tampons [29]. The transdermal combined patch has not been formally studied for heavy menstrual bleeding outcomes, but four of five users with bleeding disorders reported successful management in a cohort study [21]. Menstrual blood loss with transdermal delivery is comparable to oral and transvaginal regimens but should not be used continuously for at least more than 12 weeks, as some amount of bioaccumulation

occurs over prolonged use and safety data is not available [30].

In the setting of acute heavy menstrual bleeding, studies have only compared high-dose management strategies – there are no studies with comparisons of routine dosing. One high-dose comparison found no difference in the time to cessation of heavy bleeding between oral MPA 20 mg TID and oral combined 35 mcg EE/1 mg NET taken TID [31]. Bleeding cessation occurred by 14 days in 88% taking OCP versus 76% of MPA, with mean time to cessation 3 days in both groups ($p = 0.4$). Side effect profiles, satisfaction, and follow-up were similar in both groups, though those in the combined pill group were less likely to adhere to the treatment regimen, with approximately 20% not taking all recommended pills, likely due to side effects.

The most effective hormonal therapy for heavy menstrual bleeding currently on the market is the levonorgestrel intrauterine system (LNG-IUS). LNG-IUS is 52 mg LNG with a release rate of 20 mcg/day on a T-shaped plastic frame. Median bleeding and spotting days in the first 6 months is 18 days with irregular cycle in 20% of patients and amenorrhea by 12 months in 12% of patients [32, 33]. Several studies, including a systematic review that included five RCTs, summarize total blood loss reduction from LNG-IUS at 80–95% [34, 35].

While not studied in the acute setting, LNG-IUS is frequently utilized successfully for adolescents with chronic heavy menstrual bleeding, including those with bleeding disorders [36–39]. In randomized trials, LNG-IUS is superior treatment compared to standard dose combined and progestin-only oral hormone therapies, resulting in significantly decreased measured menstrual blood loss [35, 40–42]. Multiple medical specialty groups, including ACOG, support placement of the intrauterine device/system in adolescents at any time after menarche [43, 44]. Sedation or anxiolysis may be considered for the very young adolescent. Typically, the procedure can be accomplished without difficulty [45]. Many providers avoid penetrating cervical grasping instruments in those with suspected or confirmed bleeding disorders, favoring atraumatic instruments such as the Allis forceps. It is helpful to perform immediate ultrasound during sedation to confirm the IUS position in patients who would not otherwise tolerate a later exam.

Various cyclic progestin therapies do not demonstrate superior reduction in menstrual blood loss compared to either tranexamic acid or LNG-IUS [19, 42, 46]. Further studies are needed to compare bleeding outcomes for HMB treatment with continuously dosed progestins, lower-dose NET, subdermal implant, and comparative studies of oral progestins.

Choosing a Method

Since studies show that all hormonal therapies will aid in reducing menstrual cycle blood loss and recovery of hemoglobin, involving the adolescent in the decision-making process is a priority, as this will aid in finding a therapy the adolescent and her family is comfortable with, thereby improving compliance [47, 48].

There are many considerations a provider must take into account when choosing a method for the treatment of heavy menstrual bleeding including the patient's safety in regard to specific hormonal therapies, the patient's need for contraception, and finally the patient's tolerance for irregular breakthrough bleeding. Additionally, it is important to review the patient's medications for potential drug interactions that could result in increased breakthrough bleeding, contraceptive failure, or reduced effectiveness of the medication [49].

First, the provider must consider the patient's safety profile in regard to specific hormonal therapies. Overall, the safety and satisfaction of hormonal methods are well established for adolescents, particularly for the contraceptive methods. Much of the decision-making is relative to the risk of venous thromboembolism (VTE) with estrogen-containing hormonal therapies, though risk of other uncommon conditions in adolescents must also be considered such as risk for myocardial infarction, stroke, hypertension, and benign liver tumors [50]. The risk of venous thromboembolism in patients taking combined oral contraceptive pills is approximately twice as high as in non-users [51]. This increased risk is relative to an overall low absolute risk of venous thromboembolism. The risk of venous thromboembolism in a young healthy women rises from 1–5 per 10,000 woman-years to 3–5 per 10,000 when using a low-dose combined oral contraceptive pill, compared to the risk of VTE in pregnancy or postpartum, which is 5–20 or 40–65 per 10,000 woman-years, respectively [50, 51].

Risks are not limited to estrogen-containing medications, though progestins are overall very safe. For example, there are case reports of hepatic adenoma formation with long-term use of high-dose NETA [52].

The Centers for Disease Control and Prevention (CDC) has developed and regularly updates evidence-based guidance for contraceptive use, the US Medical Eligibility Criteria for Contraceptive Use (US MEC), that providers can reference during counseling of adolescents [17]. The four-tiered system designates the risk of specific contraceptive methods for certain patient characteristics and pre-existing medical conditions. These guidelines were developed in regard to balancing the risk of contraception with the risk of unintended pregnancy, and the risk-benefit ratio may change when considering use of these contraceptive methods for the treatment of heavy menstrual bleeding [2]. Despite this limitation, the US MEC is a useful tool when considering which hormonal therapy may be best in the treatment of heavy menstrual bleeding.

Once the provider has considered the patient's safety profile in regard to specific hormonal therapies, the provider should consider patient characteristics that will ensure selection of the ideal hormonal therapy option [53]. For example, the providers may consider if the patient also needs contraceptive benefit in addition to the treatment of heavy menstrual bleeding as different hormonal therapies have varying relative contraceptive effectiveness (Table 10.2) [54]. For example, the LNG-IUS is at least 20 times more effective for contraception than combined oral contraceptive pills with typical use [43, 55]. As 95% of the patient's final height has been achieved by menarche, the use of estrogen should not be avoided

Table 10.2 Research efficacy and user effectiveness of hormonal contraceptive methods [54]

Method	Perfect use[a]	Typical use[b]
Combination oral contraceptive pill	0.3%	9%
Norethindrone oral contraceptive pill	0.3%	9%
Contraceptive patch	0.3%	9%
Depot medroxyprogesterone acetate	0.2%	6%
Levonorgestrel 20 mcg/day intrauterine system	0.2%	0.2%
Etonogestrel contraceptive implant	0.5%	0.05%

[a]The proportion of couples who become accidentally pregnant when not stopping the method during the year and use the method of contraception in the perfect fashion

[b]The proportion of couples who become accidentally pregnant when not stopping the method during the year and use the method of contraception in the typical fashion

Table 10.3 Common myths and concerns about hormonal methods

Myth	Evidence
Hormonal methods can cause infertility	Hormonal methods do not cause infertility or significantly delay return of fertility after discontinuation of method [59]
Hormonal methods cause weight gain	No evidence exists that there is significant weight gain associated with different hormonal methods [61–63]
Hormonal methods increase the risk of breast cancer	Research studies do not support a significant risk of breast cancer with different hormonal methods during the reproductive years [60]
Hormonal methods decrease adult height	The majority of the adolescent's height is achieved by menarche and not impacted by hormonal methods [61]

in recently menarchal females due to concerns of premature closure of epiphyseal plates [3]. Likewise, there is no adverse effect on bone mineral density in adolescents with long-term use of estrogen-containing therapies [56, 57].

For adolescents, the daily dosing of oral pills can be challenging [50]. Oral contraceptive pill users can miss up to one to three doses each month [58]. It is important for providers to speak openly about the challenges of compliance with a daily regimen and evaluate whether the patient is capable of adherence [50]. Many adolescents use alarms on their personal cell phones as a technique to improve compliance with a daily pill [50].

Patient Counseling

Many patients and their families can bring preconceived notions in regard to the safety, efficacy, and side effects of hormonal therapies [50]. There are common cultural "myths" that can cause hesitance in the use of these treatments (Table 10.3). Some common "myths" that providers may encounter include that hormonal therapies cause

infertility [59], allow a buildup of menstrual blood in the body, increase risk of cancers [60], and contribute to stunted growth [61] or weight gain [50, 62, 63]. These "myths" can be counteracted by exploring the patient and her families' understanding of hormonal therapies and giving directed counseling to counteract these myths. In addition, patients and their families' religious beliefs can raise concerns when using hormonal methods for the treatment of heavy menstrual bleeding due to their corresponding contraceptive effects. Due to these preconceived notions in regard to contraceptives, a provider may choose to discuss the treatment methods as *hormonal therapies* instead of contraceptive therapies to emphasize that the intention is for the treatment of heavy menstrual bleeding versus preventing pregnancy. Effective counseling can allow shared decision-making with the provider, patient, and patient's family to select the best option for the patient's heavy menstrual bleeding.

Finally, one of the most common side effects in the first months of use of hormonal therapies is breakthrough bleeding. Typically the bleeding is light to moderate and will typically improve after about 3 months of use, so adolescents should be encouraged to wait before changing treatment method unless the breakthrough bleeding is severe and intolerable [50].

Conclusion

Overall, the available scientific literature regarding the treatment of heavy menstrual bleeding with hormonal therapies is of poor quality. There is often a lack of scientific rigor, small study sizes, short-term follow-up, and limited comparative studies for options other than IUS [48, 64]. Heavy menstrual bleeding is a common complaint with significant impact of the quality of life of patients, and further studies are needed to improve its treatment.

References

1. Wilkinson JP, Kadir RA. Management of abnormal uterine bleeding in adolescents. J Pediatr Adolesc Gynecol. 2010;23:S22–30.
2. American College of Obstetricians and Gynecologists. ACOG committee opinion no. 557: Management of acute abnormal uterine bleeding in nonpregnant reproductive-aged women. Obstet Gynecol. 2013;121:891–6.
3. Screening and management of bleeding disorders in adolescents with heavy menstrual bleeding: ACOG COMMITTEE OPINION, Number 785. Obstet Gynecol. 2019;134:e71–83.
4. Maybin JA, Critchley HO. Steroid regulation of menstrual bleeding and endometrial repair. Rev Endocr Metab Disord. 2012;13:253–63.
5. Sulak PJ, Kuehl TJ, Coffee A, Willis S. Prospective analysis of occurrence and management of breakthrough bleeding during an extended oral contraceptive regimen. Am J Obstet Gynecol. 2006;195:935–41.
6. DeVore GR, Owens O, Kase N. Use of intravenous Premarin in the treatment of dysfunctional uterine bleeding--a double-blind randomized control study. Obstet Gynecol. 1982;59:285–91.
7. Bradley LD, Gueye NA. The medical management of abnormal uterine bleeding in reproductive-aged women. Am J Obstet Gynecol. 2016;214:31–44.
8. Heinen G. Hormonal ovulation inhibition with Ovulen. Med Welt. 1964;49:2631–4.
9. Jensen JT, Garie SG, Trummer D, Elliesen J. Bleeding profile of a flexible extended regimen of ethinylestradiol/drospirenone in US women: an open-label, three-arm, active-controlled, multicenter study. Contraception. 2012;86:110–8.
10. Nakajima ST. Contemporary guide to contraception. 3rd ed. Newtown, PA: Handbooks in Health Care Co.; 2007.
11. Benson LS, Micks EA. Why stop now? Extended and continuous regimens of combined hormonal contraceptive methods. Obstet Gynecol Clin N Am. 2015;42:669–81.
12. Farquhar C, Brown J. Oral contraceptive pill for heavy menstrual bleeding. Cochrane Database Syst Rev. 2009:CD000154.
13. Fraser IS, Jensen J, Schaefers M, Mellinger U, Parke S, Serrani M. Normalization of blood loss in women with heavy menstrual bleeding treated with an oral contraceptive containing estradiol valerate/dienogest. Contraception. 2012;86:96–101.
14. Sulak PJ, Smith V, Coffee A, Witt I, Kuehl AL, Kuehl TJ. Frequency and management of breakthrough bleeding with continuous use of the transvaginal contraceptive ring: a randomized controlled trial. Obstet Gynecol. 2008;112:563–71.
15. Tepper NK, Marchbanks PA, Curtis KM. U.S. selected practice recommendations for contraceptive use, 2013. J Womens Health (Larchmt). 2014;23:108–11.
16. Stephenson J, Shawe J, Panicker S, et al. Randomized trial of the effect of tailored versus standard use of the combined oral contraceptive pill on continuation rates at 1 year. Contraception. 2013;88:523–31.
17. Curtis KM, Tepper NK, Jatlaoui TC, et al. U.S. medical eligibility criteria for contraceptive use, 2016. MMWR Recomm Rep. 2016;65:1–103.
18. Maybin JA, Critchley HO. Menstrual physiology: implications for endometrial pathology and beyond. Hum Reprod Update. 2015;21:748–61.
19. Bofill Rodriguez M, Lethaby A, Low C, Cameron IT. Cyclical progestogens for heavy menstrual bleeding. Cochrane Database Syst Rev. 2019;8:CD001016.
20. Huguelet PS, Buyers EM, Lange-Liss JH, Scott SM. Treatment of acute abnormal uterine bleeding in adolescents: what are providers doing in various specialties? J Pediatr Adolesc Gynecol. 2016;29:286–91.
21. Alaqzam TS, Stanley AC, Simpson PM, Flood VH, Menon S. Treatment modalities in adolescents who present with heavy menstrual bleeding. J Pediatr Adolesc Gynecol. 2018;31:451–8.
22. Kuhnz W, Heuner A, Humpel M, Seifert W, Michaelis K. In vivo conversion of norethisterone and norethisterone acetate to ethinyl estradiol in postmenopausal women. Contraception. 1997;56:379–85.
23. Kuhl H. Pharmacology of estrogens and progestogens: influence of different routes of administration. Climacteric. 2005;8(Suppl 1):3–63.
24. Aksu F, Madazli R, Budak E, Cepni I, Benian A. High-dose medroxyprogesterone acetate for the treatment of dysfunctional uterine bleeding in 24 adolescents. Aust N Z J Obstet Gynaecol. 1997;37:228–31.
25. Saarikoski S, Yliskoski M, Penttila I. Sequential use of norethisterone and natural progesterone in pre-menopausal bleeding disorders. Maturitas. 1990;12:89–97.
26. Santos M, Hendry D, Sangi-Haghpeykar H, Dietrich JE. Retrospective review of norethindrone use in adolescents. J Pediatr Adolesc Gynecol. 2014;27:41–4.
27. Zigler RE, McNicholas C. Unscheduled vaginal bleeding with progestin-only contraceptive use. Am J Obstet Gynecol. 2017;216:443–50.
28. Dahiya P, Dalal M, Yadav A, Dahiya K, Jain S, Silan V. Efficacy of combined hormonal vaginal ring in

comparison to combined hormonal pills in heavy menstrual bleeding. Eur J Obstet Gynecol Reprod Biol. 2016;203:147–51.

29. Terrell LR, Tanner AE, Hensel DJ, Blythe MJ, Fortenberry JD. Acceptability of the vaginal contraceptive ring among adolescent women. J Pediatr Adolesc Gynecol. 2011;24:204–10.

30. Lavelanet AF, Rybin D, White KO. The pharmacokinetics of 12-week continuous contraceptive patch use. Contraception. 2017;95:578–85.

31. Munro MG, Mainor N, Basu R, Brisinger M, Barreda L. Oral medroxyprogesterone acetate and combination oral contraceptives for acute uterine bleeding: a randomized controlled trial. Obstet Gynecol. 2006;108:924–9.

32. Nilsson CG, Luukkainen T, Diaz J, Allonen H. Clinical performance of a new levonorgestrel-releasing intrauterine device. A randomized comparison with a nova-T-copper device. Contraception. 1982;25:345–56.

33. Lethaby AE, Cooke I, Rees M. Progesterone or progestogen-releasing intrauterine systems for heavy menstrual bleeding. Cochrane Database Syst Rev. 2005.CD002126.

34. Stewart A, Cummins C, Gold L, Jordan R, Phillips W. The effectiveness of the levonorgestrel-releasing intrauterine system in menorrhagia: a systematic review. BJOG. 2001;108:74–86.

35. Kaunitz AM, Bissonnette F, Monteiro I, Lukkari-Lax E, Muysers C, Jensen JT. Levonorgestrel-releasing intrauterine system or medroxyprogesterone for heavy menstrual bleeding: a randomized controlled trial. Obstet Gynecol. 2010;116:625–32.

36. Kingman CE, Kadir RA, Lee CA, Economides DL. The use of levonorgestrel-releasing intrauterine system for treatment of menorrhagia in women with inherited bleeding disorders. BJOG. 2004;111:1425–8.

37. Schaedel ZE, Dolan G, Powell MC. The use of the levonorgestrel-releasing intrauterine system in the management of menorrhagia in women with hemostatic disorders. Am J Obstet Gynecol. 2005;193:1361–3.

38. Chi C, Huq FY, Kadir RA. Levonorgestrel-releasing intrauterine system for the management of heavy menstrual bleeding in women with inherited bleeding disorders: long-term follow-up. Contraception. 2011;83:242–7.

39. Adeyemi-Fowode OA, Santos XM, Dietrich JE, Srivaths L. Levonorgestrel-releasing intrauterine device use in female adolescents with heavy menstrual bleeding and bleeding disorders: single institution review. J Pediatr Adolesc Gynecol. 2017;30:479–83.

40. Shaaban MM, Zakherah MS, El-Nashar SA, Sayed GH. Levonorgestrel-releasing intrauterine system compared to low dose combined oral contraceptive pills for idiopathic menorrhagia: a randomized clinical trial. Contraception. 2011;83:48–54.

41. Endrikat J, Shapiro H, Lukkari-Lax E, Kunz M, Schmidt W, Fortier M. A Canadian, multicentre study comparing the efficacy of a levonorgestrel-releasing intrauterine system to an oral contraceptive in women with idiopathic menorrhagia. J Obstet Gynaecol Can. 2009;31:340–7.

42. Irvine GA, Campbell-Brown MB, Lumsden MA, Heikkila A, Walker JJ, Cameron IT. Randomised comparative trial of the levonorgestrel intrauterine system and norethisterone for treatment of idiopathic menorrhagia. Br J Obstet Gynaecol. 1998;105:592–8.

43. American College of Obstetricians and Gynecologists. ACOG Committee Opinion No. 392, December 2007. Intrauterine device and adolescents. Obstet Gynecol. 2007;110:1493–5.

44. Haamid F, Sass AE, Dietrich JE. Heavy menstrual bleeding in adolescents. J Pediatr Adolesc Gynecol. 2017;30:335–40.

45. Hillard PJ. Practical tips for intrauterine devices use in adolescents. J Adolesc Health. 2013;52:S40–6.

46. Kiseli M, Kayikcioglu F, Evliyaoglu O, Haberal A. Comparison of therapeutic efficacies of Norethisterone, tranexamic acid and Levonorgestrel-releasing intrauterine system for the treatment of heavy menstrual bleeding: a randomized controlled study. Gynecol Obstet Investig. 2016;81:447–53.

47. Matteson KA, Zaluski KM. Menstrual health as a part of preventive health care. Obstet Gynecol Clin N Am. 2019;46:441–53.

48. Uhm S, Perriera L. Hormonal contraception as treatment for heavy menstrual bleeding: a systematic review. Clin Obstet Gynecol. 2014;57:694–717.

49. Centers for Disease C, Prevention. US Medical eligibility criteria for contraceptive use, 2010. MMWR Recomm Rep. 2010;59:1–86.

50. Powell A. Choosing the right oral contraceptive pill for teens. Pediatr Clin N Am. 2017;64:343–58.

51. Practice Committee of the American Society for Reproductive Medicine, Electronic address Aao, Practice Committee of the American Society for Reproductive M. Combined hormonal contraception and the risk of venous thromboembolism: a guideline. Fertil Steril. 2017;107:43–51.

52. Brady PC, Missmer SA, Laufer MR. Hepatic adenomas in adolescents and young women with endometriosis treated with Norethindrone acetate. J Pediatr Adolesc Gynecol. 2017;30:422–4.

53. Matteson KA, Rahn DD, Wheeler TL 2nd, et al. Nonsurgical management of heavy menstrual bleeding: a systematic review. Obstet Gynecol. 2013;121:632–43.

54. Trussell J. Contraceptive failure in the United States. Contraception. 2011;83:397–404.

55. Winner B, Peipert JF, Zhao Q, et al. Effectiveness of long-acting reversible contraception. N Engl J Med. 2012;366:1998–2007.

56. Gersten J, Hsieh J, Weiss H, Ricciotti NA. Effect of extended 30 mug Ethinyl estradiol with continuous Low-dose Ethinyl estradiol and cyclic 20 mug Ethinyl estradiol oral contraception on adolescent bone density: a randomized trial. J Pediatr Adolesc Gynecol. 2016;29:635–42.

57. Jackowski SA, Baxter-Jones ADG, McLardy AJ, Pierson RA, Rodgers CD. The associations of exposure to combined hormonal contraceptive use on bone mineral content and areal bone mineral density accrual from adolescence to young adulthood: a longitudinal study. Bone Rep. 2016;5:e333–e41.
58. Chabbert-Buffet N, Jamin C, Lete I, et al. Missed pills: frequency, reasons, consequences and solutions. Eur J Contracept Reprod Health Care. 2017;22:165–9.
59. Girum T, Wasie A. Return of fertility after discontinuation of contraception: a systematic review and meta-analysis. Contracept Reprod Med. 2018;3:9.
60. Schneyer R, Lerma K. Health outcomes associated with use of hormonal contraception: breast cancer. Curr Opin Obstet Gynecol. 2018;30:414–8.
61. Beksinska ME, Smit JA, Kleinschmidt I, Milford C, Farley TM. Prospective study of weight change in new adolescent users of DMPA, NET-EN, COCs, nonusers and discontinuers of hormonal contraception. Contraception. 2010;81:30–4.
62. Gallo MF, Lopez LM, Grimes DA, Carayon F, Schulz KF, Helmerhorst FM. Combination contraceptives: effects on weight. Cochrane Database Syst Rev. 2014:CD003987.
63. Lopez LM, Ramesh S, Chen M, et al. Progestin-only contraceptives: effects on weight. Cochrane Database Syst Rev. 2016:CD008815.
64. Bitzer J, Heikinheimo O, Nelson AL, Calaf-Alsina J, Fraser IS. Medical management of heavy menstrual bleeding: a comprehensive review of the literature. Obstet Gynecol Surv. 2015;70:115–30.

Sanjay P. Ahuja, Michael Recht, and Barbara Konkle

Introduction

The medical management of heavy menstrual bleeding (HMB) in adolescent women is geared toward improving symptoms and maintaining quality of life. Unlike older adults, management of HMB in teens is not dependent on decisions around fertility preservation or considerations of pelvic pathologies as these are uncommon in the adolescent age group. Uncovering an underlying bleeding disorder is, however, a prerequisite in choosing an appropriate therapy in adolescents.

The American College of Obstetricians and Gynecologists' Committee on Adolescent Health Care recommended medical management as the first-line approach to HMB in adolescents [1]. Medical management of HMB includes hormonal combination contraceptive therapy and non-hormonal hemostatic therapies. In this chapter, non-hormonal hemostatic therapies are discussed, including anti-fibrinolytics, desmopressin, coagulation factor replacements, transfusion of blood products, and ancillary therapies such as NSAIDs (Table 11.1).

Anti-fibrinolytics

The fibrinolytic system is overly activated during the menstrual phase of the menstrual cycle in women with HMB [2]. There is evidence of increased fibrinolytic activity in menstrual fluid of those with HMB [3]. Hence, the fibrin clot that is formed to induce hemostasis during menstrual bleeding is quickly degraded leading to excessive bleeding. Inhibition of the fibrinolytic system, therefore, is an attractive medical treatment option for women and girls with HMB.

Anti-fibrinolytics are a class of medications that are inhibitors of fibrinolysis. These lysine-like drugs interfere with the formation of the fibrinolytic enzyme plasmin from its precursor plasminogen in a competitive fashion. Anti-fibrinolytics have been available as treatment for HMB outside the United States, for almost three decades. They have established efficacy in reducing menstrual blood loss (MBL) in adult women with HMB. However, limited data is available for young woman under the age of 18 years. Two choices for anti-fibrinolytics are available and approved by the US Food and Drug Administration, namely, epsilon aminocaproic

S. P. Ahuja
UH Rainbow Hemostasis & Thrombosis Center, Rainbow Babies & Children's Hospital & Case Western Reserve University, Cleveland, OH, USA

M. Recht
The Hemophilia Center at Oregon Health & Science University and American Thrombosis and Hemostasis Network, Orgeon, OR, USA

B. Konkle (✉)
Bloodworks Northwest and Department of Medicine, University of Washington, Seattle, WA, USA
e-mail: BarbaraK@BloodWorksNW.org

Table 11.1 Hemostatic therapies for HMB

Intervention	Dose	Schedule	Special considerations	References
Anti-fibrinolytics	Tranexamic acid, 1300 mg EACA, 50–100 mg/kg/dose	Three times a day for 5–7 days Every 6 hours for 5–7 days	May need to be combined with oral contraceptive therapy in bleeding disorders	[4, 5, 7, 9]
Desmopressin	Intravenous, 0.3 mcg/kg Stimate nasal spray, 1 puff <50 kg; 2 puffs >50 kg	Use once a day on days 2 and 3 of menstrual bleeding	Tachyphylaxis with more than 3–4 doses at 24-hour intervals; fluid restriction recommended	[18, 19, 21, 23]
Coagulation factor replacement	Dose as would be for other bleeding	Reports of efficacy with 1–3 days of daily treatment	Data from HMB-specific study not available rFVIIa with regulatory approval for GT	[24–32, 34, 35, 49]
Transfusions				
Platelets	HLA matched platelets; 2 single donor units usually provide >20 K functional platelets	Repeat as needed	Use only if other therapies are not effective in acute setting For GT and BSS, monitor pre-transfusion for anti-platelet receptor antibodies	[37, 38, 49]
FFP/cryoprecipitate	FFP (1 U/mL), dose to achieve level >0.2–0.3 IU/dL; cryoprecipitate 2 units/10 kg increases fibrinogen by 100 mg/dL	Repeat as needed considering factor half-life and bleeding control	Use for FV deficiency or in emergencies when virally inactivated concentrates are not available; cryoprecipitate contains >80 I.U./dL of FVIII/VWF	[39, 60]
NSAIDs	Mefenamic acid 500 mg once then 250 mg	Every 6 hours not to exceed 3 days	May be contraindicated in those with congenital or acquired bleeding disorders	[56]
	Ibuprofen 800 mg	Every 6 hours not to exceed 3 days		
	Naproxen 440 mg	Every 12 hours not to exceed 3 days		

EACA epsilon aminocaproic acid, *GT* Glanzmann thrombasthenia *BSS* Bernard-Soulier syndrome

acid and tranexamic acid (TXA). For use in HMB, most of the experience and available data is with TXA.

TXA has been shown to significantly reduce MBL in women with HMB. However, it does not reduce the length of the menstrual cycle nor does it regulate the cycle. By preventing plasmin and lysine residues from interacting, TXA reduces fibrin degradation, thereby slowing the dissolution of clots.

The reduction of MBL has ranged from 34% to 56% in adult women with HMB treated with >3 grams daily of TXA for 5 days [4]. A new oral formulation of TXA with shortened absorption time (Lysteda®) was approved by the US Food and Drug Administration in 2009 for women >18 years of age with cyclic HMB. In a pharmacokinetic study performed by the drugmaker, a dose of 3900 milligrams per day was found to be appropriate in the adolescent age group. This newer formulation was evaluated in a prospective open-label clinical study in adolescents ranging in age from 11 to 18 years [5]. A majority of the 25 subjects enrolled in the study noted significant improvement in MBL as measured by the Menorrhagia Impact Questionnaire (MIQ) and the PBAC score. TXA has also been compared to intranasal desmopressin [6], mefenamic acid [7], and placebo [8] in studies with adult women and demonstrated superior reduction in MBL in all instances. For the adolescent population, a prospective randomized crossover study [9] comparing tranexamic acid with oral contraceptives showed no difference between the two agents in terms of MBL, but only oral contraceptives shortened the length of the menstrual cycle. Commonly reported adverse events in studies have been nausea, vomiting, menstrual cramps, and headache, some of which can be attributed to the menstrual cycle itself. Although there is a theoretical risk of TXA increasing the risk of VTE, no population-based study has concluded thus. The US label recommends against combining TXA and hormonal contraceptives containing estrogen, but this is not based on data. In some patients combined treatment may be needed to control HMB. If an increased risk of thrombosis exists, it should still be very low in adolescents who overall are at low baseline risk based on age.

Even though oral contraceptive pills are first-line therapeutic option for medical management of HMB, TXA is a reasonable hemostatic alternative in adolescents with multiple barriers to the use of oral contraceptives, such as concerns of side effects, difficulties with compliance, hesitancy to commit to a daily medication, and religious or cultural hesitancy from parents with the use of birth control pills in teenagers (Table 11.1).

Desmopressin Therapy

Desmopressin or DDAVP (1-deamino-8-D-arginine vasopressin) is a synthetic vasopressin analogue that works by enhancing endogenous levels of von Willebrand factor (VWF) and factor VIII (FVIII) [10]. The increases in the plasma levels of factor VIII and VWF occur not only in defi-

cient individuals but also in individuals with normal baseline levels as well as in those who already have high levels of these factors. Desmopressin also enhances platelet adhesion to the vessel wall but has no effect on platelet count or aggregation [11]. Even though in vitro and in vivo studies have not proven a direct stimulatory effect of desmopressin on platelets, desmopressin shortens or normalizes the bleeding time in congenital platelet function defects [12]. There is usually a good response in patients with defects of platelet release function. Most patients with storage pool defects respond to desmopressin, though some do not [13]. Desmopressin also shortens the activated partial thromboplastin time and bleeding time due to unexplained causes [10]. Hence, desmopressin is indicated to treat bleeding, including HMB in hemophilia A, von Willebrand disease (VWD), and some congenital platelet function defects. As the response to desmopressin is variable among patients, a test dose is usually required to assess efficacy prior to initiating treatment.

Among adolescents and women presenting with HMB, a bleeding disorder such as VWD, congenital platelet defects, or coagulation factor deficiencies, including hemophilia, is diagnosed in up to 20% of patients, especially those with symptomatic onset at menarche and a positive family history [14–16]. Desmopressin, therefore, is a useful upfront hemostatic therapy to reduce MBL in teens and girls with a bleeding disorder presenting with HMB. However, since it corrects the unexplained prolonged aPTT and bleeding time, it can also be used in girls with HMB and prolonged aPTT without a diagnosis of a bleeding disorder [17]. It can be administered easily as a nasal spray and has shown to significantly reduce Pictorial Blood Assessment Chart (PBAC) scores [6]. The nasal spray can be administered once a day on day 2 and 3 of the menstrual bleeding (Table 11.1), keeping in mind that repeated doses may render the drug unresponsive, because the stores of VWF and FVIII are depleted [18]. The average response of FVIII drops by 30% after repeat of three to four doses of desmopressin at 24-hour intervals, as compared to the first-dose response.

Combined use of desmopressin with TXA is more effective (PBAC scores) than desmopressin alone [19]. However, as already mentioned above, when desmopressin was compared to TXA in a crossover design, TXA proved to be more effective in reduction of PBAC scores [6]. In intrauterine device (IUD)-related HMB in adults, desmopressin has been shown to be superior to mefenamic acid in reducing MBL as measured by the PBAC score [20]. A number of adverse reactions have been described with desmopressin, sometimes leading to discontinuation of the medication in up to 20% of patients [21]. Reported side effects include hyponatremia and occasionally seizures, smooth muscle cramps, vasoconstriction, and allergic reactions. As hyponatremia is a result of the anti-diuretic effect of desmopressin, fluid restriction to a maximum of maintenance total fluids over the course of 24 hours is recommended for patients, especially if multiple doses are administered over multiple days [22, 23].

Coagulation Factor Replacement

Adolescent girls and women with coagulation factor deficiencies infrequently require factor replacement therapy for HMB. Symptoms usually respond to hormonal, anti-fibrinolytic, or, if appropriate, desmopressin therapy. However, some girls and women will fail or not tolerate these therapies, and coagulation factor replacement is required (Table 11.1). This is particularly true in severe deficiencies associated with mucocutaneous bleeding such as VWD and factor VII (FVII) or factor X (FX) deficiency.

There are no published clinical trial results of factor replacement therapy in HMB, although one in VWD is underway. This is comparing recombinant VWF (rVWF) with TXA in a prospective, randomized crossover trial (VWDMin, NCT02606045). In preparation for this trial, a survey of US HTCs found that the use of VWF replacement for HMB was considered third-line therapy and was used in 13 of 816 women reported with VWD and HMB who had failed other therapies [24]. Use of plasma-derived or rVWF concentrates to treat HMB has been reported in a total of 101 women and adolescent girls as part of observational and non-randomized treatment studies of VWD [24–30]. In those reports, dosing ranged from 33 to 100 I.U./kg for 1–6 days with good results and an acceptable safety profile.

Use of factor concentrates in other inherited bleeding disorders has been reported. Adolescent girls and women with either FX or FVII deficiency can have symptoms of both mucosal and joint and muscle bleeding. A systematic review of women with FX deficiency identified 332 women, 25% of whom reported HMB [31]. Sixty-four percent of these women required blood products for treatment including fresh frozen plasma (FFP), prothrombin complex concentrates, and a plasma-derived factor X (pdFX) concentrate. The more recently available pdFX concentrate was effective in treating HMB in women with inherited FX deficiency of <0.05 I.U./dL with one to three doses at a mean dose of 24.3 I.U./kg, similar to dosing for other bleeding events [32]. This approach is now preferred for women with FX deficiency requiring replacement therapy.

While HMB is a common symptom in girls and women with FVII deficiency [33], use of rFVIIa for treatment is not common [34, 35]. In a series of ten women with FVII deficiency and HMB treated with rFVIIa, median treatment days and doses were one and two, respectively, with dosing widely varied [35]. In women with FVII deficiency and HMB unresponsive to other therapies, treatment with rFVIIa at doses (10–30 mcg/kg) used to treat other bleeding in FVII deficiency is recommended [34, 36]. rFVIIa is approved for treatment and prevention of bleeding in the autosomal recessive platelet disorder Glanzmann thrombasthenia (GT), and case reports document its use in other platelet disorders [37]. rFVIIa has not specifically been studied in HMB but, however, in the GT registry HMB was common (63/613 with moderate bleeding and 27/216 with severe bleeding), and rFVIIa overall had efficacy of 80–100% with or without co-administered anti-fibrinolytic or platelet therapy [38].

HMB is common in FXI deficiency [39]; however use of FXI concentrate for treatment has not been reported. This is likely due to the efficacy of anti-fibrinolytic therapy in FXI deficiency, as well as the limited availability of concentrates and their associated thrombotic risk.

Overall, genetic carriers of FVIII or FIX deficiency report HMB more commonly than the general population [40]. However, in a report of 15 women with moderate or severe hemophilia A or B in whom menstrual data was available, only 3/7 women with moderate hemophilia and none of the 8 women with severe hemophilia reported symptoms of heavy menses [41]. This suggests that there may be contributors to the volume of menstrual bleeding in addition to a low factor level in women with hemophilia. Other rare bleeding disorders have been reported to manifest HMB in affected girls and women [39, 42]. If specific data for treatment of HMB do not exist and the patient is not responsive or intolerant of other therapies, treatment approaches with factor replacement as used for other bleeding events should be used. In addition, there are no data to support an increased risk of thrombosis with combination therapy, such as hormonal therapy or anti-fibrinolytic therapy with replacement therapy, and a combined approach may be more effective.

Although extremely rare, severe factor V (FV) deficiency can lead to HMB. Inherited recessively, common symptoms of FV deficiency include epistaxis, easy bruising, and mucosal bleeding including HMB [43]. At this time, there is no FV concentrate available commercially. Fresh frozen plasma is the usual treatment. Interestingly, as platelets are a rich source of FV, platelet transfusions can also be used to treat or prevent bleeding in those affected by FV deficiency [44].

Factor XIII (FXIII) is also inherited in an autosomal recessive manner. Both males and females have bleeding symptoms. In addition to other bleeding symptoms, females can have HMB. Also, recurrent miscarriage is a common feature for females with severe FXIII deficiency [45]. For those with FXIII deficiency and HMB, treatment options include either plasma-derived or recombinant FXIII concentrate, cryoprecipitate, or fresh frozen plasma. Anti-fibrinolytics play an important role in controlling HMB associated with FXIII deficiency [46].

Role of Transfusion Therapy (Red Blood Cell (RBC), Platelet, FFP, Cryoprecipitate, and Others)

The most common uses of transfusion therapy [RBC, platelet, FFP, cryoprecipitate] in HMB are in treatment of acute bleeding and in specific treatment for inherited platelet disorders. Transfusion therapy is most commonly used for HMB to treat acute symptomatic anemia associated with bleeding (Table 11.1). In a study of adolescents presenting to the emergency department with HMB and symptomatic iron deficiency, 43% received RBC transfusions [47]. A comparison of factor concentrate and blood product use in adolescents versus adult women with bleeding disorders did not find a difference between the two groups [48]. While FFP and cryoprecipitate have been used to treat HMB, with increasing availability of specific virally inactivated plasma-derived or recombinant concentrates available for home use (VWF, FVIII, FIX, FX, FVIIa, FXIII, fibrinogen, PCCs), these should be made available for treatment if needed, and patients and families should be trained in self-administration to allow prompt and cost-effective treatment. In emergency situations where factor concentrates are not available, cryoprecipitate can be used for VWF, FVIII, FXIII, and fibrinogen replacement and FFP for other factor deficiencies.

Adolescent girls and women with inherited platelet disorders may require platelet transfusion for HMB if other therapies have failed. This is most likely in the severe autosomal recessive disorders Bernard-Soulier syndrome (BSS) and GT [49]. However, in non-emergency settings, patients with these disorders should receive as first- and second-line therapy other treatment approaches including hormonal therapy and/or anti-fibrinolytic therapy. Platelet transfusion is associated with a significant risk of alloimmunization and the development of platelet receptor-specific antibodies, overall reported to occur in 25–70% of transfused patients with GT [50, 51]. For this reason, platelet transfusion should be confined to use for acute menstrual bleeding with symptomatic anemia or prior to procedures, if needed. Patients with these disorders should be HLA typed so that leukocyte-depleted HLA-matched platelets can be given to reduce the risk of alloimmunization. Patients should be monitored periodically for the development of antibodies [37]. It would be prudent to HLA type pre-menarchal girls who have not previously been transfused in anticipation of heavy bleeding requiring transfusion with menarche. rFVIIa has been shown to be effective in treatment of GT, as noted above, and is an option to avoid antibody formation and to treat individuals who have already developed antibodies, particularly in patients with platelet receptor antibodies [37].

Nonsteroidal Anti-inflammatory Drugs (NSAIDs)

A rationale for the use of NSAIDs to ameliorate excessive blood loss in menstruating adolescents is supported by an accumulation of data suggesting a role for prostaglandins in the pathogenesis of HMB [52, 53]. When compared to women without HMB, the endometrium in women with HMB has been found to contain higher levels of prostaglandin E2 and prostaglandin F2α [54]. However, the exact mechanism by which the excessive blood loss occurs remains speculative. By inhibiting cyclooxygenase, NSAIDs reduce prostaglandin levels [55]. However, because drugs in this class inhibit cyclooxygenase and cyclooxygenase is required for adequate platelet function, NSAIDs have historically not been used to treat HMB in women with congenital bleeding disorders. That said, this class of medication has been demonstrated to effectively treat dysmenorrhea. A wide variety of NSAIDs, including mefenamic acid (MFA), naproxen, ibuprofen, flurbiprofen, meclofenamic acid, diclofenac, indomethacin, and acetylsalicylic acid, have been studied for this purpose (Table 11.1).

In a meta-analysis of all published studies in women without diagnosed bleeding disorders, looking at the effect of NSAIDs on HMB [56], the following could be concluded:

1. NSAIDs significantly reduced menstrual blood loss but not the number of days with menstrual bleeding compared to placebo.
2. Women's perception of "relief" from the symptoms of HMB was significantly improved in those treated with NSAIDs compared to placebo.
3. Women treated with NSAIDs had more menstrual blood loss than those treated with TXA without any effect on the number of days of menstrual bleeding.
4. There were no significant differences in reduction in menstrual blood loss in women taking NSAIDs compared to ethamsylate, oral progestogen given during the luteal phase, progesterone-releasing intrauterine devices, and oral contraception pills.
5. There was no suggestion of a differential efficacy between the different NSAIDs used across trials. In addition, there was no evidence of a difference in the safety profiles of any of the NSAIDs.

Based on the above meta-analysis, there is limited evidence for the efficacy of NSAIDs as a first-line treatment for reducing HMB in women. Other medical treatments appear to be equally effective as NSAIDs without the gastrointestinal and potential bleeding side effects. Although average menstrual blood loss is decreased in many of the trials reviewed, a significant proportion of women enrolled on the NSAID arms of the trials still had objective HMB after treatment. In addition, NSAIDs have not been studied in adolescents and women with inherited bleeding disorders and HMB.

Summary

Assessment of menstrual health is a key component of well-women and adolescent care [8]. Asking questions about the frequency, duration, regularity, and volume of menstrual bleeding will help identify individuals who experience HMB. In an online survey of over 42,000 unselected women, HMB was reported by over half of the respondents [57]. Almost 40% of the women surveyed were less active during their menses. In addition, in women with HMB, lost productivity has been estimated to exceed $2000 per person per year owing to work absence [58]. School absenteeism has been estimated to be between 10% and 60% in adolescents with HMB, with over 25% missing social activities [59]. As ~20% of young women presenting with HMB have an underlying congenital bleeding disorder, a thorough bleeding history, physical exam, and laboratory evaluation are recommended. Therapeutic options for the medical management of HMB in adolescent women has expanded greatly over the past several years. While combination birth control pills remain the first-line therapy for the vast majority of young women with congenital bleeding disorders and HMB, various second-line therapies have been demonstrated to be equally effective with a similar safety profile. Combining modalities (e.g., combination birth control pills with TXA) has also been demonstrated to be safe and effective. The choice of medical management of HMB in young women with congenital bleeding disorders will depend on a variety of factors and will be determined after discussion between the provider, the patient, and, potentially, the patient's family.

References

1. Screening and management of bleeding disorders in adolescents with heavy menstrual bleeding: ACOG Committee Opinion, number 785. Obstet Gynecol. 2019;134(3): e71–e83.
2. Gleeson N, et al. Endometrial fibrinolytic enzymes in women with normal menstruation and dysfunctional uterine bleeding. Br J Obstet Gynaecol. 1993;100(8):768–71.
3. Gleeson NC, et al. The effect of tranexamic acid on measured menstrual loss and endometrial fibrinolytic enzymes in dysfunctional uterine bleeding. Acta Obstet Gynecol Scand. 1994;73(3):274–7.
4. Bitzer J, et al. Medical management of heavy menstrual bleeding: a comprehensive review of the literature. Obstet Gynecol Surv. 2015;70(2):115–30.
5. O'Brien SH, et al. An open-label, single-arm, efficacy study of tranexamic acid in adolescents with heavy menstrual bleeding. J Pediatr Adolesc Gynecol. 2019;32(3):305–11.
6. Kouides PA, et al. Multisite management study of menorrhagia with abnormal laboratory haemostasis: a prospective crossover study of intranasal desmopressin and oral tranexamic acid. Br J Haematol. 2009;145(2):212–20.
7. Bonnar J, Sheppard BL. Treatment of menorrhagia during menstruation: randomised controlled trial of ethamsylate, mefenamic acid, and tranexamic acid. BMJ. 1996;313(7057):579–82.
8. Matteson KA, et al. Nonsurgical management of heavy menstrual bleeding: a systematic review. Obstet Gynecol. 2013;121(3):632–43.
9. Srivaths LV, et al. Oral tranexamic acid versus combined oral contraceptives for adolescent heavy menstrual bleeding: a pilot study. J Pediatr Adolesc Gynecol. 2015;28(4):254–7.
10. Mannucci PM. Desmopressin (DDAVP) in the treatment of bleeding disorders: the first 20 years. Blood. 1997;90(7):2515–21.
11. Sakariassen KS, et al. DDAVP enhances platelet adherence and platelet aggregate growth on human artery subendothelium. Blood. 1984;64(1):229–36.
12. DiMichele DM, Hathaway WE. Use of DDAVP in inherited and acquired platelet dysfunction. Am J Hematol. 1990;33(1):39–45.
13. Rao AK, et al. Mechanisms of platelet dysfunction and response to DDAVP in patients with congenital platelet function defects. A double-blind placebo-controlled trial. Thromb Haemost. 1995;74(4):1071–8.
14. Dilley A, et al. von Willebrand disease and other inherited bleeding disorders in women with diagnosed menorrhagia. Obstet Gynecol. 2001;97(4):630–6.
15. Kadir RA, et al. Frequency of inherited bleeding disorders in women with menorrhagia. Lancet. 1998;351(9101):485–9.
16. Philipp CS, et al. Platelet functional defects in women with unexplained menorrhagia. J Thromb Haemost. 2003;1(3):477–84.
17. Edlund M, Blomback M, Fried G. Desmopressin in the treatment of menorrhagia in women with no common coagulation factor deficiency but with prolonged bleeding time. Blood Coagul Fibrinolysis. 2002;13(3):225–31.
18. Mannucci PM, Bettega D, Cattaneo M. Patterns of development of tachyphylaxis in patients with haemophilia and von Willebrand disease after repeated doses of desmopressin (DDAVP). Br J Haematol. 1992;82(1):87–93.
19. Miller CH, et al. Changes in von Willebrand factor and factor VIII levels during the menstrual cycle. Thromb Haemost. 2002;87(6):1082–3.
20. Mercorio F, et al. Effectiveness and mechanism of action of desmopressin in the treatment of copper intrauterine device-related menorrhagia: a pilot study. Hum Reprod. 2003;18(11):2319–22.

21. Dunn AL, et al. Adverse events during use of intranasal desmopressin acetate for haemophilia a and von Willebrand disease: a case report and review of 40 patients. Haemophilia. 2000;6(1):11–4.
22. Mason JA, et al. Assessment and validation of a defined fluid restriction protocol in the use of subcutaneous desmopressin for children with inherited bleeding disorders. Haemophilia. 2016;22(5):700–5.
23. Federici AB. The use of desmopressin in von Willebrand disease: the experience of the first 30 years (1977–2007). Haemophilia. 2008;14(Suppl 1):5–14.
24. Ragni MV, et al. Von Willebrand factor for menorrhagia: a survey and literature review. Haemophilia. 2016;22(3):397–402.
25. Gill JC, et al. Hemostatic efficacy, safety, and pharmacokinetics of a recombinant von Willebrand factor in severe von Willebrand disease. Blood. 2015;126(17):2038–46.
26. Abshire TC, et al. Prophylaxis in severe forms of von Willebrand's disease: results from the von Willebrand Disease Prophylaxis Network (VWD PN). Haemophilia. 2013;19(1):76–81.
27. Batty P, et al. Safety and efficacy of a von Willebrand factor/factor VIII concentrate (Wilate (R)): a single centre experience. Haemophilia. 2014;20(6):846–53.
28. Berntorp E, Windyga J, European Wilate Study Group. Study, Treatment and prevention of acute bleedings in von Willebrand disease – efficacy and safety of Wilate((R)), a new generation von Willebrand factor/factor VIII concentrate. Haemophilia. 2009;15(1):122–30.
29. Holm E, et al. Changes in bleeding patterns in von Willebrand disease after institution of long-term replacement therapy: results from the von Willebrand Disease Prophylaxis Network. Blood Coagul Fibrinolysis. 2015;26(4):383–8.
30. Miesbach W, et al. Clinical use of Haemate (R) P in von Willebrand disease: a 25-year retrospective observational study. Thromb Res. 2015;135(3):479–84.
31. Spiliopoulos D, Kadir RA. Congenital factor X deficiency in women: a systematic review of the literature. Haemophilia. 2019;25(2):195–204.
32. Kulkarni R, et al. Efficacy, safety and pharmacokinetics of a new high-purity factor X concentrate in women and girls with hereditary factor X deficiency. J Thromb Haemost. 2018;16(5):849–57.
33. Kulkarni A, et al. Disorders of menstruation and their effect on the quality of life in women with congenital factor VII deficiency. Haemophilia. 2006;12(3):248–52.
34. Mariani G, Konkle BA, Ingerslev J. Congenital factor VII deficiency: therapy with recombinant activated factor VII – a critical appraisal. Haemophilia. 2006;12(1):19–27.
35. Napolitano M, et al. Women with congenital factor VII deficiency: clinical phenotype and treatment options from two international studies. Haemophilia. 2016;22(5):752–9.
36. Mariani G, et al. Recombinant, activated factor VII for surgery in factor VII deficiency: a prospective evaluation – the surgical STER. Br J Haematol. 2011;152(3):340–6.
37. Lee A, Poon MC. Inherited platelet functional disorders: general principles and practical aspects of management. Transfus Apher Sci. 2018;57(4):494–501.
38. Di Minno G, et al. The international, prospective Glanzmann Thrombasthenia registry: treatment modalities and outcomes of non-surgical bleeding episodes in patients with Glanzmann thrombasthenia. Haematologica. 2015;100(8):1031–7.
39. Peyvandi F, Garagiola I, Menegatti M. Gynecological and obstetrical manifestations of inherited bleeding disorders in women. J Thromb Haemost. 2011;9(1 S):236–45.
40. Kadir RA, et al. Assessment of menstrual blood loss and gynaecological problems in patients with inherited bleeding disorders. Haemophilia. 1999;5(1):40–8.
41. DiMichele DM, et al. Females with severe or moderate hemophilia A or B: a US study. Blood. 2007;110(11):639A.
42. Acharya SS, Coughlin A, Dimichele DM. Rare Bleeding Disorder Registry: deficiencies of factors II, V, VII, X, XIII, fibrinogen and dysfibrinogenemias. J Thromb Haemost. 2004;2(2):248–56.
43. Asselta R, Peyvandi F. Factor V deficiency. Semin Thromb Hemost. 2009;35(4):382–9.
44. Stalnaker M, Esquivel P. Managing menorrhagia in a familial case of factor V deficiency. J Pediatr Adolesc Gynecol. 2015;28(1):e9–e12.
45. Odame JE, et al. Factor XIII deficiency management: a review of the literature. Blood Coagul Fibrinolysis. 2014;25(3):199–205.
46. Sharief LA, Kadir RA. Congenital factor XIII deficiency in women: a systematic review of literature. Haemophilia. 2013;19(6):e349–57.
47. Cooke AG, et al. Iron deficiency Anemia in adolescents who present with heavy menstrual bleeding. J Pediatr Adolesc Gynecol. 2017;30(2):247–50.
48. Srivaths LV, et al. Differences in bleeding phenotype and provider interventions in postmenarchal adolescents when compared to adult women with bleeding disorders and heavy menstrual bleeding. Haemophilia. 2018;24(1):63–9.
49. Grainger JD, Thachil J, Will AM. How we treat the platelet glycoprotein defects; Glanzmann thrombasthenia and Bernard Soulier syndrome in children and adults. Br J Haematol. 2018;182(5):621–32.
50. Santoro C, et al. Prevalence of Allo-immunization anti-HLA and anti-integrin alpha IIb beta 3 in Glanzmann Thromboasthenia patients. Haemophilia. 2010;16(5):805–12.
51. Fiore M, et al. Natural history of platelet antibody formation against alpha IIb beta 3 in a French cohort of Glanzmann thrombasthenia patients. Haemophilia. 2012;18(3):e201–9.
52. Hagenfeldt K. The role of prostaglandins and allied substances in uterine haemostasis. Contraception. 1987;36(1):23–35.

53. Lopez Bernal A, et al. Meclofenamate inhibits prostaglandin E binding and adenylyl cyclase activation in human myometrium. J Endocrinol. 1991;129(3):439–45.

54. Kreutner A Jr, Johnson D, Williamson HO. Histology of the endometrium in long-term use of a sequential oral contraceptive. Fertil Steril. 1976;27(8):905–10.

55. Rees MC, et al. Leukotriene release by endometrium and myometrium throughout the menstrual cycle in dysmenorrhoea and menorrhagia. J Endocrinol. 1987;113(2):291–5.

56. Bofill Rodriguez M, Lethaby A, Farquhar C. Non-steroidal anti-inflammatory drugs for heavy menstrual bleeding. Cochrane Database Syst Rev. 2019;9:CD000400.

57. Schoep ME, et al. The impact of menstrual symptoms on everyday life: a survey among 42,879 women. Am J Obstet Gynecol. 2019;220(6):569 e1–7.

58. Frick KD, et al. Financial and quality-of-life burden of dysfunctional uterine bleeding among women agreeing to obtain surgical treatment. Womens Health Issues. 2009;19(1):70–8.

59. De Sanctis V, et al. Dysmenorrhea in adolescents and young adults: a review in different country. Acta Biomed. 2017;87(3):233–46.

60. Bolton-Maggs PHB. The rare inherited coagulation disorders. Pediatr Blood Cancer. 2013;60(1):S37–40.

Quality of Life in Female Adolescents with Bleeding Disorders

12

Anjali Pawar and Roshni Kulkarni

Introduction

Quality of Life Versus Health-Related Quality of Life

Following World War II, there were increasing awareness and recognition of social inequalities, including health, in the world [1]. In 1947, the World Health Organization (WHO) defined health as a state of complete physical, mental, and social well-being and not merely absence of disease or infirmity [2]. This provided the impetus for academic research on social indicators and subsequently for research on subjective well-being and quality of life. In the mid-1980s, the term health-related quality of life (HRQOL) was first mentioned in medical literature [3]. In 1995 WHO describes quality of life (QOL) as an individual's perception of their position in life in context of the culture and value system in which they live and in relation to their goals, expectations, standards, and concerns [4].

When QOL is considered in the context of health and disease, it is referred to as "health-related quality of life (HRQOL). The latter is a multidimensional concept that includes domains related to physical, mental, emotional, and social functioning and focuses on the impact health status has on quality of life [5]. Thus, QOL is a broader concept that covers all aspects of life, whereas HRQOL focuses on the effect of a particular illness and the impact of its treatment in an individual; the instruments used to measure it tend to be disease specific.

Inherited bleeding disorders, such as hemophilia, von Willebrand disease (VWD), deficiencies of other clotting factors, and qualitative platelet defects, all affect HRQOL. Although hemophilia being an X-linked disorder affects males, symptomatic female carriers can also experience various symptoms of bleeding [6, 7]. These bleeding disorders often disproportionately affect women and girls as they face challenges of menstruation, pregnancy, and childbirth [8].

In women and adolescent girls with bleeding disorders, heavy menstrual bleeding (HMB) is perhaps the most common manifestation/presentation. It affects daily activities as well as social functioning. In some cases, HMB may be the first/initial manifestation of an underlying bleeding disorder although many adolescents may be unaware that their menstrual cycles are heavy and require medical attention [8]. This is

A. Pawar (✉)
University of California Davis, Hemostasis and Thrombosis Center, Professor Department of Pediatrics, Hematology Oncology,
Sacramento, CA, USA
e-mail: apawar@ucdavis.edu

R. Kulkarni
Michigan State University Center for Bleeding and Clotting Disorders, Emerita Pediatric Hematology/Oncology, Department of Pediatrics and Human Development, B216 Clinical Center,
East Lansing, MI, USA

© Springer Nature Switzerland AG 2020
L. V. Srivaths (ed.), *Hematology in the Adolescent Female*,
https://doi.org/10.1007/978-3-030-48446-0_12

in sharp contrast, to the abundance of information, even in boys as young as 4 years of age, regarding HRQOL among males, with bleeding disorders [9].

Although the overall incidence of these bleeding disorders is low, they place an inordinate burden on individual patients and their family members [10, 11]. Multiple studies have reported decreased HRQOL in adult females compared to healthy controls or other females with chronic conditions, but there is a paucity of data regarding HRQOL in female adolescents with underlying bleeding disorders [12].

Assessment of HRQOL and Bleeding Severity

It is important to recognize that HMB and bleeding disorder severity/phenotype in affected women and girls impact HRQOL [13]. Therefore, in addition to HRQOL measurements, it is crucial to obtain an accurate assessment of not only blood loss during menstruation but also the bleeding severity and phenotype [14–16].

Validated standardized tools can measure menstrual blood loss and determine presence or absence of HMB. Other validated tools such as the International Society on Thrombosis and Haemostasis (ISTH) Bleeding Assessment Tool (BAT) use bleeding scores to objectively assess the severity of bleeding symptoms [17].

Tools to Assess Severity of Bleeding

International Society on Thrombosis and Hemostasis – Bleeding Assessment Tool (ISTH-BAT)

Several bleeding assessment tools were proposed and developed to translate the severities of a range of subjective bleeding symptoms into a final, summative objective bleeding score (BS). These tools went through various iterations to improve the ease of evaluation and scoring accuracy. To promote the standardiza-

tion of the available BAT, a working group was established within the framework of the ISTH/SSC Subcommittees on VWD and on Perinatal/Pediatric Hemostasis (ISTH/SSC-BAT) in 2007, and in 2010 the ISTH-BAT was published [17]. It was designed to optimize accuracy, flexibility, and ease of use in clinical or research applications. Furthermore, it accounted for bleeding frequency and severity and was suitable for use in children and adults while still maintaining a reasonable administration time. To establish the normal range of the ISTH-BAT, a bioinformatics mechanism was developed based on the ontology of bleeding symptoms used to structure the ISTH-BAT. It merged legacy data from four different bleeding questionnaires, all developed from the same original BAT. The newly established cutoffs for an abnormal BS of ≥ 4 for adult males, ≥ 6 for adult females, and ≥ 3 for children can objectively assess individuals affected by bleeding symptoms [18].

Tools to Assess Menstrual Bleeding

Table 12.1 lists some of validated instruments to measure menstrual blood loss and lists the advantages and disadvantages of the instruments.

The Pictorial Blood Assessment Chart (PBAC) is a validated semi-quantitative tool to measure menstrual blood loss and uses a pictorial chart [14]. Blood loss is calculated based on the degree to which each item of sanitary protection is soiled with blood as well as the total number of pads and tampons used. In an adult female, HMB is defined as excessive menstrual blood loss of >80 mL per cycle that interferes with a woman's physical, emotional, and social well-being and quality of life. Of these as many as 20% of women may have an inherited bleeding disorder [16].

The Centers for Disease Control and Prevention (CDC), in a US multisite cohort of 217 women with menorrhagia (PBAC ≥ 100) ages 18–50 years, evaluated a screening tool for bleeding disorders. The sensitivity of the screening tool was 89% for hemostatic defects, and sen-

Table 12.1 Tools/instruments to assess heavy menstrual bleeding (HMB)

Method	Advantages	Disadvantages	Used in adolescents
Alkaline hematin	"Gold standard" in terms of accuracy Validated for selected SAP-c towels Well suited to research setting Best used in conjunction with a pictorial method and a diary	Requires calibration curves for each product and does not take extraneous blood loss into account Patients in the clinical setting may be deterred by having to collect, store, and send sanitary products for analysis	No
PBAC score	Quick and simple Validated for selected SAP-c towels Suitable for research purposes and has potential value in the clinic	Only validated for a limited number of current products Participants must record/recall results	Yes
Menstrual pictogram	Quick and easy Validated for selected SAP-c towels Suitable for research purposes and has potential value in the clinic Differentiates between absorbency ratings of sanitary items	Only validated for a limited number of current products Participants must record/recall results	Yes
Questionnaires	Many available, ranging in complexity, with questions relating to MBL, generic or disease-specific QoL or both	Poorly validated, with a few exceptions Participants must record/recall results	Yes
Menstrual cup (Gyneseal/Mooncup)	Simple Can be used to measure effect of medical intervention	Subject to leakage during collection and therefore unsuitable for either clinical or research purposes	No
Duration of period Count of pads	Simple and easy	Participants must record/recall results Frequency of changing pads can be influenced by many variables	Yes
Self-perception	Simple Useful for clinical assessments	Does not give precise MBL measure Participants must record/recall results Individuals can be poor judges of MBL Not diagnostic	Yes

MBL menstrual blood loss, *MFL* menstrual fluid loss, *PBAC* Pictorial Blood Assessment Chart, *QoL* quality of life, *SAP-c* superabsorbent polymer-containing
Modified from Magnay et al. [47]

sitivity increased to 93% when serum ferritin ≤20 ng/mL was added and to 95% when the PBAC score was >185 [15, 16].

Tools to Measure HRQOL

These tools are in the form of questionnaires, and their results are converted to numerical value. This allows researchers to compare changes of HRQOL between patients with different disorders. The generic 36-Item Short-Form (SF-36®) Survey and the EuroQoL 5 Domain (EQ-5D) tools have the longest pedigree and form the basis for many disease-specific validated tools.

SF-36 The Short-Form Health Survey (Administration: Interview or Self)

The 36-Item Short-Form Health Survey (SF-36) was first developed by RAND corporation as part of the medical outcome study. It explained variations in patient outcomes of multi-site multi-year studies. It is a generic, self-evaluated, self-reported questionnaire for individuals 14 years and older. This validated instrument assesses QOL in eight domains: physical functioning (PF), role physical (RP), bodily pain (BP), general health (GH), vitality (VT), social functioning (SF), role emotional (RE), and mental health (MH).

Scores for each domain range from 0 to 100. The eight domains can be summarized into two measures of health: a physical component score (PCS) and a mental component score (MCS). The PCS and MCS are always norm-based and scored from all eight scales taking into account the correlation between scales. The scales most associated with MCS are mental health, role emotional, social functioning, and vitality. The scales most associated with PCS are physical functioning, role physical, bodily pain, and general health [19, 20]

SF-12 (Administration: Interview or Self)

This is a shorter 12-item version of the SF-36 that reproduced 90% of the variance in the overall physical and mental health components of the SF-36. It has been reported in different populations in women (fibroids, menorrhagia) and following various elective procedures. Lower scores compared to normal were reported in a large study of women with fibroids and HMB [21, 22]. Other studies reported improvement in scores following treatment.

EQ-5D (Administration: Interview or Self)

This is a family of instruments to describe and value health, developed by the European quality of life group. Respondents rate their health on each dimension at three levels of severity on EQ-5D 3L or 5 levels of severity on EQ-5D-5L. It is available in over 200 languages, in paper or electronic format [23].

PROMIS® Patient-Reported Outcomes Measurement Information System

The National Institute of Health (NIH) developed this measure of global health.

It consists of a set of person-centered measures that evaluates and monitors physical, men-

tal, and social health in adults and children. It can be used with the general population and in individuals of all ages living with chronic conditions [24]. The questionnaires use a 5-point Likert response scale, e.g., no days, 1 day, 2–3 days, 4–5 days, 6–7 days, not at all, little bit, quite a bit, and very much and a recall of past 7 days. PROMIS® tools are available on the HealthMeasures website [25]. The tools are available in multiple formats, e.g., paper, computer based, and smart device applications, and can easily integrate into medical documents.

HRQOL questionnaires pertaining to a disease or a condition have been validated and available for researchers. HAEMO QoL is an example of hemophilia-specific well-being index [26]. While a majority of questionnaires address adult populations, the questions must be modified for use in the pediatric population so as to be developmentally appropriate. Table 12.2 lists condition-specific instruments used to measure QOL in females with HMB.

Since 1990, pediatric questionnaires that include adolescents have become more prevalent in their use in both generic or disease-specific forms. The generic questionnaire applies to healthy as well as to any clinically affected population. In children, the most commonly used generic questionnaires are the Child Health Questionnaire (CHQ) and the Pediatric Quality of Life Inventory (PedsQL). Unlike the PEDSQL the CHQ has been cross-culturally validated in multiple languages [27].

Impact of Bleeding Disorders on QOL in Adolescent Females

Figure 12.1 lists the consequences of bleeding in women/girls with HMB regardless of the type of bleeding disorder [13]. VWD has been the flagship and most studied inherited bleeding disorder as it affects 1% of population across the world and is not gender specific. In women it causes clinical symptoms other than HMB, as von Mackensen succinctly outlined the effects of bleeding disorders on quality of life in women [28]. Using VWD as a prime example of an inherited bleeding disorder, one can easily see

Table 12.2 Instruments to assess heavy menstrual bleeding (HMB) symptoms and quality of life (QOL) in adult females

Instrument	Validated	Properties	Used in Adolescents
Menorrhagia Multi-attribute Scale (MMAS) Shaw et al. [49]	Yes, used as outcome measure for ECLIPSE study	Bleeding-specific symptom and QOL instrument. Measures impact of HMB with six items on practical difficulties, social life, mental health, physical health, work life, and family life. Responses are scored and weighted. Generates a score of 0 (most severe impact) to 100 (no impact)	No
Aberdeen Menorrhagia Severity Scale (AMSS) Also known as Ruta menorrhagia severity score Ruta et al. [50]	Yes, internally consistent and reliable health status questionnaire specific to HMB	Bleeding-specific symptom and patient-based outcome measure about HMB. It was developed in the UK and contains 15 items with a 4-point Likert scale for responses with a maximum score of 47. The score is then converted to a percentage producing a score from 0 to 100. This scale has been used in several studies and has been judged to be of good quality	No
Menorrhagia Impact Questionnaire (MIQ) Bushnell et al. [51]	Yes, developed to evaluate effectiveness of tranexamic acid in treatment of HMB	Bleeding-specific symptom and QOL instrument that measures impact of HMB with six items total on perceived amount of blood lost, impact on work, impact on physical activities, social activities, number of activities limited, and perceived impact of treatment on symptoms	No
Menstrual Bleeding Questionnaire (MBQ) AMSS + MIQ + patient input Matteson et al. [22]	Yes	Bleeding-specific symptom and QOL that measures impact of HMB with 20 items and includes perception of heaviness of bleeding, bleeding pattern, pain, and impact of symptoms including social embarrassment, fear of social embarrassment, and behavioral changes to avoid social embarrassment. Sum responses to obtain a total score and multiply score by 1.32 to scale. Zero, least impact possible; 100, worst impact possible	No

HMB heavy menstrual bleeding; *QOL* quality of life
Modified from Matteson et al. and Rahn et al. [22, 48–51]

Fig. 12.1 Consequences of bleeding. (Modified from Kulkarni [13])

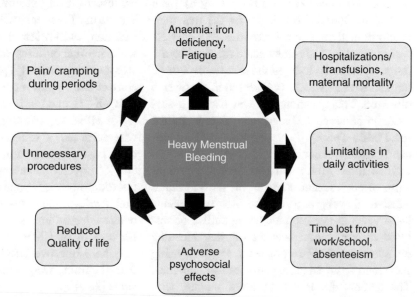

that the effects on QOL of affected individuals can be myriad. They can be as varied as effects of anemia from HMB or even recurrent epistaxis. Bleeding into joints and arthropathy can occur in patients with type 3 VWD. HMB and dysmenorrhea or mid-cycle ovulation pain exaggerated by bleeding during ovulation are known to occur among individuals with VWD. All of these signs and symptoms decrease QOL and treatment improves QOL [29, 30].

HRQOL perspectives differ in adolescents compared to adults. The WHO suggests the following domains and facets for children and adolescent quality-of-life instruments: family/social relations; physical function; psychological (internal); "physical appearance"; psychosocial relations to social and material environment; and the characteristics of the environment itself, for example, school, food, chores, spaces, and material comfort. The most commonly used QOL instruments for adolescents with menstrual problems (dysmenorrhea, HMB or oligoamenorrhea) are the SF-36 and PedsQL Teen instruments [31, 32].

Chi et al. used a questionnaire to assess QOL among adolescents with bleeding disorder and HMB. The questions, based on SF-36, included the following parameters: if during their period they felt (i) full of life, (ii) nervous[+], (iii) down in the dumps[+], (iv) calm and peaceful, (v) full of energy, (vi) downhearted and low[+], (vii) worn out[+], (viii) happy, (ix) tired[+], or (x) that their health limited their social activities[+]. All answers were scored on a six-point scale ranging from 1 (none of the time) to 6 (all the time) except those marked with a [+] which were scored in the reverse direction. This questionnaire was used to assess QOL in adolescents before and after treatment for HMB. The QOL scores improved significantly with treatment [33].

In a focus group and paper-based questionnaire of adolescents, Khair et al. showed that a substantial subgroup of the 45 respondents 9–34 years of age reported being bullied or suffered discrimination because of their bleeding disorder and 80% respondents reported being prevented from engaging in sporting activities. The authors developed the questionnaire, with

input from members of the UK Haemophilia Society, and had a shortened version for those under 16 years of age, omitting questions considered "sensitive" [34].

Pawar et al. surveyed 45 adolescents aged 15–17 years and reported on the effect of menorrhagia (as defined by a PBAC score of ≥100) on various parameters of QOL. School absenteeism and lack of awareness of HMB in respondents and their family members were common [35]. The former may have a significant impact on academic achievement in this population. Torres et al. reported that emotional dimension had the most deterioration in adolescents with HMB and in their study population; 50% of the affected adolescents missed school [36].

Adolescent/young adult females with a bleeding disorder report lower physical HRQOL when compared to men. This has been reported in women with VWD also and attributed to menorrhagia, dysmenorrhea, and pregnancy-related bleeding leading to anemia, fatigue, and pain [37–40].

Not all the current QOL/HRQOL instruments in use are culturally sensitive. There are cultural, religious, and social aspects as to how societies view menstruation let alone what constitutes country or culture-specific HRQOL. As practiced in some cultures across the globe, for an adolescent, being secluded from normal family life during the menstrual cycle, i.e., "menstrual isolation," will affect the individual's HRQOL, while in other cultures, not being able to go for a sleepover to a friend's place or participate in a competitive sport could negatively affect HRQOL. Economic impact regarding availability of effective, affordable, and hygienic products and access to toilets can affect HRQOL. The high cost of menstrual supplies can lead to "period poverty" resulting in missing school and therefore a barrier to equal opportunity in education. Adolescents are less likely to accept therapeutic interventions such as intrauterine devices for control of HMB or hormonal therapy that may help improve HRQOL. Fear of shots and fear of gaining weight may influence these decisions [38–40].

There is paucity of data and validated instruments to measure the effect of bleeding disorders on HRQOL in female adolescents. The current QOL tools do not measure the intermittent nature of the effect of HMB. There is a lack of studies in HRQOL changes during the various phases of the menstrual cycle. Efforts are underway to validate bleeding assessment tools specific to pediatric population, but it is still a work in progress [41, 42].

HRQOL Secondary to Consequences of HMB

HMB can cause iron deficiency, low ferritin, and anemia resulting in malaise, low energy, and tiredness that can affect QOL. For example, Wang et al. in their study used the Ruta menorrhagia severity score and a fatigue severity scale to compare adolescents affected by HMB to those without heavy menstrual loss. Fatigue severity scores were significantly higher in young women with HMB as compared to healthy controls [43]. As noted above, HMB is a common manifestation of inherited bleeding disorder.

The clinical effects of iron deficiency with or without anemia cover a wide spectrum. Iron deficiency without anemia is under recognized in the adolescents and young adults as noted by Johnson et al. [44]. As reported by Cooke et al. in their study, iron deficiency anemia and HMB can result in the need for urgent medical care, including ER visits, hospitalization, and blood transfusion [45]. An adolescent female with a bleeding disorder should be closely monitored to prevent iron deficiency and avoid these bad outcomes.

QOL of Family Members of Adolescent Females with Bleeding Disorders/HMB: Caregiver Burden

Taking care of an individual with a chronic health condition is demanding and can affect the caregiver's employment, finances, social connections, and other aspects of life. Many tools exist to screen for caregiver burden and determine how specific diseases affect the caregiver, e.g., for cancer, cardiac conditions, Alzheimer's disease, etc. [46]. The 36-item Hemophilia Caregiver Impact [HCI] measure is a useful new tool for clinical research composed of seven subscales assessing relevant negative aspects of caregiver impact and one subscale reflecting a positive aspect of caregiver impact. It demonstrates high reliability, good construct validity, and moderate incremental and discriminant validity. The HCI shows promise for clinical hemophilia studies as a caregiver-based tool for evaluating treatments [11]. The tool is versatile and can be used to analyze studies with very small samples. Currently there is a paucity of data regarding caregiver burden in caregivers of adolescent females with a chronic disease.

Conclusion

The most common symptom of inherited bleeding disorder in adolescents is HMB. They can experience short- and long-term consequences, especially as it relates to HRQOL. von Mackensen outlined the major reasons to assess HRQOL in women, and these same reasons apply to young girls also. Besides better understanding of what life is like for these adolescents, one can identify specific healthcare needs of this population to assess the effect of various treatment strategies and identify optimal treatment strategies to deliver appropriate care [28]. We need further research to determine if the cyclic nature of menstrual periods affects HRQOL parameters and what are the age, gender, and racial differences regarding HRQOL in persons with bleeding disorders.

References

1. https://www.britannica.com/topic/quality-of-life. Accessed 20 Sept 2019.
2. Chron World Health Organ. 1947;1(1–2):29–43. Constitution of the world health organization.
3. Torrance GW. Utility approach to measuring health -related quality of life. J Chronic Dis. 1987;40(6):593–603.

4. WHOQOL: Measuring Quality of Life. https://www. who.int/healthinfo/survey/whoqol-qualityoflife/en/. Accessed 20 Sept 2019.

5. https://www.cdc.gov/hrqol/concept.htm#2. Accessed 20 Sept 2019.

6. https://www.hemophilia.org/Community-Resources/ Women-with-Bleeding-Disorders/Women-also-Bleed. Accessed 20 Sept 2019.

7. Gilbert L, Paroskie A, Gailani D, Debaun MR, Sidonio RF. Haemophilia A carriers experience reduced health-related quality of life. Haemophilia. 2015;21:761–5.

8. Rhynders PA, Sayers CA, Presley RJ, Thierry JM. Thierry; providing young women with credible health information about bleeding disorders. Am J Prev Med. 2014;47(5):674–80.

9. Tang L, et al. Describing the quality of life of boys with haemophilia in China: Results of a multi-centre study using the CHO-KLAT. Haemophilia. 2018;24(1):113–9.

10. https://www.hemophilia.org/About-Us/Fast-Facts. Accessed 26 Sept 2019.

11. Schwartz CE, Powell VE, Eldar-Lissai A. Measuring hemophilia caregiver burden: validation of the Hemophilia Caregiver Impact measure. Qual Life Res. 2017;26:2551–62.

12. Nowak-Göttl U, Clausnizer H, Kowalski D, Limperger V, Krümpel A, Shneyder M, Reinke S, Rocke A, Juhl D, Steppat D, Krause M. Health-related quality of life in children, adolescents and adults with hereditary and acquired bleeding disorders. Blood Cells Mol Dis. 2017;67:96–101.

13. Kulkarni R. Improving care and treatment options for women and girls with bleeding disorders. Eur J Haematol. 2015;95(Suppl 81):2–10.

14. Higham JM, O'Brien PM, Shaw RW. Assessment of menstrual blood loss using a pictorial chart. Br J Obstet Gynaecol. 1990;97(8):734–9.

15. Philipp CS, Faiz A, Dowling NF, et al. Development of a screening tool for identifying women with men-orrhagia for hemostatic evaluation. Am J Obstet Gynecol. 2008;163:e1–8.

16. Philipp CS, Faiz A, Heit JA, et al. Evaluation of a screening tool for bleeding disorders in a US multi-site cohort of women with menorrhagia. Am J Obstet Gynecol. 2011;204(3):209, e1–7.

17. Rodeghiero F, Tosetto A, Abshire T, Arnold DM, Coller B, James P, Neunert C, Lillicrap D. ISTH/SSC joint VWF and Perinatal/Pediatric Hemostasis Subcommittees Working Group. ISTH/SSC bleeding assessment tool: a standardized questionnaire and a proposal for a new bleeding score for inherited bleeding disorders. J Thromb Haemost. 2010;8(9):2063–5.

18. Elbatarny M, Mollah S, Grabell J, Bae S, Deforest M, Tuttle A, Hopman W, Clark DS, Mauer AC, Bowman M, Riddel J. Normal range of bleeding scores for the ISTH-BAT: adult and pediatric data from the merging project. Blood. 2013;122:1107.

19. Ware JE Jr, Sherbourne CD. The MOS 36-item Short Form Health Survey (SF-36).I. Conceptual frame-work and item selection. Med Care. 1992;30(6):473–83. PMID:1593914.

20. https://www.rand.org/health-care/surveys_tools/mos/36-item-short-form.html. Accessed 25 Sept 2019.

21. El-Nashar SA, Hopkins MR, Barnes SA, Pruthi RK, Gebhart JB, Cliby WA. Health-related quality of life and patient satisfaction after global endometrial abla-tion for menorrhagia in women with bleeding disor-ders: a follow-up survey and systematic review. Am J Obstet Gynecol. 2010;202(4):348, e1–7.

22. Matteson KA, Scott DM, Raker CA, Clark MA. The menstrual bleeding questionnaire: development and validation of a comprehensive patient-reported outcome instrument for heavy menstrual bleeding. BJOG. 2015;122(5):681–9.

23. Buchholz I, Janssen MF, Kohlmann T, Feng YS. A systematic review of studies comparing the mea-surement properties of the three-level and five-level versions of the EQ-5D. PharmacoEconomics. 2018 Jun;36(6):645–61.

24. https://www.healthypeople.gov/sites/default/files/HRQoLWBFullReport.pdf. Accessed 20 Sept 2019.

25. http://www.healthmeasures.net/index.php. Accessed 20 Sept 2019.

26. Bullinger M, von Mackensen S, Fischer K, Khair K, Petersen C, Ravens-Sieberer U, Rocino A, Sagnier P, Tusell JM, van den Berg M, Vicariot M. Pilot testing of the 'Haemo-QoL' quality of life question-naire for haemophiliac children in six European countries. Haemophilia. 2002;8(Suppl 2):47–54. PMID:11966854.

27. Raat H, Mohangoo AD, Grootenhuis MA. Pediatric health-related quality of life questionnaires in clinical trials. Curr Opin Allergy Clin Immunol. 2006;6(3):180–5.

28. http://elearning.wfh.org/resource/quality-of-life-in-women-with-bleeding-disorders. Accessed 20 Sept 2019.

29. de Wee EM, Mauser-Bunschoten EP, Van Der Bom JG, Degenaar-Dujardin ME, Eikenboom HC, Fijnvandraat K, et al. Health-related quality of life among adult patients with moderate and severe von Willebrand dis-ease. J Thromb Haemost. 2010;8(7):1492–9.

30. Holm E, Abshire TC, Bowen J, Álvarez MT, Bolton-Maggs P, Carcao M, Federici AB, Gill JC, Halimeh S, Kempton C, Key NS, Kouides P, Lail A, Landorph A, Leebeek F, Makris M, Mannucci P, Mauser-Bunschoten EP, Nugent D, Valentino LA, Winikoff R, Berntorp E. Changes in bleeding patterns in von Willebrand disease after institution of long-term replacement therapy: results from the von Willebrand Disease Prophylaxis Network. Blood Coagul Fibrinolysis. 2015;26(4):383–8.

31. de Wee EM, Fijnvandraat K, de Goede-Bolder A, Mauser-Bunschoten EP, Eikenboom JC, et al. Impact of von Willebrand disease on health-related quality of life in a pediatric population. J Thromb Haemost. 2011;9(3):502–9.

32. Knox B, Azurah AG, Grover SR. Quality of life and menstruation in adolescents. Curr Opin Obstet Gynecol. 2015;27:309–14.

33. Chi C, Pollard D, Tuddenham EG, Kadir RA. Menorrhagia in adolescents with inherited bleeding disorders. J Pediatr Adolesc Gynecol. 2010;23(4):215–22.

34. Khair K, Holland M, Pollard D. The experience of girls and young women with inherited bleeding disorders. Haemophilia. 2013;19:e276–81.

35. Pawar A, Krishnan R, Davis K, Bosma K, Kulkarni R. Perceptions about quality of life in a school-based population of adolescents with menorrhagia: implications for adolescents with bleeding disorders. Haemophilia. 2008;14(3):579–83.

36. Torres R, Zajer C, Menéndez M, Canessa MJ, Cerda J, Wietstruck MA, Zuniga P. Heavy menstrual bleeding affects quality of life in adolescents. Rev Chil Pediatr. 2017;88(6):717–22.

37. JM ML, Munn JE, Anderson TL, Lambing A, Tortella B, Witkop ML. Predictors of quality of life among adolescents and young adults with a bleeding disorder. Health Q Life Outcomes. 2017;15(1):67. https://doi.org/10.1186/s12955-017-0643-7.

38. https://www.yourperiod.ca/normal-periods/menstruation-around-the-world/. Accessed 20 Sept 2019.

39. Coast E, Lattof SR, Strong J. Puberty and menstruation knowledge among young adolescents in low- and middle-income countries: a scoping review. Int J Public Health. 2019;64(2):293–304.

40. Van Eijk AM, Zulaika G, Lenchner M, Mason L, Sivakami M, Nyothach E, Unger H, Laserson K, Phillips-Howard PA. Menstrual cup use, leakage, acceptability, safety, and availability: a systematic review and meta-analysis. Lancet Public Health. 2019;4(8):e376–93.

41. Peters B, Stokhuijzen E, Cnossen M, Biss T, Peters M, Suijker M, Silva M, Blanchette V, James P, Rand M, Fijnvandraat K. Ichec: refining the pediatric bleeding assessment tool. https://academy.isth.org/isth/2019/melbourne/264026/karin.fijnvandraat.ichec.refining.the.pediatric.bleeding.assessment.tool.html. Accessed 20 Sept 2019.

42. Limperg PF, Terwee CB, Young NL, Price VE, Gouw SC, Peters M, Grootenhuis MA, Blanchette V, Haverman L. Health-related quality of life questionnaires in individuals with haemophilia: a systematic review of their measurement properties. Haemophilia. 2017;23(4):497–510.

43. Wang W, Bourgeois T, Klima J, Berlan ED, Fischer AN, O'Brien SH. Iron deficiency and fatigue in adolescent females with heavy menstrual bleeding. Haemophilia. 2013;19(2):225–30.

44. Johnson S, Lang A, Sturm M, O'Brien SH. Iron deficiency without anemia: a common yet under-recognized diagnosis in young women with heavy menstrual bleeding. J Pediatr Adolesc Gynecol. 2016;29(6):628–31.

45. Cooke AG, McCavit TL, Buchannan GR, Powers JM. Iron deficiency anemia in adolescents who present with heavy menstrual bleeding. J Pediatr Adolesc Gynecol. 2017;30(2):247–50.

46. Adelman RD, Tmanova LL, Delgado D, Dion S, Lachs MS. Caregiver burden: a clinical review. JAMA. 2014;311(10):1052–60.

47. Magnay JL, O'Brien S, Gerlinger C, Seitz C. A systematic review of methods to measure menstrual blood loss. BMC Womens Health. 2018;18(1):142.

48. Rahn DD, Abed H, Sung VW, Matteson KA, Rogers RG, Morrill MY, Barber MD, Schaffer JI, Wheeler TL II, Balk EM, Uhlig K. Systematic review highlights difficulty interpreting diverse clinical outcomes in abnormal uterine bleeding trials. J Clin Epidemiol. 2011;64(3):293–300.

49. Shaw RW, Brickley MR, Evans L, Edwards MJ. Perceptions of women on the impact of menorrhagia on their health using multi-attribute utility assessment. BJOG. 1998;105:1155–9.

50. Ruta DA, Garratt AM, Chadha YC, Flett GM, Hall MH, Russell IT. Assessment of patients with menorrhagia: how valid is a structured clinical history as a measure of health status? Qual Life Res. 1995;4(1):33–40. PMID:7711689.

51. Bushnell DM, Martin ML, Moore KA, Richter HE, Rubin A, Patrick DL. Menorrhagia Impact Questionnaire: assessing the influence of heavy menstrual bleeding on quality of life. Curr Med Res Opin. 2010;26(12):2745–55. PMID: 21043553.

Part II

Thromboembolism in the Adolescent Female

Prevalence and Risk Factors of Adolescent Venous Thromboembolism

13

Arash Mahjerin, Julie Jaffray, and Brian Branchford

Prevalence and Patient Characteristics

Venous thromboembolism (VTE), consisting of deep venous thrombosis (DVT) and pulmonary embolism (PE), has been increasingly recognized as a serious and potentially fatal occurrence in hospitalized children [1, 2]. Children diagnosed with a VTE are at risk for developing VTE progression, embolic stroke, recurrent VTE (up to 21%), and post-thrombotic syndrome (chronic limb swelling secondary to venous insufficiency) in 26% of cases [2–4]. The mortality rate in children directly related to VTE is 2% [5].

The overall incidence of VTE in children of all ages is estimated to be 0.05–0.14 per 10,000 children, but rates specifically in hospitalized children are remarkably higher, up to 30–60 per 10,0000 hospital admissions [1, 6–9]. The rate of hospital-acquired (HA) VTE has increased over the last two decades by 70–200% [1, 2].

The distribution of pediatric VTE incidence is bimodal, with the highest peak occurring under 1 year of age and the second peak during adolescence [5, 6]. After adjusting for number of admissions per age group, one study found the rate of hospital-acquired VTE was highest in older adolescents and young adults compared to all other age groups [6]. The incidence of VTE in female adolescents who are not hospitalized is 0.11 to 3 per 10,000, although the rate of HA-VTE is higher, up to 94 per 10,000 hospital admissions [1, 8, 10]. VTEs diagnosed in young adults and adolescents are more likely to be hospital-acquired rather than community-acquired [6]. Studies have revealed a male predominance in HA-VTE for all children, but the rate of DVT was found to be twice as high in adolescent females as compared to males [8, 11].

Risk Factors

Many VTE risk factors are common among children of all ages, such as decreased mobility, a central venous catheter (CVC), diagnosis with pro-thrombotic conditions such as cancer or an inflammatory disease, or thrombophilia (discussed in a separate chapter). But certain characteristics are unique to the adolescent subpopulation (Table 13.1), such as hormonal exposure through contraception or pregnancy as well as obesity and tobacco use. Many of these factors represent aspects of Virchow's Triad of VTE risk factors, as seen in Fig. 13.1.

A. Mahjerin (✉)
Children's Hospital Orange County, University of California – Irvine, Irvine, CA, USA
e-mail: AMahajerin@choc.org

J. Jaffray
Children's Hospital Los Angeles, University of Southern California Keck School of Medicine, Los Angeles, CA, USA

B. Branchford
Children's Hospital Colorado, University of Colorado School of Medicine, Aurora, CO, USA

© Springer Nature Switzerland AG 2020
L. V. Srivaths (ed.), *Hematology in the Adolescent Female*,
https://doi.org/10.1007/978-3-030-48446-0_13

Table 13.1 Published risk factors for venous thromboembolism specifically studied and reported for adolescents

Risk factors	Conclusions	References
Hospitalization	94 cases of adolescent VTE out of 10,0000 hospitalized children After adjusting for number of admissions per age group, incidence of HA-VTE is highest in older adolescents and young adults	Raffini et al. [1], Takemoto et al. [6]
Central venous catheters	Noncritically ill older children (≥10 years) with a CVC	Smitherman et al. [18]
Malignancy	Adolescents with ALL treated with asparaginase and steroids Adolescents with leukemia, lymphoma, and sarcomas over brain tumors	Grace et al. [21], Tuckuviene et al. [22], O'Brien et al. [23]
Surgery	Children >15 years having surgery	Sherrod et al. [15]
Trauma	Trauma patients requiring hospitalization who are adolescent Increased incidence in those 17–21 years	Takemoto et al. [6], Yen et al. [51], O'Brien et al. [49]
Oral contraception	Estrogen from OCPs	Hennessey et al. [10]
Pregnancy	27% of adolescents with a VTE found to be pregnant Pregnant adolescents have twice the VTE rate compared to nonpregnant adolescents	Stein et al. [8]
Family history	35% of adolescents taking OCPs and diagnosed with a VTE also had a family history of VTE	Pillai et al. [58]
Thrombophilia	15% of adolescents taking OCPs and diagnosed with a VTE were found to have an inherited thrombophilia	Pillai et al. [58]
NSAIDs	Unknown if VTE risk is directly from NSAIDs or underlying inflammatory condition	Bergendal et al. [62]
Obesity	Obesity was the 2nd most common VTE risk factor in adolescents taking OCPs	Abdollahi et al. [86]

VTE venous thromboembolism, *CVC* central venous catheter, *ALL* acute lymphoblastic leukemia, *OCP* oral contraceptive pill, *NSAIDs* nonsteroidal anti-inflammatory drugs

Fig. 13.1 Modified Virchow's Triad. 3 broad categories of thrombotic risk factors, with representative examples pertinent to the adolescent female

Hypercoagulability
Inflammatory conditions
Genetic and acquired thrombophilia
Malignancy
Increased estrogen exposure
Obesity
Substance abuse

Endothelial Injury
Surgery
Trauma
Central venous catheter

VTE Risk

Stasis of Flow
Post-operative state
Decreased mobility
Central venous catheter
Dehydration

Hospitalization

Hospitalization plays the largest role in VTE development due to frequent comorbid risk factors such as acute illness or surgery, immobilization, or mechanical ventilation. Hospitalized adolescents in particular have an incident rate ratio that is nearly eightfold of developing a VTE compared to children aged 2–9 years [6].

A retrospective case-control study found increased risk of HA-VTE risk in children with bacteremia, presence of a CVC, ICU admission, hospitalization ≥7 days, immobilization for more than 72 hours, and use of oral contraception [12]. One systematic review and meta-analysis of risk factors for VTE in hospitalized children identified admission in an intensive care unit (ICU), prolonged hospital stay, mechanical ventilation, and CVCs as the most statistically significant independent variables [13]. For critically ill children, CVC, length of hospital stay ≥4 days, and a serious infection were found to significantly increase risk of VTE [14]. When evaluating complex chronic conditions (CCCs) in hospitalized children with a VTE, 67% of those less than 1 year of age had a cardiac diagnosis compared to the adolescent age group who were primarily trauma patients [6].

Children with HA-VTE often have a recent history of surgery, and those older than 15 years have a higher risk of postoperative VTE than children of younger ages [6, 11, 15]. Cardiothoracic and general surgery are the most common surgeries prior to VTE diagnosis in all children, and median time from surgery to VTE diagnosis is 9 days [15]. Few studies have evaluated VTE risk specifically in postoperative adolescent patients, although one study of 2783 adolescents undergoing knee arthroscopy found a VTE incidence of 0.25% that occurred on average 8.8 days after their procedure [16].

Central Venous Catheters

After hospitalization, CVCs are the next most prominent risk factor for VTE in children of all ages [11, 13, 17]. This is likely due to the vascular trauma associated with CVC placement, as well as the turbulent flow around the catheter and upstream stasis of flow due to the decreased effective vessel caliber. Children with various underlying medical conditions require a CVC for life-sustaining treatment, ranging from those with malignancy, congenital heart disease, parental nutrition, and mitochondrial or metabolic disorders.

There is great heterogeneity in studies regarding CVC-associated VTE in children due to differences in patient population, inclusion of asymptomatic VTEs, as well as CVC types (peripherally inserted central catheters versus tunneled lines, totally implanted devices, or temporary lines). As a result, identifying the least thrombogenic catheter type or insertion technique is difficult. According to the national pediatric VTE registry in the Netherlands, almost all VTEs are CVC-associated in neonates compared to adolescents in which only one third are CVC-associated VTE [9], although another study evaluating CVC-associated VTE in noncritically ill children found an increased incidence in older children (≥10 years) and females [18].

Disease-Related

Malignancy

Cancer is a well-known risk factor for VTE in both children and adults due to the hypercoagulable state of malignancy itself, chemotherapeutic agents, surgeries, immobilization, and CVCs [19]. L-asparaginase and steroids are the chemotherapeutics most identified with VTE risk in children. L-asparaginase causes disruption of both the physiological pro- and anticoagulation system within the liver, as well as platelet activation [20]. Adolescents in particular are at a significantly increased risk of VTE when treated with protocols containing both asparaginase and steroids for high-risk (due to age) acute lymphoblastic leukemia [21, 22].

The Pediatric Health Information System (PHIS) database revealed the incidence of VTE in adolescents and young adults with cancer is 5.3%, with an increased risk in those 18–20 years of age compared to those 15–17 years old [23]. PHIS data also revealed adolescents and young adults with leukemia, lymphoma, and sarcomas had a higher risk of VTE compared to those with brain tumors. A single institution study found the VTE incidence in adolescents and young adults with sarcoma is 16%, although only 60% of the VTE cases were symptomatic [24]. Tumor compression added to thrombosis risk in half of the patients and the majority of patients had distant metastasis at the time of VTE diagnosis.

Inflammatory Conditions

A complex interplay exists among inflammation, innate immunity, and the coagulation system [25]. Mounting evidence suggests the inflammatory response may be a cause, as well as consequence, of VTE. Current anticoagulation treatment regimens, however, are not designed to inhibit inflammation. In fact, many established clinical VTE risk factors such as surgery, obesity, cystic fibrosis, sepsis, systemic infection, cancer, inflammatory bowel disease, and lupus likely modulate thrombosis through a common pathway of inflammatory mediators. The key event in the initiation of VTE formation is most likely vein wall inflammation, though the contribution of specific immune modulators has not yet been elucidated. It has been recently demonstrated that a probable association exists between VTE and several other markers of inflammation such as C-reactive protein (CRP), IL-6, IL-8, and tumor necrosis factor alpha [26–30]. These pro-inflammatory cytokines play an important role in VTE by promoting a procoagulant state primarily by inducing tissue factor expression. Several immune system components (cytokines, chemokines, and various leukocyte subtypes) are involved in the underlying inflammatory process of VTE, as is very well-described in a recent review from Saghazadeh et al. [31]. Additionally, it has been recently described that inflammatory mediators such as polyphosphates, bradykinin, and others may directly activate the contact system and initiate the extrinsic coagulation pathway [32–34]. A growing body of evidence suggests inflammation is a major contributor to the pathophysiology of VTE [35], likely by enhancing the hypercoagulable state and increasing endothelial damage. Activation of endothelial cells, platelets, and leukocytes, with subsequent initiation of inflammation and microparticle formation, triggers the coagulation system through induction of tissue factor, which likely contributes to the hypercoagulable state featured in Virchow's Triad [26, 36, 37]. Both formation and resolution of thrombosis have been associated with a series of inflammatory cascades [38, 39]. Moderate to severe inflammation (inflammatory infiltrates throughout the thrombi, mostly composed of lymphocytes, with some mixing with other components including plasma cells, neutrophils, and eosinophils) [40] was found in approximately 15% of thrombus specimens from pulmonary thromboendarterectomy [31], and immunity/inflammatory genes constitute nearly 10% of those genes whose expressions are substantially altered under the influence of VTE [40, 41].

Polyphosphate (polyP) is present in human platelet dense granules and is released upon platelet activation, assisting with coagulation by increasing activation of factor V, decreasing tissue factor pathway inhibitor activity, and delaying clot lysis by activating thrombin-activatable fibrinolysis inhibitor [42–45]. PolyP is also a potent pro-inflammatory signal when released from mast cells during a hypersensitivity reaction, for example [43]. Additionally, histones have been shown to be increased in sepsis and other inflammatory conditions along with nucleosomes (DNA + histones) and are toxic to the endothelium. Activated protein C inactivates histones, protecting the endothelium in the process. Extracellular DNA fibers extruded from neutrophils (neutrophil extracellular traps, NETs) are produced in response to infection to allow neutrophils to trap and destroy invading microorganisms. Fibrin formation and deposition, important processes for trapping organisms and controlling infections, are stimulated by NETs. NETs also increase platelet adhesion and are linked to VTE in experimental models [46]. Moreover, platelets have been shown to stimulate NET production [47]. A lot of work remains to fully detail the role of inflammation in VTE, but new mechanistic insights may allow for additional diagnostic biomarker discovery and/or therapeutic augmentation.

Trauma

Trauma is frequently identified as a risk factor for thrombosis in both pediatric and adult populations – primarily in hospitalized patients. Data regarding pediatric VTE in the trauma setting come from a disparate group of sources including single-institution studies, national trauma registries, and administrative data sets. The incidence in the general trauma population has been reported to vary from 0.1% to 1.2% [48] with higher incidence noted in older age groups, 2.1% in 17–21-year-old patients [49].

Several risk factors have been identified to have independent risk for VTE in the trauma setting. The first clinical risk assessment model (RAM) for VTE in children was derived from the National Trauma Data Bank (NTDB) and identified independent risk with Glasgow Coma Scale score ≤12, age <1 or ≥10 (with risk increasing with increasing age beyond 10 years of age), female sex, ICU admission, intubation, transfusion of blood products, CVC placement, pelvic or lower extremity fractures, and major surgery [50]. An additional RAM derived using single-institution data combined with data from the NTDB identified older age, surgery, transfusion, higher Injury Severity Score, and lower Glasgow Coma Scale score as independently associated with VTE [51].

The Injury Severity Score (ISS) is an anatomical scoring system to detail extent of injury in patients with multiple injuries [52]. The ISS has been shown to be predictive of VTE. In unselected populations, an ISS >25 was strongly associated with VTE, whereas children in the ICU have shown independent risk with an ISS >9 [53]. Additional factors have a putative association with VTE in the trauma population but have not shown consistent independent risk: spinal cord injury, thoracic or abdominal injury, obesity, mechanical ventilation, and immobilization [54]. Challenges that vex studies of VTE risk in trauma include difficulty determining which factors are proxies for overall severity of illness/injury and the extent to which pathophysiologic processes, e.g., fibrinolysis shutdown [55], modulate and/or interact with the clinical risk factors and how these interactions impact the pediatric population.

Hormonal

Estrogen is a well-established risk factor for thrombosis in females, which may be due to increased resistance to activated protein C, elevated factor VIII activity, and increased levels of D-dimer [56, 57], although in adolescent females, estrogen may not be the only risk factor for VTE. Examination of the PHIS database revealed 96% of female adolescents diagnosed with a VTE had other risk factors besides only estrogen exposure [10]. A single-institution study evaluating adolescent females diagnosed with a VTE while using hormonal contraception found 50% of the patients are obese, 35% have a positive family history of VTE, and 15% were found to have an inherited thrombophilia [58].

Pregnancy has also been linked to increased VTE risk, due to the development of a hypercoagulable state. In adult females, the risk of VTE was found to increase fivefold in pregnancy. A review of adolescent females with a DVT found 27% of the patients to be pregnant [8]. The DVT incidence of those who were pregnant was 109 per 100,000 adolescent females/year compared to 10.2 per 100,000 adolescent females/year in those who were not pregnant, with a rate ratio of 10.6 [8].

Mental Health

Mental health disorders, including depression and anxiety, affect adolescent females, and an association exists between these disorders and VTE, according to the United Kingdom's (UK) Million Women Study [59]. Women in this study who reported antidepressant use had a significantly higher risk of VTE than women who reported neither depression nor use of psychotropic drugs. A recent meta-analysis showed that both the underlying disorder itself and the medication used to treat it are associated with elevated VTE risk [60]. Subjects taking antidepressants in this study were 27% more likely to have VTE than those not taking antidepressants. In the studies comparing patients with depression compared to those without depression, the risk of VTE was increased by 31%. Interestingly, a causative relationship between VTE and subsequent mental health problems has also been investigated [61]. The trauma from potential life-threatening nature of VTE, in addition to complications with long-term morbidity such as post-thrombotic syndrome and chronic thromboembolic pulmonary embolism, can lead to adverse mental health effects.

Nonsteroidal Anti-inflammatory Drugs

A class of medications used frequently by adolescent females is nonsteroidal anti-inflammatory drugs (NSAIDs), which have been independently linked to VTE risk [62].

It is unclear whether this increase risk is a direct effect of the drug itself or if driven by an underlying inflammatory condition that may have led to its use. A recent meta-analysis of European studies demonstrated a pooled VTE risk ratio of nearly twofold among NSAID users [63]. It appears that risk was primarily driven by COX-2 inhibition (likely due to combined effect of antagonizing prostacyclins and stimulating the release of thromboxane from activated platelets), whereas aspirin (a COX-1 inhibitor) has been used in some cases for VTE prevention. Similarly a population-based case-control study of the National Patient Registry in Denmark demonstrated that the use of nonselective NSAIDs or COX-2 inhibitors was associated with a twofold or more increased risk of VTE [64].

Family History

Obtaining family history is a critical part of assessing risk for thrombosis. Epidemiologic studies have identified a relatively lower risk of VTE until approximately ages 45–55, at which point the incidence begins increasing sharp, particularly for those over 80 years of age [65]. One study showed that a positive family history (defined as first-degree relative with VTE and "strong" if at least one family member was affected before the age of 50 or multiple first-degree relatives affected) independently increased risk of VTE by more than twofold regardless of presence of acquired risk factors or known thrombophilia [66]. The risk increased if the family history was "strong." Additional studies have confirmed increased risk of VTE in first-degree relatives even if thrombophilia testing is negative [67, 68].

It is common practice to ask about family history of thrombotic events, particularly if these events happened in relatives under the ages of 45–55. However, additional studies are needed to delineate, if possible, contributors to the increase in risk with such a positive family history given a positive family history impacts medical care, particularly prescription of oral contraceptives [69] and use of VTE prophylaxis [70].

Lifestyle

Obesity

Obesity in adolescent females is becoming a more prevalent problem, and the incidence of VTE and obesity in children has been increasing in parallel over the last 20 years. A case-control study of pediatric inpatients demonstrated a doubling of the VTE risk in obese children (>95% BMI) compared to children with normal weight (BMI <85%) [71].

Central obesity is associated with increased intra-abdominal pressure and decreased venous return in the lower extremities promoting venostasis [72, 73]. This association with waist circumference was further evaluated in a study from Brazil that indicated the association with VTE was attenuated after adjustment for IL-6 levels, suggesting a potential role of this interleukin in mediating the link between abdominal obesity and VTE [74]. Obese individuals tend to have elevated levels of plasminogen activator inhibitor

[75], factor VII, factor VIII, fibrinogen, and von Willebrand factor [76], all of which increase the risk of thrombosis. In fact, a study from Stockholm demonstrated a correlation between obesity and thrombin generation in women, with increased levels of fibrinogen and prothrombin [77]. Other abnormalities associated with obesity presumed to contribute to the hypercoagulable state include a chronic low-grade inflammatory state, platelet activation, and endothelial dysfunction [78].

Obesity has also been associated with high fibrinogen levels and changes of the thrombin generation assay suggestive of hypercoagulability (shorter lag time, shorter time to peak, higher endogenous thrombin potential) [79]. Interestingly, these laboratory abnormalities resolved in the obese children whose weight returned to normal after lifestyle interventions [80]. Existence of a hypercoagulable state in an obese individual is evidenced by the presence of elevated factor VIII level, thrombin, and thrombin-antithrombin complexes, tissue factor procoagulant activity, fibrinogen concentration, and platelet activation [81, 82].

Obesity is an independent VTE risk factor and is commonly observed in association with hormonal contraceptive-associated VTE in adolescents [58]. More than 31% of children aged 2–19 years in the United States are considered overweight, almost 17% are considered obese, and these numbers continue to increase [83]. One single-institution pediatric study that involved 26 hormonal contraception (HC)-associated VTEs revealed that obesity was the most common additional VTE risk factor in women aged 12–21 years who developed a VTE. Obese women have twice the VTE risk of the general population, and obese women using HCs have up to a tenfold increased VTE risk compared with the general population [84]. Obesity is also associated with earlier onset of puberty, which could result in earlier use of HC agents [85]. It is difficult to truly understand the HC-associated VTE risk in all overweight and obese adolescents because women younger than 18 years of age are often excluded from HC studies.

The risks of all contraceptive methods are lower than the risks of pregnancy and the post-partum period for overweight and obese adolescents. The main concern with the use of estrogen-containing contraceptives in obese adolescents is the risk of venous thromboembolism (VTE) given that obesity is an independent risk factor for VTE [86]. However, VTE is an exceedingly rare event in children and adolescents, even among those with significant risk factors for clotting. For example, patients with hypercoagulable conditions do not typically present with a clot until after the age of 20 years [87]. The *US Medical Eligibility Criteria for Contraceptive Use* gives all contraceptives a classification of either "safe for use with no restrictions" (category 1) or "advantages generally outweigh theoretical or proven risks" (category 2) for obese adolescents from menarche to 18 years without other medical conditions [88].

Alcohol

By late adolescence, 78.2% of US adolescents had consumed alcohol, 47.1% had reached regular drinking levels defined by at least 12 drinks within a given year, and 15.1% met criteria for lifetime abuse [89], and the median age at onset was 14 years for alcohol abuse with or without dependence. A recent prospective, population-based cohort study from Sweden interestingly demonstrated that high alcohol consumption and alcohol dependence were associated with increased VTE risk in males, but not in females [90]. Another Swedish study demonstrated an increased risk of VTE in subjects with alcohol use disorders, even in the absence of alcohol-related somatic complications, but sex differences were not specifically explored [91]. A study from Taiwan revealed a strong media effect on alcohol use in adolescents [92], and another study from this country demonstrated an increased incidence of VTE of more than threefold observed among patients with heavy intake, after adjustment for age, sex, and comorbidities [93].

Smoking

Tobacco smoking is a well-established risk factor for atherosclerotic disease, but its role as an independent risk factor for VTE remains controversial. Further analysis from the UK's Million

Women Study demonstrated adjusted relative risk of VTE of 1.4 in smokers compared to non-smokers [94]. A recent meta-analysis corroborated this, demonstrating a relative VTE risk of just over 1.2 for current smokers compared to nonsmokers, and further showed that the risk increased by more than 10% for each additional ten cigarettes smoked each day [95]. Two recent additional studies confirmed that smoking does indeed increase VTE risk, but only if other risk factors are present. A Norwegian single-center, prospective, population-based, cohort trial demonstrated a higher VTE risk for heavy smokers compared with nonsmokers but only regarding provoked VTE [96]. The risk for VTE increases with the number of risk factors; smoking adds to the risk but only in conjunction with other established risk factors.

A pertinent contemporary consideration is the rise of electronic cigarettes (e-cigarettes), which are also associated with increased platelet activation and thrombosis. Typical users of e-cigarettes are between 14 and 30 years, and 56 percent of users are female. Due to the perception that these e-cigarettes are safer or less harmful than conventional cigarettes, their usage, particularly in the adolescent age group, has increased tremendously during the past decade. A recent study demonstrated that platelets from e-cigarette-exposed mice demonstrate a more reactive phenotype (hyperactive, with enhanced aggregation, dense and α-granule secretion, activation of the αIIbβ3 integrin, phosphatidylserine expression, and Akt and ERK activation), when compared with clean air-exposed platelets, and are also more resistant to inhibition by prostacyclin, findings which were also correlated with faster thrombus formation and shorter bleeding times [97].

Other Drugs

Drug use was reported by 42.5% of American adolescents and drug abuse by 16.4%, in a study that also reported the median age at onset was 14 years for drug abuse with dependence and 15 years for drug abuse without dependence [89]. The prevalence of previous VTE in users of opioids was 13.9% with an annual incidence rate of 3.2% (approximately 100-fold higher than the general population), and the risk was independently elevated by factors such as increasing age, female sex, sex-worker status, and intravenous drug delivery [98]. Similar to tobacco smoke in its traditional association with arterial thrombosis, cocaine has also been implicated in case reports of upper extremity deep vein thrombosis.

Conclusion/Summary

VTE is a rising concern for pediatrics and adolescents in particular. There are several established and emerging risk factors along with burgeoning evidence on the role of inflammation. One of the challenges of assessing risk for VTE in pediatrics remains the low quality of evidence, lack of prospective studies (particularly validation studies for RAMs), and overall lower incidence than VTE in adults. The Children's Hospital-Acquired Thrombosis (CHAT) Consortium aims to overcome many of these limitations via retrospective derivation of RAMs for pediatric VTE with prospective validation [11]. A focus on hospital-acquired thrombosis with efforts aimed at better risk prediction to inform potential prophylactic strategies coupled with education campaigns regarding risk associated with over-the-counter medications and lifestyle factors will significantly reduce the burden of this disease for adolescent females.

References

1. Raffini L, Huang YS, Witmer C, Feudtner C. Dramatic increase in venous thromboembolism in children's hospitals in the United States from 2001 to 2007. Pediatrics. 2009;124(4):1001–8.
2. Carpenter SL, Richardson T, Hall M. Increasing rate of pulmonary embolism diagnosed in hospitalized children in the United States from 2001 to 2014. Blood Adv. 2018;2(12):1403–8.
3. Goldenberg NA, Donadini MP, Kahn SR, Crowther M, Kenet G, Nowak-Gottl U, et al. Post-thrombotic syndrome in children: a systematic review of frequency of occurrence, validity of outcome measures, and prognostic factors. Haematologica. 2010;95(11):1952–9.
4. Journeycake JM, Manco-Johnson MJ. Thrombosis during infancy and childhood: what we know and

what we do not know. Hematol Oncol Clin North Am. 2004;18(6):1315–38, viii–ix.

5. Monagle P, Adams M, Mahoney M, Ali K, Barnard D, Bernstein M, et al. Outcome of pediatric thromboembolic disease: a report from the Canadian Childhood Thrombophilia Registry. Pediatr Res. 2000;47(6):763–6.

6. Takemoto CM, Sohi S, Desai K, Bharaj R, Khanna A, McFarland S, et al. Hospital-associated venous thromboembolism in children: incidence and clinical characteristics. J Pediatr. 2014;164(2):332–8.

7. Andrew M, David M, Adams M, Ali K, Anderson R, Barnard D, et al. Venous thromboembolic complications (VTE) in children: first analyses of the Canadian Registry of VTE. Blood. 1994;83(5):1251–7.

8. Stein PD, Kayali F, Olson RE. Incidence of venous thromboembolism in infants and children: data from the National Hospital Discharge Survey. J Pediatr. 2004;145(4):563–5.

9. van Ommen CH, Heijboer H, Buller HR, Hirasing RA, Heijmans HS, Peters M. Venous thromboembolism in childhood: a prospective two-year registry in The Netherlands. J Pediatr. 2001;139(5):676–81.

10. Hennessey CA, Patel VK, Tefera EA, Gomez-Lobo V. Venous thromboembolism in female adolescents: patient characteristics. J Pediatr Adolesc Gynecol. 2018;31(5):503–8.

11. Jaffray J, Mahajerin A, Young G, Goldenberg N, Ji L, Sposto R, et al. A multi-institutional registry of pediatric hospital-acquired thrombosis cases: the Children's Hospital-Acquired Thrombosis (CHAT) project. Thromb Res. 2018;161:67–72.

12. Sharathkumar AA, Mahajerin A, Heidt L, Doerfer K, Heiny M, Vik T, et al. Risk-prediction tool for identifying hospitalized children with a predisposition for development of venous thromboembolism: Peds-Clot clinical Decision Rule. J Thromb Haemost. 2012;10(7):1326–34.

13. Mahajerin A, Branchford BR, Amankwah EK, Raffini L, Chalmers E, van Ommen CH, et al. Hospital-associated venous thromboembolism in pediatrics: a systematic review and meta-analysis of risk factors and risk-assessment models. Haematologica. 2015;100(8):1045–50.

14. Arlikar SJ, Atchison CM, Amankwah EK, Ayala IA, Barrett LA, Branchford BR, et al. Development of a new risk score for hospital-associated venous thromboembolism in critically-ill children not undergoing cardiothoracic surgery. Thromb Res. 2015;136(4):717–22.

15. Sherrod BA, McClugage SG 3rd, Mortellaro VE, Aban IB, Rocque BG. Venous thromboembolism following inpatient pediatric surgery: analysis of 153,220 patients. J Pediatr Surg. 2019;54(4):631–9.

16. Murphy RF, Heyworth B, Kramer D, Naqvi M, Miller PE, Yen YM, et al. Symptomatic venous thromboembolism after adolescent knee arthroscopy. J Pediatr Orthop. 2019;39(3):125–9.

17. Massicotte MP, Dix D, Monagle P, Adams M, Andrew M. Central venous catheter related thrombo-sis in children: analysis of the Canadian Registry of Venous Thromboembolic Complications. J Pediatr. 1998;133(6):770–6.

18. Smitherman AB, Alexander T, Connelly M, Snavely AC, Weston BW, Liles EA, et al. The incidence of catheter-associated venous thrombosis in noncritically ill children. Hosp Pediatr. 2015;5(2):59–66.

19. Rickles FR. Mechanisms of cancer-induced thrombosis in cancer. Pathophysiol Haemost Thromb. 2006;35(1–2):103–10.

20. Goyal G, Bhatt VR. L-asparaginase and venous thromboembolism in acute lymphocytic leukemia. Future Oncol. 2015;11(17):2459–70.

21. Grace RF, Dahlberg SE, Neuberg D, Sallan SE, Connors JM, Neufeld EJ, et al. The frequency and management of asparaginase-related thrombosis in paediatric and adult patients with acute lymphoblastic leukaemia treated on Dana-Farber Cancer Institute consortium protocols. Br J Haematol. 2011;152(4):452–9.

22. Tuckuviene R, Ranta S, Albertsen BK, Andersson NG, Bendtsen MD, Frisk T, et al. Prospective study of thromboembolism in 1038 children with acute lymphoblastic leukemia: a Nordic Society of Pediatric Hematology and Oncology (NOPHO) study. J Thromb Haemost. 2016;14(3):485–94.

23. O'Brien SH, Klima J, Termuhlen AM, Kelleher KJ. Venous thromboembolism and adolescent and young adult oncology inpatients in US children's hospitals, 2001 to 2008. J Pediatr. 2011;159(1):133–7.

24. Paz-Priel I, Long L, Helman LJ, Mackall CL, Wayne AS. Thromboembolic events in children and young adults with pediatric sarcoma. J Clin Oncol. 2007;25(12):1519–24.

25. Branchford BR, Carpenter SL. The role of inflammation in venous thromboembolism. Front Pediatr. 2018;6:142.

26. Poredos P, Jezovnik MK. The role of inflammation in venous thromboembolism and the link between arterial and venous thrombosis. Int Angiol. 2007;26(4):306–11.

27. Matos MF, Lourenco DM, Orikaza CM, Bajerl JA, Noguti MA, Morelli VM. The role of IL-6, IL-8 and MCP-1 and their promoter polymorphisms IL-6 -174GC, IL-8 -251AT and MCP-1 -2518AG in the risk of venous thromboembolism: a case-control study. Thromb Res. 2011;128(3):216–20.

28. Mahemuti A, Abudureheman K, Aihemaiti X, Hu XM, Xia YN, Tang BP, et al. Association of interleukin-6 and C-reactive protein genetic polymorphisms levels with venous thromboembolism. Chin Med J. 2012;125(22):3997–4002.

29. Gao Q, Zhang P, Wang W, Ma H, Tong Y, Zhang J, et al. The correlation analysis of tumor necrosis factor-alpha-308G/A polymorphism and venous thromboembolism risk: a meta-analysis. Phlebology. 2016;31(9):625–31.

30. Folsom AR, Lutsey PL, Astor BC, Cushman M. C-reactive protein and venous thromboembo-

lism. A prospective investigation in the ARIC cohort. Thromb Haemost. 2009;102(4):615–9.

31. Saghazadeh A, Hafizi S, Rezaei N. Inflammation in venous thromboembolism: cause or consequence? Int Immunopharmacol. 2015;28(1):655–65.

32. Long AT, Kenne E, Jung R, Fuchs TA, Renne T. Contact system revisited: an interface between inflammation, coagulation, and innate immunity. J Thromb Haemost. 2016;14(3):427–37.

33. van Montfoort ML, Meijers JC. Recent insights into the role of the contact pathway in thrombo-inflammatory disorders. Hematology Am Soc Hematol Educ Program. 2014;2014(1):60–5.

34. Wu Y. Contact pathway of coagulation and inflammation. Thromb J. 2015;13:17.

35. Wakefield TW, Myers DD, Henke PK. Mechanisms of venous thrombosis and resolution. Arterioscler Thromb Vasc Biol. 2008;28(3):387–91.

36. Date K, Ettelaie C, Maraveyas A. Tissue factor-bearing microparticles and inflammation: a potential mechanism for the development of venous thromboembolism in cancer. J Thromb Haemost. 2017;15(12):2289–99.

37. Manly DA, Boles J, Mackman N. Role of tissue factor in venous thrombosis. Annu Rev Physiol. 2011;73:515–25.

38. Kroegel C, Reissig A. Principle mechanisms underlying venous thromboembolism: epidemiology, risk factors, pathophysiology and pathogenesis. Respiration. 2003;70(1):7–30.

39. Meissner MH, Wakefield TW, Ascher E, Caprini JA, Comerota AJ, Eklof B, et al. Acute venous disease: venous thrombosis and venous trauma. J Vasc Surg. 2007;46(Suppl S):25S–53S.

40. Bernard J, Yi ES. Pulmonary thromboendarterectomy: a clinicopathologic study of 200 consecutive pulmonary thromboendarterectomy cases in one institution. Hum Pathol. 2007;38(6):871–7.

41. Cheng KB, Wang LM, Gao HJ, Hu Y. An study on screening the gene clusters associated with pulmonary embolism-deep venous thrombosis by oligo microarray. Zhonghua Yi Xue Za Zhi. 2007;87(34):2420–2.

42. Choi SH, Smith SA, Morrissey JH. Polyphosphate accelerates factor V activation by factor XIa. Thromb Haemost. 2015;113(3):599–604.

43. Docampo R. Polyphosphate: a target for thrombosis attenuation. Blood. 2014;124(22):3177–8.

44. Morrissey JH, Choi SH, Smith SA. Polyphosphate: an ancient molecule that links platelets, coagulation, and inflammation. Blood. 2012;119(25):5972–9.

45. Travers RJ, Smith SA, Morrissey JH. Polyphosphate, platelets, and coagulation. Int J Lab Hematol. 2015;37(Suppl 1):31–5.

46. Fuchs TA, Brill A, Wagner DD. Neutrophil extracellular trap (NET) impact on deep vein thrombosis. Arterioscler Thromb Vasc Biol. 2012;32(8):1777–83.

47. Esmon CT, Xu J, Lupu F. Innate immunity and coagulation. J Thromb Haemost. 2011;9(Suppl 1):182–8.

48. Petty JK. Venous thromboembolism prophylaxis in the pediatric trauma patient. Semin Pediatr Surg. 2017;26(1):14–20.

49. O'Brien SH, Klima J, Gaines BA, Betz S, Zenati MS. Utilization of low-molecular-weight heparin prophylaxis in pediatric and adolescent trauma patients. J Trauma Nurs. 2012;19(2):117–21.

50. Connelly CR, Laird A, Barton JS, Fischer PE, Krishnaswami S, Schreiber MA, et al. A clinical tool for the prediction of venous thromboembolism in pediatric trauma patients. JAMA Surg. 2016;151(1):50–7.

51. Yen J, Van Arendonk KJ, Streiff MB, McNamara L, Stewart FD, Conner KG, et al. Risk factors for venous thromboembolism in pediatric trauma patients and validation of a novel scoring system: the risk of clots in kids with trauma score. Pediatr Crit Care Med. 2016;17(5):391–9.

52. Palmer C. Major trauma and the injury severity score–where should we set the bar? Annu Proc Assoc Adv Automot Med. 2007;51:13–29.

53. Cyr C, Michon B, Pettersen G, David M, Brossard J. Venous thromboembolism after severe injury in children. Acta Haematol. 2006;115(3–4):198–200.

54. Mahajerin A, Petty JK, Hanson SJ, Thompson AJ, O'Brien SH, Streck CJ, et al. Prophylaxis against venous thromboembolism in pediatric trauma: a practice management guideline from the Eastern Association for the Surgery of Trauma and the Pediatric Trauma Society. J Trauma Acute Care Surg. 2017;82(3):627–36.

55. Moore HB, Moore EE, Liras IN, Gonzalez E, Harvin JA, Holcomb JB, et al. Acute fibrinolysis shutdown after injury occurs frequently and increases mortality: a multicenter evaluation of 2,540 severely injured patients. J Am Coll Surg. 2016;222(4):347–55.

56. Westhoff CL, Eisenberger A, Tang R, Cremers S, Grossman LV, Pike MC. Clotting factor changes during the first cycle of oral contraceptive use. Contraception. 2016;93(1):70–6.

57. Tans G, Bouma BN, Buller HR, Rosing J. Changes of hemostatic variables during oral contraceptive use. Semin Vasc Med. 2003;3(1):61–8.

58. Pillai P, Bonny AE, O'Brien SH. Contraception-related venous thromboembolism in a pediatric institution. J Pediatr Adolesc Gynecol. 2013;26(3):186–8.

59. Parkin L, Balkwill A, Sweetland S, Reeves GK, Green J, Beral V, et al. Antidepressants, depression, and venous thromboembolism risk: large prospective study of UK women. J Am Heart Assoc. 2017;6(5):e005316.

60. Kunutsor SK, Seidu S, Khunti K. Depression, antidepressant use, and risk of venous thromboembolism: systematic review and meta-analysis of published observational evidence. Ann Med. 2018;50(6):529–37.

61. Hunter R, Noble S, Lewis S, Bennett P. Long-term psychosocial impact of venous thromboembolism: a qualitative study in the community. BMJ Open. 2019;9(2):e024805.

62. Bergendal A, Adami J, Bahmanyar S, Hedenmalm K, Larfars G, Persson I, et al. Non-steroidal anti-inflammatory drugs and venous thromboembolism in women. Pharmacoepidemiol Drug Saf. 2013;22(6):658–66.

63. Ungprasert P, Srivali N, Wijarnpreecha K, Charoenpong P, Knight EL. Non-steroidal anti-inflammatory drugs and risk of venous thromboembolism: a systematic review and meta-analysis. Rheumatology (Oxford). 2015;54(4):736–42.

64. Schmidt M, Christiansen CF, Horvath-Puho E, Glynn RJ, Rothman KJ, Sorensen HT. Non-steroidal anti-inflammatory drug use and risk of venous thromboembolism. J Thromb Haemost. 2011;9(7):1326–33.

65. Cushman M. Epidemiology and risk factors for venous thrombosis. Semin Hematol. 2007;44(2):62–9.

66. Bezemer ID, van der Meer FJ, Eikenboom JC, Rosendaal FR, Doggen CJ. The value of family history as a risk indicator for venous thrombosis. Arch Intern Med. 2009;169(6):610–5.

67. Couturaud F, Leroyer C, Julian JA, Kahn SR, Ginsberg JS, Wells PS, et al. Factors that predict risk of thrombosis in relatives of patients with unprovoked venous thromboembolism. Chest. 2009;136(6):1537–45.

68. Sørensen HT, Riis AH, Diaz LJ, Andersen EW, Baron JA, Andersen PK. Familial risk of venous thromboembolism: a nationwide cohort study. J Thromb Haemost. 2011;9(2):320–4.

69. Zöller B, Ohlsson H, Sundquist J, Sundquist K. Family history of venous thromboembolism is a risk factor for venous thromboembolism in combined oral contraceptive users: a nationwide case-control study. Thromb J. 2015;13:34.

70. Calhoon MJ, Ross CN, Pounder E, Cassidy D, Manco-Johnson MJ, Goldenberg NA. High prevalence of thrombophilic traits in children with family history of thromboembolism. J Pediatr. 2010;157(3):485–9.

71. Stokes S, Breheny P, Radulescu A, Radulescu VC. Impact of obesity on the risk of venous thromboembolism in an inpatient pediatric population. Pediatr Hematol Oncol. 2014;31(5):475–80.

72. Willenberg T, Schumacher A, Amann-Vesti B, Jacomella V, Thalhammer C, Diehm N, et al. Impact of obesity on venous hemodynamics of the lower limbs. J Vasc Surg. 2010;52(3):664–8.

73. van Rij AM, De Alwis CS, Jiang P, Christie RA, Hill GB, Dutton SJ, et al. Obesity and impaired venous function. Eur J Vasc Endovasc Surg. 2008;35(6):739–44.

74. Matos MF, Lourenco DM, Orikaza CM, Gouveia CP, Morelli VM. Abdominal obesity and the risk of venous thromboembolism among women: a potential role of interleukin-6. Metab Syndr Relat Disord. 2013;11(1):29–34.

75. Alessi MC, Juhan-Vague I. PAI-1 and the metabolic syndrome: links, causes, and consequences. Arterioscler Thromb Vasc Biol. 2006;26(10):2200–7.

76. Steffen LM, Cushman M, Peacock JM, Heckbert SR, Jacobs DR Jr, Rosamond WD, et al. Metabolic syndrome and risk of venous thromboembolism: longitudinal investigation of thromboembolism etiology. J Thromb Haemost. 2009;7(5):746–51.

77. Sonnevi K, Tchaikovski SN, Holmstrom M, Antovic JP, Bremme K, Rosing J, et al. Obesity and thrombin-generation profiles in women with venous thromboembolism. Blood Coagul Fibrinolysis. 2013;24(5):547–53.

78. Darvall KA, Sam RC, Silverman SH, Bradbury AW, Adam DJ. Obesity and thrombosis. Eur J Vasc Endovasc Surg. 2007;33(2):223–33.

79. Fritsch P, Kleber M, Rosenkranz A, Fritsch M, Muntean W, Mangge H, et al. Haemostatic alterations in overweight children: associations between metabolic syndrome, thrombin generation, and fibrinogen levels. Atherosclerosis. 2010;212(2):650–5.

80. Fritsch P, Kleber M, Schlagenhauf A, Laschnik B, Fritsch M, Muntean W, et al. Normalization of haemostatic alterations in overweight children with weight loss due to lifestyle intervention. Atherosclerosis. 2011;216(1):170–3.

81. Samad F, Ruf W. Inflammation, obesity, and thrombosis. Blood. 2013;122(20):3415–22.

82. Lovely R, Hossain J, Ramsey JP, Komakula V, George D, Farrell DH, et al. Obesity-related increased gamma' fibrinogen concentration in children and its reduction by a physical activity-based lifestyle intervention: a randomized controlled study. J Pediatr. 2013;163(2):333–8.

83. Ogden CL, Carroll MD, Kit BK, Flegal KM. Prevalence of obesity in the United States, 2009–2010. NCHS Data Brief. 2012;82:1–8.

84. Murthy AS. Obesity and contraception: emerging issues. Semin Reprod Med. 2010;28(2):156–63.

85. Anderson SE, Dallal GE, Must A. Relative weight and race influence average age at menarche: results from two nationally representative surveys of US girls studied 25 years apart. Pediatrics. 2003;111(4 Pt 1):844–50.

86. Abdollahi M, Cushman M, Rosendaal FR. Obesity: risk of venous thrombosis and the interaction with coagulation factor levels and oral contraceptive use. Thromb Haemost. 2003;89(3):493–8.

87. Lensen RP, Rosendaal FR, Koster T, Allaart CF, de Ronde H, Vandenbroucke JP, et al. Apparent different thrombotic tendency in patients with factor V Leiden and protein C deficiency due to selection of patients. Blood. 1996;88(11):4205–8.

88. Curtis KM, Tepper NK, Jatlaoui TC, Berry-Bibee E, Horton LG, Zapata LB, et al. U.S. medical eligibility criteria for contraceptive use, 2016. MMWR Recomm Rep. 2016;65(3):1–103.

89. Swendsen J, Burstein M, Case B, Conway KP, Dierker L, He J, et al. Use and abuse of alcohol and illicit drugs in US adolescents: results of the National Comorbidity Survey-Adolescent Supplement. Arch Gen Psychiatry. 2012;69(4):390–8.

90. Johansson M, Johansson L, Wennberg M, Lind M. Alcohol consumption and risk of first-time venous thromboembolism in men and women. Thromb Haemost. 2019;119(6):962–70.

91. Zoller B, Ji J, Sundquist J, Sundquist K. Alcohol use disorders are associated with venous thromboembolism. J Thromb Thrombolysis. 2015;40(2):167–73.

92. Chen CY, Huang HY, Tseng FY, Chiu YC, Chen WJ. Media alcohol advertising with drinking behav-

iors among young adolescents in Taiwan. Drug Alcohol Depend. 2017;177:145–52.

93. Shen CJ, Kao CH, Hsu TY, Chen CY, Lin CL, Shih HM. Effect of alcohol intoxication on the risk of venous thromboembolism: a nationwide retrospective cohort study. Medicine (Baltimore). 2017;96(42):e8041.

94. Sweetland S, Parkin L, Balkwill A, Green J, Reeves G, Beral V, et al. Smoking, surgery, and venous thromboembolism risk in women: United Kingdom cohort study. Circulation. 2013;127(12):1276–82.

95. Cheng YJ, Liu ZH, Yao FJ, Zeng WT, Zheng DD, Dong YG, et al. Current and former smoking and risk for venous thromboembolism: a systematic review and meta-analysis. PLoS Med. 2013;10(9):e1001515.

96. Enga KF, Braekkan SK, Hansen-Krone IJ, le Cessie S, Rosendaal FR, Hansen JB. Cigarette smoking and the risk of venous thromboembolism: the Tromso Study. J Thromb Haemost. 2012;10(10):2068–74.

97. Qasim H, Karim ZA, Silva-Espinoza JC, Khasawneh FT, Rivera JO, Ellis CC, et al. Short-term E-cigarette exposure increases the risk of thrombogenesis and enhances platelet function in mice. J Am Heart Assoc. 2018;7(15):e009264.

98. Cornford CS, Mason JM, Inns F. Deep vein thromboses in users of opioid drugs: incidence, prevalence, and risk factors. Br J Gen Pract. 2011;61(593):e781–6.

Diagnosis, Prevention, and Management of Venous Thromboembolism in the Adolescent Female

14

Lauren E. Amos, Mukta Sharma, and Shannon L. Carpenter

Diagnosis

The hemostatic system is designed to regulate vessel patency and integrity. This process is achieved by maintaining balance between pro- and anticoagulant factors. When this balance is shifted by factors well-described in Virchow's triad of endothelial damage, venous stasis, and hypercoagulability, thrombosis can occur [1]. Clinical presentation of VTE is dependent on location of thrombosis [2]. Symptoms are a result of venous hypertension which develops from the thrombus obstructing venous outflow [3]. Risk factors for the development of VTE in adolescents have been previously discussed (see Chap. 13).

Presentation, Laboratory Evaluation, and Diagnostic Imaging Modalities

Presentation and Imaging

Venous thrombosis of the extremities is classified by either superficial or deep vessel involvement. Superficial venous thrombosis can occur in any vascular location but typically presents in the upper or lower extremities. Upper extremity superficial venous thrombosis is often caused by venipuncture, intravenous catheter placement or infusions, or trauma [4]. Presenting symptoms include a palpable cord, pain, and erythema at the site of the thrombosed superficial vessel [5]. Venous ultrasound with Doppler is typically used to confirm the diagnosis and exclude deep vessel involvement.

Acute deep venous thrombosis (DVT) of the extremities is the most common location of thrombosis in adolescents. It often presents with swelling, erythema, warmth, and pain of the affected limb. If the DVT is associated with a central venous catheter (CVC), the presenting symptom may be catheter malfunction [3]. For patients with upper extremity DVT, extension can occur into the superior vena cava (SVC) and cause SVC syndrome which is associated with swelling and erythema of the neck and face and can be a medical emergency. Patients with chronic DVTs may present with vascular prominence, edema,

L. E. Amos (✉)
Division of Hematology/Oncology/BMT, Children's Mercy Kansas City, Kansas City, MO, USA
e-mail: lamos@cmh.edu

M. Sharma · S. L. Carpenter
University of Missouri Kansas City, Kansas City, MO, USA

© Springer Nature Switzerland AG 2020
L. V. Srivaths (ed.), *Hematology in the Adolescent Female*,
https://doi.org/10.1007/978-3-030-48446-0_14

pain, or rarely even skin ulceration [2]. Venous ultrasound with Doppler is the preferred imaging modality to confirm an extremity DVT [1].

Although pulmonary embolism (PE) is rare in children, it may occur more frequently in adolescent females than any other pediatric age group [6]. PE in adolescent females may have a more subtle presentation than in adults. In addition, physicians may have a lower diagnostic suspicion for PE in younger adolescents leading to lack of recognition and increased mortality [7]. Symptoms may include pleuritic chest pain, dyspnea, and cough [8]. Patients may also have an associated extremity DVT most commonly located in the lower extremity with the signs and symptoms listed above. Depending on the extent and location of the PE, vital sign instability with fever, tachycardia, tachypnea, hypoxia, and hypotension may be present. Historically, ventilation/perfusion (V/Q) scans were considered the standard to diagnose PE. However, computed tomography (CT) pulmonary angiography is now commonly used for first-line imaging in the pediatric population due to its increased diagnostic sensitivity, comparable radiation dose, and shorter time to diagnosis [9]. Chest x-ray is unlikely to be helpful in the diagnosis of PE. Alternative diagnostic methods include echocardiogram, cardiac angiography, and conventional angiography, but these are rarely used in the initial evaluation of PE [7]. Once a PE is diagnosed, electrocardiogram and echocardiogram may be used to determine the severity of the PE by revealing right heart strain or decreased cardiac output.

Cerebral sinus venous thrombosis (CSVT) refers to thrombus formation in either the superficial venous system, deep venous structures, or dural venous sinuses in the brain [10]. CSVT tends to occur more frequently in neonates and younger children, but also presents in adolescence. Risk factors for CSVT are age dependent [11]. When CSVT occurs in healthy young adults, it is often the result of head and neck infections such as sinusitis and mastoiditis, dehydration, prothrombotic states, or head trauma. CSVT in adolescents is also associated with chronic diseases such as leukemia especially after treatment with L-asparaginase,

congenital heart disease, inflammatory bowel disease, autoimmune diseases such as systemic lupus erythematosus, and nephrotic syndrome [12]. Clinical signs and symptoms of CSVT depend on the location and extent of the thrombus and may include headache, vomiting, altered consciousness, focal neurologic deficits such as cranial nerve palsies, and seizures [13]. Seizures are the most common presenting symptom in all pediatric age groups. Prompt diagnosis and treatment are important in CSVT as delayed diagnosis can lead to adverse neurologic outcomes and death [10]. Imaging to diagnose CSVT includes CT venography and magnetic resonance (MR) venography. CT venography allows for a more rapid diagnosis but has the disadvantage of exposure to contrast and ionizing radiation. MR venography imaging may be less accessible and take longer to obtain but is considered the most sensitive imaging modality. Conventional angiography is rarely used due to the ability to diagnose CSVT with CT or MR venography but can be useful if those imaging techniques fail to give a definitive diagnosis.

Laboratory Evaluation

Initial laboratory testing is not likely to be helpful in establishing a diagnosis of VTE in adolescent females. In adults, D-dimer assays have demonstrated high sensitivity and negative predictive value and are useful in ruling out VTE [14]. The role of D-dimer in pediatric and adolescent patients is less clear and may be sensitive but less specific as compared to adults [15]. Laboratory evaluation should be undertaken after the diagnosis of VTE is established in order to determine bleeding risk and end-organ function prior to initiation of anticoagulation therapy. These laboratory tests include complete blood count (CBC), basic metabolic panel, liver function tests, prothrombin time (PT), activated partial thromboplastin time (PTT), and fibrinogen [8]. The decision to obtain testing and recommended laboratory evaluation for inherited and acquired thrombophilias has been discussed elsewhere (see Chap. 15).

Acute Treatment of VTE

Acute management of VTE is tailored to the individual patient. Physicians must determine the clinical stability of the patient, need for possible urgent or emergent invasive procedures, and presence of bleeding or bleeding risk in order to select anticoagulation therapy. Anticoagulation should be initiated if the risk associated with the thrombotic event is greater than the bleeding risk [16]. The therapeutic goals of anticoagulation are to decrease VTE propagation and recurrence risk, decrease embolization, and decrease long-term complications such as venous insufficiency and post-thrombotic syndrome (PTS) [2].

Thrombolysis

Thrombolytic therapy is indicated for life- or limb-threatening VTE such as massive PE with cardiovascular instability, obstructive SVC syndrome, acute iliofemoral thrombosis with decreased limb perfusion, and CSVT with neurologic deterioration [16, 17]. In adolescent patients, recombinant tissue-type plasminogen activator (tPA) is used most frequently when thrombolysis is indicated. As indicated by its name, tPA activates plasminogen which increases fibrinolysis by converting plasminogen to plasmin [18]. Standard contraindications to giving tPA have been established, and tPA is not typically used if those contraindications are present (Table 14.1).

Thrombolysis is administered either systemically using an intravenous infusion or via an

Table 14.1 Major contraindications to tPA administration: International Society of Thrombosis and Hemostasis Guidelines [17]

Major surgery or hemorrhage within 10 days of therapy
Severe asphyxial event within 7 days of therapy
Seizures within 48 hours of therapy
Prematurity <32 weeks' gestation
Severe sepsis
Active bleeding at the time of therapy
Inability to maintain platelets >50–100,000/μL or fibrinogen >100 mg/dL despite transfusion support

endovascular catheter in a site-directed approach [19]. Regardless of approach, unfractionated heparin (UFH) should be infused intravenously at a low dose of 5–10 units/kg/hr, while the tPA is given in order to prevent new thrombus formation. Systemic tPA is given using either a low-dose regimen of 0.03 mg/kg to 0.06 mg/kg per hour for 6–72 hours or a high-dose regimen of 0.1–0.5 mg/kg per hour for 6 hours with maximum dosing of 2 mg/hour for either regimen. Site-directed thrombolysis is given with an initial bolus tPA dose of 0.1–0.3 mg/kg (maximum dose of 10 mg) followed by 0.01–0.03 mg/kg/hour for up to 72–96 hours with maximum dose of 1–2 mg/hour [20]. Laboratory monitoring with CBC, PT, aPTT, fibrinogen, and D-dimer should be performed at regular intervals during the tPA infusion. Platelet count should be maintained above 100,000/μL and fibrinogen above 100 mg/dL [21]. TPA is metabolized by the liver and has a very short half-life of approximately 5 minutes [18]. As the risk of major bleeding is estimated at up to 15% and minor bleeding at 50%, tPA should only be given under supervision of a hematologist. Efficacy rates as defined by full resolution of the thrombus are reported at 79% for systemic tPA and 76% for site-directed tPA [19].

Clinically Unstable Patients

For patients who do not meet criteria for thrombolysis but are critically ill, may require emergent or invasive procedures, or have an increased bleeding risk, choice of initial anticoagulant is determined based upon individual patient characteristics [22]. The agents most frequently used in these situations are unfractionated heparin (UFH) or direct thrombin inhibitors such as bivalirudin or argatroban due to intravenous administration and shorter half-life as compared to other anticoagulants [23].

Unfractionated Heparin

Unfractionated heparin is widely considered the first-line anticoagulant for critically ill adolescents [2]. UFH primarily exerts its anti-coagulant effect by potentiating antithrombin which inactivates factor Xa and thrombin. For therapeutic anticoagulation, it is administered via a continuous intravenous infusion. The half-life of UFH ranges from 30 to 60 minutes. UFH can be monitored using the activated PTT (aPTT) or anti-activated factor X activity (anti-Xa) [1]. UFH offers the advantages of significant clinical experience in the pediatric population, minimal renal clearance, and its ability to be fully reversed by protamine sulfate. Disadvantages of heparin include its dependence on circulating antithrombin to exert therapeutic effect and unreliable pharmacokinetics making dosing and therapeutic stability difficult in some patients [2]. Adverse effects of UFH include bleeding and heparin-induced thrombocytopenia (HIT). HIT occurs due to the development of antibodies against the heparin and platelet factor 4 complex on the platelet surface. HIT occurs rarely in pediatric patients including adolescents but should be considered if a patient on heparin develops new-onset thrombocytopenia [24].

Direct Thrombin Inhibitors

Direct thrombin inhibitors (DTIs) such as argatroban and bivalirudin are safe and effective alternatives to UFH in critically ill adolescent patients or patients with HIT or heparin resistance. DTIs are not antithrombin dependent and achieve therapeutic anticoagulation rapidly and more consistently than UFH. Argatroban and bivalirudin have been studied in pediatric patients and have established dosing and monitoring parameters [25, 26]. Both are parenterally administered and monitored using the activated PTT. Argatroban is hepatically excreted and has a half-life of 39–51 minutes [27]. Bivalirudin is primarily cleared by proteolysis in the blood with 20% renal clearance [28]. The major adverse effect of DTIs is bleeding. Currently, no reversal agents are available for argatroban or bivalirudin [29].

Clinically Stable Patients

Low Molecular Weight Heparin

Low molecular weight heparin (LMWH) is fractionated from UFH and predominantly exerts anticoagulant effect by inhibition of factor Xa [30]. LMWH is administered by subcutaneous injection every 12 hours and is advantageous compared to UFH due to more stable pharmacokinetics, less frequent therapeutic monitoring, and ability to be given as an outpatient [23]. Due to differences in pediatric metabolism, therapeutic drug monitoring is recommended using the anti-Xa assay [31]. Enoxaparin is the most frequently used LMWH in adolescent patients [32]. Due to its longer half-life of 4.5–7 hours and ability to be only partially reversed by protamine, LMWH is used for initial anticoagulation in patients who are not critically ill. In addition, LMWH is largely renally cleared, so is not an appropriate choice for adolescents with acute kidney injury or renal failure. Bleeding and injection site reactions are the most common side effects of LMWH [33].

Vitamin K Antagonists

Vitamin K antagonists (VKA) have historically been the only oral anticoagulant available for use in adolescent patients. Warfarin is the VKA most frequently used in these patients. Warfarin inhibits vitamin K epoxide reductase causing depletion of reduced vitamin K which is a cofactor for the γ carboxylation of the vitamin K-dependent factors II, VII, IX, and X and proteins C and S [34]. Warfarin is hepatically metabolized and has a half-life of 35–40 hours. It offers the advantages of once-daily dosing and is available as a tablet. Significant disadvantages include its narrow therapeutic window which is affected by genetic polymorphisms in the genes CYP2C9 and VKORC1, dietary intake of vitamin K, and drug interactions which can lead to supratherapeutic levels and major bleeding [2]. Warfarin is monitored by using the internationalized normalized ratio (INR) [3]. Warfarin can be reversed by using vitamin K, prothrombin complex concentrate, or fresh frozen plasma. The most common adverse events are bleeding and rarely skin necrosis or osteoporosis [34]. Due to warfarin's inhibition of proteins C and S, an additional anticoagulant such as UFH or LMWH must be started with initiation of warfarin and continued for at least 5 days until warfarin is therapeutic [3] (Table 14.2).

Direct Oral Anticoagulants

Direct oral anticoagulants (DOACs) are FDA approved and used frequently as first-line therapy for anticoagulation in adults with VTE [35]. Two pharmacologic classes of DOACs exist. There are direct factor Xa inhibitors such as rivaroxaban and apixaban and the direct thrombin inhibitor dabigatran. These drugs offer numerous advantages for adolescent patients including oral administration, no food or drug interactions, stable and predictable pharmacokinetics allowing for no therapeutic drug monitoring, and increased therapeutic window with potentially less bleeding risk as compared to conventional anticoagulation [36]. Adult data has shown limitations to DOAC use in certain patient populations such as prosthetic or mechanical valves and anti-phospholipid antibody syndrome due to increased thrombotic and bleeding risks [37, 38]. DOACs should not be used in patients with severe renal or hepatic failure [36]. FDA-approved reversal agents for DOACs include idarucizumab for dabigatran and andexanet alfa for rivaroxaban and apixaban [39].

Duration of Anticoagulation

Duration of anticoagulation therapy in adolescents is primarily based upon adult evidence and depends on whether the VTE was provoked by an identified risk factor [1]. The 2012 American College of Chest Physicians pediatric guidelines recommend initial anticoagulation therapy for unprovoked VTE for a duration of 6–12 months. For patients with a provoked VTE in whom the risk factor contributing to VTE development has resolved, a duration of 3 months of treatment with anticoagulation is recommended. For patients with ongoing risk factors, treatment is recommended beyond 3 months until the risk factor resolves. Repeat imaging of the VTE is typically done at 3 months and, if VTE still present, at the end of therapy [16, 40].

VTE and Thrombophilia

For an adolescent female with acute VTE in whom an underlying thrombophilia is identified, the initial management is the same as discussed above. The decision to extend the duration of anticoagulation therapy is multi-factorial and depends on risk of VTE recurrence and risk of bleeding [41]. Patients with two or more inherited thrombophilias are at highest risk for recurrent VTE, and most clinicians recommend treating these patients with lifelong anticoagulation. Antithrombin

Table 14.2 Summary of adolescent anticoagulants [3, 29]

Anticoagulant	Route of administration and dosing	Therapeutic monitoring	Half-life	Reversal agent
UFH	IV 28 units/kg/hr (age <1 year) 20 units/kg/hr (age ≥1 year)	aPTT or anti-Xa level	30 minutes	Protamine sulfate
Argatroban	IV 0.75 mcg/kg/min	aPTT	40 minutes	No
Bivalirudin	IV 0.25–0.5 mg/kg/hr	aPTT	25 minutes	No
Enoxaparin	Subcutaneous 1.5 mg/kg/dose (age <2 months) q 12 hours 1 mg/kg/dose (age ≥2 months) q 12 hours	Anti-Xa level	6 hours	Partially reversed by protamine sulfate
Warfarin	Oral 0.1 mg/kg/day	INR	36–40 hours	Vitamin K or prothrombin complex concentrates

deficiency, protein C deficiency, and protein S deficiency are considered high-risk thrombophilias. Patients with these conditions have the next highest recurrence risk after patients with two inherited thrombophilias and are also often managed with lifelong anticoagulation. For patients with lower-risk thrombophilias such as Factor V Leiden or Prothrombin gene 20210A mutations, decision to extend anticoagulation is made on an individual patient basis [23, 42].

Anti-phospholipid Antibody Syndrome

Current management of adolescent patients with VTE and anti-phospholipid antibody syndrome (APS) is largely based upon adult guidelines [43]. However, key differences exist between pediatric and adult patients with APS. Patients less than 18 years of age with APS are most likely to have a lower extremity DVT as their initial thrombotic event [44]. These patients are also at increased risk of recurrent VTE as compared to adults with APS [45]. 2017 European guidelines recommend chronic anticoagulation for pediatric and adolescent patients with APS and VTE [46]. This is consistent with management of VTE in adult patients with APS and VTE who are treated with indefinite anticoagulation. In adult patients with triple positive APS and VTE, use of rivaroxaban as compared to warfarin resulted in increased thrombotic and bleeding events [38]. Traditionally, adolescents with APS are treated with warfarin or LMWH [43].

Challenges of Anticoagulation in Adolescent Females

Ensuring adherence to therapeutic anticoagulation in adolescent patients can be very difficult. Teenagers may be resistant to anticoagulation due to activity limitations such as contact sports due to bleeding risk and interruption in daily life due to medication administration, lab monitoring, and physician appointments [43]. Adolescents represent a unique developmental group as they are struggling to achieve autonomy and may resent medication therapy especially involving injections and lab draws, leading to non-adherence [47]. Adolescent females may also experience heavy menstrual bleeding while on therapeutic anticoagulation which negatively impacts their quality of life and contributes to non-adherence [48]. Understanding these challenges is imperative for physicians treating adolescent females for VTE with either acute or potentially lifelong anticoagulation.

VTE Sequelae

Recurrent VTE

Adolescents have been shown to have the highest VTE recurrence rate among pediatric patients [32]. Overall recurrence for pediatric VTE is estimated at 7.5–21% with adolescent recurrence as high as 37% [3, 32, 40]. Patients with a recurrent, unprovoked VTE are treated with indefinite anticoagulation. Patients with a recurrent VTE with a reversible risk factor are treated with anticoagulation until the risk factor is no longer present [16]. Examples of this would be continuing therapeutic anticoagulation in patients with a VTE and CVC until catheter removal or with VTE and active malignancy.

Post-thrombotic Syndrome

Post-thrombotic syndrome (PTS) develops due to chronic venous insufficiency after VTE occurrence and is the most common chronic complication of VTE in adolescents [49]. Incidence of PTS in children and adolescents ranges widely from 3% to 70% of patients. Patients at increased risk for PTS development include those with recurrent VTE, persistence or extension of VTE after 3–6 months of treatment, and multiple vessels involved by the VTE [3]. Adolescents also have a higher risk due to age as compared to younger children [49]. Clinical signs and symptoms of PTS include pain, swelling, numbness or tingling, increased limb circumference, pitting edema, venous stasis dermatitis, and, in severe cases, skin ulceration [3, 50]. The two instruments used most commonly in pediatrics to assess for PTS are the Manco-Johnson Instrument and the modified Villalta score [50]. PTS is not diagnosed until 6 months after VTE occurrence to allow for acute symptoms to subside [51]. Unfortunately, there are no effective strategies in pediatrics to prevent or treat PTS. Compression stockings are used as some data has shown efficacy in managing PTS in adult patients [50].

VTE Prevention

VTE prevention in hospitalized adolescent females focuses on identifying patients at risk for VTE and instituting appropriate thromboprophylaxis. As these patients are at higher risk of VTE due to age alone, presence of additional risk factors should prompt consideration of mechanical thromboprophylaxis such as sequential compression devices or pharmacologic prophylaxis with LMWH [52]. Evidence-based guidelines regarding pharmacologic thromboprophylaxis in adolescents are lacking [53]. Despite standardized guidelines, certain adolescent patient populations should be considered for pharmacologic prophylaxis. This includes patients hospitalized due to trauma or post-operatively with limited mobility [54]. Patients with chronic medical conditions such as complex congenital heart disease, cardiac failure, inflammatory bowel disease, total parenteral nutrition dependence, cystic fibrosis, autoimmune disease, nephrotic syndrome, and active malignancy are also at high risk of VTE while hospitalized and may benefit from pharmacologic prophylaxis depending on bleeding risk [53, 55, 56]. Patients with history of CVC-associated VTE should be considered for chemical prophylaxis if new risk factors develop such as hospitalization with limited mobility or placement of a new CVC [52]. In patients where pharmacologic prophylaxis is contraindicated, use of mechanical prophylaxis should be implemented.

References

1. Radulescu VC. Management of venous thrombosis in the pediatric patient. Pediatr Health Med Ther. 2015;6:111–9.
2. Betensky M, Bittles MA, Colombani (Monagle), et al. How we manage pediatric deep venous thrombosis. Semin Intervent Radiol. 2017;34:35–49.
3. Jaffray J, Young G. Deep vein thrombosis in pediatric patients. Pediatr Blood Cancer. 2017;65:e26881.
4. Beyer-Westendorf J. Controversies in venous thromboembolism: to treat or not to treat superficial venous thrombosis. Hematology Am Soc Hematol Educ Program. 2017;1:223–30.
5. Scott G, Mahdi AJ, Alikhan R. Superficial vein thrombosis: a current approach to management. Br Jr Hematol. 2015;168:639–45.
6. Carpenter SL, Richardson T, Hall M. Increasing rate of pulmonary embolism diagnosed in hospitalized children in the United States from 2001 to 2014. Blood Adv. 2018;2:1403–8.
7. Biss TT, Brandao LR, Kahr WH, et al. Clinical features and outcome of pulmonary embolism in children. Br Jr Hematol. 2008;142:808–18.
8. Zaidi AU, Hutchins KK, Rajpurkar M. Pulmonary embolism in children. Front Pediatr. 2017;5:170.
9. Victoria T, Mong A, Altes T, et al. Evaluation of pulmonary embolism in a pediatric population with high clinical suspicion. Pediatr Radiol. 2008;39:35–41.
10. Hedlund GL. Cerebral sinovenous thrombosis in pediatric practice. Pediatr Radiol. 2013;43:173–88.
11. DeVeber G, Andrew M, Adams C, et al. Cerebral sinovenous thrombosis in children. N Engl J Med. 2001;345:417–23.
12. Ichord R. Cerebral sinovenous thrombosis. Front Ped. 2017;5:1–7.
13. Ichord RN, Benedict SL, Chan AK, et al. Paediatric cerebral sinovenous thrombosis: findings of the International Paediatric Stoke Study. Arch Dis Child. 2014;100:1174–9.
14. Prisco D, Grifoni E. The role of D-dimer testing in patients with suspected venous thromboembolism. Semin Thromb Hemost. 2009;35:50 9.
15. Strouse JJ, Tamma P, Kickler TS, et al. D-Dimer for the diagnosis of venous thromboembolism in children. Am J Hematol. 2008;84:62–3.
16. Monagle P, Chan AK, Goldenberg NA, et al. Antithrombotic therapy in neonates and children: antithrombotic therapy and prevention of thrombosis, 9th ed: American College of Chest Physicians evidence-based clinical practice guidelines. Chest. 2012;141(2 Suppl):e737S–801S.
17. Manco-Johnson MJ, Grabowski EF, Hellgreen M, et al. Recommendations for tPA thrombolysis in children. On behalf of the Scientific Subcommittee on Perinatal and Pediatric Thrombosis of the Scientific and Standardization Committee of the International Society of Thrombosis and Haemostasis. Thromb Haemost. 2002;88:157–8.
18. Goel R, Vedantham S, Goldenberg NA. Antithrombotic therapies anticoagulation and thrombolysis. Pediatr Clin N Am. 2013;60:1463–74.
19. Mahajerin A, Betensky M, Goldenberg NA. Thrombosis in children approach to anatomic risks, thrombophilia, prevention, and treatment. Hematol Oncol Clin N Am. 2019;33:439–53.
20. Tarango C, Manco-Johnson MJ. Pediatric thrombolysis: a practical approach. Front Pediatr. 2017;5:260.

21. Goldenberg NA, Branchford B, Wang M, et al. Percutaneous mechanical and pharmacomechanical thrombolysis for occlusive deep venous thrombosis of the proximal limb in adolescents: findings from an institution-based prospective inception cohort study of pediatric venous thromboembolism. J Vasc Interv Radiol. 2011;22:121–32.

22. Monagle P, Newall F. Management of thrombosis in children and neonates: practical use of anticoagulants in children. Hematology Am Soc Hematol Educ Program. 2018:399–404.

23. Kerlin BA. Current and future management of pediatric venous thromboembolism. Am J Hematol. 2012;87:S68–74.

24. Risch L, Huber AR, Schmugge M. Diagnosis and treatment of heparin-induced thrombocytopenia in neonates and children. Thromb Res. 2006;118:123–35.

25. Young G, Boshkov LK, Sullivan JE, et al. Argatroban therapy in pediatric patients requiring nonheparin anticoagulation: an open-label, safety, efficacy, and pharmacokinetic study. Pediatr Blood Cancer. 2011;56:1103–9.

26. O'Brien SH, Yee DL, Lira J, et al. UNBLOCK: an open-label, dose-finding, pharmacokinetic and safety study of bivalirudin in children with deep vein thrombosis. J Thromb Haemost. 2015;13:1615–22.

27. Hursting MJ, Dubb J, Verme-Gibboney CN. Argatroban anticoagulation in pediatric patients. J Pediatr Hematol Oncol. 2006;28:4–10.

28. Buck ML. Bivalirudin as an alternative to heparin for anticoagulation in infants and children. J Pediatr Pharmacol Ther. 2015;20:408–17.

29. Young G. Anticoagulants in children and adolescents. Hematology Am Soc Hematol Educ Program. 2015:111–6.

30. Punzalan RC, Hillery CA, Montgomery RR, et al. Low-molecular weight heparin in thrombotic disease in children and adolescents. J Pediatr Hematol Oncol. 2000;22:137–42.

31. Klassen ILM, Sol JJ, Suijker MH, et al. Are low-molecular weight heparins safe and effective in children? A systematic review. Blood Rev. 2019;33:33–42.

32. Raffini L, Huang YS, Witmer C, et al. Dramatic increase in venous thromboembolism in children's hospitals in the United States from 2001 to 2007. Pediatrics. 2009;124:1001–8.

33. Schobess R, During C, Bidlingmaier C, et al. Long-term safety and efficacy data on childhood venous thrombosis treated with a low molecular weight heparin: an open-label pilot study of once-daily versus twice-daily enoxaparin administration. Haematologica. 2006;91:1701–4.

34. Dabbous MK, Sakr FR, Malaeb DM. Anticoagulant therapy in pediatrics. J Basic Clin Pharm. 2014;5:27–33.

35. Cohen AT, Bauersachs R. Rivaroxaban and the EINSTEIN clinical trial programme. Blood Coagul Fibrinolysis. 2019;30:85–95.

36. Male C, Thom K, O'Brien SH. Direct oral anticoagulants: what will be their role in children? Thromb Res. 2019;173:178–85.

37. Burnett AE, Mahan CE, Vazquez SR, et al. Guidance for the practical management of the direct oral anticoagulants (DOACs) in VTE treatment. J Thromb Thrombolysis. 2016;41:206–32.

38. Pengo V, Denas G, Zoppellar G, et al. Rivaroxaban vs. warfarin in high-risk patients with antiphospholipid antibody syndrome. Blood. 2018;132:1365–71.

39. Cuker A, Burnett A, Triller D, et al. Reversal of direct oral anticoagulants: guidance from the anticoagulation forum. Am J Hematol. 2019;94:697–709.

40. Tarango C, Schulman S, Betensky M, et al. Duration of anticoagulant therapy in pediatric venous thromboembolism: current approaches and updates from randomized controlled trials. Expert Rev Hematol. 2018;11:37–44.

41. Van Ommen CH, Nowak-Gottl U. Inherited thrombophilia in pediatric venous thromboembolic disease: why and who to test. Front Pediatr. 2017;5:50.

42. Young G, Albisetti M, Bonduel M, et al. Impact of inherited thrombophilia on venous thromboembolism in children: a systematic review and meta-analysis of observational studies. Circulation. 2008;118:1373–82.

43. Wincup C, Ioannou Y. The differences between childhood and adult onset antiphospholipid syndrome. Front Pediatr. 2018;6:362.

44. Avcin T, Cimaz R, Silverman ED, et al. Pediatric antiphospholipid syndrome: clinical and immunologic features of 121 patients in an international registry. Pediatrics. 2008;122:1100–7.

45. Berkun Y, Padeh S, Barash J, et al. Antiphospholipid syndrome and recurrent thrombosis in children. Arthritis Rheum. 2006;55:850–5.

46. Groot N, de Graeff N, Avcin T, et al. European evidence-based recommendations for the diagnosis and treatment of paediatric antiphospholipid syndrome: the SHARE initiative. Ann Rheum Dis. 2017;76:1637–41.

47. Monagle P, Newall F. Anticoagulation in children. Thromb Res. 2012;130:142–6.

48. Boonyawat K, O'Brien SH, Bates SM. How I treat heavy menstrual bleeding associated with anticoagulants. Blood. 2017;130:2603–9.

49. Goldenberg NA, Donadini MP, Kahn SR. Post-thrombotic syndrome in children: a systematic review of frequency of occurrence, validity of outcome measures, and prognostic factors. Haematologica. 2010;95:1952–9.

50. Betensky M, Goldenberg NA. Post-thrombotic syndrome in children. Thromb Res. 2018;164:129–35.

51. Rajpurkar M, Sharathkumar A, Williams S, et al. Recommendations for the assessment of non-extremity venous thromboembolism outcomes: communication from the SCC of the ISTH. J Thromb Haemost. 2015;13:477–80.

52. Raffini L, Trimarchi T, Beliveau J, et al. Thromboprophylaxis in a pediatric hospital: a patient-safety and quality-improvement initiative. Pediatrics. 2011;127:1326–32.

53. Srivaths L, Dietrich JE. Prothrombotic risk factors and preventative strategies in adolescent venous thromboembolism. Clin Appl Thromb Hemost. 2016;22:512–9.

54. Mahajerin A, Petty JK, Hanson SJ, et al. Prophylaxis against venous thromboembolism in pediatric trauma: a practice management guideline from the Eastern Association for the Surgery of Trauma and the Pediatric Trauma Society. J Trauma Acute Care Surg. 2016;82:627–36.

55. Lyle CA, Sidonio RF, Goldenberg NA. New developments in pediatric venous thromboembolism and anticoagulation, including the target-specific oral anticoagulants. Curr Opin Pediatr. 2015;27:18–25.

56. Biss T, Alikhan R, Payne J, et al. Venous thromboembolism occurring during adolescence. Arch Dis Child. 2016;101:427–32.

Thrombophilia and Hormonal Therapy in Adolescents

Shannon M. Bates, Tazim Dowlut-McElroy,
and Kelley McLean

Introduction

Thromboembolic events in children and adolescents show an age-related bimodal distribution, with the highest risks in neonates less than 1 year of age and in adolescents more than 13 years of age [1]. Use of combined oral contraceptives (COCs) is likely a major driver of the heightened risk of venous thromboembolism (VTE) in adolescence as compared to late childhood. The findings of a case-control study of children and adolescents in which current or recent use COC was the most significant risk factor for pulmonary embolism (PE) (odds ratio [OR] 14.667, 95% confidence interval [CI] 3.001–71.678, $P < 0.001$) in an emergency department setting highlight the role of COCs in VTE risk in this population [2]. The risk of contraceptive-related VTE is compounded in adolescents who have an underlying thrombophilia (an inher-ited or acquired laboratory abnormality associated with an increased risk of thrombosis) [1]. These abnormalities are very common, and collectively, inherited thrombophilias are present in at least 15% of the population [2]. Acquired risk factors (e.g., tobacco use, age, obesity) further affect the risk of contraceptive-related VTE. While the additive risk of underlying thrombophilia in the context of combined hormonal contraception (CHC) use has not been specifically studied in adolescents, the increased risk for VTE in young adult women has been well-described, with CHC use and underlying thrombophilia having a synergistic effect on thrombosis risk [3, 4]. This risk increase applies not only to VTE but also to cerebral sinus thrombosis and, to a lesser extent, ischemic stroke risk [5–7].

The following sections will first provide a review of inherited and acquired thrombophilias, as well as a brief discussion on screening for thrombophilias. The remainder of the chapter will then focus on thrombosis risk associated with the various contraceptive options in thrombophilic adolescent girls and young women.

S. M. Bates
Thrombosis and Atherosclerosis Research Institute
and Department of Medicine, McMaster University,
Hamilton, ON, Canada

T. Dowlut-McElroy
Department of Obstetrics and Gynecology, University
of Missouri-Kansas City School of Medicine,
Kansas City, MO, USA

K. McLean (✉)
Department of Obstetrics, Gynecology and
Reproductive Medicine, University of Vermont,
Burlington, VT, USA
e-mail: kelley.mclean@uvmhealth.org

Thrombophilias

Inherited Thrombophilias

The first identified inherited thrombophilias were the deficiencies of the natural anticoagulants, antithrombin, protein C, and protein S. These are

© Springer Nature Switzerland AG 2020
L. V. Srivaths (ed.), *Hematology in the Adolescent Female*,
https://doi.org/10.1007/978-3-030-48446-0_15

relatively uncommon disorders that are inherited in an autosomal dominant fashion and have an estimated prevalence in the general population of less than 0.2%, less than 0.5%, and less than 0.2%, respectively [8, 9]. Antithrombin is a serine protease inhibitor (SERPIN) that primarily acts to inactivate factors IIa (thrombin) and Xa, in addition to factors IXa, XIa, and XIIa [10]; while proteins C and S are vitamin K-dependent glycoproteins that act together to inactivate factors Va and VIIIa [11, 12].

Deficiencies of antithrombin, protein C, and protein S are either quantitative (decreased antigenic levels) or qualitative (a functional deficiency in which activity levels are decreased more than antigenic levels). While antithrombin and protein C deficiencies are classified as type I (quantitative) and type II (qualitative), there are three types of protein S deficiency. Type I and III are quantitative with decreased levels of both total and free protein S antigen and free protein S antigen only, respectively; while type II deficiency is qualitative with decreased activity but normal antigen levels. Most patients with inherited antithrombin deficiency are heterozygous; homozygous antithrombin deficiency is very rare and usually fatal in utero or early in life [13]. Protein C and S deficiencies are also typically heterozygous; homozygous or compound heterozygous forms are much less common [14, 15]. While antithrombin deficiency appears to increase the risk of a first venous thromboembolic event approximately 16-fold, the increased risks with protein C and S deficiency are less, at 7.5- and 5.4-fold, respectively [8, 16]. As a group, deficiencies of the natural anticoagulants are estimated to have an annual risk of VTE of 1.5% per year (95% CI, 0.7–2.8%) [9].

Factor V Leiden is the most common inherited thrombophilia, with approximately 5% of those with European ancestry carrying the heterozygous form of this thrombophilia, although it is rarely found in African and Asian individuals [17]. The frequency of homozygosity for factor V Leiden is estimated to be approximately 1 in 5000 persons. Factor V Leiden is characterized by a single nucleotide substitution in the factor V gene that changes arginine to glutamine at posi-

tion 506, the normal initial cleavage site in factor V for activated protein C, resulting in slower inactivation of activated factor V [18]. While homozygosity for the factor V Leiden mutation is considered a high-risk thrombophilia with an 11-fold increase in risk for a first VTE (estimated annual risk of 1.8%; 95% CI, 0.1–4.0%), the heterozygous state is associated with a more modest 3- to five-fold risk increase (estimated annual risk of 0.5%, 95% CI, 0.1–1.3%) [8, 9].

The prothrombin gene mutation, in which adenine substitutes for guanine at position 2010 in a noncoding portion of the gene, resulting in an increase in prothrombin protein levels, is found in approximately 2% of Caucasians and is rare in other populations [19]. Heterozygosity for the prothrombin gene mutation is a low-risk thrombophilia, increasing the risk of a first venous thromboembolic event 2- to three-fold, for an estimated annual risk of 0.4% (95% CI, 0.1–1.1%) [8, 9], while homozygosity for the prothrombin gene mutation is associated with an estimated 6.7 fold (95% CI, 2.19–20.72) risk increase [20].

Acquired Thrombophilias

Antiphospholipid antibodies are antibodies directed against phospholipids, proteins bound to phospholipids, and protein-phospholipid complexes. The best known of these includes lupus anticoagulants, anticardiolipin antibodies (IgG and IgM isotypes), and anti-beta-2 glycoprotein I antibodies (IgG and IgM isotypes) [21]. Transient antibodies are common in the healthy population. Antiphospholipid antibodies are present in 2–5% of the population, with no increased risk of adverse clinical events [22–24]. However, the presence of persistent moderate- or high-titer antiphospholipid antibodies and, in particular, positivity on multiple different assays is associated with increased risk of venous and arterial thrombosis [25]. Other complications associated with these antibodies include pregnancy loss, immune thrombocytopenia, Libman-Sacks endocarditis, and livedo reticularis. Those with antiphospholipid antibodies that meet specific laboratory testing criteria who experience venous or arterial thrombosis or specific obstetrical complications (unexplained death of a morphologically normal fetus at or beyond 10 weeks or 3 or more unexplained, consecutive spontaneous abortions before 10 weeks gestation, or premature birth of a morphologically normal neonate before 34 weeks gestation as a result of eclampsia, preeclampsia, or placental insufficiency) are said to have antiphospholipid antibody syndrome [21].

Screening for Thrombophilia

The benefit of thrombophilia screening remains controversial. Although testing to identify inherited thrombophilias in groups felt to be at increased risk of VTE has become commonplace, there are few data on the potential benefits of thrombophilia testing. Screening is useful only when results will affect management decisions and when the potential benefits justify the potential drawbacks of testing, which include cost, negative psychological effects, difficulties with insurability, bleeding risks with primary prophylaxis, additional medical expenditures, false reassurance from a negative test result, and the effect of incorporating this information into important life decisions including pregnancy, surgery, and contraceptive choice [26–29]. Screening is not useful when treatment is indicated for other risk factors or there are no data to support intervention. Given these limitations, the potential benefits and drawbacks of screening should be discussed with the patient before testing is undertaken.

It has been suggested that thrombophilia testing of asymptomatic individuals will allow them the opportunity to avoid or mitigate risk factors for VTE, including contraceptive therapy. The Thrombosis Risk and Economic Assessment of Thrombophilia Screening (TREATS) study showed that routine thrombophilia testing in young women considering COC therapy is not practical or cost-effective [30]. However, testing women who have a first-degree relative with a history of VTE or those with a family history highly suggestive of a thrombophilia (history of

VTE at less than 40–50 years of age, particularly if unprovoked or associated with weak provoking risk factors) may help in informed decision-making [31].

That said, a family history of VTE is a rather poor predictor for the presence of a thrombophilia but is associated with a two- to fourfold increase in the risk of VTE [32, 33]. Therefore, when counseling women from families with a history of VTE and/or thrombophilia, it is important to note that the risk of thrombosis is increased even in those who test negative for the thrombophilia [34]. For example, COC users from families with deficiencies of the natural anticoagulants who test negative still have an elevated risk compared with users from the general population (0.48–0.7% versus 0.04% per year of pill use) [35, 36]. The same holds true for those from families with the factor V Leiden or prothrombin gene mutation (0.19% versus 0.04% per year of pill use) [37]. Therefore, those with positive family histories who are unwilling to accept any additional increased risk of VTE do not necessarily require thrombophilia testing and should avoid contraceptive options associated with an increased risk of thrombosis.

Contraceptive Therapy in Adolescents with Thrombophilia

In adolescents, hormonal therapy is commonly used for contraceptive, as well as noncontraceptive indications that include acne, heavy menstrual bleeding, dysmenorrhea, irregular menstrual cycles, and hormone replacement therapy in the setting of primary ovarian insufficiency. The following sections will provide an overview of the different hormonal contraceptive classes as they relate to adolescents and young women with thrombophilia. The most efficacious and lowest-risk methods (i.e., long-acting reversible contraceptives, LARC) are discussed first.

As contraceptives are most commonly used to avoid unplanned pregnancies, it is important to place the risks of contraceptive-related VTE in the context of the risks of pregnancy-associated VTE risk. Population-based studies have shown the relative risk of VTE in pregnancy to be increased fivefold over the nonpregnant state, with an even more pronounced risk in the postpartum period [38, 39]. A systematic review reported that the risk in the first 6 weeks postpartum was increased 21.5- to 84-fold compared with that in nonpregnant, non-postpartum women [39, 40]. As a result, the VTE risk in a non-thrombophilic pregnant or postpartum woman is higher than in a nonpregnant woman with heterozygosity for the factor V Leiden or prothrombin gene mutation who uses CHCs. This point was well-illustrated in a large retrospective family cohort study in which the VTE risk during COC use and pregnancy/postpartum was assessed in 798 adolescents and women with a first-degree relative with VTE and thrombophilia who were heterozygous, double heterozygous, or homozygous for the factor V Leiden or prothrombin gene mutation. In women heterozygous for the factor V Leiden or prothrombin gene mutation, the absolute risk of VTE on CHCs was 0.47 (CI, 0.18–1.07) per 100 person-years but was 0.73 (95% CI: 0.3–1.51) in pregnant/postpartum women without thrombophilia. As shown in Table 15.1, the findings of this study also emphasize the increased VTE risk with pregnancy in thrombophilic women, as well as the risk difference in women with heterozygous single mutations, versus those with compound factor V Leiden and prothrombin gene mutations, or homozygosity for either mutation [41].

In the United States, approximately 80% of pregnancies in adolescents (ages 15–19 years) are unintended [42]. In the context of the increased

Table 15.1 Absolute VTE risk per 100 person-years (95% CI) during COC use and in pregnancy in women with factor V Leiden or prothrombin gene mutations [41]

Thrombophilia testing	Overall	COC use	Pregnancy and postpartum
Negative	0.13 (0.08–0.21)	0.19 (0.07–0.41)	0.73 (0.3–1.51)
Single gene mutation	0.35 (0.22–0.53)	0.49 (0.18–1.07)	1.97 (0.94–3.63)
Double gene mutation	0.94 (0.47–1.67)	0.86 (0.11–3.11)	7.65 (3.08–15.76)

risk of thrombosis associated with pregnancy, including in those with thrombophilia, such a high unintended pregnancy rate underscores the importance of providing efficacious contraception that is acceptable to the patient.

Flexibility in shared decision-making is fundamentally important and should include consideration of an individual's thrombotic risk profile, based on her specific thrombophilia, personal history of VTE, family history of VTE, smoking, obesity, and/or other underlying chronic medical conditions. As is discussed in the most recent American Academy of Pediatrics (AAP) policy statement on "Contraception for Adolescents," frequent follow-up for support and to encourage contraceptive continuation and adherence is particularly important in adolescents [43].

Long-Acting Reversible Contraceptives (LARC) in Adolescents and Young Women with Thrombophilia

The intrauterine device (IUD) and the etonogestrel implant are two options for LARCs. LARC methods have higher efficacy, higher continuation rates, and higher satisfaction in adolescents compared to short-acting methods [44, 45]. As such, both the American College of Obstetricians and Gynecologists (ACOG) and the AAP recommend LARC as first-line contraceptives in adolescents [43, 46]. Given the current evidence detailed below, the same should be true for adolescents with thrombophilia.

The Centers for Disease Control and Prevention (CDC)'s adaptation of the World Health Organization's (WHO) Medical Eligibility Criteria for Contraceptive Use (MEC) for use in the United States was updated in 2016 [47]. The CDC MEC uses four categories to classify medical conditions affecting eligibility for the use of each type of contraception (see Table 15.2). All LARC methods are safe (either Category 1 or 2) for use in women with a history of VTE and/or those with an underlying thrombophilia. As the copper IUD results in no hormone exposure, the USMEC classifies its use in women with prior VTE and/or thrombophilia as Category 1. Both

Table 15.2 U.S. Medical Eligibility Criteria categories for classifying intrauterine devices and hormonal contraceptives [47]

Category	Definition
1	A condition for which there is no restriction for the use of the contraceptive method
2	A condition for which the advantages of using the method generally outweigh the theoretical or proven risks
3	A condition for which the theoretical or proven risks usually outweigh the advantages of using the method
4	A condition that represents an unacceptable health risk if the contraceptive method is used

the levonorgestrel IUD (LNG-IUD) and the etonogestrel subdermal implant are classified as Category 2 (a condition for which the advantages of using the method generally outweigh the theoretical or proven risks). This classification reflects the results of early studies that inconsistently suggest a possible small increase in VTE risk with progestin-only contraceptives [48–51]. However, more recent studies and meta-analyses have found no association between progesterone-based LARC and VTE [52, 53]. Further, a large Swedish case-control study showed no increase in VTE with use of the subdermal implant or the LNG-IUD for contraception in women with the factor V Leiden mutation [54].

Taken together, all LARC options should be considered first-line contraceptives for adolescents and young women with thrombophilia. Because LARC methods each variably alter uterine bleeding volume and/or patterns, it is important to set expectations at the time of placement and to provide ongoing, developmentally appropriate education and counseling.

Progestin-Only Pills (POPS) and Depot Medroxyprogesterone Acetate (DMPA) in Adolescents and Young Women with Thrombophilia

As is the case with the progestin-based LARC methods, the USMEC classifies POPs and DMPA as Category 2 in women with a history of VTE and/or thrombophilia. As noted previously, inconsistent results from studies published in the 1990s demonstrated a possible small increase in VTE risk with progesterone-only contraceptives [48–51]. However, as was the case with the LNG-IUD and the etonogestrel implant, more recent studies and meta-analyses have found no association between POP-based contraception and VTE [52, 53, 55]. There appears, however, to be a dose-response relationship between progestins and thrombotic risk. A recent systematic review of progestin-only contraception and VTE risk identified two studies showing increased odds of VTE with noncontraceptive, therapeutic use of progestin-only pills (one study with POPs, the other with unspecified progesterone only contraception) [53]. The current literature specific to DMPA is also suggestive of a dose-response relationship in terms of VTE risk. DMPA results in higher plasma concentrations of progestin than do POPs and unlike POPs, DMPA has been shown to increase VTE risk approximately two-fold [52, 54]. That said, the data are sparse, and an accurate assessment of absolute VTE risk increase in women using DMPA is currently not possible.

There is very little published literature specific to POPs and DMPA in women with thrombophilia. However, the previously cited Swedish case-control study which showed no increase in VTE in women with the factor V Leiden mutation using either the subdermal implant or the LNG-IUD also showed no increased risk with POP use, but showed a considerable increase in the odds of VTE with DMPA use (though with a wide CI relating to small numbers) (OR 16.7; 95% CI, 2.4–714) [54]. Despite these reports of a possible increase in VTE risk in women taking DMPA, along with a possible further increase in thrombophilic DMPA users, the U.S. MEC makes no distinction between the safety of DMPA compared to other progestin-only contraceptives, and they are all classified as Category 2. DMPA may be a preferred method of contraception by adolescents as a result of the convenient dosing schedule and improved opportunity for confidentiality, though it should be noted that some experts advise against the use of DMPA in those at increased risk of VTE [56].

As adolescents and women using DMPA show reduction in bone mineral density (BMD), caution should be exercised when using DMPA as a long-term contraceptive in adolescents and young women. This is particularly true for adolescents because they have not yet attained their peak bone mass. Multiple studies have shown that the reduction in BMD associated with DMPA use is fully reversible in all age groups, including in adolescents, and the ACOG identifies DMPA as a good contraceptive choice for many adolescents [46, 57]. There are no studies assessing the impact of DMPA on BMD in concert with anticoagulants (including those that may also affect BMD, such as heparin) in adolescents, however.

Combined Hormonal Contraceptives (CHC) in Adolescents and Young Women with Thrombophilia

Although VTE is rare in adolescents, the risk of VTE increases in users of CHCs containing ethinyl estradiol (EE) and various types of progestins. In users of CHCs, the risk of VTE is 3–15/10,000 woman-years compared to 1–5/10,000 woman-years in nonusers [58]. The risk of VTE is greater during the first year of use of CHCs, in obese women, and increases with age [58]. In general, CHCs are classified into five categories as per Table 15.3.

COCs, which are currently the most popular hormonal contraceptive method in adolescents, and non-oral (vaginal ring and transdermal patch) combined contraceptives increase the baseline risk of thrombosis and appear to act synergistically in women with an underlying thrombophilia [43]. All estrogen-containing contraceptives are categorized as a single group by the USMEC. In women with thrombophilia, the USMEC classifies all CHCs as Category 4, irrespective of whether they have a personal history of VTE (see Table 15.1 for USMEC classifications).

Data regarding the actual VTE risk with various CHCs remain controversial. While the overall risk of VTE in users of COCs is increased approximately three- to fivefold, the risk appears to vary

Table 15.3 Categories of combined hormonal contraceptives

CHC category	CHC formulation
First-generation oral	50 µg EE (+ 1 of various progestins)
Second-generation oral	<50 µg EE + norethindrone and derivatives including levonorgestrel
Third-generation oral	<50 µg EE + desogestrel and gestodene (formulated to be less androgenic than second-generation progestins). Norgestimate is a third-generation progestin but differs from other third-generation progestins in that its bioactivity is mediated though levonorgestrel
Fourth-generation oral	<50 µg EE + drospirenone (derived from spironolactone and has anti-androgenic activity)
Non-oral	Transdermal patch, vaginal ring

CHC combined hormonal contraceptive, *EE* ethinyl estradiol

according to dose of estrogen and type of progestin. In a 2014 Cochrane review, use of a 50 µg EE pill-containing levonorgestrel was associated with a relative risk (RR) of VTE of 2.1 (95% CI, 1.4–3.2) and 2.3 (95% CI, 1.3–4.2), compared to use of a 30 µg and 20 µg EE pill with the same progesterone, respectively [59]. Other studies have not found that reducing the EE dose to <50 µg lowers the risk of VTE, and there is no evidence that decreasing the dose to less than 35 µg EE further decreases this risk [58]. In terms of the type of progestin, observational studies suggest a higher VTE risk with third- and fourth-generation progestins. A meta-analysis of 23 studies reported a 50% to 80% increase in the RR of VTE among users third generation or drospirenone COCs, compared to users of levonorgestrel COCs at the same EE dose (30–35 µg) [59]. The RR of VTE with third generation compared to second-generation progestins was 1.3 (95% CI, 1.0–1.8). Norgestimate, a type of third-generation progestin, is an exception, with a RR of VTE similar to that with the second-generation progestin, levonorgestrel. However, there are no randomized trials large enough to compare the VTE risk in patients using different types of COCs. Reported differences in VTE risk between second- and third-generation progestins and drospirenone may be due to confounding factors such as increased risk of VTE among new users, obesity, increasing age, and family history of VTE. If there is an increased risk of VTE with third- and fourth-generation progestins, the absolute increase in risk is small. In one meta-analysis that included 25 studies, the absolute risk of VTE with third- and fourth-generation progestins was 10–15/10,000 women-year compared with 8/10,000 women-years with levonorgestrel and 2/10,000 women-years with no use [60]. As such, the choice of COC should not be based solely on the type of progestin.

There also appears to be substantial variation in VTE risk with COCs depending upon individual underlying risk factors [41, 58, 61]. For women with underlying thrombophilia, the risk of VTE appears to be increased with COC use, but as noted in the section, *Screening for Thrombophilia*, the estimates of the magnitude of this risk increase vary by type of thrombophilia [41, 62, 63] and, as reported in the TREATS systematic review, between individual studies [63]. Despite this variation in risk estimates, it appears that heterozygosity for the two most prevalent thrombophilias, the factor V Leiden and prothrombin gene mutations, carries a lower COC-associated VTE risk (approximately 0.49% [95% CI, 0.18–1.07%] per year of use [37]) than do homozygosity or compound heterozygosity for these mutations or a deficiency of one of the natural anticoagulants, protein C, protein S, or antithrombin, with two family cohort studies reporting risks of 4.3% (95% CI, 1.4–9.7%) and 4.62% (95% CI, 2.4–7.9%) per year of use in this latter group [35, 36]. These women should avoid COC use. Whether or not COC use is acceptable in patients with lower-risk thrombophilias depends on the presence of additional risk factors (which will increase thrombotic risk), as well as patient values and preferences.

Compared to that for COCs, there is relatively little data on VTE risk with non-oral CHCs and no published data specifically focused on thrombophilic women. Current data regarding the risk of VTE with use of the contraceptive vaginal ring or contraceptive patch are limited and some-

times conflicting. The vaginal ring (NuvaRing ®, Merck) contains 11.7 mg etonogestrel (the biologically active metabolite of desogestrel) and 2.7 mg EE and releases approximately 120 µg etonogestrel and 15 µg EE daily [64]. The transdermal patch contains 6 mg norelgestromin (the active metabolite of norgestimate) and 0.75 mg EE and delivers approximately 150 µg norelgestromin and 20 µg EE daily [65]. While both the transdermal patch and the vaginal contraceptive ring increase the risk of thrombosis compared to nonusers, whether they increase thrombotic risk beyond that of second-generation and norgestimate-containing COCs is controversial. There are both pharmacokinetic and biomarker data suggesting increased thrombotic risk with non-oral CHCs, particularly the transdermal patch. Despite lower maximum EE levels, mean EE exposure is greatest with patch use [66]. Users of the vaginal ring have lower maximum levels and lower overall exposure to EE [66]. Whether the different levels of EE achieved by non-oral routes of delivery correlate with the risk of thrombosis remains unclear. A retrospective cohort study of four Danish registries found an increased risk of VTE among users of the vaginal ring compared to users of levonorgestrel-containing COCs (RR 1.9; 95% CI 1.3–2.7) [67]. In contrast, a large prospective observational study performed in the United States and five European countries found no increased risk of VTE among users of the vaginal ring as compared to COC users (HR 0.8; 95% CI 0.5–1.5) [68]. Similarly, conflicting results have been published regarding the risk of VTE with use of the transdermal patch as compared to COCs. A case-control study evaluating the thromboembolic outcomes of users of the transdermal patch found a twofold increase risk of VTE relative to norgestimate-containing COCs (OR 2.0; 95% CI 1.2–3.3) [69]. Another case-control study reported a more than twofold increase in the VTE rate (incidence rate ratio 2.2, 95% CI 1.3–3.8) among transdermal patch users compared to users of norgestimate-containing COCs [70]. In contrast, a large retrospective cohort study using databases of four US health plans found no difference in VTE risk among users of the vaginal ring and COCs containing ≤35 μg EE [71]. The incidence of VTE among patch and ring users has been reported as 8–10 per 10,000 woman-years [67, 68]. The authors of a 2017 systematic review of non-oral CHCs and VTE, which demonstrated the generally conflicting results on VTE risk with the patch and/or ring as compared to COC use, concluded that "any potential elevated risk likely represents a small number of events on a population level." [72]

In the context of variable VTE risk estimates in adolescents and women with thrombophilia taking CHCs, some have recommended consideration of CHCs in thrombophilic women with lower VTE risk, particularly given the much higher risk of VTE associated with pregnancy and the puerperium [41]. In the context of higher failure rates, less perfect use, and high discontinuation rates compared to LARC in adolescents, however, the decision to use CHC instead of LARC comes with a higher risk of unintended pregnancies. Thus, the circumstance in which it may be most reasonable to consider CHC use in adolescents and young women with thrombophilia is the need for the noncontraceptive, therapeutic benefits of CHC, including in the context of treating adolescents with various gonadal disorders including Turner syndrome and primary ovarian insufficiency hormone replacement therapy, in those who decline more physiologic dosing of estrogen replacement therapy. Prescription of CHC to thrombophilic adolescents and young women should be restricted to those with lower-risk thrombophilias who have been counseled on the possible increased risk of VTE associated with these formulations and are accepting of them.

Hormonal Contraception in Thrombophilic Adolescents and Young Women Receiving Anticoagulant Therapy

With the awareness of a high rate of unintended pregnancies in adolescents and young women, healthcare providers caring for thrombophilic patients not infrequently confront decisions about

whether to start, continue, or discontinue contraceptives when anticoagulants are initiated. In the specific case of women receiving anticoagulants for at least 3 months for VTE, with or without thrombophilia, the USMEC includes the following clarification: "women using anticoagulant therapy are at risk for gynecologic complications of therapy, such as hemorrhagic ovarian cysts and severe menorrhagia. Hormonal contraceptive methods can be of benefit in preventing or treating these complications. When a contraceptive method is used as a therapy, rather than solely to prevent pregnancy, the risk/benefit ratio might differ and should be considered on a case-by-case basis." [47] Theoretically, the prothrombotic effect of any hormonal therapy is likely to be suppressed by therapeutic dose anticoagulation. On this basis, a 2012 Clinical Guideline published by the Scientific Subcommittee of the International Society on Thrombosis and Haemostasis suggested that hormonal therapy can be continued in selected patients with VTE, as long as anticoagulant therapy is continued for the duration of hormonal therapy and, of course, is well-managed [73]. The safety of this approach was subsequently confirmed using data from randomized, controlled, phase 3 studies in patients with acute VTE treated with either one of the direct oral anticoagulants (rivaroxaban [Xarelto®, Janssen Pharmaceuticals]) or low-molecular weight heparin bridging to warfarin that showed no difference in the risk of recurrent VTE between women continuing or starting hormonal therapy and those discontinuing or without hormonal therapy [74]. The number of thrombophilic patients included in this analysis is unknown; however, most common thrombophilias are not associated with resistance to long-term anticoagulant therapy.

Hormonal Contraception in Thrombophilic Adolescents and Young Women with a History of VTE

As noted above, ongoing well-managed anticoagulant therapy may mitigate the risk of recurrence associated with hormonal therapy in patients with a history of VTE [74]. However, in the absence of anticoagulation, contraceptives associated with an increased risk of VTE should be avoided in those with a prior history of deep vein thrombosis or PE.

Research Gaps and Conclusions

The current standard in adolescent contraception counseling, recommended by both the AAP and the ACOG, is to begin with a discussion of the most effective contraceptive options, which are the LARC methods. LARC methods, including the copper IUD, the LNG-IUD, and the etonogestrel subdermal implant, are the only contraceptive options that combine low to no increased VTE risk with high contraceptive efficacy, including with typical, real-world use. For the vast majority of adolescents and young women with thrombophilia, LARC methods should be the first-line contraceptive choice.

Cases in which the adolescent declines LARC methods but wishes to take a CHC, and/or the adolescent requires noncontraceptive, therapeutic use of CHC, highlight the need for a better understanding of the relative and absolute risks associated with CHC use for each type of thrombophilia. Adolescents and young women with an acquired or genetic thrombophilia are often counseled to avoid CHC both for contraceptive and noncontraceptive purposes. However, it is important that clinicians caring for such patients understand the relative and absolute thrombotic risk not only of different CHC doses, formulations, and routes of administration but also understand thrombotic risk, relative efficacy, and failure rates of other forms of contraception, including progestin-only pills, implants, and intrauterine devices. Of equal importance is consideration of an individual's specific thrombophilia, as the currently identified thrombophilias have been associated with different relative increases in VTE risk at baseline, in the context of hormonal contraception and in pregnancy and

puerperium, as well as an individual's tolerance for increased VTE risk.

Precise understanding of the relationship between different thrombophilias and CHC use, DMPA use, and during pregnancy and the postpartum period remains a research gap to be filled. Further, a more complete understanding and description of individual risk profiles, based not only on type of thrombophilia but also on personal and family history of VTE, obesity, and smoking status, is needed. The substantial difference in magnitude of VTE risk in adolescents and young women with different thrombophilias, with further differences in the response to exogenous hormonal and pregnancy-related challenges, makes the concept of risk-based clinical action thresholds appealing. Such models, which are based on combining individual risk factors to create risk levels, are now the basis for cervical cancer screening in the United States. Management is based on the specific risk level, under the principle "equal management of equal risks," and the need to balance benefits and harms. [75] Creation of similar risk-based models to better equate individual VTE risk factor combinations in thrombophilic women would allow better assessment of the added risk of hormonal contraceptives and of pregnancy.

Finally, there is very little known about safety of continuation and/or initiation of different contraceptive methods in adolescents and women on anticoagulant therapy. The frequency and degree of menorrhagia and hemorrhagic ovarian cysts in anticoagulated women (including those receiving hormonal contraception) is not well-described, and whether adolescents have similar side-effect profiles as older women is unknown. There are no published studies specifically evaluating the risk of recurrent VTE in adolescents or thrombophilic patients using CHCs, DMPA, and other progestin-based methods while on anticoagulant therapy. Data regarding the safety of placement of an IUD or the subdermal implant and/or use of the copper IUD with anticoagulation are also lacking.

References

1. Chan AK, Deveber G, Monagle P, Brooker LA, Massicotte PM. Venous thrombosis in children. J Thromb Haemost. 2003;1(7):1443–55.
2. Wang CY, Ignjatovic V, Francis P, et al. Risk factors and clinical features of acute pulmonary embolism in children from the community. Thromb Res. 2016;138:86–90.
3. Dayan N, Holcroft CA, Tagalakis V. The risk of venous thrombosis, including cerebral vein thrombosis, among women with thrombophilia and oral contraceptive use: a meta-analysis. Clin Aappl Thromb Hemost. 2011;17(6):E141–52.
4. Hugon-Rodin J, Horellou MH, Conard J, Gompel A, Plu-Bureau G. Type of combined contraceptives, factor V Leiden mutation and risk of venous thromboembolism. Thromb Haemost. 2018;118(5):922–8.
5. de Bruijn SF, Stam J, Koopman MM, Vandenbroucke JP. Case-control study of risk of cerebral sinus thrombosis in oral contraceptive users and in [correction of who are] carriers of hereditary prothrombotic conditions. The Cerebral Venous Sinus Thrombosis Study Group. BMJ. 1998;316(7131):589–92.
6. Dulicek P, Ivanova E, Kostal M, et al. Analysis of risk factors of stroke and venous thromboembolism in females with oral contraceptives use. Clin Appl Thromb Hemost. 2018;24(5):797–802.
7. Martinelli I, Battaglioli T, Burgo I, Di Domenico S, Mannucci PM. Oral contraceptive use, thrombophilia and their interaction in young women with ischemic stroke. Haematologica. 2006;91(6):844–7.
8. Freed J, Bauer KA. Thrombophilia: clinical and laboratory assessment and management. In: Kitchens CS, Kessler C, Konkle BA, Streiff BM, Garcia DA, editors. Consultative hemostasis and thrombosis. 4th ed. Philadelphia, PA: Elsevier. p. 242–65.
9. Middeldorp S, van Hylckama Vlieg A. Does thrombophilia testing help in the clinical management of patients? Br J Haematol. 2008;143(3):321–35.
10. Maclean PS, Tait RC. Hereditary and acquired antithrombin deficiency: epidemiology, pathogenesis and treatment options. Drugs. 2007;67(10):1429–40.
11. Esmon CT, Vigano-D'Angelo S, D'Angelo A, Comp PC. Anticoagulation proteins C and S. Adv Exp Med Biol. 1987;214:47–54.
12. Griffin JH, Evatt B, Zimmerman TS, Kleiss AJ, Wideman C. Deficiency of protein C in congenital thrombotic disease. J Clin Invest. 1981;68(5):1370–3.
13. Rodgers GM. Role of antithrombin concentrate in treatment of hereditary antithrombin deficiency. An update. Thromb Haemost. 2009;101(5):806–12.
14. Inoue H, Terachi SI, Uchiumi T, et al. The clinical presentation and genotype of protein C deficiency with double mutations of the protein C gene. Pediatr Blood Cancer. 2017;64(7):1–6. https://doi.org/10.1002/pbc.26404.
15. Mahasandana C, Suvatte V, Marlar RA, Manco-Johnson MJ, Jacobson LJ, Hathaway WE. Neonatal purpura fulminans associated with homozygous protein S deficiency. Lancet (London, England). 1990;335(8680):61–2.
16. Di Minno MN, Ambrosino P, Ageno W, Rosendaal F, Di Minno G, Dentali F. Natural anticoagulants deficiency and the risk of venous thromboembolism: a meta-analysis of observational studies. Thromb Res. 2015;135(5):923–32.
17. Rees DC, Cox M, Clegg JB. World distribution of factor V Leiden. Lancet (London, England). 1995;346(8983):1133–4.
18. Bertina RM, Koeleman BP, Koster T, et al. Mutation in blood coagulation factor V associated with resistance to activated protein C. Nature. 1994;369(6475):64–7.
19. Rosendaal FR, Doggen CJ, Zivelin A, et al. Geographic distribution of the 20210 G to A prothrombin variant. Thromb Haemost. 1998;79(4):706–8.
20. Simone B, De Stefano V, Leoncini E, et al. Risk of venous thromboembolism associated with single and combined effects of factor V Leiden, prothrombin 20210A and methylenetetrahydrofolate reductase C677T: a meta-analysis involving over 11,000 cases and 21,000 controls. Eur J Epidemiol. 2013;28(8):621–47.
21. Miyakis S, Lockshin MD, Atsumi T, et al. International consensus statement on an update of the classification criteria for definite antiphospholipid syndrome (APS). J Thromb Haemost. 2006;4(2):295–306.
22. Manukyan D, Rossmann H, Schulz A, et al. Distribution of antiphospholipid antibodies in a large population-based German cohort. Clin Chem Lab Med. 2016;54(10):1663–70.
23. Petri M. Epidemiology of the antiphospholipid antibody syndrome. J Autoimmun. 2000;15(2):145–51.
24. Vila P, Hernandez MC, Lopez-Fernandez MF, Batlle J. Prevalence, follow-up and clinical significance of the anticardiolipin antibodies in normal subjects. Thromb Haemost. 1994;72(2):209–13.
25. Mustonen P, Lehtonen KV, Javela K, Puurunen M. Persistent antiphospholipid antibody (aPL) in asymptomatic carriers as a risk factor for future thrombotic events: a nationwide prospective study. Lupus. 2014;23(14):1468–76.
26. Cohn DM, Vansenne F, Kaptein AA, De Borgie CA, Middeldorp S. The psychological impact of testing for thrombophilia: a systematic review. J Thromb Haemost. 2008;6(7):1099–104.
27. Green MJ, Botkin JR. "Genetic exceptionalism" in medicine: clarifying the differences between genetic and nongenetic tests. Ann Intern Med. 2003;138(7):571–5.
28. Homsma SJ, Huijgen R, Middeldorp S, Sijbrands EJ, Kastelein JJ. Molecular screening for familial hypercholesterolaemia: consequences for life and disability insurance. Eur J Hum Genet. 2008;16(1):14–7.
29. Lerman C, Croyle RT, Tercyak KP, Hamann H. Genetic testing: psychological aspects and implications. J Consult Clin Psychol. 2002;70(3):784–97.

30. Wu O, Robertson L, Twaddle S, et al. Screening for thrombophilia in high-risk situations: a meta-analysis and cost-effectiveness analysis. Br J Haematol. 2005;131(1):80–90.

31. Connors JM. Thrombophilia testing and venous thrombosis. N Engl J Med. 2017;377(23):2298.

32. Bezemer ID, van der Meer FJ, Eikenboom JC, Rosendaal FR, Doggen CJ. The value of family history as a risk indicator for venous thrombosis. Arch Intern Med. 2009;169(6):610–5.

33. van Sluis GL, Sohne M, El Kheir DY, Tanck MW, Gerdes VE, Buller HR. Family history and inherited thrombophilia. J Thromb Haemost. 2006;4(10):2182–7.

34. Middeldorp S. Is thrombophilia testing useful? Hematology Am Soc Hematol Educ Program. 2011;2011:150–5.

35. Simioni P, Sanson BJ, Prandoni P, et al. Incidence of venous thromboembolism in families with inherited thrombophilia. Thromb Haemost. 1999;81(2):198–202.

36. van Vlijmen EF, Brouwer JL, Veeger NJ, Eskes TK, de Graeff PA, van der Meer J. Oral contraceptives and the absolute risk of venous thromboembolism in women with single or multiple thrombophilic defects: results from a retrospective family cohort study. Arch Intern Med. 2007;167(3):282–9.

37. van Vlijmen EF, Wiewel-Verschueren S, Monster TB, Meijer K. Combined oral contraceptives, thrombophilia and the risk of venous thromboembolism: a systematic review and meta-analysis. J Thromb Haemost. 2016;14(7):1393–403.

38. Heit JA, Kobbervig CE, James AH, Petterson TM, Bailey KR, Melton LJ 3rd. Trends in the incidence of venous thromboembolism during pregnancy or postpartum: a 30-year population-based study. Ann Intern Med. 2005;143(10):697–706.

39. Jackson E, Curtis KM, Gaffield ME. Risk of venous thromboembolism during the postpartum period: a systematic review. Obstet Gynecol. 2011;117(3):691–703.

40. James AH. Venous thromboembolism in pregnancy. Arterioscler Thromb Vasc Biol. 2009;29(3):326–31.

41. van Vlijmen EF, Veeger NJ, Middeldorp S, et al. Thrombotic risk during oral contraceptive use and pregnancy in women with factor V Leiden or prothrombin mutation: a rational approach to contraception. Blood. 2011;118(8):2055–61. quiz 2375

42. Finer LB, Zolna MR. Declines in unintended pregnancy in the United States, 2008–2011. N Engl J Med. 2016;374(9):843–52.

43. Ott MA, Sucato GS, Committee on A. Contraception for adolescents. Pediatrics. 2014;134(4):e1257–81.

44. Hubacher D. Long-acting reversible contraception acceptability and satisfaction is high among adolescents. Evid Based Med. 2017;22(6):228–9.

45. Usinger KM, Gola SB, Weis M, Smaldone A. Intrauterine contraception continuation in ado-lescents and young women: a systematic review. J Pediatr Adolesc Gynecol. 2016;29(6):659–67.

46. Committee on Adolescent Health C. Committee Opinion No. 710: counseling adolescents about contraception. Obstet Gynecol. 2017;130(2):e74–80.

47. Curtis KM, Tepper NK, Jatlaoui TC, et al. U.S. medical eligibility criteria for contraceptive use, 2016. MMWR Recomm Rep. 2016;65(3):1–103.

48. Cardiovascular disease and use of oral and injectable progestogen-only contraceptives and combined injectable contraceptives. Results of an international, multicenter, case-control study. World Health Organization Collaborative Study of Cardiovascular Disease and Steroid Hormone Contraception. Contraception. 1998;57(5):315–24.

49. Barsoum MK, Heit JA, Ashrani AA, Leibson CL, Petterson TM, Bailey KR. Is progestin an independent risk factor for incident venous thromboembolism? A population-based case-control study. Thromb Res. 2010;126(5):373–8.

50. Heinemann LA, Assmann A, DoMinh T, Garbe E. Oral progestogen-only contraceptives and cardiovascular risk: results from the transnational study on oral contraceptives and the health of young women. Eur J Contracept Reprod Health Care. 1999;4(2):67–73.

51. Vasilakis C, Jick H, del Mar Melero-Montes M. Risk of idiopathic venous thromboembolism in users of progestagens alone. Lancet (London, England). 1999;354(9190):1610–1.

52. Mantha S, Karp R, Raghavan V, Terrin N, Bauer KA, Zwicker JI. Assessing the risk of venous thromboembolic events in women taking progestin-only contraception: a meta-analysis. BMJ. 2012;345:e4944.

53. Tepper NK, Whiteman MK, Marchbanks PA, James AH, Curtis KM. Progestin-only contraception and thromboembolism: a systematic review. Contraception. 2016;94(6):678–700.

54. Bergendal A, Persson I, Odeberg J, et al. Association of venous thromboembolism with hormonal contraception and thrombophilic genotypes. Obstet Gynecol. 2014;124(3):600–9.

55. Le Moigne E, Tromeur C, Delluc A, et al. Risk of recurrent venous thromboembolism on progestin-only contraception: a cohort study. Haematologica. 2016;101(1):e12–4.

56. Bistervels IM, Scheres LJJ, Hamulyak EN, Middeldorp S. Sex matters: practice 5P's when treating young women with venous thromboembolism. J Thromb Haemost. 2019;17(9):1417–29.

57. Scholes D, LaCroix AZ, Ichikawa LE, Barlow WE, Ott SM. Change in bone mineral density among adolescent women using and discontinuing depot medroxyprogesterone acetate contraception. Arch Pediatr Adolesc Med. 2005;159(2):139–44.

58. Practice Committee of the American Society for Reproductive Medicine. Electronic address Aao, Practice Committee of the American Society for Reproductive M. Combined hormonal contraception

and the risk of venous thromboembolism: a guideline. Fertil Steril. 2017;107(1):43–51.

59. de Bastos M, Stegeman BH, Rosendaal FR, et al. Combined oral contraceptives: venous thrombosis. Cochrane Database Syst Rev. 2014;3:CD010813.

60. Martinez F, Ramirez I, Perez-Campos E, Latorre K, Lete I. Venous and pulmonary thromboembolism and combined hormonal contraceptives. Systematic review and meta-analysis. Eur J Contracept Reprod Health Care. 2012;17(1):7–29.

61. Lidegaard O, Nielsen LH, Skovlund CW, Skjeldestad FE, Lokkegaard E. Risk of venous thromboembolism from use of oral contraceptives containing different progestogens and oestrogen doses: Danish cohort study, 2001-9. BMJ. 2011;343:d6423.

62. Maxwell WD, Jacob M, Spiryda LB, Bennett CL. Selection of contraceptive therapy for patients with thrombophilia: a review of the evidence. J Womens Health (Larchmt). 2014;23(4):318–26.

63. Wu O, Robertson L, Twaddle S, et al. Screening for thrombophilia in high-risk situations: systematic review and cost-effectiveness analysis. The Thrombosis: Risk and Economic Assessment of Thrombophilia Screening (TREATS) study. Health Technol Assess. 2006;10(11):1–110.

64. Timmer CJ, Mulders TM. Pharmacokinetics of etonogestrel and ethinylestradiol released from a combined contraceptive vaginal ring. Clin Pharmacokinet. 2000;39(3):233–42.

65. Abrams LS, Skee DM, Natarajan J, Wong FA, Lasseter KC. Multiple-dose pharmacokinetics of a contraceptive patch in healthy women participants. Contraception. 2001;64(5):287–94.

66. van den Heuvel MW, van Bragt AJ, Alnabawy AK, Kaptein MC. Comparison of ethinylestradiol pharmacokinetics in three hormonal contraceptive formulations: the vaginal ring, the transdermal patch and an oral contraceptive. Contraception. 2005;72(3):168–74.

67. Lidegaard O, Nielsen LH, Skovlund CW, Lokkegaard E. Venous thrombosis in users of non-oral hormonal contraception: follow-up study, Denmark 2001-10. BMJ. 2012;344:e2990.

68. Dinger J, Mohner S, Heinemann K. Cardiovascular risk associated with the use of an etonogestrel-containing vaginal ring. Obstet Gynecol. 2013;122(4):800–8.

69. Dore DD, Norman H, Loughlin J, Seeger JD. Extended case-control study results on thromboembolic outcomes among transdermal contraceptive users. Contraception. 2010;81(5):408–13.

70. Cole JA, Norman H, Doherty M, Walker AM. Venous thromboembolism, myocardial infarction, and stroke among transdermal contraceptive system users. Obstet Gynecol. 2007;109(2 Pt 1):339–46.

71. Sidney S, Cheetham TC, Connell FA, et al. Recent combined hormonal contraceptives (CHCs) and the risk of thromboembolism and other cardiovascular events in new users. Contraception. 2013;87(1):93–100.

72. Tepper NK, Dragoman MV, Gaffield ME, Curtis KM. Nonoral combined hormonal contraceptives and thromboembolism: a systematic review. Contraception. 2017;95(2):130–9.

73. Baglin T, Bauer K, Douketis J, et al. Duration of anticoagulant therapy after a first episode of an unprovoked pulmonary embolus or deep vein thrombosis: guidance from the SSC of the ISTH. J Thromb Haemost. 2012;10(4):698–702.

74. Martinelli I, Lensing AW, Middeldorp S, et al. Recurrent venous thromboembolism and abnormal uterine bleeding with anticoagulant and hormone therapy use. Blood. 2016;127(11):1417–25.

75. Massad LS, Einstein MH, Huh WK, et al. 2012 updated consensus guidelines for the management of abnormal cervical cancer screening tests and cancer precursors. J Low Genit Tract Dis. 2013;17(5 Suppl 1):S1–S27.

Heavy Menstrual Bleeding and Anticoagulation

16

Angela C. Weyand and Janice M. Staber

Heavy menstrual bleeding (HMB), defined as bleeding greater than 7 days or blood loss greater than 80 mL per menses, is a common complaint among adolescents. Up to 40% of females experience HMB during adolescence [1, 2]. To guide clinicians in the underlying diagnosis of HMB and abnormal uterine bleeding in all patients, the International Federation of Gynecology and Obstetrics (FIGO) Executive Board approved the FIGO (PALM-COEIN) classification system. PALM-COEIN divides causes into two groups: structural (*p*olyps, *a*denomyosis, *l*eiomyoma, and *m*alignancy) and nonstructural (*c*oagulopathy, *o*vulatory, *e*ndometrial, *i*atrogenic, and *n*ot yet classified) [3]. In adolescence, nonstructural causes are more common. Medication-induced HMB is categorized as a nonstructural (iatrogenic) cause. Medications, which can cause HMB, include anticoagulation, hormonal contraceptives (such as depot medroxyprogesterone), SSRIs, antipsychotics, tamoxifen, and herbals. Here, we will discuss epidemiology, evaluation, and management of anticoagulation-induced HMB.

Epidemiology of HMB in an Adolescent on Anticoagulation

Limited data is available investigating the rate of HMB in adolescents on anticoagulants. A large portion of the current data investigates rates of vaginal bleeding due to anticoagulation (specifically low-molecular weight heparin, LMWH) during pregnancy and/or postpartum hemorrhage. An additional difficulty to determine the rate of HMB in adolescents on anticoagulation is that the age range includes but is not limited to adolescents, for example, 14–55 or 18–55 years of age. Given the limited data, studies investigating either adolescents alone or adolescents and adult women treated with anticoagulants for treatment of venous thromboembolism or other causes are included in our discussion here.

HMB increases in adolescents after starting anticoagulation. In a study of 68 adolescents (9–21 years old) who all received anticoagulation due to thromboembolism (67/68) and/or cardiac (4/68) reasons, 76% of patients had HMB [4]. Thirteen of the 68 (19%) noted development of HMB after starting anticoagulation [4]. This study included the anticoagulants: enoxaparin, warfarin, unfractionated heparin, alteplase, fondaparinux, and/or aspirin.

A. C. Weyand
Division of Hematology and Oncology, Department of Pediatrics, University of Michigan Medical School, Ann Arbor, MI, USA

J. M. Staber (✉)
Division of Hematology, Oncology, and BMT, Stead Family Department of Pediatrics, University of Iowa Carver College of Medicine, Iowa City, IA, USA
e-mail: janice-staber@uiowa.edu

© Springer Nature Switzerland AG 2020
L. V. Srivaths (ed.), *Hematology in the Adolescent Female*,
https://doi.org/10.1007/978-3-030-48446-0_16

To investigate the risk of HMB when using warfarin alone, a retrospective chart review of adolescent females was conducted. Twenty-four (30%) of 81 adolescent females on warfarin were referred to gynecology due to HMB and 19 of the 24 patients required treatment [5]. To quantify this further, the Royal Free Hospital in London investigated changes in menstrual bleeding while on warfarin. Fifty-three women between 14 and 50 years old completed questionnaires including a pictorial blood assessment chart (PBAC) before and after initiating oral anticoagulation (warfarin) [6]. Forty-seven of the 53 completed the PBAC and revealed that after starting oral anticoagulation, the duration of menstruation increased from 5 to 7 days. Additionally, PBAC scores were increased over 100 in 31 of the 47 women after starting anticoagulation [6].

Although the age range does not specify that it included adolescents, a study in Pakistan had similar conclusions regarding the risk of HMB while taking warfarin. In 85 women of reproductive age (mean 30.13 ± 7.69 years) on warfarin due to prosthetic valve replacement, the mean PBAC score was elevated (162.8 ± 24.86, mean ± SD). Forty-six (54.1%) had continuous vaginal bleeding, 33 (38.8%) had HMB, 4 (4.7%) had intermenstrual bleeding, and 2 (2.4%) had HMB and polymenorrhea [7].

When the direct oral anticoagulants initiated clinical trials and then subsequently came to market, the community anticipated that these new agents would potentially decrease bleeding risk. In adults, the new oral anticoagulants result in decreased all-cause mortality and intracranial hemorrhage [8]. To further understand the risk of bleeding in women, Beyer-Westendorf and colleagues investigated the rate of HMB and vaginal bleeding using direct oral anticoagulants (DOACs) [9]. In 178 women (mean 39 ± 12 years) on apixaban (18, 10.1%), edoxaban (4, 2.2%), or rivaroxaban (156, 87.6%), 57 women reported vaginal bleeding. Of the vaginal bleeding events, HMB was the most common (59 of 72 events) in the 57 women. The rate of vaginal bleeding events was spread evenly among the DOACs (women effect/total women 6/18 apixaban, 1/4 edoxaban, and 50/156 rivaroxaban) [9].

Therefore, like the other anticoagulants, DOACs increase HMB.

With the development of the new anticoagulants, recent studies have sought to understand the differences in HMB rates between DOACs and warfarin. From a post-hoc analysis of the Hokusai-VTE study, 665 women less than 50 years old were taking warfarin, and 628 women less than 50 years old were taking edoxaban [10]. Abnormal vaginal bleeding was calculated as person-years and was found to be present in 9/100 person-years when taking warfarin and 15/100 person-years when taking edoxaban [10]. When edoxaban was compared to warfarin, the overall risk for major vaginal bleeding was increased (OR 2.8, edoxaban> warfarin).

Results from AMPLIFY were used to compare the incidence of abnormal vaginal bleeding between patients taking apixaban and warfarin including 1122 women on apixaban with a mean age of 46 years and 1106 women on warfarin with a mean age of 44 years [11]. Twenty-eight (2.5%) of those taking apixaban had clinically relevant nonmajor (CRNM) vaginal bleeding, and 24 (2.1%) of those taking warfarin had CRNM vaginal bleeding (OR 1.2, 95% CI 0.7–2.0). Although the absolute numbers were similar, the percentage of CRNM bleeding events related to vaginal bleeding was higher in the apixaban group. The total CRNM bleeding events in the apixaban group were 62, and 28 (40%) of those were related to vaginal bleeding. The total CRNM bleeding events in the warfarin group were 120 and 24 (20%) of those were related to vaginal bleeding. When apixaban was compared to warfarin, the risk of vaginal bleeding was significantly increased (OR 3.4, 95%CI 1.8–6.7) [11].

Bryk et al. and Cohen et al. have compared the rate of HMB between rivaroxaban and warfarin [12, 13]. In women (18–55 years old) taking rivaroxaban, 31 (41%) of 76 had HMB. This was compared to women (18–55 years old) taking vitamin K antagonists (VKAs) of which 8 (18%) of 45 women had HMB. Overall the risk of HMB was increased in women taking rivaroxaban compared to VKAs (OR 3.2, 95% CI 1.4–8.2; $p = 0.0009$) [12]. Additionally, a higher percentage of women required an intervention for HMB when taking rivaroxaban (29/76) compared to VKAs (6/45), $p = 0.004$ [12]. Additionally, through a retrospective questionnaire, Cohen et al. reported that rivaroxaban had a significant effect on menstrual bleeding compared to VKAs [13]. In women ages 14–55 years ($n = 52$ in each group), rivaroxaban was compared to VKA. Rivaroxaban was more likely to prolong menstrual bleeding ($p = 0.017$), has increased intermenstrual bleeding, and has increased average menstrual bleeding time compared to VKA [13]. Rivaroxaban increased the duration of menses from 5 to 6 days ($p = 0.001$) compared to no change in the VKA group [13].

The findings that edoxaban, rivaroxaban, and apixaban have a higher rate of HMB compared to warfarin lead to investigation of HMB in women taking dabigatran compared to warfarin. In a post-hoc analysis of the RE-COVER and RE-MEDY trials, 1280 between the ages of 18–50 years were randomized between dabigatran (643 patients) and warfarin (637 patients) [14]. Overall the rate of abnormal uterine bleeding was 8.1% (99/1280) [14]. Of those treated with warfarin, 61 (9.6%) had AUB compared to 38 (5.9%) in those treated with dabigatran (OR 0.59, 95% CI 0.39–0.90) [14]. Majority of the AUB in both groups were due to HMB and most of these were deemed mild in nature.

In summary, across studies DOACs (rivaroxaban, apixaban, edoxaban) compared to warfarin, direct Xa inhibitors had higher risk of abnormal uterine bleeding [10–13, 15]. Dabigatran was no different compared to VKA [14].

Evaluation of a Patient with HMB on Anticoagulation

HMB in women on anticoagulation is likely underrecognized as patients often do not report their change in bleeding pattern. A detailed menstrual bleeding history should be specifically sought in all women on anticoagulation. Symptoms predictive of HMB include a requirement to change sanitary pads or tampons more often than hourly, greater than 1-inch clots, and

a low ferritin level [16]. An underlying bleeding disorder should be considered in patients with long-standing HMB, other bleeding symptoms, and/or a suggestive family history. To determine and treat the underlying etiology of a woman's HMB, a stepwise approach is typically used. First, the provider should collect a thorough history with focus on medical, surgical, obstetric, gynecologic, family, hematologic, trauma, and medication histories. Physical examination should include vital sign assessment, cardiovascular, pulmonary, abdominal, and pelvic examinations. Laboratory evaluation should include urine or serum beta-human chorionic gonadotropin, complete blood count, type and cross (in case of need for transfusion), and iron studies to assess for deficiency. For women on anticoagulation, initial assessment should include an evaluation of whether the medication is truly needed and appropriately dosed. Concomitant medications that may exacerbate bleeding should also be reviewed. Laboratory evaluation is dependent on the specific anticoagulant used: an INR for patients on warfarin, creatinine clearance for patients on DOAC, and an anti-Xa level for patients on unfractionated or low-molecular weight heparin. Assessment of the necessity of continuing anticoagulant therapy is ideally made in collaboration with the physicians who originally prescribed the medication.

Management of HMB in a Patient on Anticoagulation

The goal of treating HMB is to decrease menstrual blood loss and its associated complications, such as iron deficiency anemia. Initial treatment decisions should be centered on the urgency of the situation. Specific treatment algorithms have been proposed [17–20].

Emergent

In the setting of acute severe bleeding, discontinuation of anticoagulation should be considered, versus discontinuation and utilization of a reversal agent. This decision ultimately depends on the individual patient's overall risk. In patients with hemodynamic instability, withholding anticoagulation, in addition to pharmacologic reversal, may be required. In patients with a recent venous thromboembolism (VTE) history (<1 month), continuation of some form of anticoagulation should be attempted [17]. In many patients with acute HMB, specific hormonal therapy is usually needed in addition to anticoagulation management in order to control bleeding. At this time, there is no data on the risk of thrombosis with hormonal therapy for acute HMB although high-dose estrogen therapy is likely to confer an elevated risk of thrombosis. Antifibrinolytics may be used acutely to improve hemostasis [17]. In the emergency setting, tranexamic acid can be given in a single IV dose of 10 mg/kg and repeated as required for bleeding every 6–8 hours. Experts have recommended this option be considered in patients with a remote VTE event (>3 months) due to lower recurrence risk [17]. ε-Aminocaproic acid [21] and ulipristal acetate [22] are two other treatment options that can be considered in the acute setting, although more research is needed. Surgical treatment is rarely necessary, but a consultation with gynecology to consider surgical options should be performed early in the evaluation. Cessation of bleeding can typically be achieved with intrauterine balloon tamponade, with inflation of a Foley balloon to the point of resistance (~30 mL) which is left in place from 2–48 hours [23, 24]. Dilation and curettage can be helpful diagnostically but their therapeutic efficacy is unknown. Endometrial ablation is effective in controlling HMB in 82–97% [19] although further surgery may be required in up to 8.5% [25]. Additionally, in a retrospective cohort study, it was found to be no more effective than the levonorgestrel intrauterine system (LNG-IUS) [26]. Uterine artery embolization is another less invasive option but has only been studied in the presence of fibroids, where it has been shown to decrease menstrual blood loss by up to 90% [27, 28]. Although hysterectomy is the definitive treatment for HMB, it is quite invasive and asso-

ciated with significant complications including bleeding and thrombosis. Experts recommend elective surgery be avoided for 6 months after an acute VTE. Beyond this 6-month period, patients with VTE history can receive perioperative anticoagulation prophylaxis if they are no longer on anticoagulation or have their anticoagulation temporarily interrupted [19].

Routine Management

The majority of HMB related to anticoagulation is minor and can be managed conservatively [20]. Patients with iron deficiency should receive iron therapy, in addition to treatments specific to HMB. Conservative management may entail a change in or initiation of hormonal therapy or temporary interruption or dose reduction of anticoagulation.

Anticoagulation Management

Dose reduction should be considered in patients who are stable and on anticoagulation for secondary prevention. In patients in the acute phase of venous thromboembolism, the risk of thromboembolic complications is high, and dose alteration may not be a safe option. With the increasing use of DOACs, dose reduction and temporary interruption have become more practical options. Data from the EINSTEIN CHOICE trial suggests that rivaroxaban 10 mg reduces menstrual bleeding without any increased thrombotic risk compared to the 20 mg dose. A small observational study reported seven patients with HMB who switched from rivaroxaban to apixaban, with five of these patients reporting resolution of symptoms [29]. Vitamin K antagonists have been demonstrated to confer a lower risk of HMB than the direct oral factor Xa inhibitors [9–13, 15] so an anticoagulation class switch could also be considered. However, this may not be wholly effective as Vitamin K antagonists are associated with higher rates of HMB compared with no anticoagulation [30, 31].

Hormonal Therapies

Combined hormonal contraceptives (CHC) significantly decrease menstrual blood loss in women with HMB, in turn increasing hemoglobin levels [32, 33]. CHCs have not been studied in women on anticoagulation, and historically, the thrombotic risk associated with CHCs has deterred their use in this population [34]. However, more recent evidence suggests that therapeutic-dose anticoagulation sufficiently overcomes the thrombotic risk associated with CHCs. Post-hoc analyses of the EINSTEIN deep venous thrombosis (DVT) and pulmonary embolism (PE) studies demonstrated similar risk of recurrent VTE in women receiving hormonal therapy (CHCs and progestin-only contraceptives) compared with those not receiving hormonal therapy (adjusted hazard ratio 0.56 (95% CI: 0.23–1.39)) [35]. These results reiterate guidelines from the International Society on Thrombosis and Hemostasis which support continuation of hormonal therapy in selected patients after anticoagulation initiation [36]. It is important to note that this increased thrombotic risk is overcome by treatment (not prophylactic) anticoagulation and any agents associated with increased thrombotic risk should be discontinued before discontinuation or de-escalation of anticoagulation.

Low-dose progestin-only contraceptives (POC), i.e., 0.5 mg norethindrone, have not been studied in HMB but are effective for contraception. A short course of higher dose POCs (10–15 mg daily of norethindrone, divided, for 7–11 days) has been studied for HMB but was found to be inferior to tranexamic acid, danazol, and the LNG-IUS [37]. A longer course (taken on days 5–26 of menstrual cycle) was also found to be inferior to these treatments but similar reduction in menstrual blood loss when compared to the combined vaginal ring [37]. Neither of these regimens has been studied in patients on anticoagulation.

Depot medroxyprogesterone acetate (DMPA) is an effective contraceptive and has also been used for HMB, with amenorrhea reported in 50% of normally menstruating women during the first year of use [38]. There is limited evidence to suggest increased odds of VTE with the use of DMPA, and this minimal increased risk is likely abrogated by therapeutic anticoagulation [39].

The LNG-IUS is extremely effective for HMB [40, 41] and has been recommended as the first-line option for HMB in women who also desire contraception [42]. There is evidence for the efficacy of the LNG-IUS for the treatment of HMB in women on anticoagulation. Multiple observational studies demonstrate decreased duration and amount of menstrual bleeding [43–45]. A randomized trial comparing women with HMB receiving VKAs assigned patients to LNG-IUS versus no treatment. Patients in the LNG-IUS group experienced a significant decrease in the number of bleeding days per cycle at 3 and 6 months, as well as an increase in mean hemoglobin and ferritin levels at 3 months [46]. The thrombotic risk of LNG-IUS is unknown, but general consensus is that in women with a history of VTE or thrombophilia, the benefits outweigh the risks [47].

There are many hormonal options available for the management of HMB in women on anticoagulation. An additional consideration when choosing a hormonal option is the risk of corpus luteum hemorrhage. Although the incidence of this complication is unknown, it can be fatal in up to 11% [48] and recur in up to 31% of patients [49]. Ovulation suppression should be considered and can be achieved with CHCs and DMPA. Progestin-only pills and LNG-IUS do not consistently suppress ovulation.

Antifibrinolytics

Tranexamic acid, an antifibrinolytic agent that inhibits clot breakdown, has been shown to be an effective treatment for HMB in women not receiving anticoagulation. Although it appears to be more effective than placebo, NSAIDs, oral luteal progestogens, ethamsylate, and herbal remedies, tranexamic acid may be less effective than the LNG-IUS [50]. The product monograph indicates a contraindication in patients with current or prior VTE, due to a post-marketing report suggesting an increased risk of thromboembolic events; however, this theoretical thrombotic risk has not held up in multiple studies [51, 52]. Further, most studies of antifibrinolytics in HMB did not specifically include thromboembolism as an outcome. Current evidence and general consensus support using tranexamic acid in women experiencing HMB on anticoagulation. Prospective studies are needed to confirm this consensus.

HMB in women on AC is a common yet underrecognized complication. Anticipatory guidance and prompt recognition may prevent catastrophic bleeding.

References

1. Barr F, Brabin L, Agbaje S, Buseri F, Ikimalo J, Briggs N. Reducing iron deficiency anaemia due to heavy menstrual blood loss in Nigerian rural adolescents. Public Health Nutr. 1998;1(4):249–57.
2. Friberg B, Orno AK, Lindgren A, Lethagen S. Bleeding disorders among young women: a population-based prevalence study. Acta Obstet Gynecol Scand. 2006;85(2):200–6.
3. Munro MG, Critchley HO, Broder MS, Fraser IS, FIGO Working Group on Menstrual Disorders. FIGO classification system (PALM-COEIN) for causes of abnormal uterine bleeding in nongravid women of reproductive age. Int J Gynaecol Obstet. 2011;113(1):3–13.
4. Soni H, Kurkowski J, Guffey D, Dietrich JE, Srivaths LV. Gynecologic bleeding complications in postmenarchal female adolescents receiving antithrombotic medications. J Pediatr Adolesc Gynecol. 2018;31(3):242–6.
5. Peake LJ, Grover SR, Monagle PT, Kennedy AD. Effect of warfarin on menstruation and menstrual management of the adolescent on warfarin. J Paediatr Child Health. 2011;47(12):893–7.
6. Huq FY, Tvarkova K, Arafa A, Kadir RA. Menstrual problems and contraception in women of reproductive age receiving oral anticoagulation. Contraception. 2011;84(2):128–32.
7. Nadeem S, Abbas S, Jalal A. The effect of oral progesterone for the treatment of abnormal uterine bleeding in women taking warfarin following prosthetic valve replacement. Pak J Med Sci. 2019;35(4):887–92.
8. Ruff CT, Giugliano RP, Braunwald E, Hoffman EB, Deenadayalu N, Ezekowitz MD, et al. Comparison of the efficacy and safety of new oral anticoagulants with warfarin in patients with atrial fibrillation: a meta-analysis of randomised trials. Lancet. 2014;383(9921):955–62.
9. Beyer-Westendorf J, Michalski F, Tittl L, Hauswald-Dorschel S, Marten S. Vaginal bleeding and heavy menstrual bleeding during direct oral anti-Xa inhibitor therapy. Thromb Haemost. 2016;115(6):1234–6.
10. Scheres L, Brekelmans M, Ageno W, Ay C, Buller HR, Eichinger S, et al. Abnormal vaginal bleeding in women of reproductive age treated with edoxaban or warfarin for venous thromboembolism: a post hoc analysis of the Hokusai-VTE study. BJOG. 2018;125(12):1581–9.
11. Brekelmans MP, Scheres LJ, Bleker SM, Hutten BA, Timmermans A, Buller HR, et al. Abnormal vaginal bleeding in women with venous thromboembolism treated with apixaban or warfarin. Thromb Haemost. 2017;117(4):809–15.
12. Bryk AH, Pirog M, Plens K, Undas A. Heavy menstrual bleeding in women treated with rivaroxaban and vitamin K antagonists and the risk of recurrent venous thromboembolism. Vasc Pharmacol. 2016;87:242–7.
13. Cohen H, Arachchillage DR, Beyer-Westendorf J, Middeldorp S, Kadir RA. Direct oral anticoagulants and women. Semin Thromb Hemost. 2016;42(7):789–97.
14. Huisman MV, Ferreira M, Feuring M, Fraessdorf M, Klok FA. Less abnormal uterine bleeding with dabigatran than warfarin in women treated for acute venous thromboembolism. J Thromb Haemost: JTH. 2018;16(9):1775–8.
15. De Crem N, Peerlinck K, Vanassche T, Vanheule K, Debaveye B, Middeldorp S, et al. Abnormal uterine bleeding in VTE patients treated with rivaroxaban compared to vitamin K antagonists. Thromb Res. 2015;136(4):749–53.
16. Warner PE, Critchley HO, Lumsden MA, Campbell-Brown M, Douglas A, Murray GD. Menorrhagia I: measured blood loss, clinical features, and outcome in women with heavy periods: a survey with follow-up data. Am J Obstet Gynecol. 2004;190(5):1216–23.
17. Boonyawat K, O'Brien SH, Bates SM. How I treat heavy menstrual bleeding associated with anticoagulants. Blood. 2017;130(24):2603–9.
18. James AH. Heavy menstrual bleeding: work-up and management. Hematology Am Soc Hematol Educ Program. 2016;2016(1):236–42.
19. Rivara A, James AH. Managing heavy menstrual bleeding in women at risk of thrombosis. Clin Obstet Gynecol. 2018;61(2):250–9.
20. Beyer-Westendorf J, Michalski F, Tittl L, Hauswald-Dorschel S, Marten S. Management and outcomes of vaginal bleeding and heavy menstrual bleeding in women of reproductive age on direct oral anti-factor Xa inhibitor therapy: a case series. Lancet Haematol. 2016;3(10):e480–e8.
21. Kasonde JM, Bonnar J. Effect of ethamsylate and aminocaproic acid on menstrual blood loss in women using intrauterine devices. Br Med J. 1975;4(5987):21–2.
22. Maybin JA, Critchley HO. Medical management of heavy menstrual bleeding. Women's Health (Lond, Engl). 2016;12(1):27–34.

23. Hamani Y, Ben-Shachar I, Kalish Y, Porat S. Intrauterine balloon tamponade as a treatment for immune thrombocytopenic purpura-induced severe uterine bleeding. Fertil Steril. 2010;94(7):2769.e13–5.

24. Goldrath MH. Uterine tamponade for the control of acute uterine bleeding. Am J Obstet Gynecol. 1983;147(8):869–72.

25. Fergusson RJ, Lethaby A, Shepperd S, Farquhar C. Endometrial resection and ablation versus hysterectomy for heavy menstrual bleeding. Cochrane Database Syst Rev. 2013;(11):Cd000329.

26. Bhattacharya S, Middleton LJ, Tsourapas A, Lee AJ, Champaneria R, Daniels JP, et al. Hysterectomy, endometrial ablation and Mirena(R) for heavy menstrual bleeding: a systematic review of clinical effectiveness and cost-effectiveness analysis. Health Technol Assess (Winch, Engl). 2011;15(19):iii–xvi, 1–252.

27. Walker WJ, Pelage JP. Uterine artery embolisation for symptomatic fibroids: clinical results in 400 women with imaging follow up. BJOG. 2002;109(11):1262–72.

28. Khaund A, Moss JG, McMillan N, Lumsden MA. Evaluation of the effect of uterine artery embolisation on menstrual blood loss and uterine volume. BJOG. 2004;111(7):700–5.

29. Myers B, Webster A. Heavy menstrual bleeding on Rivaroxaban – Comparison with Apixaban. Br J Haematol. 2017;176(5):833–5.

30. Sjalander A, Friberg B, Svensson P, Stigendal L, Lethagen S. Menorrhagia and minor bleeding symptoms in women on oral anticoagulation. J Thromb Thrombolysis. 2007;24(1):39–41.

31. van Eijkeren MA, Christiaens GC, Haspels AA, Sixma JJ. Measured menstrual blood loss in women with a bleeding disorder or using oral anticoagulant therapy. Am J Obstet Gynecol. 1990;162(5):1261–3.

32. Fraser IS, Romer T, Parke S, Zeun S, Mellinger U, Machlitt A, et al. Effective treatment of heavy and/or prolonged menstrual bleeding with an oral contraceptive containing estradiol valerate and dienogest: a randomized, double-blind Phase III trial. Hum Reprod (Oxford, Engl). 2011;26(10):2698–708.

33. Lethaby A, Wise MR, Weterings MA, Bofill Rodriguez M, Brown J. Combined hormonal contraceptives for heavy menstrual bleeding. Cochrane Database Syst Rev. 2019;2:Cd000154.

34. WHO Guidelines Approved by the Guidelines Review Committee. Medical eligibility criteria for contraceptive use. Geneva: World Health Organization; 2015. Copyright (c) World Health Organization 2015.

35. Martinelli I, Lensing AW, Middeldorp S, Levi M, Beyer-Westendorf J, van Bellen B, et al. Recurrent venous thromboembolism and abnormal uterine bleeding with anticoagulant and hormone therapy use. Blood. 2016;127(11):1417–25.

36. Baglin T, Bauer K, Douketis J, Buller H, Srivastava A, Johnson G. Duration of anticoagulant therapy after a first episode of an unprovoked pulmonary embolus or deep vein thrombosis: guidance from the SSC of the ISTH. J Thromb Haemost: JTH. 2012;10(4):698–702.

37. Bofill Rodriguez M, Lethaby A, Low C, Cameron IT. Cyclical progestogens for heavy menstrual bleeding. Cochrane Database Syst Rev. 2019;8:Cd001016.

38. Hubacher D, Lopez L, Steiner MJ, Dorflinger L. Menstrual pattern changes from levonorgestrel subdermal implants and DMPA: systematic review and evidence-based comparisons. Contraception. 2009;80(2):113–8.

39. Tepper NK, Whiteman MK, Marchbanks PA, James AH, Curtis KM. Progestin-only contraception and thromboembolism: a systematic review. Contraception. 2016;94(6):678–700.

40. Lethaby A, Hussain M, Rishworth JR, Rees MC. Progesterone or progestogen-releasing intrauterine systems for heavy menstrual bleeding. Cochrane Database Syst Rev. 2015;(4):Cd002126.

41. Stewart A, Cummins C, Gold L, Jordan R, Phillips W. The effectiveness of the levonorgestrel-releasing intrauterine system in menorrhagia: a systematic review. BJOG. 2001;108(1):74–86.

42. National Collaborating Centre for Women's and Children's Health (UK). National Institute for Health and Clinical Excellence: Guidance. Heavy menstrual bleeding. London: RCOG Press, National Collaborating Centre for Women's and Children's Health; 2007.

43. Vilos GA, Tureanu V, Garcia M, Abu-Rafea B. The levonorgestrel intrauterine system is an effective treatment in women with abnormal uterine bleeding and anticoagulant therapy. J Minim Invasive Gynecol. 2009;16(4):480–4.

44. Lukes AS, Reardon B, Arepally G. Use of the levonorgestrel-releasing intrauterine system in women with hemostatic disorders. Fertil Steril. 2008;90(3):673–7.

45. Pisoni CN, Cuadrado MJ, Khamashta MA, Hunt BJ. Treatment of menorrhagia associated with oral anticoagulation: efficacy and safety of the levonorgestrel releasing intrauterine device (Mirena coil). Lupus. 2006;15(12):877–80.

46. Kilic S, Yuksel B, Doganay M, Bardakci H, Akinsu F, Uzunlar O, et al. The effect of levonorgestrel-releasing intrauterine device on menorrhagia in women taking anticoagulant medication after cardiac valve replacement. Contraception. 2009;80(2):152–7.

47. Curtis KM, Tepper NK, Jatlaoui TC, Berry-Bibee E, Horton LG, Zapata LB, et al. U.S. medical eligibility criteria for contraceptive use, 2016. MMWR Recomm Rep. 2016;65(3):1–103.

48. Ho WK, Wang YF, Wu HH, Tsai HD, Chen TH, Chen M. Ruptured corpus luteum with hemoperitoneum: case characteristics and demographic changes over time. Taiwan J Obstet Gynecol. 2009;48(2):108–12.

49. Peters WA 3rd, Thiagarajah S, Thornton WN Jr. Ovarian hemorrhage in patients receiving anticoagulant therapy. J Reprod Med. 1979;22(2):82–6.

50. Bryant-Smith AC, Lethaby A, Farquhar C, Hickey M. Antifibrinolytics for heavy menstrual bleeding. Cochrane Database Syst Rev. 2018;4:Cd000249.

51. Long B, April MD. Does tranexamic acid affect risk of venous and arterial thrombosis or mortality in nonsurgical patients? Ann Emerg Med. 2020;75(4):535–7.

52. Chornenki NLJ, Um KJ, Mendoza PA, Samienezhad A, Swarup V, Chai-Adisaksopha C, et al. Risk of venous and arterial thrombosis in non-surgical patients receiving systemic tranexamic acid: a systematic review and meta-analysis. Thromb Res. 2019;179:81–6.

Part III

Anemia in the Adolescent Female

Iron Deficiency Anemia

Amanda E. Jacobson-Kelly, Ruchika Sharma, and Jacquelyn M. Powers

Introduction

Role of Iron

Iron, the fourth most common element on earth, is biologically essential for every living organism [1]. While the majority of the body's iron resides within the hemoglobin of circulating red blood cells and in the muscle protein myoglobin, high levels can also be found in the macrophages, liver, and brain [2–4]. Iron is critical for the delivery of oxygen to the tissues, the formation of enzymes involved in both electron transfer, oxidation-reduction reactions related to cellular growth and differentiation, as well as energy metabolism [5]. Myelin formation is also dependent on iron, and iron homeostasis is critical for normal brain function, especially in learning and memory [3, 6, 7].

Epidemiology

The World Health Organization (WHO) defines anemia as a condition in which the number of red blood cells or their oxygen-carrying capacity is insufficient to meet physiologic needs. Iron deficiency is the leading cause of anemia worldwide, affecting over one billion people [8]. Both the prevalence and severity of IDA are higher and more pronounced in women, with those of childbearing age comprising the greatest proportion of affected individuals [8]. In the United States (US), it is estimated that 9–11% of girls between 12 and 19 years of age are iron deficient based on data extracted from the National Health and Nutrition Examination Survey [9]. An analysis of the Pediatric Hospital Information System database from 2012 to 2015 found that hundreds of adolescent girls are admitted annually to US children's hospitals due to severe IDA [10].

Outcomes

Iron deficiency, with or without anemia, impairs tissue oxygen delivery and results in significant physical and cognitive symptoms (Table 17.1) [11].

Amanda E. Jacobson-Kelly and Ruchika Sharma contributed equally with all other contributors.

A. E. Jacobson-Kelly
Department of Pediatrics, Division of Hematology/Oncology/BMT, Nationwide Children's Hospital/The Ohio State University College of Medicine, Columbus, OH, USA

R. Sharma
Department of Pediatrics, Medical College of Wisconsin, Milwaukee, WI, USA

J. M. Powers (✉)
Department of Pediatrics, Baylor College of Medicine, Texas Children's Cancer and Hematology Center, Houston, TX, USA
e-mail: jacquelyn.powers@bcm.edu

© Springer Nature Switzerland AG 2020
L. V. Srivaths (ed.), *Hematology in the Adolescent Female*,
https://doi.org/10.1007/978-3-030-48446-0_17

Table 17.1 Non-hematologic effects of iron deficiency in adolescent girls

Common effects
Fatigue
Loss of hair
Muscle weakness, exercise intolerance
Difficulty concentrating
Cognitive deficits
Restless legs, sleep disturbances
Learning impairment
Headaches
Depression, mood disturbances
Rare effects
Reduced immune response
Koilonychia
Plummer-Vinson syndrome (atrophic glossitis, esophageal webs/strictures)
Anemic retinopathy [59, 60]
Ischemic stroke, cerebral venous sinus thrombosis

Impaired health-related quality of life, fatigue, sleep disturbance, muscle weakness, cognitive impairment, and poorer school performance have been reported [11, 12]. A study that randomized over 600 non-anemic iron-deficient adolescent girls to oral iron supplementation or placebo demonstrated improved scores on tests of verbal learning and memory in the group treated with iron [11]. Additional studies have demonstrated effects of iron deficiency on attention span and sensory perception functions [11]. Exercise performance is attenuated in persons with iron deficiency, and supplementation has demonstrated improved endurance capacity and aerobic adaptation during exercise in those affected [12]. Iron deficiency has been shown to impact immune status as well as morbidity from infection [13]. Finally, during pregnancy, IDA increases perinatal risks for mothers and is associated with increased overall infant mortality [14].

Iron Homeostasis

In healthy adults, typical iron losses of approximately 1 mg per day are balanced by the absorption of 1–2 mg of dietary iron daily, maintaining a net iron balance. Absorption of iron occurs within the duodenum [15]. While the mechanism of heme iron absorption is not well understood, non-heme iron absorption has been well characterized. From the luminal surface of the duodenal enterocyte, non-heme iron in the ferric ($^{+3}$) form is reduced by ferrireductase to the ferrous ($^{+2}$) form and then transported into the cell across divalent metal transporter 1 (DMT1) [2]. Inside the enterocyte, iron may be stored as ferritin or, in states of iron deficiency, will be transported across the transmembrane iron exporter ferroportin into the plasma [16]. There, iron is oxidized and then bound by transferrin for transport to tissues such as the bone marrow for erythropoiesis or other storage sites. Ferritin is the major iron storage protein and located predominantly in macrophages of the spleen, liver, bone marrow, and skeletal muscle [16]. Limited iron absorption is required in persons with normal iron status due to the efficient recycling of iron from circulating erythrocytes. At the end of their lifespan, erythrocytes are catabolized by macrophages, releasing iron. Iron is then exported, also by the transmembrane protein ferroportin, with the aid of the ferroxidase ceruloplasmin, into the plasma and transported in a similar manner by transferrin.

Iron homeostasis is regulated primarily by hepcidin, a hepatic peptide hormone [15]. Hepcidin acts on ferroportin, causing its endocytosis and internal degradation, at the sites of absorption (enterocytes of the duodenum), storage (primarily hepatocytes of the liver), and recycling (macrophages of the reticuloendothelial system). Many physiologic and pathophysiologic conditions affect the expression of hepcidin [17]. However, its production is particularly sensitive to iron status. In response to increased iron levels, hepcidin synthesis is increased, which results in a decrease in the release of iron from tissues. Conversely, iron deficiency states result in the downregulation of hepcidin, allowing for more efficient iron absorption. Mutations in the *TMPRSS6* gene, encoding a transmembrane serine protease that suppresses hepcidin production, have been implicated in the rare condition of iron-refractory iron deficiency anemia (IRIDA) [18, 19].

Pathophysiology of Iron Deficiency

Iron deficiency results when either iron losses or requirements, or both, exceed absorption. Multiple etiologies place adolescent girls at high risk for iron deficiency including a low iron diet, increased iron requirement associated with growth, menstrual blood loss, gastrointestinal blood loss and/or impaired absorption, and potential inflammation from underlying medical conditions.

Low Iron Diet/Rapid Growth

Growing adolescents are at increased risk for iron deficiency due to increased growth velocity (i.e., growth spurts) [20]. In addition to growth, dietary habits typical of adolescents such as erratic eating or skipped meals may lead to lower iron consumption. Eating disorders are also highly prevalent in this population, with peak age of onset between 13 and 18 years of age, and may contribute to the development of nutritional deficiencies [21].

The types of iron consumed (heme versus non-heme) is also important to consider given differences in bioavailability. Heme iron, derived predominantly from hemoglobin and myoglobin in meats, is better absorbed. Non-heme iron found in both meat and plant foods is highly insoluble, and its bioavailability can be affected by other dietary components. Therefore, any adolescent girl following a restrictive diet, including a vegan or vegetarian diet, should make a concerted effort to incorporate iron-rich foods from non-heme sources and be mindful of consuming other foods that aid iron absorption rather than impair it.

Menstrual Blood Loss

Menstrual blood loss is a significant risk factor for the development of iron deficiency in adolescent girls and young women. Post-menarchal females have lower iron stores at baseline and are susceptible to both iron deficiency and pro-gression to IDA [22]. Abnormal uterine bleeding, specifically heavy menstrual bleeding (HMB), defined as excessive or prolonged menstruation leading to >80 mL blood loss per cycle, places adolescent girls at even higher risk [20]. All young women presenting with HMB should be screened for iron deficiency with a serum ferritin and treated with iron therapy as needed to prevent serious complications such as severe IDA [23].

Other Etiologies

Athlete's Anemia

Iron deficiency is widely reported in athletes, particularly female and high-endurance athletes. In at least one study, the prevalence of iron deficiency or depletion (i.e., low ferritin) and IDA in young female athletes was 86% and 53%, respectively [24]. Potential mechanisms include increased plasma volume, occult gastrointestinal bleeding, acute inflammation, and tissue injury. Exercise-induced or "foot-strike" hemolysis is typically seen as mild intravascular hemolysis during physical exercise in athletes. Direct mechanical injury caused by forceful contact with the ground, repeated muscle contractile activity, or vasoconstriction in internal organs are potential sources of exercise-induced hemolysis in athletes [25].

GI Blood Loss/Impaired GI Absorption

IDA in an adolescent female without a history of poor diet or HMB, diet should prompt evaluation for gastrointestinal (GI) blood loss. Anemia, due to a combination of iron deficiency and/or acute blood loss, is the most common extra-intestinal symptom, and often a presenting symptom, of inflammatory bowel disease (IBD) [26, 27]. IBD, both Crohn's disease and ulcerative colitis, has a peak incidence at 15–30 years of age. Thus, it should be in the differential diagnosis for IDA in adolescent and young adult women even in the absence of overt GI symptoms [28].

Additional potential causes of GI blood loss, though less frequent in this age group, include infection, gastritis, gastric or duodenal ulcers, GI polyps, or malignancies. *Helicobacter pylori* (*H. pylori*) is a common infectious cause of gastritis and upper GI ulcers, especially in patients from endemic populations [29]. *H. pylori*-related gastritis as well as autoimmune gastritis can interfere with iron absorption. Given its rising prevalence, 1% in most Western populations, celiac disease should also be considered as it can cause significant IDA due to poor absorption, even in the absence of symptoms [30, 31]. Proton pump inhibitors for acid reflux can also reduce non-heme iron absorption, rendering oral iron therapy less effective.

sis in which iron is present but unavailable for utilization, leading to decreased iron availability for the production of red blood cells [32]. AI is often multifactorial. Altered iron metabolism from upregulation of hepcidin, decreased erythropoietin production, and/or poor response to erythropoietin all contribute [33]. While AI can mimic IDA, it is important to remember that many patients may have both AI and functional iron deficiency, and such patients may benefit from treatment, specifically with intravenous iron. Iron deficiency in patients with inflammatory disorders can be challenging to diagnose because typical iron laboratory parameters may be inaccurate in the setting of inflammation (Table 17.2).

Anemia of Inflammation (AI)/Mixed AI/IDA

Chronic inflammatory states seen in patients with chronic kidney disease, rheumatologic disorders, IBD, or heart failure may result in development of anemia of inflammation (AI) or chronic disease. AI is a form of iron-restricted erythropoie-

Diagnosis

Clinical History

Clinical history is critically important in identifying the underlying etiology or etiologies of IDA in adolescent girls. The presence of certain risk factors should increase your index of suspi-

Table 17.2 Iron parameters for adolescent females based on iron status

Parameter	Iron deficiency without anemia	Iron deficiency anemia (IDA)	Anemia of inflammation (AI)	Mixed AI/IDA	Limitations
Hemoglobin concentration	≥12 g/dL	≥9 to <12 g/dL (mild) <9 g/dL (moderate/severe)	<12 g/dL	<12 g/dL	Inflammation may transiently decrease hemoglobin
Mean corpuscular volume (MCV)	Normal (>80 fL)	Decreased	Decreased	Decreased	Presence of thalassemia, hemoglobin E, or hemoglobin C trait will lower MCV MCV may be normal if IDA is mixed with another nutritional deficiency like folate or B12 deficiency or initially normal with acute blood loss
Serum ferritin	Decreased (<15 ng/dL)	Decreased	Normal or elevated	Normal or elevated	Ferritin is an acute phase reactant and will be falsely normal or elevated in inflammatory states
Serum iron	Normal or decreased	Decreased (<30 mcg/dL)	Normal	Decreased or normal	Varies by time of day and recent iron ingestion

Table 17.2 (continued)

Parameter	Iron deficiency without anemia	Iron deficiency anemia (IDA)	Anemia of inflammation (AI)	Mixed AI/ IDA	Limitations
Transferrin saturation	Normal or decreased (<15–20%)	Decreased	Decreased	Decreased	Calculated measure of serum iron and TIBC (thus, anything affecting those measures will impact transferrin saturation)
Total iron binding capacity (TIBC)	Elevated (>450 mcg/ dL)	Elevated	Normal or decreased	Normal or decreased	May be normal in early iron deficiency Inflammation, liver disease, protein loss, and hemolysis may lower value Hormonal contraceptives and pregnancy may increase value
Soluble transferrin receptor (sTfR)	Elevated (>2.5 mg/L)	Elevated	Normal	Elevated	Can be elevated in high-turnover states (hemolytic anemia) Not widely available, typically a send-out Reference ranges often not available for patients <18 years
sTfR-ferritin index[a]	Elevated (>1.5)	Elevated	Normal	Elevated	Not widely available, typically a send-out Reference ranges often not available for patients <18 years
Reticulocyte hemoglobin content (CHr) or equivalent (RET-He) [61]	Decreased (<27 pg)	Decreased	Decreased	Decreased	Will also be decreased if thalassemia or thalassemia trait is present, though to a greater extent than IDA alone
Hepcidin	Decreased	Decreased	Increased	Increased	Not yet widely clinically available, typically only performed on research basis

[a]sTfR-ferritin index = sTfR in mg/L ÷ Log(ferritin in ng/mL)

cion and guide testing. All girls should be asked about a previous history of iron deficiency, overall diet including dietary restrictions or disordered eating, HMB, and GI blood loss or symptoms. The patient's growth chart may provide evidence of being underweight or obese, both of which are risk factors for iron deficiency. A detailed menstrual history is key as patients in this age group may not report or recognize HMB. Adolescent girls should be asked specifically about menses lasting >7 days, bleeding that soaks through 1 or more tampons/pads within 1 hour for several hours in a row, needing to wear "double protection" (i.e., a pad and a tampon or two pads to prevent leaking), having to change products overnight due to bleeding, or passing blood clots larger than a quarter [34, 35].

In girls 16 years of age or older, a history of blood donation may also place them at risk for iron deficiency. It is also prudent to assess for additional risk factors such as long-distance running or other high-endurance sports, as well as any concomitant chronic illness [36]. Pica, the craving and/or consumption of non-food items, can also be a sign of iron deficiency. Pica for ice (pagophagia) is a common form that is strongly associated with iron deficiency, particularly in Western cultures [37]. Other common symptoms include fatigue, exercise intolerance, headaches, orthostatic dizziness, poor concentration, and restless legs [38, 39].

Laboratory Assessment

In an otherwise healthy female adolescent, the diagnosis of iron deficiency should be straightforward. A microcytic anemia with a clinical history consistent with IDA, in addition to characteristic findings on peripheral smear, is sufficient for the diagnosis [32]. In patients without anemia or those with less convincing clinical histories, iron studies may be obtained. While there is no gold standard test, a low serum ferritin (<15 ng/mL) is always consistent with iron deficiency. Identifying iron deficiency in patients with chronic disease can be challenging because typical iron laboratory parameters may be inaccurate in the setting of inflammation. Absence of stainable iron on a bone marrow biopsy is considered the definitive marker for iron deficiency, but it is prohibitively invasive, particularly in children. Assessment of the serum soluble transferrin receptor (sTfR) and/or the sTfR-ferritin index (sTfR/log ferritin) may be helpful in distinguishing between IDA and AI or mixed anemia (IDA + AI) as sTfR concentration is less affected by inflammation [40–43]. A combination of ferritin and transferrin saturation (also called iron saturation in some labs) may also be used to make the diagnosis of AI. Consensus recommendations on identifying iron deficiency in the setting inflammation in adults suggest using a serum ferritin threshold of <100 ng/mL or a transferrin saturation of <20% and when the serum ferritin is >100 but <300 ng/mL to identify iron deficiency [44]. Table 17.2 demonstrates laboratory parameters for iron based on iron status, as well as limitations associated with each specific test.

Therapy

Dietary Counseling

All adolescent girls with IDA should be provided dietary counseling. For those girls who are not vegetarian or vegan, heme iron found in meats (including poultry and red meat) may be encouraged due to their higher bioavailability. For those girls with religious and/or personal oppositions, counseling should be provided to identify iron-rich non-heme sources that can be incorporated into the diet.

Oral Iron

For the majority of adolescent females, initial treatment for IDA should be oral iron therapy in addition to dietary counseling to improve iron intake. Iron salts, specifically ferrous sulfate tablets, are generally the first line for treatment as they are more effectively absorbed compared to ferric forms of iron and are generally well-tolerated [45]. We recommend tablets over enteric-coated capsules as the latter may result in suboptimal absorption. Other oral iron supplements include ferrous fumarate, ferrous gluconate, ferrous citrate, and polysaccharide-iron complex.

Dosing

All oral iron dosing should be based on elemental iron content with a recommended daily dose of 65–130 mg administered once daily (not divided). This dose, approximately 1–2 tablets of iron, should be sufficient for the majority of affected adolescents. In girls with newly diagnosed moderate to severe IDA, two tablets (130 mg) may be considered initially followed by a decreased dose to one tablet (65 mg) as the anemia improves. Higher or more frequent dosing may increase side effects and decrease subsequent fractional absorption of oral iron [46]. Every other day dosing can be considered in adolescents with non-anemic iron deficiency or in IDA patients in whom the hemoglobin concentration has normalized, as this strategy maximizes the fractional absorption of iron and decreases side effects [47]. To facilitate absorption, oral iron should be taken 2 hours before or 4 hours after ingestion of antacids and separate from calcium supplements or milk products, which can both significantly inhibit absorption.

Safety and Adverse Effects

Oral iron therapy is not tolerated by all patients. Common GI complaints include nausea, "upset" stomach, and constipation, and typically, such side effects are dose-related (i.e., increase with higher doses of elemental iron). Taking iron with food can also reduce side effects but, as noted earlier, may impair absorption. Adding concomitant administration of ascorbic acid may help ameliorate this impact on absorption [48].

Response

In patients with moderate to severe IDA (Hgb <9 g/dL) who have initiated oral iron therapy, a complete blood count (CBC), including hemoglobin concentration (Hgb) and red blood cell indices, along with a reticulocyte count should be reassessed in 7–10 days. Reticulocytosis along with an increase in Hgb by ≥1 g/dL marks an appropriate response. For patients with mild anemia, the Hgb should rise by at least 1 g/dL, or ideally normalize, within 4 weeks of iron therapy initiation. All patients should be assessed again with both a CBC and serum ferritin at the 3-month time point to determine whether the IDA is fully resolved or if additional iron is required to replenish iron stores. This approach ensures that iron therapy is not discontinued too early, a common cause for recurrent IDA.

Intravenous Iron

Indications

Due to high cost and perceived risk of adverse events, intravenous iron therapy is typically considered a second-line treatment for IDA in most adolescent females. Yet, side effects of oral iron may contribute to poor adherence and persistent iron deficiency. Therefore, for any patient who is intolerant of, or unresponsive to, oral iron, intravenous iron administration may be considered [49]. Additional indications include poor GI absorption (i.e., IBD, newly diagnosed celiac disease, or celiac disease with poor adherence to gluten-free diet), ongoing GI blood loss, need for rapid anemia correction (prior to surgery), and functional iron deficiency or AI (i.e., inflammatory arthritis, systemic lupus erythematosus, or chronic kidney disease, [*see previous section on AI*]) [50]. Intravenous iron should be considered in these affected patients, regardless of the degree of anemia [51].

Preparations and Dosing

Five intravenous iron preparations have been approved by the US Food and Drug Administration (FDA) for use in adults (Table 17.3). All intravenous iron products are colloids of spherical iron-carbohydrate nanoparticles [50]. The strength of

Table 17.3 Intravenous iron preparations, labeled indications, and adolescent dosing in the United States

Generic name	Ferric gluconate	Iron sucrose	Low-molecular weight iron dextran	Ferumoxytol	Ferric carboxymaltose
Trade name	Ferrlecit	Venofer	INFeD	Feraheme	Injectafer
FDA indication (Adult)	Patients with chronic kidney disease on dialysis + erythropoiesis-stimulating agents	Patients with chronic kidney disease	Patients in whom oral iron administration is unsatisfactory or impossible	Patients with chronic kidney disease	Patients with intolerance or unsatisfactory response to oral iron; non-dialysis dependent chronic kidney disease
FDA approved (Pediatric)	Yes, >6 years	Yes, >2 years	Yes, >4 months	No	No
Pediatric dosing per infusion (Max)	1.5 mg/kg (125 mg)	5–7 mg/kg (300 mg)	Calculate deficit (100 mg)[a]	Adult dosing only 510 mg	Adult dosing only 15 mg/kg (750 mg)
Infusion time	60 minutes	2–5 minutes	60 minutes	15–60 minutes	15–60 minutes
Test dose required	No	No	Yes (25 mg)	No	No
Black box warning	No	No	Yes	Yes	No
Iron concentration	12.5 mg/mL	20 mg/mL	50 mg/mL	30 mg/mL	50 mg/mL

[a]Off-label total dose iron dextran up to 1000 mg has been reported in pediatrics [54]

the iron-carbohydrate complex directly affects the amount of iron that can be safely administered during a single infusion with higher amounts resulting in toxicity due to the release of free iron. Newer preparations have stronger complexes that allow for a slower release of iron, which results in less toxicity and allows for larger doses to be administered via smaller number of infusions [50]. All forms of intravenous iron are more costly than available oral iron therapies, with newer preparations being the most expensive. Obtaining insurance approval and discussing costs with families are important aspects to consider for this treatment option.

Regardless of the preparation, the total iron dose required by any individual patient should be the same. To calculate the iron deficit (to determine total dose of iron needed), the Ganzoni formula can be used: total iron deficit in mg = weight [kg] × ([target hemoglobin [g/dL] – actual hemoglobin [g/dL]) × 2.4 + iron stores ([mg] 500 mg for adults and children >35 kg) [52]. Once both the total iron dose required and intravenous iron product are determined, then the approximate number of infusions needed to achieve that dose can be determined.

Ferric gluconate and iron sucrose both have FDA labeling for use in children with chronic kidney disease (Table 17.3) [49]. These formulations have excellent safety profiles but are limited by the maximum dose of iron that can be given in a single infusion [53]. Low-molecular weight iron dextran (LMWID) is approved for children who are intolerant to oral iron therapy. The FDA-labeled maximum dose is 100 mg, although data exists to support the off-label administration of up to 1000 mg in a single infusion [54]. Both ferumoxytol and ferric carboxymaltose are FDA approved for the treatment of IDA in adults. They both allow for larger infusions to be administered compared to earlier generations of intravenous iron (510 mg for ferumoxytol and 15 mg/kg or 750 mg for ferric carboxymaltose, with some data on the use of these products in children [55, 56].

Safety and Adverse Effects
Historical concerns for high rates of anaphylaxis are predominantly related to older, less stable intravenous iron preparations [51]. Newer preparations in the last two decades have markedly improved safety profiles although LMWID and ferumoxytol carry black box warnings, with the former requiring a test-dose prior to full-dose administration. Recent literature supports that all currently available intravenous iron formulations are safe and efficacious, and the risk of serious adverse events such as anaphylaxis is low [50, 51]. Patients receiving ferric carboxymaltose should have phosphorus monitoring performed due to reports of transient hypophosphatemia in treated adults [57]. Any patient receiving intravenous iron therapy should be monitored closely during infusion to minimize the risk of extravasation, which can result in permanent darkening of staining of the subcutaneous tissue.

Response
Patients receiving intravenous iron therapy should have repeat hematologic testing 4–6 weeks following administration to assess for efficacy. Patients at risk for recurrent iron deficiency including those with ongoing GI blood loss or HMB should be reassessed periodically to evaluate for recurrence of IDA and the need for ongoing treatment.

Red Cell Transfusion

Allogenic packed red blood cell transfusions should be reserved for adolescents with symptomatic anemia, hemodynamic instability, and/or evidence of end-organ ischemia. Typically, this does not occur until hemoglobin concentration is <7 g/dL [58]. In patients with severe anemia, transfusions should be administered in small aliquots to minimize the risk of heart failure, which may develop with rapid transfusion or larger transfusion volumes.

Summary

Iron deficiency, with or without anemia, is common in adolescent girls. Clinical risk factors include low iron diet and menstrual blood loss.

Girls with GI conditions, chronic inflammation, or who participate in high-endurance activities and/or sports are also at higher risk for developing IDA. Understanding the clinical risk factors and available laboratory assessments can support accurate diagnosis. Iron therapy with oral or intravenous iron may be offered based on the patient's underlying etiology, risk factors, as well as patient and family preferences.

References

1. Denic S, Agarwal MM. Nutritional iron deficiency: an evolutionary perspective. Nutrition. 2007;23(7-8):603–14.
2. Andrews NC, Fleming MD, Levy JE. Molecular insights into mechanisms of iron transport. Curr Opin Hematol. 1999;6(2):61–4.
3. Youdim MB, Ben-Shachar D, Yehuda S. Putative biological mechanisms of the effect of iron deficiency on brain biochemistry and behavior. Am J Clin Nutr. 1989;50(Suppl):607–15.
4. Camaschella C. Iron-deficiency anemia. N Engl J Med. 2015;372(19):1832–43.
5. Lieu PT, Heiskala M, Peterson PA, Yang Y. The roles of iron in health and disease. Mol Asp Med. 2001;22(1-2):1–87.
6. Youdim MB, Ben-Shachar D, Yehuda S, Riederer P. The role of iron in the basal ganglion. Adv Neurol. 1990;53:155–62.
7. Gerlach M, Ben-Shachar D, Riederer P, Youdim MB. Altered brain metabolism of iron as a cause of neurodegenerative diseases? J Neurochem. 1994;63(3):793–807.
8. Kassebaum NJ, Jasrasaria R, Naghavi M, et al. A systematic analysis of global anemia burden from 1990 to 2010. Blood. 2014;123(5):615–24.
9. Looker AC, Dallman PR, Carroll MD, Gunter EW, Johnson CL. Prevalence of iron deficiency in the United States. JAMA. 1997;277(12):973–6.
10. Powers JM, Stanek JR, Srivaths L, Haamid FW, O'Brien SH. Hematologic considerations and management of adolescent girls with heavy menstrual bleeding and anemia in U.S. children's hospitals. J Pediatr Adolsec Gynecol. 2018;31(5):446–50.
11. Bruner AB, Joffe A, Duggan AK, Casella JF, Brandt J. Randomised study of cognitive effects of iron supplementation in non-anaemic iron-deficient adolescent girls. Lancet. 1996;348(9033):992–6.
12. Hinton PS, Giordano C, Brownlie T, Haas JD. Iron supplementation improves endurance after training in iron-depleted, nonanemic women. J Appl Physiol. 2000;88(3):1103–11.
13. Jonker FA, Boele van Hensbroek M. Anaemia, iron deficiency and susceptibility to infections. J Infect. 2014;69(Suppl 1):S23–7.
14. World Health Organization. Iron deficiency anaemia: assessment, prevention, and control. A guide for programme managers. Geneva: World Health Organization; 2001.
15. Nemeth E, Ganz T. The role of hepcidin in iron metabolism. Acta Haematol. 2009;122(2-3):78–86.
16. Andrews NC. Disorders of iron metabolism. N Engl J Med. 1999;341(26):1986–95.
17. Girelli D, Nemeth E, Swinkels DW. Hepcidin in the diagnosis of iron disorders. Blood. 2016;127(23):2809–13.
18. De Falco L, Sanchez M, Silvestri L, et al. Iron refractory iron deficiency anemia. Haematologica. 2013;98(6):845–53.
19. Buchanan GR, Sheehan RG. Malabsorption and defective utilization of iron in three siblings. J Pediatr. 1981;98(5):723–8.
20. Diaz A, Laufer MR, Breech LL. Menstruation in girls and adolescents: using the menstrual cycle as a vital sign. Pediatrics. 2006;118(5):2245–50.
21. Campbell K, Peebles R. Eating disorders in children and adolescents: state of the art review. Pediatrics. 2014;134(3):582–92.
22. Hallberg L, Hulthen L, Garby L. Iron stores and haemoglobin iron deficits in menstruating women. Calculations based on variations in iron requirements and bioavailability of dietary iron. Eur J Clin Nutr. 2000;54(8):650–7.
23. Haamid F, Sass AE, Dietrich JE. Heavy menstrual bleeding in adolescents. J Pediatr Adolesc Gynecol. 2017;30(3):335–40.
24. Shoemaker ME, Gillen ZM, McKay BD, Koehler K, Cramer JT. High prevalence of poor iron status among 8- to 16-year-old youth athletes: interactions among biomarkers of iron, dietary intakes, and biological maturity. J Am Coll Nutr. 2019;24:1–8.
25. Lippi G, Sanchis-Gomar F. Epidemiological, biological and clinical update on exercise-induced hemolysis. Ann Transl Med. 2019;7(12):270.
26. Rosen MJ, Dhawan A, Saeed SA. Inflammatory bowel disease in children and adolescents. JAMA Pediatr. 2015;169(11):1053–60.
27. Wiskin AE, Fleming BJ, Wootton SA, Beattie RM. Anaemia and iron deficiency in children with inflammatory bowel disease. J Crohns Colitis. 2012;6(6):687–91.
28. Johnston RD, Logan RF. What is the peak age for onset of IBD? Inflamm Bowel Dis. 2008;14(Suppl 2):S4–5.
29. Chey WD, Wong BC. Practice Parameters Committee of the American College of Gastroenterology guideline on the management of Helicobacter pylori infection. Am J Gastroenterol. 2007;102(8):1808–25.

30. Repo M, Lindfors K, Maki M, et al. Anemia and iron deficiency in children with potential celiac disease. J Pediatr Gastroenterol Nutr. 2017;64(1):56–62.

31. Lebwohl B, Ludvigsson JF, Green PH. Celiac disease and non-celiac gluten sensitivity. BMJ. 2015;351:h4347.

32. Powers JM, O'Brien SH. How I approach iron deficiency with and without anemia. Pediatr Blood Cancer. 2019;66(3):e27544.

33. Theurl I, Mattle V, Seifert M, Mariani M, Marth C, Weiss G. Dysregulated monocyte iron homeostasis and erythropoietin formation in patients with anemia of chronic disease. Blood. 2006;107(10):4142–8.

34. Kadir RA, Economides DL, Sabin CA, Pollard D, Lee CA. Assessment of menstrual blood loss and gynaecological problems in patients with inherited bleeding disorders. Haemophilia. 1999;5(1):40–8.

35. James AH, Kouides PA, Abdul-Kadir R, et al. Von Willebrand disease and other bleeding disorders in women: consensus on diagnosis and management from an international expert panel. Am J Obstet Gynecol. 2009;201(1):12 e11–8.

36. Iron requirements and iron deficiency in adolescents 2018. www.uptodate.com. Accessed 28 June 2019.

37. Rector WG Jr. Pica: its frequency and significance in patients with iron-deficiency anemia due to chronic gastrointestinal blood loss. J Gen Intern Med. 1989;4(6):512–3.

38. Sharma R, Stanek JR, Koch TL, Grooms L, O'Brien SH. Intravenous iron therapy in non-anemic iron-deficient menstruating adolescent females with fatigue. Am J Hematol. 2016;91(10):973–7.

39. Murray-Kolb LE, Beard JL. Iron treatment normalizes cognitive functioning in young women. Am J Clin Nutr. 2007;85(3):778–87.

40. Punnonen K, Irjala K, Rajamaki A. Serum transferrin receptor and its ratio to serum ferritin in the diagnosis of iron deficiency. Blood. 1997;89(3):1052–7.

41. Abitbol V, Borderie D, Polin V, et al. Diagnosis of iron deficiency in inflammatory bowel disease by transferrin receptor-ferritin index. Medicine. 2015;94(26):e1011.

42. Mucke V, Mucke MM, Raine T, Bettenworth D. Diagnosis and treatment of anemia in patients with inflammatory bowel disease. Ann Gastroenterol. 2017;30(1):15–22.

43. Harms K, Kaiser T. Beyond soluble transferrin receptor: old challenges and new horizons. Clin Endocrinol Metab. 2015;29(5):799–810.

44. Cappellini MD, Comin-Colet J, de Francisco A, et al. Iron deficiency across chronic inflammatory conditions: international expert opinion on definition, diagnosis, and management. Am J Hematol. 2017;92(10):1068–78.

45. Powers JM, Buchanan GR, Adix L, Zhang S, Gao A, McCavit TL. Effect of low-dose ferrous sulfate vs iron polysaccharide complex on hemoglobin concentration in young children with nutritional iron-deficiency anemia: a randomized clinical trial. JAMA. 2017;317(22):2297–304.

46. Moretti D, Goede JS, Zeder C, et al. Oral iron supplements increase hepcidin and decrease iron absorption from daily or twice-daily doses in iron-depleted young women. Blood. 2015;126(17):1981–9.

47. Stoffel NU, Cercamondi CI, Brittenham G, et al. Iron absorption from oral iron supplements given on consecutive versus alternate days and as single morning doses versus twice-daily split dosing in iron-depleted women: two open-label, randomised controlled trials. Lancet Haematol. 2017;4(11):e524–33.

48. Teucher B, Olivares M, Cori H. Enhancers of iron absorption: ascorbic acid and other organic acids. Int J Vitam Nutr Res. 2004;74(6):403–19.

49. Auerbach M, Adamson JW. How we diagnose and treat iron deficiency anemia. Am J Hematol. 2016;91(1):31–8.

50. Mantadakis E. Advances in pediatric intravenous Iron therapy. Pediatr Blood Cancer. 2016;63(1):11–6.

51. Munoz M, Gomez-Ramirez S, Besser M, et al. Current misconceptions in diagnosis and management of iron deficiency. Trasfusione del sangue. 2017;15(5):422–37.

52. Ganzoni AM. Intravenous iron-dextran: therapeutic and experimental possibilities. Schweiz Med Wochenschr. 1970;100(7):301–3.

53. Crary SE, Hall K, Buchanan GR. Intravenous iron sucrose for children with iron deficiency failing to respond to oral iron therapy. Pediatr Blood Cancer. 2011;56(4):615–9.

54. Plummer ES, Crary SE, McCavit TL, Buchanan GR. Intravenous low molecular weight iron dextran in children with iron deficiency anemia unresponsive to oral iron. Pediatr Blood Cancer. 2013;60(11):1747–52.

55. Hassan N, Boville B, Reischmann D, Ndika A, Sterken D, Kovey K. Intravenous ferumoxytol in pediatric patients with iron deficiency anemia. Ann Pharmacother. 2017;51(7):548–54.

56. Powers JM, Shamoun M, McCavit TL, Adix L, Buchanan GR. Intravenous ferric carboxymaltose in children with iron deficiency anemia who respond poorly to oral iron. J Pediatr. 2017;180:212–6.

57. Wolf M, Chertow GM, Macdougall IC, Kaper R, Krop J, Strauss W. Randomized trial of intravenous iron-induced hypophosphatemia. JCI Insight. 2018;3(23):e124486.

58. Salpeter SR, Buckley JS, Chatterjee S. Impact of more restrictive blood transfusion strategies on clinical outcomes: a meta-analysis and systematic review. Am J Med. 2014;127(2):124–131 e123.

59. Weiss LM. Anemic retinopathy. Pa Med. 1966;69(6):35–6.

60. Coskun M, Sevencan NO. The evaluation of ophthalmic findings in women patients with iron and vitamin B12 deficiency anemia. Transl Vis Sci Technol. 2018;7(4):16.

61. Ullrich C, Wu A, Armsby C, et al. Screening healthy infants for iron deficiency using reticulocyte hemoglobin content. JAMA. 2005;294(8):924–30.

Vitamin B$_{12}$ Deficiency

Jennifer Davila and Maria C. Velez-Yanguas

Introduction

Vitamin B$_{12}$ is recognized as an essential molecule for DNA synthesis. Its deficiency results in megaloblastic anemia usually accompanied by leukopenia and thrombocytosis. However, the cellular alterations seen with vitamin B$_{12}$ deficiency are not limited to the blood and bone marrow cells. All rapidly proliferating cells are affected including epithelial cells lining the gastrointestinal tract (buccal mucosa, tongue, small intestine), cervix, vagina, and uterus [1]. Manifestations in the central nervous system range from irritability and failure to thrive (in young children) and paresthesia to more severe symptoms including weakness, unsteady gait, and psychosis. These changes are not found in all patients. Hematological and epithelial cell changes are reversed after adequate treatment [2]. However, long-term neurological sequelae have been documented in some studies [3–5].

In the nineteenth century, the association between morphologically abnormal blood cells and pernicious anemia (PA) was initially reported in the medical literature. Since these original publications by Combe [6] and Addison [7], the medical community has learned and continues to better understand the complex manifestations of vitamin B$_{12}$ deficiency. The history of pernicious anemia, vitamin B$_{12}$ deficiency, and the complex clinical spectrum of symptoms have been elegantly reviewed, and the authors encourage the reader to refer to these publications by M.M. Wintrobe, I. Chanarin, and D. Watkins et al. [8–10].

Physiology of Cobalamin (Vitamin B$_{12}$)

Cobalamin is the largest and most complex chemical structure of the vitamins [11]. It is synthesized exclusively by bacteria. Humans receive cobalamin solely from the diet. Dietary sources of vitamin B$_{12}$ are primarily meat, fish, and dairy products. The liver has the greatest amount of vitamin B$_{12}$. Shellfish, which ingest bacteria, are also a good source of dietary vitamin B$_{12}$ [12]. Plants do not synthesize or accumulate cobalamin; an exclusively vegetarian diet contains no vitamin B$_{12}$. Cobalamin, contrary to folate, is stable to high-temperature cooking. Inadequate intake of vitamin B$_{12}$ causes deficiency. The recommended daily intake of cobalamin for adolescent and young females is listed in Table 18.1 [13].

J. Davila (✉)
Hemophilia and Thrombosis Center at Montefiore, The Children's Hospital at Montefiore, Albert Einstein College of Medicine, Bronx, NY, USA
e-mail: JEDAVILA@montefiore.org

M. C. Velez-Yanguas
Hemophilia Treatment Center, Hemostasis and Thrombosis Program, Louisiana State University Health Sciences Center and Children's Hospital of New Orleans, New Orleans, LA, USA

© Springer Nature Switzerland AG 2020
L. V. Srivaths (ed.), *Hematology in the Adolescent Female*,
https://doi.org/10.1007/978-3-030-48446-0_18

Table 18.1 Recommended dietary allowances and adequate intakes of vitamin B_{12}

	Age group	μg/d
Females	9–13 y	1.8
	14–18 y	2.4
	19–30 y	2.4
Pregnancy	14–18 y	2.6
	19–30 y	2.6
Lactation	14–18 y	2.8
	19–30 y	2.8

Vitamin B_{12} is an essential nutrient important in transferring the methyl group in a methionine synthase-requiring reaction, which converts homocysteine to methionine. This reaction activates folate, which can be utilized in DNA synthesis. Cobalamin is also needed in the synthesis of myelin and thus the maintenance and repair of neural axons. In addition, cobalamin is essential for the synthesis of energy in mitochondria and for erythropoiesis in bone marrow [14].

Cobalamin and its binding proteins, intrinsic factor (IF), transcobalamin II (TC II), and haptocorrin (transcobalamin I or TC I), form the required cobalamin-protein complex to effectively transport cobalamin into the cells via the receptors on the cell surface and through its cellular membrane. Cobalamin in the ingested food is protein-bound. It binds to salivary or gastric haptocorrin after it is released in the acidic environment of the stomach. Once in the duodenum, the pancreatic proteases release cobalamin allowing it to bind to IF (produced in the parietal cells of the stomach). The IF-cobalamin complex binds to receptors in the distal ileum and is internalized by endocytosis. Cobalamin then binds TC II (holotranscobalamin [holo-TC]) facilitating the entrance of cobalamin into a variety of cell types. For a detailed description of the physiology of cobalamin, the authors recommend Carmel R et al. [15].

Table 18.2 Common causes of vitamin B12 deficiency in adolescent females

Nutritional factors (decreased intake)
Strict vegetarian/vegan/macrobiotic diet by choice or cultural preferences
Children on restricted diets due to developmental or behavioral disabilities
Access to food in poverty areas
Caregiver nutritional ignorance or misinformation
Breast-fed infants of mothers with unrecognized vitamin B_{12} deficiency due to vegan diet, gastric bypass, pernicious anemia
Gastrointestinal
Abnormal absorption
Intrinsic factor (IF) deficiency
Autoimmune pernicious anemia
Juvenile pernicious anemia with multiple endocrinopathies
Status post partial gastric resection/bariatric surgery
Congenital deficiency of IF (autosomal recessive)
Mutations in GIF (intrinsic factor gene)
Pancreatic insufficiency
Decreased gastric acid
Long-term therapy with proton pump inhibitors, H2 blockers
Failure of intestinal absorption (ileal surface)
Crohn's disease
Celiac disease
Regional ileitis
Surgical procedures involving ileum (resection)
Abnormal ileal receptor (Imerslund-Gräsbeck disease)
Competition for vitamin B12
Syndrome of bacterial overgrowth in the small intestine
Parasitic infection (fish tapeworm found in raw seafood)
Inborn errors of B12 transport and metabolism
Defective transport
Congenital deficiency of transcobalamin II (TC II)
Mutations in TC II
Defects in metabolism
Inherited disorders

Causes of Vitamin B_{12} Deficiency

Although it was thought that the incidence of vitamin B_{12} deficiency in children and adolescents was low, studies have shown that this deficiency is more common than previously recognized [16–19]. The following table (Table 18.2) highlights the common causes of vitamin B_{12} deficiency with emphasis in adolescent females.

Vitamin B$_{12}$ deficiency with or without megaloblastic anemia is a worldwide problem including in the United States. In publication from the World Health Organization (WHO), the data about the prevalence of vitamin B$_{12}$ and/or folate deficiency are derived from relatively small, local, or national surveys and studies from few countries suggesting that these deficiencies may be a public health problem [20].

In the developing countries, difficulties in adequate access to food may lead to nutritional deficiencies including vitamin B$_{12}$. In developed countries restricted diets due to personal or parental choices or due to medical conditions including children and adolescents with developmental and behavioral problems account for possible causes for this deficiency.

Special attention needs to be considered for adolescents who choose a vegan or strict vegetarian diet. Many times they are not familiar with the nutritional needs or available food options that provide the necessary vitamins and micronutrients especially if they grew up in a non-vegan household. Parents and primary care physicians need to be aware of the reasons behind these choices since many adolescent females decide on a vegan or vegetarian diet as a method of weight control and could mask a potential eating disorder. These adolescent females should be supported and educated in following a diet that offers the needed nutrition while it provides the health benefits from their dietary choice [21]. Children and adolescents on atypical diets may develop vitamin B$_{12}$ deficiency. Severe neurologic manifestations had been reported in an adolescent with vitamin B$_{12}$ deficiency associated with a strict vegetarian diet [22]. Several publications have reported low vitamin B$_{12}$ levels in vegans with low or no evidence of megaloblastic anemia [5, 14, 17, 23].

Adolescent mothers who followed a strict vegetarian or vegan diet require vitamin B$_{12}$ supplementation during breastfeeding to prevent vitamin B$_{12}$ deficiency in their infants with its potential neurological complications [3, 17, 21].

Reports of low vitamin B$_{12}$ levels in obese children, adolescents, and adults bring the concern for potential complications related to this and other possible micronutrient deficiencies in this growing population [24–27]. However, further studies are needed to establish appropriate guidelines and recommendations.

Stabler and Allen [28] summarized several studies about the relative frequency and prevalence of pernicious anemia (PA) in the United States. In one study the incidence of PA was 49.2 per 100,000 in women and 25.1 per 100,000 for men per year [29]. In terms of racial distribution, Carmel and Johnson reported 47% of the patients were defined as European (descendants from several European countries), 33% African American, and 31% Latinos. The age was lower in African American and Latino female patients with PA when compared with Europeans [30].

Pernicious anemia, an autoimmune phenomenon against the gastric parietal cells and against intrinsic factor, may be associated with other autoimmune disorders, including chronic autoimmune thyroiditis, insulin-dependent diabetes mellitus, Addison's disease, Graves' disease, vitiligo, myasthenia gravis, and possibly Sjögren's syndrome. These patients are at increased risk for carcinoma of the stomach [10].

Clinical Manifestations of Vitamin B$_{12}$ Deficiency

Signs and symptoms of vitamin B$_{12}$ deficiency reflect the effects in the involved systems: hematological, gastrointestinal, and neurological. Table 18.3 summarizes these clinical manifestations [17, 31, 32].

Hematologic Findings

The period of high proliferation rates during erythropoiesis makes the erythroid progenitor cells more susceptible than other types of cells to the impaired DNA synthesis in folate or vitamin B12 deficiency [33]. Megaloblastic anemia is a term that refers to anemia in which the process of nucleic acid metabolism is impaired, resulting in nuclear-cytoplasmic dyssynchrony, reduced number of cell divisions in the bone marrow, and nuclear abnormalities in both myeloid and erythroid precursors (see Fig. 18.1). A rise in the mean corpuscular volume (MCV) and mean corpuscular hemoglobin (MCH) may be noted even with a normal hemoglobin level. However, these initial changes may be masked by concomitant iron deficiency or thalassemia trait making the early suspicion more challenging [15].

Another early manifestation preceding anemia is hypersegmentation of the neutrophils, defined as more than 5% of neutrophils containing more than five lobes or a single neutrophil containing more than six lobes (see Fig. 18.2). The changes in the neutrophils are a more specific feature of megaloblastic changes than is macrocytosis [12].

Table 18.3 Clinical manifestations of vitamin B$_{12}$ deficiency in children and adolescents

Hematological	Neurological/ psychiatric	General/ gastrointestinal
Hypersegmented neutrophils	Paresthesia	Glossitis
Macrocytosis	Developmental delay/regression	Anorexia/weight loss
Anemia	Ataxia	Failure to thrive/ poor weight gain
Thrombocytopenia	Depression	Icterus
Leukopenia	Psychosis/ dementia	Fatigue
Pancytopenia	Memory loss	Irritability
	Poor school performance	Weakness
	Personality changes	Skin hyperpigmentation
	Impaired vibratory and proprioceptive sense	Infertility

As the anemia worsens, other hematological changes including thrombocytopenia and leukopenia are noted. Pancytopenia as a clinical presentation of megaloblastic anemia may mimic severe aplastic anemia. An elevated serum lactate dehydrogenase (LDH) and indirect hyperbilirubinemia, due to ineffective myelopoiesis and erythropoiesis with a shortened red cell half-life (T1/2) of 16–21 days and intramedullary hemolysis as part of the hematological manifestations of PA, can help the clinician in the differential diagnosis [12, 15].

Neurologic Manifestations

Vitamin B$_{12}$ deficiency and its most severe complication, megaloblastic anemia, have an impact on the central nervous system and its myelination process. Subacute combined degeneration

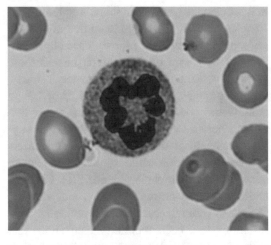

Fig. 18.2 Hypersegmented neutrophil. (Courtesy of Dr. Stephanie Moss)

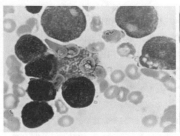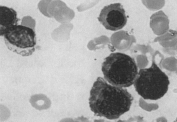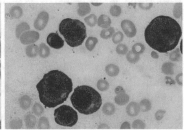

Fig. 18.1 Megaloblastic changes in the bone marrow. (Courtesy of Dr. Stephanie Moss)

of the spinal cord (SCDSC) consists of demyelination and degeneration of the posterior and lateral columns of the spinal cord, along with a peripheral neuropathy that is more severe in the lower than the upper extremities [10]. Neurologic changes can occur without hematologic abnormalities. Please refer to Table 18.3 for a list of neurologic and psychiatric manifestations [4, 5, 17, 34].

Gastrointestinal and Other General Manifestations

Most often patients complain of gradual onset of fatigue and weakness with decreased exercise tolerance related to the anemia. Loss of appetite, weight loss, and sore tongue (glossitis) are often reported. Skin hyperpigmentation is noted in non-white patients.

Diagnosis of B12 Deficiency

Mean cell volume and blood film examination Two major effects on hematopoiesis in B$_{12}$ deficiency include macrocytic red blood cells and hypersegmentation of neutrophils. An elevated MCV on routine CBC evaluation, with or without anemia, should prompt smear review and testing for B$_{12}$ deficiency. However, in a review by Oosterhuis and colleagues, in patients with confirmed B$_{12}$ deficiency, only 17% had an elevated MCV. When anemia was present in addition to the confirmed B$_{12}$ deficiency, 30% had macrocytic erythrocytes [35]. Therefore, if the suspicion for B$_{12}$ deficiency is strong enough, testing should be pursued despite the presence of normocytic RBCs.

Vitamin B$_{12}$ level (serum) A serum cobalamin level is currently the standard initial routine diagnostic test. An extremely low level (<100 pg per milliliter [<73.8 pmpl per liter]) is usually associated with clinical deficiency [36]. Periodic monitoring of vitamin B$_{12}$ levels may be appropriate in individuals with intestinal disorders that might

affect absorption of vitamin B$_{12}$ (i.e., inflammatory bowel disease, short gut syndrome, celiac disease). Physicians should use caution when interpreting laboratory results in patients with alcoholism, liver disease, or cancer because of decreased hepatic clearance of transport proteins and resultant higher circulating levels of vitamin B$_{12}$. Testing for pernicious anemia with anti-intrinsic factor antibodies should be considered in patients with vitamin B$_{12}$ deficiency whose history and physical examination do not suggest an obvious dietary or malabsorptive etiology.

Metabolite testing (Plasma total homocysteine (tHcy) and plasma methylmalonic acid (MMA) Deficiency of cobalamin results in elevation of plasma tHcy and MMA (See Table 18.4). tHcy is a sensitive biomarker of cobalamin deficiency and increases early in the course of the deficiency, sometimes preceding symptoms, and progresses as the deficiency worsens [37]. Plasma MMA is elevated in cobalamin deficiency with a >95% sensitivity [38]. MMA is not elevated in folic acid deficiency. MMA can also be elevated with normal B$_{12}$ levels in renal failure and methylmalonic aciduria.

Evaluation of Bone marrow (generally not indicated) Vitamin B$_{12}$ deficiency is a well-recognized and reversible cause of bone marrow failure [39]. A bone marrow aspirate and biopsy are not required to evaluate for vitamin B$_{12}$ deficiency. Should a bone marrow be performed to rule out myelodysplastic syndrome (MDS) or malignancy in an individual with vitamin B$_{12}$ or folate deficiency, it is likely to reveal a markedly hypercellular marrow with megaloblastic erythroid hyperplasia, giant metamyelocytes, and frequent mitoses. Increased chromosome breakage with

Table 18.4 Interpretation of metabolite testing

MMA and homocysteine normal	No deficiency of vitamin B$_{12}$ or folate
MMA and homocysteine elevated	Deficiency of vitamin B$_{12}$
MMA normal, homocysteine elevated	No deficiency of vitamin B$_{12}$ Consistent with deficiency of folate

other alterations in chromosome structure in vitamin B_{12} has been described in adult and in children [40, 41].

Treatment of B_{12} Deficiency

Vitamin B_{12} deficiency can be treated with intramuscular injections of cyanocobalamin or oral vitamin B_{12} therapy. Approximately 10% of the standard injectable dose of 1 mg is absorbed, which allows for rapid replacement in patients with severe deficiency or severe neurologic symptoms [42]. Patients with an irreversible cause should be treated indefinitely. Those with a reversible cause should be treated until resolution of symptoms. Vegans and strict vegetarians should be counseled to consume fortified cereals or supplements to prevent deficiency. The American Society for Metabolic and Bariatric Surgery recommends that patients who have had bariatric surgery take 1 mg of oral vitamin B12 per day indefinitely [43].

References

1. Anthony AC. Megaloblastic anemias. In: Hoffman R, Benz EJ, Shattil SJ, et al., editors. Hematology: basic principles and practice. New York: Churchill Livingstone; 1991. p. 392–422.
2. Chanarin I. The megaloblastic anaemias. London: Blackwell Scientific Publications; 1979. p. 225–6.
3. Graham SM, Arvela OM, Wise GA. Long-term neurological consequences of nutritional vitamin B_{12} deficiency in infants. J Pediatr. 1992;121:710–4.
4. Evim MS, Erdöl S, et al. Long-term outcome in children with vitamin B_{12} deficiency. Turk J Hematol. 2011;28:286–93.
5. Kapoor A, Baig M, et al. Neuropsychiatric and neurological problems among Vitamin B_{12} deficient young vegetarians. Neurosciences. 2017;22(3):228–32.
6. Combe JS. History of a case of anaemia. Trans Med Chir Soc Edin. 1824;1:194.
7. Addison T. Anaemia: disease of the supra-renal capsules. London Med Gaz. 1849;43:517.
8. Wintrobe MM. Hematology, the blossoming of a science: a story of inspiration and effort. Philadelphia: Lea & Febiger; 1985.
9. Chanarin I. A history of pernicious anaemia. Br J Haematol. 2000;111:407–15.
10. Watkins D, Whitehead VM, Rosenblatt DS. Megaloblastic anemia. In: Orkin SH, et al., editors. Nathan and Oski: Hematology of Infancy and Childhood. 7th ed. Philadelphia: Saunders Elsevier; 2009. p. 467–520.
11. Smith E. Purification of anti-pernicious anemia factors from liver. Nature. 1948;161:638–9.
12. Kamen BA, Meyers P. Megaloblastic anemias. In: Miller DR, Miller LP, et al., editors. Blood disease of infancy and childhood: in the tradition of CH smith. 7th ed: Mosby; 1995. p. 220–39.
13. http://nationalacademies.org/hmd/~/media/Files/Report%20Files/2019/DRI-Tables-2019/2_RDAAIVVE.pdf?la=en.
14. Pawlak R, Parrott SJ, et al. How prevalent is vitamin B_{12} deficiency among vegetarians? Nutr Rev. 2013;71(2):110–7.
15. Carmel R, Watkins D, Rosenblatt DS. Megaloblastic anemia. In: Orkin SH, et al., editors. In Nathan and Oski: Hematology of Infancy and Childhood. 8th ed. Philadelphia: Elsevier Saunders; 2015. p. 308–56.
16. Wright JD, Bialostosky K, Gunter EW, Carroll MD, Najjar MF, Bowman BA, et al. Blood folate and vitamin B_{12}: United States, 1988–94. Vital Health State. 1998;11:1–78.
17. Rasmussen SA, Fernhoff PM, et al. Vitamin B_{12} deficiency in children and adolescents. J Pediatr. 2001;138(1):10–7.
18. Verma S. Vitamin B_{12} and folate deficiency amongst adolescents. Int J Contemp Med Res. 2017;4(8):1755–7.
19. Kirby M, Danner E. Nutritional deficiencies in children on restricted diets. Pediatr Clin N Am. 2009;56:1085–103.
20. Moilanen BC. Vegan Diets in Infants. Children and Adolescents Pediatrics in Review. May 2004;25(5):174–6.
21. Conclusions of a WHO Technical Consultation on folate and vitamin B_{12} deficiencies. Food Nutr Bull. 29(2 supplement) © 2008, The United Nations University S238–44.
22. Ashkenazi S, Weitz R, et al. Vitamin B_{12} deficiency due to a strictly vegetarian diet in adolescence. Clin Pediatr (Phila). 1987;26:662–3.
23. Bar-Sella P, Rakover Y, Ratner D. Vitamin B_{12} and folate levels in long term vegans. Isr J Med Sci. 1990;26:309–12.
24. Pinhas-Hamiel O, Doron-Panush N, et al. Obese children and adolescents: a risk group for low vitamin B_{12} concentration. Arch Pediatr Adolesc Med. 2006;160:933–6.
25. Ho M, Halim JH, et al. Vitamin B_{12} in obese adolescents with clinical features of insulin resistance. Nutrients. 2014;6(12):5611–8.
26. Sun Y, Sun M, et al. Inverse association between serum vitamin B_{12} concentration and obesity among adults in the United States. Front Endocrinol. 2019; https://doi.org/10.3389/fendo.2019.00414.

27. Baltaci D, Kutlucan A, et al. Association of vitamin B$_{12}$ with obesity, overweight, insulin resistance and metabolic syndrome and body fat composition: primary care-based study. Med Glas (Zenica). 2013 Aug;10(2):203–10.

28. Stabler SP, Allen RH. Vitamin B$_{12}$ deficiency as a worldwide problem. Annu Rev Nutr. 2004;24:299–326.

29. Furszyfer J, WM MC, et al. On the increased association of Graves'disease with pernicious anemia. Mayo Clin Proc. 1971;46:37–9.

30. Carmel RC, Johnson CS. Racial patterns in pernicious anemia. Early age at onset and increased frequency of intrinsic-factor antibody in black women. N Engl J Med. 1978;298:647–50.

31. Singh C, Pukhraj G, et al. A prospective, cross sectional open label clinicoepidemiological study of vitamin B$_{12}$ deficiency in adolescent children. Int J Contemp Pediatr. 2018 Jul;5(4):1468–73.

32. Stabler SP. Vitamin B$_{12}$ Deficiency. N Engl J Med. 2013;368:149–60.

33. Koury MJ, Ponka P. New insights into erythropoiesis: the roles of folate, vitamin B$_{12}$, and iron. Annu Rev Nutr. 2004;24:105–31.

34. Dietary reference intakes for thiamin, riboflavin, niacin, vitamin B6, folate, vitamin B$_{12}$, pantothenic acid, biotin, and choline. Washington, DC: National Academy Press. 1998, p. 306–356, http://www.nap.edu/catalog/6015.html.

35. Oosterhuis WP, et al. Diagnostic value of the mean corpuscular volume in the detection of vitamin B$_{12}$ deficiency. Scand J Clin Lab Invest. 2000;60(1):9–18.

36. Stabler SP. Clinical practice. Vitamin B$_{12}$ deficiency. N Engl J Med. 2013;368(2):149–60.

37. Devalia V, et al. Guidelines for the diagnosis and treatment of cobalamin and folate disorders. Br J Haematol. 2014;166(4):496–513.

38. Oberley MJ, Yang DT. Laboratory testing for cobalamin deficiency in megaloblastic anemia. Am J Hematol. 2013;88(6):522–6.

39. Randhawa J, et al. What should I know before ordering a bone marrow aspiration/biopsy in patients with vitamin B12 deficiency? BMJ Case Rep. 2013;2013:bcr2013010200.

40. Chintagumpala MM, Dreyer ZA, Steuber CP, et al. Pancytopenia with chromosomal fragility: vitamin B$_{12}$ deficiency. J Pediatr Hematol Oncol. 2013;1996:166–70.

41. Heath CW Jr. Cytogenetic observations in vitamin B$_{12}$ and folate deficiency. Blood. 1966;27(6):800–15.

42. Langan RC, Goodbred AJ. Vitamin B$_{12}$ deficiency: recognition and management. Am Fam Physician. 2017;96(6):384–9.

43. Mechanick JI, et al. Clinical practice guidelines for the perioperative nutritional, metabolic, and nonsurgical support of the bariatric surgery patient–2013 update: cosponsored by American Association of Clinical Endocrinologists, The Obesity Society, and American Society for Metabolic & Bariatric Surgery. Obesity (Silver Spring). 2013;21(Suppl 1):S1–27.

Stephanie A. Fritch Lilla, Sylvia T. Singer, and Elliott P. Vichinsky

Introduction

When thalassemia was first described by Dr. Thomas Cooley in the mid-1920s [1], most individuals did not live past early childhood. A century later the treatment has advanced significantly. Curative options through allogeneic bone marrow transplant are available, and more recently novel treatments of gene manipulation and gene therapy are emerging [2]. With advancements in care, many individuals with thalassemia, in areas with access to specialized care, live to be adults and face new challenges as they age. For adolescents with severe forms of thalassemia, adherence to conventional therapy of transfusion and chelation is essential for prolonging survival and improving quality of life as well as remaining eligible for novel therapies and curative options. Adolescent girls and women with thalassemia face specific challenges related to puberty and reproductive health. In this chapter, we provide an overview of thalassemia and concentrate on issues affecting adolescent girls and young women.

The thalassemias are an inherited group of disorders caused by absent or abnormal globin chain synthesis and insufficient hemoglobin production [3]. The imbalanced synthesis of α and β globin chains leads to ineffective erythropoiesis and chronic hemolytic anemia as well as secondary effects including compensatory hematopoiesis, skeletal changes, iron overload (both intestinal absorption and transfusion mediated) with resultant organ damage, and coagulopathy [4]. As a group, thalassemias are the most common monogenic disorder [3]. Thalassemia affects approximately 1–5% of the population globally [4]. Due to global immigration patterns, thalassemia is widespread, though historically it was most prevalent along the malaria belt, as a result of relative resistance of the heterozygous state against infection with *Plasmodium falciparum* [4, 5].

Clinically, the genotype and phenotype do not always align. This has led to transitioning to clinical classification of thalassemia over the past decade [4]. Individuals who require regular transfusions (previously referred to as "thalassemia major") and are not able to produce sufficient hemoglobin for survival are considered to have transfusion-dependent thalassemia (TDT). TDT diagnosis may include β-thalassemia major, severe HbE/β-thalassemia, non-deletional HbH, and surviving Hb Bart's hydrops. Individuals with non-transfusion-dependent thalassemia (NTDT) (previously referred to as "thalassemia

S. A. Fritch Lilla (✉)
Children's Hospitals and Clinics of Minnesota, Minneapolis, MN, USA
e-mail: stephanie.fritchlilla@childrensmn.org

S. T. Singer · E. P. Vichinsky
UCSF Benioff Children's Hospital Oakland, Oakland, CA, USA

© Springer Nature Switzerland AG 2020
L. V. Srivaths (ed.), *Hematology in the Adolescent Female*,
https://doi.org/10.1007/978-3-030-48446-0_19

intermedia") may require intermittent transfusion or regular transfusions for periods of time but do not require lifelong transfusions [4]. Some NTDT patients, however, become transfusion-dependent as they age or develop complications that are better managed with regular transfusions.

Beta Thalassemia

Beta thalassemia is most common in countries around the Mediterranean Sea, Middle East, India, and Southeast Asia [4]. Over 350 mutations of the β-globin gene have been reported having a clinical phenotype of TDT or NTDT [6]. Individuals with β-thalassemia trait are heterozygous, carrying one abnormal copy β-globin gene, and are typically asymptomatic but may have clinical symptoms of mild to moderate thalassemia if the mutation behaves as a dominant one or if in conjunction with excess alpha globin chains (alpha triplication). With the exception of rare dominant forms, the majority of individuals with TDT and NTDT are compound heterozygous or homozygous. β⁰-thalassemia mutations produce no β-globin chains, and β⁺-thalassemia mutations have decreased production of β-globins [7]. Hemoglobin E-β-thalassemia is a distinct but common type of β-thalassemia [8]. Individuals with hemoglobin E-β-thalassemia inherit a β-thalassemia allele from one parent and a structural hemoglobin variant, HbE, from the other parent. Both β-thalassemia and hemoglobin E are present in high frequencies in many Asian countries such that globally hemoglobin E-β-thalassemia is responsible for approximately 50% of clinically severe transfusion-dependent β-thalassemia [9]. Hemoglobin E-β hemoglobin variant produces slightly reduced rate of β-globin [10], which is mildly unstable and has increased sensitivity to oxidant injury [9].

Alpha Thalassemia

Alpha thalassemia is most common in Southeast Asia and China, where in some regions of Southern Asia, nearly 100% individuals carry at least one α-globin gene mutation [3]. Over 100 genetic forms of α-thalassemia have been identified thus far [3]. As each individual carries four alpha genes, the clinical phenotype is generally predictable based on the number of deleted α-globin genes: [3] Silent carrier, α-thalassemia trait, hemoglobin H disease, or hemoglobin Bart's hydrops fetalis syndrome correlate to one, two, three, and four gene deletions, respectively [11]. When a total of three of the four genes are deleted, an individual has hemoglobin H disease. If two alpha genes are deleted in combination with a third non-deletional mutation such as Constant Spring, it is named hemoglobin H-Constant Spring. Hemoglobin H is produced when excess β-globin forms tetramers. Hemoglobin H β tetramers can precipitate damaging the RBC membrane and lead to shortened RBC life span from hemolysis [11]. Generally individuals with hemoglobin H have a mild phenotype with mild to moderate anemia and are at risk of requiring intermittent transfusions during periods of stress due to oxidative damage causing hemolysis [12]. Some non-deletional mutations, including hemoglobin Constant Spring, result in production of an elongated α-chain, a highly unstable hemoglobin variant that is often associated with a more severe anemia with some individuals requiring chronic transfusions and managed similar to β-thalassemia TDT [5]. Since α-globins are produced early in embryonic development, they can lead to severe anemia in utero if a child has four gene deletions, hydrops fetalis syndrome, often resulting in fetal demise unless identified early in pregnancy and fetal transfusions given.

Diagnosis

Due to the inherited nature of thalassemia and known high-risk populations, many countries offer premarital, neonatal, and newborn screening (NBS). Hemoglobin Bart's, a gamma chain tetramer, can be detected on NBS, allowing for early detection of individuals with α-thalassemia, hemoglobin H disease. For individuals with hemoglobin Bart's hydrops fetalis in utero, prenatal diagnosis is essential to allow for intervention with fetal transfusions and assuring safe pregnancy and delivery for both fetus and mother [3]. Other forms of thalassemia diagnosed in the post-natal period are identified on NBS or through standard blood testing that includes complete blood count and methods to diagnose a hemoglobinopathy such as hemoglobin electrophoresis and through DNA analysis [13, 14]. Peripheral smear morphology is often notable for hypochromic and microcytic red blood cells with anisocytosis and poikilocytosis [13]. Hemoglobin electrophoresis shows elevated fetal hemoglobin for age, increase A_2 in β-thalassemia, possibly decreased A_2 in individuals with α-thalassemia, as well as HbH and other variants such as HbE [14].

Pathogenesis and Disease Complications

Ineffective Erythropoiesis

Ineffective erythropoiesis develops as the body attempts to increase production of RBC but fails due to premature cell death from abnormal hemoglobin production [15]. In individuals with β-thalassemia, ineffective erythropoiesis is a result of α-globin tetramers that accumulate and precipitate forming inclusion bodies in erythroid precursors [4, 7]. These inclusion bodies bind to the RBC membrane skeleton and cause oxidative membrane damage, leading to premature apoptosis at sites of erythropoiesis [4, 7]. Ineffective erythropoiesis in individuals with α-thalassemia is similar to those with β-thalassemia but occurs to a lesser extent [16]. Individuals with α-thalassemia have excess β-globins that form soluble tetramers (hemoglobin H) that precipitate, forming insoluble inclusions (Heinz bodies) which lead to RBC membrane damage [4]. The hypoxic stress from ineffective erythropoiesis leads to increased intestinal iron absorption mediated by hepcidin, which contributes, along with transfusional iron, to the overall iron overload in individuals with thalassemia [4, 15]. Ineffective erythropoiesis leads to medullary expansion and subsequent bone deformities including frontal bossing and maxillary hyperplasia. Bone health is impacted, leading to an increased risk of osteopenia, bone demineralization, and increased risk of fractures [15]. Compensatory extramedullary hematopoiesis is most common in the spleen and liver, but pseudotumors can develop in any tissue including the spinal canal [4]. Splenomegaly from increased erythropoietic activity may lead to splenic sequestration leading to further decline in hemoglobin [15].

Iron Overload

Iron overload is a common complication in thalassemia resulting from transfusion-related iron overload, increased gastrointestinal iron absorption driven by ineffective erythropoicsis, as well as the lack of a physiologic mechanism for removal of excess iron [17]. The rate of iron loading for each individual is variable and related to their underlying clinical phenotype (NTDT V TDT), presence of transfusions, increased dietary absorption, and access to iron chelation therapy. In addition, different organs within an individual may load iron at different rates [17]. Individuals with TDT and NTDT are at risk of developing liver fibrosis, cirrhosis, and osteoporosis secondary to iron overload. Individuals with TDT are more likely than NTDT individuals to develop cardiac siderosis with left ventricular heart failure, viral hepatitis, and endocrine complications including hypothyroidism, hypoparathyroidism, growth retardation, hypogonadism, and diabetes mellitus as a result of iron overload [17]. As a result of the mechanism of iron loading with transfusion, individuals with TDT tend to develop iron overload in the first 1–2 years of life (10–20 transfusions), whereas NTDT does not develop iron overload until later in life at 10–15 years old [17].

Chronic Anemia

In addition to ineffective erythropoiesis and iron overload, individuals with NTDT are subject to sequelae of chronic anemia [18]. Chronic anemia for NTDT individuals is a result not only of ineffective erythropoiesis but also peripheral hemolysis. Peripheral hemolysis places NTDT individuals at higher risk of pulmonary hypertension with secondary heart failure and increased risk of thrombosis [18]. In addition, individuals with NTDT have been found to have increased rates of extramedullary hematopoiesis and leg ulcers when compared to TDT. Females with NTDT in the OPTIMAL CARE study, which assessed complications and management of NTDT, were found to have increased risk of osteoporosis, hypogonadism, and cholelithiasis [18].

Management

There is significant molecular and phenotypic variance among the thalassemias. NTDT individuals are able to produce sufficient hemoglobin and do not require regular transfusions as individuals with TDT do. For individuals with TDT, regular transfusions work by suppressing ineffective erythropoiesis preventing subsequent pathophysiologic complications [2, 4]. NTDT individuals intermittently require transfusions during periods of stress with surgery, pregnancy, or infections. Iron overload management with chelation therapy is essential for individuals with both TDT and NTDT. Hydroxyurea, aimed to increase fetal and total hemoglobin, has been used to improve hemoglobin levels in individuals with thalassemia. Splenectomy is reserved for severe cases with massive splenomegaly or refractory iron overload as spleen removal increases the risk four- to fivefold of severe complications including thrombosis, pulmonary hypertension, leg ulcers, and silent stroke [4].

Until recently, allogeneic bone marrow transplantation was the only curative therapy. With the development of novel targeted therapeutics, options to cure or improve treatment through reducing the transfusion need and iron toxicity are currently in clinical trials. These include gene therapy for a curative goal, erythroid maturation agents including luspatercept (ACE-536) and sotatercept (ACE011), JAK 2 inhibitors, hepcidin, and hepcidin mimetics. Other gene manipulation approaches are also being studied.

Transfusion and Iron Chelation Therapy

Transfusion therapy with iron chelation remains the conventional treatment in thalassemia. RBC transfusions are essential to the management of TDT with a goal to improve symptomatic anemia and suppress ineffective erythropoiesis. Most TDT individuals start regular transfusion during the first year of life. In less severe individuals where the molecular diagnosis and clinical phenotype do not correlate, the decision to start a chronic transfusion program can be complex and involves discussions of the care team with the patient and family. Clinical symptoms that help guide the need to initiate a transfusion program include hemoglobin level (<7 g/dL on at least two occasions at least 2 weeks apart), poor growth velocity, bone changes from medullary expansion, significant extramedullary hematopoiesis including massive splenomegaly, pulmonary hypertension or cardiac failure, and unacceptable quality of life [19]. Most individuals require transfusions every 2–5 weeks to maintain a goal hemoglobin nadir prior to transfusion of 9–10.5 g/dL. A higher pre-transfusion hemoglobin (>11 g/dL) might be required by adult patients. All patients should receive phenotypically matched and leukocyte-depleted RBC units [19].

Iron overload, a result of transfusion therapy along with increased dietary iron absorption, is the primary cause of morbidity and mortality. Iron chelation is an essential part of transfusion therapy. Currently there are three iron chelators commercially available in the USA: two oral chelators, deferiprone and deferasirox, and the third is a parenterally administered chelator, deferoxamine. Each chelator can be used as monotherapy for individuals with acceptable iron burden or in combination for individuals with severe iron burden or organ toxicity [20]. Each chelation medication has side effects and requires close monitoring for toxicity.

Issues for Adolescent and Young Adult Females with Thalassemia

Thalassemia as a group of disorders is heterogeneous, in which TDT individuals who have severe iron overload experience the most significant comorbidities. This section focuses on common challenges facing adolescents, highlighting issues affecting adolescent females, including endocrinopathies, nutrition, and psychosocial issues affecting quality of life and transition of care.

Endocrine Dysfunction

As iron overload progresses in individuals with thalassemia, transferrin becomes fully saturated, and non-transfusion-bound iron (NTBI) increases [21]. NTBI and its active form, labile plasma iron (LPI), enter non-hematopoietic cells, damaging cells and forming reactive oxygen species that further harm cells [22]. The endocrine system is particularly sensitive to iron overload, and even well-chelated individuals experience complications over time, including delayed sexual maturation, impaired fertility, impaired glucose tolerance, diabetes, hypothyroidism, hypoparathyroidism, growth hormone deficiency, and low bone density [22].

Hypogonadism and Delayed Puberty

Hypogonadism is the most common endocrinopathy in individuals with TDT, reported to affect >50% and up to 80% of in some studies [21, 23]. Clinically for adolescent females, this leads to delayed puberty and amenorrhea or abnormal menstrual cycles [24]. In females delayed puberty is defined as absent pubertal development by age 13, and hypogonadism is the absence of breast development by age 16 [21]. The primary cause of hypogonadism in the thalassemias is iron deposition in the pituitary gland [21, 24]. Twenty-five percent of TDT individuals were found to have severe pituitary iron overload in the 1st decade of life. Pituitary iron deposition acceler-

ates during adolescence, and clinically significant volume loss was observed in the 2nd decade of life. Both iron overload and gland shrinkage were found to be independently predictive of hypogonadism [23]. Iron deposition impacts the pituitary gland cells at different rates; gonadotropes are the most sensitive, with iron overload causing decreased synthesis of luteinizing hormone (LH) and follicle-stimulating hormone (FSH) [21]. Iron deposition in the gonads may also contribute in severe iron overload cases. Leptin and ghrelin, which have been found to be low in individuals with thalassemia, are also believed to play a role in delayed puberty [25].

Pituitary iron assessment by MRI is not routinely performed; however, strong correlation with pancreatic iron and cardiac iron was reported [23]. Close monitoring of LH/FSH/estradiol levels, changes in menstrual pattern, as well as increase in cardiac and/or pancreatic iron levels should prompt a discussion about impending deleterious iron effect on the reproductive system, and considerations for intensifying iron chelation therapy should be taken.

Farmaki et al. reported that after successful therapy with intensive combined chelation therapy, partial reversal of both primary and secondary hypogonadism may be possible [26]. Additionally, a longitudinal study (median 6.5 years) showed that chelation with oral deferasirox resulted in lower incidence of new occurring hypogonadism, suggesting possible better chelation ability of deferasirox coupled with improved compliance [27]. Both studies are encouraging and stress the importance of iron chelation for prevention and possibly for treatment of hypogonadism. For those who are not able to prevent or reverse hypogonadism, hormone replacement therapy (HRT) is generally recommended with a goal of maintenance of normal puberty and induction of fertility when desired [21, 24].

There are multiple estrogen formulations available for hormone replacement, including oral estradiol, oral conjugated estrogens, transdermal estrogen patches, and gel. The majority of providers favor use of ethinyl estradiol, which follows the recommendations of the Thalassemia

International Federation [21, 24]. Significant side effects from HRT do occur including venous and arterial thrombosis, hypertension, dyslipidemia, and hepatic dysfunction [24]. Prior to initiation of HRT, providers should consider risk factors including history of splenectomy, impaired glucose tolerance or diabetes, migraine with aura, and personal or family history of inherited thrombophilia [24].

Fertility

Early introduction of the topic of fertility is important for adolescent girls even before they are young women contemplating pregnancy. Since poor compliance with iron chelation treatment is prevalent in this age group, increasing awareness of the long-term consequences of high iron levels on the reproductive system is essential [28]. If hypogonadism persists, it leads to fertility problems, and the thalassemia care team should address reproduction and family planning early on.

For many years pregnancy was difficult to attain for TDT women due to hypogonadism and lack of ovulation as well as concerns of maternal safety. Pregnancy was considered high risk due to concerns of progressive or new-onset cardiac dysfunction, hyperglycemia, bone pain, and thrombosis risk. In recent decades >200 successful pregnancies in TDT women have been described. Moreover, thanks to improved management and likely a lower incidence of iron-induced hypogonadism, a higher percentage of spontaneous pregnancies not requiring gonadotrophin-induced ovulation were reported [29, 30].

When hypogonadotropic hypogonadism persists, it results in infertility. The relationship of gonadotropin levels and pituitary iron and volume with reproductive status is not always informative or predictive concerning ovarian or testicular function [23]. An additional iron effect on the gonads may also exist, in particular in severe iron overload cases, but it has only been partially studied [31, 32]. Disruption of reproductive tissue in women with TDT is believed to occur via similar mechanisms to the physiologic decline in fertility with aging, a result of increased oxidative stress. Increased levels of redox activity in the follicular fluid from a TDT individual were demonstrated, as well as hemosiderin in the endometrial tissue, suggesting iron-induced oxidative tissue injury and impairment of blastocyst implantation and female reproduction [31, 33, 34].

Despite these findings, in well-managed women, even in those suffering from primary or secondary amenorrhea, ovarian function is generally preserved. This is evidenced by successful pregnancies after hormonal stimulation for ovulation induction. Since abnormalities in ovulation are common, reported in 30–80% of women [35–37], ovulation induction is not always successful, and some women require further treatments with assisted reproductive technology (ART) that involves manipulation of eggs or embryos in vitro [38].

Evaluation of reproductive potential requires several tests that can be repeated annually or more often when applicable. LH/FSH and estradiol have poor predictive values of female reproductive potential. Ultrasound measure of ovarian antral follicle counts (AFC) can provide more specific information. Anti-Mullerian hormone (AMH) produced by granulosa cells of the preantral and antral follicles correlates with AFC and is a good measure of ovarian reserve. AMH is an ideal biomarker as it is obtained by a simple blood test and does not change through the menstrual cycle, nor is it affected by LH/FSH levels, which are often reduced in these women. AMH levels were shown to provide information on ovarian reserve in thalassemia; levels were significantly lower in women with thalassemia compared to those in controls and inversely correlated to ferritin levels [39–41].

Impaired Glucose Tolerance and Diabetes

Impaired glucose tolerance and diabetes are a result of multifactorial interactions including iron overload, zinc deficiency, individual sensitivity to iron damage, beta cell failure, and increased collagen deposition [42]. Prevalence of diabetes mellitus (DM) was reported at 6.54% for individuals with TDT β-thalassemia, and impaired glucose tolerance (IGT) was present in 12.46% of individuals [43]. IGT and DM are uncommon in young children with thalassemia, but risk increases during adolescence and for young adults [44]. Healthy diet, good chelation, and close monitoring are important in adolescents with thalassemia to decrease the risk of IGT and DM. Monitoring should include periodic measure of fasting glucose as well as a fructosamine level which is used in place of hemoglobin A1C, which isn't reliable in transfused patients. Oral glucose tolerance test is also performed periodically.

Growth

Individuals with thalassemia are at risk of poor growth due to multiple risk factors including iron overload, endocrinopathies, chronic anemia, zinc deficiency, and chelation therapy [45, 46]. Improved transfusion and chelation therapy have decreased but have not eliminated the risk of short stature for individuals with thalassemia [45]. Both TDT and NTDT individuals may be impacted with 7–46% of NTDT β-thalassemia having short stature (2 SD below mean height for age) [47, 48]. Origa et al. reviewed short stature among individual cohorts according to chelation medications that were available during their treatment course. In individuals born prior to chelation availability, 80% had short stature; among those born when hypertransfusion with a pre-transfusion hemoglobin goal of 11 g/dL was recommended and desferrioxamine was newly available, 68% had short stature. Only 19% of individuals who had goal pre-hemoglobin of 9–10.5 g/dL and were treated with chelators early in childhood had short stature [7]. These findings support the idea that both transfusions and chelation are important in decreasing the risk of short stature. With appropriate therapy, children may grow as expected until 9–10 years of age when growth velocity declines and they have reduced

or absent pubertal growth spurt [46]. Complete growth plate fusion may not occur until the second decade of life in individuals with thalassemia [46]. In addition to well-managed transfusions and chelation therapy, it is important to assess for other endocrinopathies and consider growth hormone (GH) therapy if growth hormone deficiency is detected.

Bone Health

Individuals with thalassemia are at high risk of abnormal bone health due to risk related to complications from increased bone turnover, medullary marrow expansion, iron toxicity, chelator toxicity, vitamin D deficiency, reduced physical activity, and hormonal deficiency [6, 49]. As a result reduced bone density, fractures, bone deformity, and pain are common [49]. Adolescence is a critical period of bone development that is limited in adolescents with thalassemia due to the increased bone turnover preventing positive bone accrual and limiting optimal peak bone mass [6, 50]. Females with thalassemia are at risk of having low progesterone and estrogen levels, which leads to increased osteoclast activity and subsequent decrease in bone formation.

In attempt to overcome the anemia, the medullary cavity expands, which leads to thinning of the bone cortex and places individuals at increased risk of fractures [6]. Fractures were reported in 30–50% of individuals prior to implementation of effective transfusion and chelation therapy [51–53]. Current rates of fractures have ranged from approximately 10% up to 36%. Individuals with α-thalassemia have lower rates of fractures compared with TDT and NTDT β-thalassemia, and individuals with HbE-β-thalassemia have intermediate rates [49].

Despite transfusion programs that maintained Hb >9 g/dL, individuals >12 years of age were still found to have decreased bone mineral density [54]. Due to the continuous bone resorption that young adults display, therapeutic intervention with exercise, calcium supplementation, hormone replacement, and bisphosphonates is important [55]. Further nutritional support including sufficient vitamin D, calcium, vitamin K, zinc, and strontium (where available) is also important in maximizing bone health [56]. Physical activity can be more challenging for individuals with thalassemia due to the degree of intermittent anemia and cardiac complications. Fung et al. found that increased levels of physical activity have a positive impact on lean mass and bone health [57]. Overall females with thalassemia have been found to have significant lean mass deficits compared to healthy controls [58]. They also found that total calcium intake has a negative impact on body fat and lean and total weight [57]. For patients who are unable to participate in physical activity due to cardiac contraindications, preliminary evidence showed that whole-body vibration therapy was found to be beneficial when utilized for 20 minutes/day for adults [59]. In addition, HRT has been found to improve bone density [60].

Nutrition

Individuals with thalassemia are at increased risk of nutritional deficiencies which may contribute to poor growth, delayed puberty, and decreased immune function [61]. Nutritional deficiencies are believed to be multifactorial as a result of insufficient dietary intake, increased losses, as well as increased endogenous requirement [61]. Goldberg et al. evaluated a cohort of relatively well-nourished individuals with thalassemia, who received care at UCSF Benioff Children's Hospital Oakland, and found that many had nutritional deficiencies. Zinc deficiencies were present in 40%, vitamin D deficiency in 35%, and copper and vitamin C deficiency in 20% of individuals with thalassemia [61]. They proposed increased nutritional requirements for individuals with thalassemia including zinc >10 mg/day (25% higher than general population), copper 1 mg/day (42% higher than general population), and vitamin C at 100 mg/day (33% higher than general population). Unfortunately, nutritional supplementation can be challenging, and individuals prescribed 400–1000 IU vitamin D per

day often continue to have insufficient or deficient vitamin D levels. Outcomes improved with high-dose 50,000 IU of vitamin D_2 given at 3-week intervals, which could be given at the time of transfusion [62]. Optimal nutritional status is important for adolescents who are at a critical phase of bone health and growth.

Psychosocial Considerations and Quality of Life

Thalassemia, like many other chronic medical conditions, can have a significant psychological and quality of life (QOL) impact. The challenges that face individuals with chronic disease are particularly challenging for adolescents as they develop a sense of identity and independence [63]. A study of adolescents in Thailand aged 13–18 years showed that individuals with thalassemia had lower QOL scores compared with age-matched controls, especially in psychosocial and school functioning [64]. There were concerns that limitations on social and school activities lead to poor self-esteem, negative feelings, and poor body image [64]. They also found that ferritin level and comorbidities impacted QOL [64]. A QOL study done on individuals with thalassemia living in the USA, UK, and Canada similarly showed that lower iron burden was associated with improved mental and physical QOL [28]. This study also showed decreased adherence to chelation therapy during adolescence and young adult years, which improved when they were 35 years or older [28]. Foe et al. assessed the factors related to iron chelation therapy adherence in young adults with thalassemia and found that the individual's desire was to minimize the impact of thalassemia in their lives [65]. Thus chelation adherence improved if chelation therapy was viewed as a facilitator of normalcy and decreased if it was perceived as a departure from normalcy [65]. They identified four driving factors including integration of thalassemia into the individual's life, low perceived burden of chelation, perceived independence, self-motivation of the chelation process, and understanding the necessity of chelation in minimizing iron burden [65]. Working from this framework, providers may encourage compliance by reviewing individuals' iron burden in response to chelation therapy, aiming for independence with chelation, and limiting barriers to care [65].

Chronic pain has also been reported to decrease QOL in those affected. Reports of pain more than doubled from 30% of 12–17 year olds to 66% in 18–24 year olds and up to 79% in those ≥35 years old [66]. Lower back pain is most common, followed by legs, head, hips, and upper or mid back [67]. Low hemoglobin has been reported as a trigger, with pain improved following blood transfusion [67].

While one would generally expect that individuals with a more severe disease burden would have a lower quality of life (QOL), Musallam and colleagues showed that individuals with NTDT reported lower QOL than TDT. While they were unable to evaluate the association between clinical complications and QOL, they reported that the individuals with NTDT suffered more clinical complications including serious cardiovascular complication (VTE and PHTN), endocrinological, hepatic, and/or skeletal when compared with TDT individuals. Additionally, they considered the timing of diagnosis with the TDT individuals being diagnosed earlier in childhood and allowing more time to adapt to living with thalassemia compared to NTDT [68].

Studies on treatment intervention to improve psychological issues in thalassemia are limited. Cognitive behavioral therapy (CBT) is a short-term psychological therapy aimed at changing patterns of thinking or behavior to ultimately change the way they feel. Mohamadian et al. assessed the impact of CBT on individuals with thalassemia. They randomly assigned individuals with thalassemia to receive or not receive CBT and found that there was a decline in both anxiety and depression in the individuals who underwent CBT [63].

Transition of Care

As the life span for individuals with thalassemia has extended into adulthood, providers caring for thalassemia patients have been faced with the challenge of managing adults with thalassemia or

transitioning the care to an adult care team. This transition from pediatric to adult care comes at a high-risk time for patients living with chronic illness who are also facing the normal developmental challenges of adolescence. During this time adolescents and young adults with chronic illness are at risk of decreased utilization of preventive healthcare, loss to follow-up, and poor overall health outcomes [69]. Some thalassemia centers continue to provide care to adult patients, while others transition to an adult program. Both options have benefits and challenges. Pediatric centers are often ill equipped to address adult complications such as reproductive health but have expertise in providing care to patients with childhood chronic illnesses [70]. Adult centers may lack the expertise to provide care to what was previously a childhood illness and may not have patient numbers and staff to develop expertise. The Hospital for Sick Children and Toronto General Hospital developed a program utilizing a transition navigator (TN) for their patients with thalassemia and sickle cell. There was also a joint visit with both the pediatric and adult care providers and TN prior to transition to the adult center. The TN followed patients from age 12 to 1 year following transition which results in decreased number of individuals lost to follow-up from 29% to 7% [69]. Improvement in appointment attendance (≥90%) was seen along with an improvement in medication adherence with hydroxyurea and chelation medications [69]. Transition goals have been developed for many chronic illnesses including thalassemia to help ease the transition process, even if a formal transition navigator is not available.

References

1. Cooley TB, Witwer ER, Lee P. Anemia in children with splenomegaly and peculiar changes in the bones: report of cases. JAMA Pediatr. 1927;34(3): 347–63.
2. Rund D. Thalassemia 2016: modern medicine battles an ancient disease. Am J Hematol. 2016;91(1):15–21.
3. Piel FB, Weatherall DJ. The alpha-thalassemias. N Engl J Med. 2014;371(20):1908–16.
4. Taher AT. Thalassemia. Hematol Oncol Clin North Am. 2018;32(2):xv–xvi.

5. Farashi S, Harteveld CL. Molecular basis of alpha-thalassemia. Blood Cells Mol Dis. 2018;70:43–53.
6. De Sanctis V, Soliman AT, Elsefdy H, Soliman N, Bedair E, Fiscina B, et al. Bone disease in beta thalassemia patients: past, present and future perspectives. Metabolism. 2018;80:66–79.
7. Origa R. beta-Thalassemia. Genet Med. 2017;19(6):609–19.
8. Algiraigri AH, Kassam A. Hydroxyurea for hemoglobin E/beta-thalassemia: a systematic review and meta-analysis. Int J Hematol. 2017;106(6):748–56.
9. Fucharoen S, Weatherall DJ. The hemoglobin E thalassemias. Cold Spring Harb Perspect Med. 2012;2(8):a011734.
10. Frischer H, Bowman J. Hemoglobin E, an oxidatively unstable mutation. J Lab Clin Med. 1975;85(4):531–9.
11. Marengo-Rowe AJ. The thalassemias and related disorders. Proc (Bayl Univ Med Cent). 2007;20(1):27–31.
12. Harewood J, Azevedo AM. Alpha Thalassemia (Hemoglobin H Disease). In: StatPearls. Treasure Island (FL): StatPearls Publishing LLC; 2019.
13. Choudhry VP. Thalassemia minor and major: current management. Indian J Pediatr. 2017;84(8):607–11.
14. Brancaleoni V, Di Pierro E, Motta I, Cappellini MD. Laboratory diagnosis of thalassemia. Int J Lab Hematol. 2016;38(Suppl 1):32–40.
15. Rivella S. Iron metabolism under conditions of ineffective erythropoiesis in beta-thalassemia. Blood. 2019;133(1):51–8.
16. Schrier SL. Pathophysiology of thalassemia. Curr Opin Hematol. 2002;9(2):123–6.
17. Taher AT, Saliba AN. Iron overload in thalassemia: different organs at different rates. Hematology Am Soc Hematol Educ Program. 2017;2017(1):265–71.
18. Taher AT, Musallam KM, Karimi M, El-Beshlawy A, Belhoul K, Daar S, et al. Overview on practices in thalassemia intermedia management aiming for lowering complication rates across a region of endemicity: the OPTIMAL CARE study. Blood. 2010;115(10):1886–92.
19. Franchini M, Forni GL, Liumbruno GM. Is there a standard-of-care for transfusion therapy in thalassemia? Curr Opin Hematol. 2017;24(6):558–64.
20. Kwiatkowski JL. Current recommendations for chelation for transfusion-dependent thalassemia. Ann N Y Acad Sci. 2016;1368(1):107–14.
21. Srisukh S, Ongphiphadhanakul B, Bunnag P. Hypogonadism in thalassemia major patients. J Clin Transl Endocrinol. 2016;5:42–5.
22. Nienhuis AW, Nathan DG. Pathophysiology and clinical manifestations of the beta-thalassemias. Cold Spring Harb Perspect Med. 2012;2(12):a011726.
23. Noetzli LJ, Panigrahy A, Mittelman SD, Hyderi A, Dongelyan A, Coates TD, et al. Pituitary iron and volume predict hypogonadism in transfusional iron overload. Am J Hematol. 2012;87(2):167–71.
24. De Sanctis V, Soliman AT, Daar S, Di Maio S, Yassin MA, Canatan D, et al. The experience of a tertiary unit on the clinical phenotype and management of hypogonadism in female adolescents and young adults with transfusion dependent thalassemia. Acta Biomed. 2019;90(1):158–67.
25. Moshtaghi-Kashanian GR, Razavi F. Ghrelin and leptin levels in relation to puberty and reproductive function in patients with beta-thalassemia. Hormones (Athens). 2009;8(3):207–13.
26. Farmaki K, Tzoumari I, Pappa C, Chouliaras G, Berdoukas V. Normalisation of total body iron load with very intensive combined chelation reverses cardiac and endocrine complications of thalassaemia major. Br J Haematol. 2010;148(3):466–75.
27. Casale M, Citarella S, Filosa A, De Michele E, Palmieri F, Ragozzino A, et al. Endocrine function and bone disease during long-term chelation therapy with deferasirox in patients with β-thalassemia major. Am J Hematol. 2014;89(12):1102–6.
28. Trachtenberg FL, Gerstenberger E, Xu Y, Mednick L, Sobota A, Ware H, et al. Relationship among chelator adherence, change in chelators, and quality of life in thalassemia. Qual Life Res. 2014;23(8):2277–88.
29. Carlberg KT, Singer ST, Vichinsky EP. Fertility and pregnancy in women with transfusion-dependent thalassemia. Hematol Oncol Clin North Am. 2018;32(2):297–315.
30. Cassinerio E, Baldini IM, Alameddine RS, Marcon A, Borroni R, Ossola W, et al. Pregnancy in patients with thalassemia major: a cohort study and conclusions for an adequate care management approach. Ann Hematol. 2017;96(6):1015–21.
31. Reubinoff BE, Simon A, Friedler S, Schenker JG, Lewin A. Defective oocytes as a possible cause of infertility in a beta-thalassaemia major patient. Hum Reprod. 1994;9(6):1143–5.
32. Birkenfeld A, Goldfarb AW, Rachmilewitz EA, Schenker JG, Okon E. Endometrial glandular haemosiderosis in homozygous beta-thalassaemia. Eur J Obstet Gynecol Reprod Biol. 1989;31(2):173–8.
33. Roussou P, Tsagarakis NJ, Kountouras D, Livadas S, Diamanti-Kandarakis E. Beta-thalassemia major and female fertility: the role of iron and iron-induced oxidative stress. Anemia. 2013;2013:617204.
34. Reubinoff BE, Har-El R, Kitrossky N, Friedler S, Levi R, Lewin A, et al. Increased levels of redox-active iron in follicular fluid: a possible cause of free radical-mediated infertility in beta-thalassemia major. Am J Obstet Gynecol. 1996;174(3):914–8.
35. Chatterjee R, Katz M, Cox TF, Porter JB. Prospective study of the hypothalamic-pituitary axis in thalassaemic patients who developed secondary amenorrhoea. Clin Endocrinol. 1993;39(3):287–96.
36. Bronspiegel-Weintrob N, Olivieri NF, Tyler B, Andrews DF, Freedman MH, Holland FJ. Effect of age at the start of iron chelation therapy on gonadal function in beta-thalassemia major. N Engl J Med. 1990;323(11):713–9.
37. Skordis N, Gourni M, Kanaris C, Toumba M, Kleanthous M, Karatzia N, et al. The impact of iron overload and genotype on gonadal function in women with thalassaemia major. Pediatr Endocrinol Rev. 2004;2(Suppl 2):292–5.

38. Origa R, Piga A, Quarta G, Forni GL, Longo F, Melpignano A, et al. Pregnancy and beta-thalassemia: an Italian multicenter experience. Haematologica. 2010;95(3):376–81.

39. Singer ST, Vichinsky EP, Gildengorin G, van Disseldorp J, Rosen M, Cedars MI. Reproductive capacity in iron overloaded women with thalassemia major. Blood. 2011;118(10):2878–81.

40. Uysal A, Alkan G, Kurtoglu A, Erol O, Kurtoglu E. Diminished ovarian reserve in women with transfusion-dependent beta-thalassemia major: is iron gonadotoxic? Eur J Obstet Gynecol Reprod Biol. 2017;216:69–73.

41. Chang HH, Chen MJ, Lu MY, Chern JP, Lu CY, Yang YL, et al. Iron overload is associated with low anti-mullerian hormone in women with transfusion-dependent beta-thalassaemia. BJOG. 2011;118(7):825–31.

42. Li MJ, Peng SS, Lu MY, Chang HH, Yang YL, Jou ST, et al. Diabetes mellitus in patients with thalassemia major. Pediatr Blood Cancer. 2014;61(1):20–4.

43. He LN, Chen W, Yang Y, Xie YJ, Xiong ZY, Chen DY, et al. Elevated prevalence of abnormal glucose metabolism and other endocrine disorders in patients with beta-thalassemia major: a meta-analysis. Biomed Res Int. 2019;2019:6573497.

44. Delvecchio M, Cavallo L. Growth and endocrine function in thalassemia major in childhood and adolescence. J Endocrinol Investig. 2010;33(1):61–8.

45. Origa R, Danjou F, Orecchia V, Zappu A, Dessi C, Foschini ML, et al. Current growth patterns in children and adolescents with thalassemia major. Blood. 2016;128(21):2580–2.

46. Kyriakou A, Skordis N. Thalassaemia and aberrations of growth and puberty. Mediterr J Hematol Infect Dis. 2009;1(1):e2009003.

47. De Sanctis V, Tangerini A, Testa MR, Lauriola AL, Gamberini MR, Cavallini AR, et al. Final height and endocrine function in thalassaemia intermedia. J Pediatr Endocrinol Metab. 1998;11(Suppl 3):965–71.

48. Inati A, Noureldine MA, Mansour A, Abbas HA. Endocrine and bone complications in beta-thalassemia intermedia: current understanding and treatment. Biomed Res Int. 2015;2015:813098.

49. Wong P, Fuller PJ, Gillespie MT, Milat F. Bone disease in thalassemia: a molecular and clinical overview. Endocr Rev. 2016;37(4):320–46.

50. Vogiatzi MG, Macklin EA, Fung EB, Cheung AM, Vichinsky E, Olivieri N, et al. Bone disease in thalassemia: a frequent and still unresolved problem. J Bone Miner Res. 2009;24(3):543–57.

51. Dines DM, Canale VC, Arnold WD. Fractures in thalassemia. J Bone Joint Surg Am. 1976;58(5):662–6.

52. Exarchou E, Politou C, Vretou E, Pasparakis D, Madessis G, Caramerou A. Fractures and epiphyseal deformities in beta-thalassemia. Clin Orthop Relat Res. 1984;189:229–33.

53. Finsterbush A, Farber I, Mogle P, Goldfarb A. Fracture patterns in thalassemia. Clin Orthop Relat Res. 1985;192:132–6.

54. Doulgeraki A, Athanasopoulou H, Voskaki I, Tzagaraki A, Karabatsos F, Fragodimitri C, et al. Bone health evaluation of children and adolescents with homozygous beta-thalassemia: implications for practice. J Pediatr Hematol Oncol. 2012;34(5): 344–8.

55. Voskaridou E, Kyrtsonis MC, Terpos E, Skordili M, Theodoropoulos I, Bergele A, et al. Bone resorption is increased in young adults with thalassaemia major. Br J Haematol. 2001;112(1):36–41.

56. Fung EB. The importance of nutrition for health in patients with transfusion-dependent thalassemia. Ann N Y Acad Sci. 2016;1368(1):40–8.

57. Fung EB, Xu Y, Kwiatkowski JL, Vogiatzi MG, Neufeld E, Olivieri N, et al. Relationship between chronic transfusion therapy and body composition in subjects with thalassemia. J Pediatr. 2010;157(4):641–7, 647.e641–642.

58. Fung EB, Vichinsky EP, Kwiatkowski JL, Huang J, Bachrach LK, Sawyer AJ, et al. Characterization of low bone mass in young patients with thalassemia by DXA, pQCT and markers of bone turnover. Bone. 2011;48(6):1305–12.

59. Fung EB, Gariepy CA, Sawyer AJ, Higa A, Vichinsky EP. The effect of whole body vibration therapy on bone density in patients with thalassemia: a pilot study. Am J Hematol. 2012;87(10):E76–9.

60. Anapliotou ML, Kastanias IT, Psara P, Evangelou EA, Liparaki M, Dimitriou P. The contribution of hypogonadism to the development of osteoporosis in thalassaemia major: new therapeutic approaches. Clin Endocrinol. 1995;42(3):279–87.

61. Goldberg EK, Neogi S, Lal A, Higa A, Fung E. Nutritional deficiencies are common in patients with transfusion-dependent thalassemia and associated with Iron overload. J Food Nutr Res (Newark). 2018;6(10):674–81.

62. Fung EB, Aguilar C, Micaily I, Haines D, Lal A. Treatment of vitamin D deficiency in transfusion-dependent thalassemia. Am J Hematol. 2011;86(10).871–3.

63. Mohamadian F, Bagheri M, Hashemi MS, Komeili SH. The effects of cognitive behavioral therapy on depression and anxiety among patients with thalassemia: a randomized controlled trial. J Caring Sci. 2018;7(4):219–24.

64. Boonchooduang N, Louthrenoo O, Choeyprasert W, Charoenkwan P. Health-related quality of life in adolescents with thalassemia. Pediatr Hematol Oncol. 2015;32(5):341–8.

65. Foe M, Treadwell M, Yamashita R, Lal A. Factors related to iron chelation therapy adherence in young adults with thalassemia: a framework from the patient perspective. Blood. 2017;130:2080.

66. Haines D, Martin M, Carson S, Oliveros O, Green S, Coates T, et al. Pain in thalassaemia: the effects of age on pain frequency and severity. Br J Haematol. 2013;160(5):680–7.

67. Lal A. Assessment and treatment of pain in thalassemia. Ann N Y Acad Sci. 2016;1368(1):65–72.

68. Musallam KM, Khoury B, Abi-Habib R, Bazzi L, Succar J, Halawi R, et al. Health-related quality of life in adults with transfusion-independent thalassaemia intermedia compared to regularly transfused thalassaemia major: new insights. Eur J Haematol. 2011;87(1):73–9.

69. Allemang B, Allan K, Johnson C, Cheong M, Cheung P, Odame I, et al. Impact of a transition program with navigator on loss to follow-up, medication adherence, and appointment attendance in hemoglobinopathies. Pediatr Blood Cancer. 2019;66(8): e27781.

70. Levine L, Levine M. Health care transition in thalassemia: pediatric to adult-oriented care. Ann N Y Acad Sci. 2010;1202:244–7.

Sickle Cell Disease in the Adolescent Female

20

Nelda Itzep and Vivien Sheehan

Introduction

Sickle cell disease (SCD) is the most common inherited blood disorder in the world. It affects over 100,000 Americans and millions more worldwide [1]. SCD is a severe monogenic disorder marked by significant morbidity and mortality, affecting every organ in the body [2]. The term sickle cell disease refers to all genotypes that cause sickling; the most common are the homozygous hemoglobin SS (HbSS) and compound heterozygotes hemoglobin SC (HbSC), hemoglobin S-beta thalassemia⁰ (HbSβ⁰), and hemoglobin S-beta thalassemia⁺ (HbSβ⁺), although HbS and several rarer hemoglobin variants such as HbS/O Arab and HbS/D Punjab can also cause sickle cell disease [3]. SCD is most commonly found in individuals of African heritage but also affects Hispanics and people of Middle Eastern and subcontinent Indian heritage [4]. The distribution of the HbS overlaps with the distribution of malaria; this is because HbS carriers, or individual with sickle cell trait (SCT),

have protection against malaria [5]. This chapter reviews the pathophysiology of SCD, common clinical complications, and available therapies, as they apply to adolescent females with SCD.

Pathophysiology

HbS is the result of a substitution of valine for glutamic acid in the sixth amino acid of the β-globin chain [6]. The change from a hydrophilic to a hydrophobic amino acid causes the hemoglobin molecules to stack or polymerize when deoxygenated. This rigid rod of hemoglobin distorts the cell, producing the characteristic crescent or sickle shape that gives the disease its name [7]. The sickle red cell is very abnormal; it is rigid and dense and lacks the deformability needed to navigate the microvasculature [8]. Blood flow blockages in the microvasculature result in ischemia, causing painful vaso-occlusive episodes that are the hallmark of the disease, as well as damage to the spleen, kidneys, and liver [9].

The sickle red cell is also fragile, with a lifespan of only approximately 20 days compared to 120 days in a normal individual [7]. Frequent red cell hemolysis results in anemia and the release of free hemoglobin, which both scavenges nitric oxide, and impairs production of more nitric oxide, which is essential for vasodilatation [10]. This contributes to vascular dysfunction and the

N. Itzep
Department of Pediatrics, University of Texas MD Anderson Cancer Center, Department of Pediatric Hematology Oncology, Houston, TX, USA

V. Sheehan (✉)
Department of Pediatrics, Baylor College of Medicine, Division of Hematology/Oncology, Houston, TX, USA
e-mail: vxsheeha@texaschildrens.org

© Springer Nature Switzerland AG 2020
L. V. Srivaths (ed.), *Hematology in the Adolescent Female*,
https://doi.org/10.1007/978-3-030-48446-0_20

increased risk of stroke and other organ damage over time [11]. If untreated, the natural course of sickle cell anemia is mortality in early childhood [12]. However, in countries with newborn screening and penicillin prophylaxis given to prevent death from overwhelming bacterial sepsis, survival into adulthood is the norm. In the USA, average life expectancy is 47 years for females with HbSS and HbSβ⁰ genotypes.

One of the most challenging aspects of SCD is its clinical variability. While in general, HbSS and HbSβ⁰ genotypes are the most severe, some patients with HbSC and HbSβ⁺ have significant sickle cell related complications and a clinical course similar to that of a HbSS patient [13]. A great deal of this clinical variability cannot yet be explained, but some can be attributed to endogenous fetal hemoglobin (HbF) levels [14, 15]. The degree of HbF varies widely between individuals from zero to 20–30%, with a median of 10% [16]. When HbF is added to the HbS polymer, it prevents further extension of the rigid hemoglobin rod or fiber. Red cells with significant amounts of HbF are less likely to sickle or hemolyze and live longer in circulation, leading to higher total body hemoglobin. Individuals who produce more HbF have a milder course, in general [17].

Clinical Complications

Pain Crises

In SCD, vaso-occlusive pain events may be common, often beginning in early childhood [15]. There is a great deal of variability in pain symptoms between individuals and within individuals at various times in their lives [18]. The frequency and severity of pain events are modulated by HbF levels, alpha thalassemia status (alpha thalassemia co-inheritance may increase pain event frequency), SCD genotypes, and therapies like hydroxyurea, L-glutamine, crizanlizumab or chronic transfusion therapy [15, 19]. Personal mental health factors, such as psychosocial stressors, anxiety, and depression, also contribute to the frequency of pain events [20]. Environmental pain event triggers include expo-

sure to cold water, windy or cold weather, temperature changes, and extreme temperatures [21].

Acute management of pain episodes involves nonsteroidal anti-inflammatory medications, hydration, and oral opioids, and when hospitalization is required, IV opioids, often delivered via patient-controlled analgesia (PCA) pumps [22]. As SCD patients become teenagers and young adults, some experience an increased frequency of pain episodes, with fewer pain-free days, or a failure to return to baseline before the next pain crisis occurs [23]. This is characteristic of emerging chronic pain [24].

Menstruation as a Trigger for Vaso-Occlusive Crisis (VOC)

The landmark multicenter Cooperative Study of Sickle Cell Disease (CSSCD) found a sex difference in rates of acute pain crises, with women experiencing more VOCs throughout their lives compared to men [15]. The higher rate of VOC observed in women is observed throughout the lifespan, but the peak difference in VOC frequency between men and women corresponds to womens' reproductive years, starting in adolescence. Many young women report that VOC crises are temporally related to their menstruation, either prior to or during their cycle. This recurring pattern may implicate hormones as a trigger for pain crises in young women. Several studies have shown a reduction in pain when women were treated with hormonal therapy, typically progesterone only medications such as Depo-Provera [25, 26], and conversely, an increase in pain during pregnancy or in the postpartum period [27]. The exact mechanism for hormonal influence on pain crises is unknown, but the effects of progesterone on rates of hemolysis are under investigation [28].

Chronic Pain

Chronic pain is a significant problem in adult SCD patients, with up to 85% reporting pain on most days [23, 29]. Emerging chronic pain, with acute VOC becoming closer and closer in time, eventually without a pain-free interval in between, often begins in adolescence [24]. The development of chronic pain may be reduced by early and aggressive treatment of acute pain events, as well as the use of hydroxyurea to reduce the number of pain events. Many adult sickle cell patients with chronic pain are treated with daily opioids [30]; this practice may paradoxically contribute to chronic pain by causing opioid induced hyperalgesia [31–33]. Given the significant side effects of chronic opioid use sedation, respiratory depression, itching, nausea, and impairment of function and quality of life, non-opioid therapies are under intense investigation [34]. Many chronic pain patients have symptoms of neuropathic pain and may benefit from neuropathic agents like gabapentin or amitriptyline, both to reduce opioid use and to more effectively treat chronic neuropathic pain, which is known to respond poorly to opioids [35].

Pulmonary Complications

Acute chest syndrome (ACS) is defined as an acute respiratory illness characterized by fever, shortness of breath, a new oxygen requirement, and a new pulmonary infiltrate on chest X-ray. ACS is the leading cause of death in individuals with SCD [2]. ACS is treated with simple or exchange transfusions, antibiotics, and supportive care [36]. In the pediatric age range, ACS is often caused by a bacterial or viral pneumonia; in adults, fat emboli may contribute to ACS. All age ranges are particularly vulnerable to ACS in the third day of hospitalization with a pain event, as atelectasis from shallow breathing and sedation from opioids can contribute to a hypoxic environment, potentiating sickling. All patients hospitalized with a SCD complication should have an incentive spirometer at the bedside to prevent ACS [37].

Thrombotic Events

SCD is also a pro-thrombotic condition; rates of venous thromboembolism (VTE) in children with SCD is approximately 2% higher than the

VTE rate in children with trauma and lower-extremity fractures (0.05–0.2%). Adolescent females with SCD are particularly high risk and may have levels approaching that of adults, which may be as high as 25%. The prevalence of pulmonary emboli in patients less than 40 with SCD is 3.5× higher than age and race-matched healthy controls [38]. DVT prophylaxis should be strongly considered for hospitalized adolescent females with SCD, and estrogen containing birth control avoided, as it increases thrombotic risk.

Abdominal Pain

Patients with SCD are at risk for developing gallstones in adolescence due to chronic hemolysis, which releases bilirubin, potentially leading to bilirubin gallstones. If asymptomatic, gallstones and gallbladder sludge should be observed; 40% of patients with gallbladder sludge do not develop gallstones [39].

Most patients with SCD have nonfunctional atrophic state of SCD. However, acute splenic sequestration may still occur; splenic sequestration is when red cells are trapped in the splenic sinuses and must be ruled out in an adolescent sickle cell patient with abdominal pain accompanied by dropping platelets and red cells, especially in milder subtypes like HbSC that often have splenic function preserved onto adolescence and adulthood [40].

Stroke

Individuals with SCD have a high lifetime risk for stroke; without any disease-specific intervention, 11% of patients with SCD will experience an overt stroke by the age of 20 [41]. Many more may have silent infarcts that impair neurocognitive abilities, particularly executive functioning, processing speed, and mathematical ability [42]. A major advance in sickle cell care includes screening for stroke risk through transcranial Doppler ultrasound (TCD) [43]. This screening tool has reduced the incidence of stroke to 1%. However, TCDs typically cannot be performed after the age of 16 years due to changes in the skull.

Disease-Specific Therapies

Penicillin Prophylaxis

In high-resource countries with newborn screening, the initiation of penicillin prophylaxis has dramatically altered the natural history of the disease, allowing the majority of patients to reach adulthood [44]. Penicillin prophylaxis is usually discontinued at age 5; however, individuals who have undergone surgical splenectomy or have had pneumococcal sepsis on penicillin prophylaxis may remain on penicillin to age 18 or beyond [30].

Blood Transfusion

The most common indication for chronic, i.e., scheduled, blood transfusion is stroke prevention. Patients who have had an overt stroke may be placed on chronic blood transfusion indefinitely. Patients also may be identified as being at high risk for stroke by TCD and placed on chronic transfusion therapy and transitioned to hydroxyurea at a later date, according to the discretion of the hematology care provider [43, 45]. Monthly chronic transfusions typically have a goal of suppressing the % HbS to 30–50. Patients may also be placed on chronic transfusion therapy to prevent splenic sequestration, ACS, or frequent VOC, although there is less evidence to support these practices.

Hydroxyurea

The most widely used pharmacologic therapy for SCD is hydroxyurea [46]. A significant portion of the benefit of hydroxyurea stems from its induction of HbF [16]. The level of HbF needed to achieve clinical improvement is not known, but in vitro assays suggest 20% HbF is needed to prevent sickling [47]. Hydroxyurea likely has other disease-modifying effects as well, reduction of white blood cell count and reticulocyte count, and reduction of red cell adhesion to the endothelium among them [48]. Hydroxyurea is given daily and dosed to maximum-tolerated dose for the individual by following the absolute neutrophil count (ANC). HbF response to hydroxyurea has been shown to decline in late adolescence [49], contributing to the observed increase in disease severity and early mortality in the transition age period [50]. Hydroxyurea is a teratogen in animal models and should be used along with effective birth control in sexually active patients.

Hematopoietic Stem Cell Transplant

The only curative therapy for SCD is hematopoietic stem cell transplant (HSCT) [51]. Transplant use is limited by availability of matched sibling donors, and even at experienced centers has a small risk for mortality, graft rejection, and graft versus host disease. Consensus on disease complications for which transplant is recommended is also lacking [52]. A potentially curative alternative to HSCT is gene based therapy, in which the patient's own stem cells are altered; these clinical trials in SCD are ongoing [53].

Unique Challenges for Female Adolescents with SCD

Effect of SCD on Puberty and Growth

Adolescent girls with SCD may experience delayed puberty based on Tanner staging. Studies have described a delay in menarche of over 2 years for girls with HbSS and a delay of half a year for those with HbSC [54]. The delay in puberty shows the negative effect of SCD on growth and development. In the CSSCD study, girls with SCD were on a lower percentile for height and weight than the published norms for black girls. SCD therefore likely has a constitutional effect on sexual maturation rather than altering endocrine function directly [55].

Dysfunctional Uterine Bleeding in Adolescents with SCD

Dysfunctional uterine bleeding (DUB) is common among adolescent girls with a reported rate of up to 45% of the general population [56]. DUB may be underdiagnosed in women and girls with SCD, because underlying anemia masks anemia from DUB and thus delays the proper workup and diagnosis. Worsening anemia, particularly accompanied by declining MCV and widening red cell distribution width (RDW), often alerts the clinician to additional blood loss; these cues may be obscured in SCD, however. A commonly used medication in SCD, hydroxyurea, may also confound the diagnosis of blood loss as it causes macrocytosis and also widens the RDW. Co-inheritance of alpha thalassemia or the compound heterozygote state of HbSβ thalassemia may cause microcytosis; however, RDW should be narrow in the absence of blood loss. It is therefore important that the clinician has a systematic and comprehensive approach, including detailed menstrual bleeding history and physical examination, for evaluating menstruation at comprehensive SCD visits with adolescent girls.

Effect of SCD on Fertility

SCD presents several challenges for women of reproductive age, including infertility and increased risk of maternal and fetal morbidity/mortality [57]. Fertility in women and girls with SCD may be compromised due to chronic inflammation, ovarian injury from ischemic insults, and iron overload from chronic transfusions [58]. Furthermore, the conditioning regimen for HSCT may cause a loss of fertility. Although there is a push for less aggressive conditioning regimens in nonmalignant HSCT, many still contain alkylating agents and/or total body irradiation which can lead to premature ovarian failure [58]. Female patients considering gene-based therapies must also be made aware of the potential loss of fertility even in the lower-dose autologous transplant regimens. Lastly, it has been suggested that chronic opioid use can suppress the hypothalamic-

pituitary-gonadal axis which can also lead to irregular menses and decreased fertility [59].

Pregnancy in SCD

Pregnancy in SCD is automatically considered high risk, and SCD-related conditions such as pulmonary hypertension, cardiomyopathy, neurologic deficits after stroke, and renal insufficiency may increase the risk level of pregnancy. The added metabolic demand due to pregnancy can be particularly taxing on the young adolescent body. Progesterone can increase total pulmonary resistance and thus unmask underlying cardiopulmonary dysfunction. Blood pH changes during pregnancy may also precipitate sickling crises [57]. Pregnancy in the setting of chronic hemolytic anemia can result in intrauterine growth restriction, premature birth, or even fetal demise [57]. Additionally, increased levels of coagulation factors and activated endothelium during pregnancy can increase existing thrombotic risk in a pregnant woman with SCD. This can manifest as stroke or placental thrombi, which can be fatal for the fetus as well as the mother [57]. Multidisciplinary care is of utmost importance for a pregnant woman with SCD. She should receive early and frequent prenatal care and consult with a hematologist, obstetrician, and other specialists depending on her comorbid conditions.

Reproductive Counseling

Important for all adolescent girls, and in particular those with chronic conditions such as SCD, is reproductive counseling to decrease the risk of unintended pregnancies. Combined hormonal contraception poses an increased risk of venous thromboembolism for healthy women due to the estrogen component [60]. Progesterone-only contraceptives have been found to be safe and effective in SCD women [61], and in some studies, it was even found to decrease the number of pain crises [25]. The mode of inheritance of SCD should also be explained to adolescents with

SCD and the importance of knowing the sickle cell trait or disease status of a partner.

Medication Noncompliance

Although disease-modifying medications like hydroxyurea can be life changing for girls with SCD, long-term medication compliance is challenging, particularly in the adolescent age range. They may see the prospect of lifelong medication as too overwhelming, not understand the importance of HU and not prioritize it during their daily routine, or may feel well in the present moment and feel HU is not necessary. A study examining hydroxyurea adherence in adolescents with SCD identified low adherence in over half of the participants [62].

Pain medication, including opioids, is commonly prescribed for adolescents with SCD, and these have the potential for abuse. Adolescents may be tempted to treat their anxiety and/or depression with opioid medications or take opioids daily because they theorize it will prevent VOC. This can lead to opioid-induced hyperalgesia, dependency, and poorer quality of life. Limiting the number of physicians who prescribe opioids to the patient and investigating pharmacy fill records are tools to combat improper use. Medication compliance should be addressed regularly at routine visits with special care taken to understand barriers to proper compliance.

Transition of Care

Previously a disease of childhood, SCD, is now a chronic illness with an estimated 94–98% of SCD patients reaching adulthood in high-resource countries [50]. Thus, the majority of SCD patients must transition from pediatric to adult care—a move that occurs during a vulnerable time in life, often without adequate health-care support [63]. Transition age SCD patients are susceptible to medical complications and early mortality, which coincides with their decreased use of life-prolonging therapies and increased use of emergency care [50, 64].

Unfortunately, despite the clear need for transition to occur in a coordinated and smooth manner, many SCD patients suffer a high-risk period during transition characterized by high risk of mortality and poorer clinical outcomes including more frequent SCD complications like pain, pulmonary disease, and infection, high emergency department reliance, and less frequent use of hydroxyurea and transfusion therapy [50, 65]. There is a paucity of information regarding transition outcomes, in part due to a lack of communication between pediatric and adult providers of patients with SCD, and difficulty in locating and surveying patients who did not successfully establish care with an adult health-care provider [66].

Mental Health Issues in SCD

Psychological Complications

A significant percentage of pediatric SCD patients suffer from psychological complications, including anxiety, adjustment-related concerns, pica, and depression [67, 68]. In a survey of Medicaid data from South Carolina, 46% of pediatric SCD patients were diagnosed with a depressive disorder [67]. Untreated depression was associated with lower quality of life and poor clinical outcomes [69]. SCD patients with comorbid depressive disorder were 2.8 fold more likely to become high utilizers of acute care [68]. The mean age of diagnosis of dysthymia in patients with SCD is 9 years; the mean age of diagnosis of major depression is 14 years [67].

Delayed Independence

Adolescence is often a time for developing independence from parents, spending more time with peers, possibly beginning to join the workforce, and taking on more self-care responsibilities. Because SCD requires frequent medical care such as daily medication administration and frequent clinic visits for wellness checks, laboratory assessments, and blood transfusions, it can be very difficult for an adolescent to manage all this without their parents. As a result, parents are often heavily involved in their medical care thus delaying or preventing the development of this aspect of their independence. It is imperative that both medical providers and parents are aware of this and make attempts to help adolescents develop this important life skill. Missed days of school and lack of socialization with peers due to hospitalizations for SCD complications may further delay independence.

Body Image Dissatisfaction

As previously mentioned, SCD can cause a delay in puberty and sexual maturation. This can be very distressing to adolescent girls who are witnessing their peers mature. Adolescents with SCD are more likely to report body dissatisfaction than their non SCD peers [70], and this dissatisfaction can be exacerbated by frequent pain crises [71]. Lower body weight, common in adolescents with SCD, may also contribute to body dissatisfaction, and scleral icterus from hemolysis may be a source of embarrassment. Physical, psychological, and emotional distress from living with the chronic illness of SCD can contribute to depression or suicidal ideation. It is important that clinicians assess mental health during well visits to ensure timely referral and treatment if necessary.

References

1. Weatherall D, Hofman K, Rodgers G, Ruffin J, Hrynkow S. A case for developing North-South partnerships for research in sickle cell disease. Blood. 2005;105:921–3.
2. Platt OS, Brambilla DJ, Rosse WF, et al. Mortality in sickle cell disease. Life expectancy and risk factors for early death. N Engl J Med. 1994;330:1639–44.
3. Rees DC, Williams TN, Gladwin MT. Sickle-cell disease. Lancet. 2010;376:2018–31.
4. Flint J, Harding RM, Boyce AJ, Clegg JB. The population genetics of the haemoglobinopathies. Baillieres Clin Haematol. 1998;11:1–51.
5. Allison AC. The distribution of the sickle-cell trait in East Africa and elsewhere, and its apparent relation-

ship to the incidence of subtertian malaria. Trans R Soc Trop Med Hyg. 1954;48:312–8.
6. Bunn HF. Pathogenesis and treatment of sickle cell disease. N Engl J Med. 1997;337:762–9.
7. Brittenham GM, Schechter AN, Noguchi CT. Hemoglobin S polymerization: primary determinant of the hemolytic and clinical severity of the sickling syndromes. Blood. 1985;65:183–9.
8. Ballas SK, Dover GJ, Charache S. Effect of hydroxyurea on the rheological properties of sickle erythrocytes in vivo. Am J Hematol. 1989;32:104–11.
9. Frenette PS. Sickle cell vaso-occlusion: multistep and multicellular paradigm. Curr Opin Hematol. 2002;9:101–6.
10. Reiter CD, Wang X, Tanus-Santos JE, et al. Cell-free hemoglobin limits nitric oxide bioavailability in sickle-cell disease. Nat Med. 2002;8:1383–9.
11. Nouraie M, Lee JS, Zhang Y, et al. The relationship between the severity of hemolysis, clinical manifestations and risk of death in 415 patients with sickle cell anemia in the US and Europe. Haematologica. 2013;98:464–72.
12. Serjeant GR. The natural history of sickle cell disease. Cold Spring Harb Perspect Med. 2013;3:a011783.
13. Serjeant GR. Natural history and determinants of clinical severity of sickle cell disease. Curr Opin Hematol. 1995;2:103–8.
14. Falusi AG, Olatunji PO. Effects of alpha thalassaemia and haemoglobin F (HbF) level on the clinical severity of sickle-cell anaemia. Eur J Haematol. 1994;52:13–5.
15. Platt OS, Thorington BD, Brambilla DJ, et al. Pain in sickle cell disease. Rates and risk factors. N Engl J Med. 1991;325:11–6.
16. Steinberg MH, Voskaridou E, Kutlar A, et al. Concordant fetal hemoglobin response to hydroxyurea in siblings with sickle cell disease. Am J Hematol. 2003;72:121–6.
17. Perrine RP, Brown MJ, Clegg JB, Weatherall DJ, May A. Benign sickle-cell anaemia. Lancet. 1972;2:1163–7.
18. Serjeant GR, Ceulaer CD, Lethbridge R, Morris J, Singhal A, Thomas PW. The painful crisis of homozygous sickle cell disease: clinical features. Br J Haematol. 1994;87:586–91.
19. Niihara Y, Miller ST, Kanter J, et al. A phase 3 trial of l-glutamine in sickle cell disease. N Engl J Med. 2018;379:226–35.
20. Gil KM, Carson JW, Porter LS, Scipio C, Bediako SM, Orringer E. Daily mood and stress predict pain, health care use, and work activity in African American adults with sickle-cell disease. Health Psychol. 2004;23:267–74.
21. Jones S, Duncan ER, Thomas N, et al. Windy weather and low humidity are associated with an increased number of hospital admissions for acute pain and sickle cell disease in an urban environment with a maritime temperate climate. Br J Haematol. 2005;131:530–3.

22. Resar LM, Oski FA. Cold water exposure and vaso-occlusive crises in sickle cell anemia. J Pediatr. 1991;118:407–9.

23. Darbari DS, Ballas SK, Clauw DJ. Thinking beyond sickling to better understand pain in sickle cell disease. Eur J Haematol. 2014;93:89–95.

24. Hollins M, Stonerock GL, Kisaalita NR, Jones S, Orringer E, Gil KM. Detecting the emergence of chronic pain in sickle cell disease. J Pain Symptom Manag. 2012;43:1082–93.

25. de Abood M, de Castillo Z, Guerrero F, Espino M, Austin KL. Effect of Depo-Provera or Microgynon on the painful crises of sickle cell anemia patients. Contraception. 1997;56:313–6.

26. De Ceulaer K, Gruber C, Hayes R, Serjeant GR. Medroxyprogesterone acetate and homozygous sickle-cell disease. Lancet. 1982;2:229–31.

27. Baum KF, Dunn DT, Maude GH, Serjeant GR. The painful crisis of homozygous sickle cell disease. A study of the risk factors. Arch Intern Med. 1987;147:1231–4.

28. Haddad LB, Curtis KM, Legardy-Williams JK, Cwiak C, Jamieson DJ. Contraception for individuals with sickle cell disease: a systematic review of the literature. Contraception. 2012;85:527–37.

29. Ballas SK, Lusardi M. Hospital readmission for adult acute sickle cell painful episodes: frequency, etiology, and prognostic significance. Am J Hematol. 2005;79:17–25.

30. Yawn BP, Buchanan GR, Afenyi-Annan AN, et al. Management of sickle cell disease: summary of the 2014 evidence-based report by expert panel members. JAMA. 2014;312:1033–48.

31. Arout CA, Edens E, Petrakis IL, Sofuoglu M. Targeting opioid-induced hyperalgesia in clinical treatment: neurobiological considerations. CNS Drugs. 2015;29:465–86.

32. Aslaksen PM, Lyby PS. Fear of pain potentiates nocebo hyperalgesia. J Pain Res. 2015;8:703–10.

33. Bannister K. Opioid-induced hyperalgesia: where are we now? Curr Opin Support Palliat Care. 2015;9:116–21.

34. Ballas SK, Darbari DS. Neuropathy, neuropathic pain, and sickle cell disease. Am J Hematol. 2013;88:927–9.

35. Brandow AM, Farley RA, Dasgupta M, Hoffmann RG, Panepinto JA. The use of neuropathic pain drugs in children with sickle cell disease is associated with older age, female sex, and longer length of hospital stay. J Pediatr Hematol Oncol. 2015;37:10–5.

36. Castro O, Brambilla DJ, Thorington B, et al. The acute chest syndrome in sickle cell disease: incidence and risk factors. The cooperative study of sickle cell disease. Blood. 1994;84:643–9.

37. Howard J, Hart N, Roberts-Harewood M, et al. Guideline on the management of acute chest syndrome in sickle cell disease. Br J Haematol. 2015;169:492–505.

38. Kumar R, Stanek J, Creary S, Dunn A, O'Brien SH. Prevalence and risk factors for venous thromboembolism in children with sickle cell disease: an administrative database study. Blood Adv. 2018;2:285–91.

39. Walker TM, Hambleton IR, Serjeant GR. Gallstones in sickle cell disease: observations from The Jamaican Cohort study. J Pediatr. 2000;136:80–5.

40. Brousse V, Buffet P, Rees D. The spleen and sickle cell disease: the sick(led) spleen. Br J Haematol. 2014;166:165–76.

41. Ohene-Frempong K, Weiner SJ, Sleeper LA, et al. Cerebrovascular accidents in sickle cell disease: rates and risk factors. Blood. 1998;91:288–94.

42. DeBaun MR, Gordon M, McKinstry RC, et al. Controlled trial of transfusions for silent cerebral infarcts in sickle cell anemia. N Engl J Med. 2014;371:699–710.

43. Adams RJ, Brambilla DJ, Granger S, et al. Stroke and conversion to high risk in children screened with transcranial Doppler ultrasound during the STOP study. Blood. 2004;103:3689–94.

44. Adamkiewicz TV, Sarnaik S, Buchanan GR, et al. Invasive pneumococcal infections in children with sickle cell disease in the era of penicillin prophylaxis, antibiotic resistance, and 23-valent pneumococcal polysaccharide vaccination. J Pediatr. 2003;143:438–44.

45. Ware RE, Davis BR, Schultz WH, et al. Hydroxycarbamide versus chronic transfusion for maintenance of transcranial doppler flow velocities in children with sickle cell anaemia-TCD With Transfusions Changing to Hydroxyurea (TWiTCH): a multicentre, open-label, phase 3, non-inferiority trial. Lancet. 2016;387:661–70.

46. Charache S. Mechanism of action of hydroxyurea in the management of sickle cell anemia in adults. Semin Hematol. 1997;34:15–21.

47. Noguchi CT, Rodgers GP, Serjeant G, Schechter AN. Levels of fetal hemoglobin necessary for treatment of sickle cell disease. N Engl J Med. 1988;318:96–9.

48. Jiang J, Jordan SJ, Barr DP, Gunther MR, Maeda H, Mason RP. In vivo production of nitric oxide in rats after administration of hydroxyurea. Mol Pharmacol. 1997;52:1081–6.

49. Green NS, Manwani D, Qureshi M, Ireland K, Sinha A, Smaldone AM. Decreased fetal hemoglobin over time among youth with sickle cell disease on hydroxyurea is associated with higher urgent hospital use. Pediatr Blood Cancer. 2016;63:2146–53.

50. Quinn CT, Rogers ZR, McCavit TL, Buchanan GR. Improved survival of children and adolescents with sickle cell disease. Blood. 2010;115:3447–52.

51. Hsieh MM, Kang EM, Fitzhugh CD, et al. Allogeneic hematopoietic stem-cell transplantation for sickle cell disease. N Engl J Med. 2009;361:2309–17.

52. King A, Shenoy S. Evidence-based focused review of the status of hematopoietic stem cell transplantation as treatment of sickle cell disease and thalassemia. Blood. 2014;123:3089–94; quiz 210.

53. Ribeil JA, Hacein-Bey-Abina S, Payen E, et al. Gene therapy in a patient with sickle cell disease. N Engl J Med. 2017;376:848–55.
54. Serjeant GR, Singhal A, Hambleton IR. Sickle cell disease and age at menarche in Jamaican girls: observations from a cohort study. Arch Dis Child. 2001;85:375–8.
55. Platt OS, Rosenstock W, Espeland MA. Influence of sickle hemoglobinopathies on growth and development. N Engl J Med. 1984;311:7–12.
56. Deligeoroglou E, Karountzos V, Creatsas G. Abnormal uterine bleeding and dysfunctional uterine bleeding in pediatric and adolescent gynecology. Gynecol Endocrinol. 2013;29:74–8.
57. Boga C, Ozdogu H. Pregnancy and sickle cell disease: a review of the current literature. Crit Rev Oncol Hematol. 2016;98:364–74.
58. Ghafuri DL, Stimpson SJ, Day ME, James A, DeBaun MR, Sharma D. Fertility challenges for women with sickle cell disease. Expert Rev Hematol. 2017;10:891–901.
59. Reece AS, Thomas MR, Norman A, Hulse GK. Dramatic acceleration of reproductive aging, contraction of biochemical fecundity and healthspan-lifespan implications of opioid-induced endocrinopathy-FSH/LH ratio and other interrelationships. Reprod Toxicol. 2016;66:20–30.
60. Reid RL, Westhoff C, Mansour D, et al. Oral contraceptives and venous thromboembolism consensus opinion from an international workshop held in Berlin, Germany in December 2009. J Fam Plann Reprod Health Care. 2010;36:117–22.
61. Legardy JK, Curtis KM. Progestogen-only contraceptive use among women with sickle cell anemia: a systematic review. Contraception. 2006;73:195–204.
62. Badawy SM, Thompson AA, Liem RI. Beliefs about hydroxyurea in youth with sickle cell disease. Hematol Oncol Stem Cell Ther. 2018;11:142–8.
63. Hemker BG, Brousseau DC, Yan K, Hoffmann RG, Panepinto JA. When children with sickle-cell disease become adults: lack of outpatient care leads to increased use of the emergency department. Am J Hematol. 2011;86:863–5.
64. Blinder MA, Vekeman F, Sasane M, Trahey A, Paley C, Duh MS. Age-related treatment patterns in sickle cell disease patients and the associated sickle cell complications and healthcare costs. Pediatr Blood Cancer. 2013;60:828–35.
65. Blinder MA, Duh MS, Sasane M, Trahey A, Paley C, Vekeman F. Age-related emergency department reliance in patients with sickle cell disease. J Emerg Med. 2015;49:513–22. e1.
66. Travis K, Wood A, Yeh P, et al. Pediatric to adult transition in sickle cell disease: survey results from young adult patients. Acta Haematol. 2020;143(2):163–75.
67. Jerrell JM, Tripathi A, McIntyre RS. Prevalence and treatment of depression in children and adolescents with sickle cell disease: a retrospective cohort study. Prim Care Companion CNS Disord. 2011;13(2):e1–7.
68. Jonassaint CR, Jones VL, Leong S, Frierson GM. A systematic review of the association between depression and health care utilization in children and adults with sickle cell disease. Br J Haematol. 2016;174:136–47.
69. Graves JK, Hodge C, Jacob E. Depression, anxiety, and quality of life in children and adolescents with sickle cell disease. Pediatr Nurs. 2016;42:113–9, 44.
70. Bhatt-Poulose K, James K, Reid M, Harrison A, Asnani M. Increased rates of body dissatisfaction, depressive symptoms, and suicide attempts in Jamaican teens with sickle cell disease. Pediatr Blood Cancer. 2016;63:2159–66.
71. Jacob E. The pain experience of patients with sickle cell anemia. Pain Manage Nurs. 2001;2:74–83.

Immune Thrombocytopenia in Adolescents

21

Anna Griffith and Alice D. Ma

Introduction

Immune thrombocytopenia (ITP) is defined as an isolated platelet count of <100,000/microL with a normal white blood cell count and hemoglobin concentration in the absence of identifiable and specific precipitants. In children, the presenting platelet count is typically less than 30,000/microL, and 45% of children have a platelet count of less than 10,000/microL [1–3]. The etiology is often unknown but can be triggered by a virus or other immune trigger. Primary ITP makes up about 80% of all causes of ITP and is characterized by an isolated thrombocytopenia with no other apparent etiology. Secondary ITP is an immune-mediated thrombocytopenia with an underlying cause (i.e., drugs, systemic autoimmune disease, or viral infection).

The International ITP Working Group established terminology to characterize the duration and severity of the illness [4]. Newly diagnosed ITP refers to the first 3 months from the initial diagnosis. Persistent ITP is a disease lasting from months 3–12 after the diagnosis. Chronic ITP is a disease lasting beyond 12 months. Severity of disease is often used to determine the need for treatment. Severe ITP is characterized by clinically relevant bleeding and requires treatment.

A. Griffith · A. D. Ma (✉)
Division of Hematology Oncology, University of North Carolina at Chapel Hill, Chapel Hill, NC, USA
e-mail: alice_ma@med.unc.edu

Refractory ITP is defined as severe thrombocytopenia after splenectomy.

Pathogenesis

This process was previously called idiopathic thrombocytopenic purpura (ITP) but has been renamed based on a better understanding of the pathogenesis of the disease process. Autoantibodies, usually immunoglobulin G (IgG), are directed against platelet membrane antigens (e.g., glycoprotein IIb/IIIa complex). Platelets coated with antibodies are then cleared by macrophages, resulting in a shortened half-life and resulting thrombocytopenia [5]. Contributing to platelet destruction are cytotoxic T-cells which are implicated in the pathogenesis of chronic ITP [6]. In addition to increased destruction, thrombocytopenia is compounded by impaired megakaryocytopoeisis [7].

Epidemiology

ITP is a common disorder, occurring in roughly 8 per 100,000 children and 12 per 100,000 adults [8]. There is a female predominance in the age range from 15 to 39 and 40 to 59 and a male predominance in patients ager >70 [9]. Studies have shown that one-fifth to one-third of patients are asymptomatic at the time of diagnosis [10].

Historically, ITP has been associated with female patients in the young adult years (ages 18–45), and some have postulated that there is a relationship between estrogen and autoimmunity.

Initial Evaluation

Evaluation of the patient with thrombocytopenia should begin with a complete history and physical exam with close attention to clinical evidence of bleeding as well as constitutional symptoms such as fevers, night sweats, and weight loss, which may suggest an alternative diagnosis. Laboratory evaluation should include a CBC with differential, smear review, type and screen, reticulocyte count, direct antiglobulin testing, and a complete metabolic panel. Examination of the blood smear to search for schistocytes, blasts, and spherocytes is imperative to rule out alternative diagnosis. Careful attention to platelet size is also helpful in supporting a diagnosis of ITP, as platelets are often large in ITP as the bone marrow attempts to compensate for the low platelet count. HIV and hepatitis C virus should be ruled out. Hepatitis B serologies should be obtained as a part of the initial workup to determine if the patient has chronic hepatitis B virus (HBV) infection, as the treatment of ITP sometimes requires immunosuppression that puts patients with chronic HBV at risk for reactivation. Administration of intravenous immunoglobulin (IVIg) prior to testing can confound serology results.

ITP is a clinical diagnosis and should be considered in patients with isolated thrombocytopenia with a platelet count of <100,000/microL and no evidence of blasts or hemolysis on the blood smear. The diagnosis is confirmed by response to ITP-specific treatment. Generally speaking, testing for antibodies to specific platelet glycoproteins is not recommended [4, 11]. A bone marrow biopsy is not necessary to diagnose ITP, although there is debate regarding if a bone marrow biopsy is necessary in patients who do not respond to first line therapy [11]. Any atypical clinical or laboratory features that are not consistent with ITP and suggest malignancy or bone marrow failure warrant further workup with a bone marrow biopsy.

General Management Guidelines

There are several general management principles that are specific to the adolescent population. The decision for treatment versus watchful waiting will be addressed in the next section but is an important one in the adolescent population as these patients have a higher risk of relapse or chronic disease than children, but in time, many adolescents do achieve a lasting remission. Additionally, the adolescent age group tends to be very physically active. There is variation in clinical practice, but the provider must advise patients regarding participation in athletics, and some providers recommend avoiding contact sports entirely due to the risk of bleeding. All patients should be educated about avoiding anticoagulant and antiplatelet medications including NSAIDs. Providers should rely on treatment with acetaminophen and celecoxib for management of pain and fever requiring pharmacologic treatment. Additionally, attention must be paid to menses in adolescent females to prevent severe menorrhagia in girls with thrombocytopenia. Attempts should be made to control or inhibit menses with either hormonal therapy or fibrinolytics to control bleeding.

Monitoring frequency is largely dependent upon the trajectory of the platelet count. Patients should be followed with serial labs and clinical evaluations for bleeding. Typically, we recommend starting with once weekly labs and increasing the interval between laboratory checks based on the platelet trends. Active monitoring should occur until the platelet count has normalized (>150,000/microL) and remains stable without treatment.

Lastly, efforts should be made to educate both the adolescent patient and their caregivers regarding symptoms suggestive of recurrent thrombocytopenia and resulting anemia including severe bleeding, bruising, melena, menorrhagia, and hematuria. Patients should be educated regarding the risk of intracerebral hemorrhage in the setting of severe thrombocytopenia and cautioned to seek medical care for severe headache.

Deciding When to Treat

The overall goal in treating ITP is adequate hemostasis, not a normal platelet count. There is robust evidence that the majority of pediatric patients may be managed with observation in the outpatient setting [4, 11, 12]. 50–70% of children recover within 3–6 months of presentation with or without treatment [2, 3, 13]. Younger children with less severe bleeding are more likely to recover spontaneously than adolescents [14, 15]. Increasing age is a risk factor for bleeding, so while adolescents have a lower chance of spontaneous recovery than younger children, they do represent a unique population that should not simply be treated as adults [16]. In a patient with minimal or no bleeding, there is no indication for treatment, regardless of the platelet count. Conversely, prompt treatment is clearly indicated for severe life-threatening bleeding, such as intracranial hemorrhage, gastrointestinal hemorrhage, and pulmonary hemorrhage with cardiopulmonary compromise. The incidence of intracranial hemorrhage in pediatric patients with ITP is 0.1–0.8% [17, 18], and combination therapy is more effective at quickly increasing the platelet count. Platelet transfusions should also be used for life-threatening bleeding until the other treatments successfully raise the platelet count. Severe non-life- threatening bleeding can include internal hemorrhage, mucosal bleeding, and severe epistaxis and pulmonary hemorrhage without cardiopulmonary compromise and muscle or joint hemorrhage. The risk of severe non-life-threatening bleeding in children is about 3%, and this clinical scenario also warrants treatment, often with combination therapy [17–19].

Treatment Strategies: First Line

Selection of therapy is dependent upon the clinical scenario. First-line treatment strategies include steroids, IVIG, and anti-D immunoglob-

ulin. A randomized multicenter trial from China established dexamethasone as the preferred strategy for treatment of newly diagnosed primary ITP in adults [20]. This study compared the efficacy and safety of high-dose dexamethasone (40 mg daily for 4 days) with prednisone 1 mg/kg for 4 weeks, then tapered, and found equal efficacy and improved tolerability. The median time to response in the dexamethasone group was 3 days (range 1–9) and in the prednisone group was 6 days (range 2–24). Long-term steroids are associated with significant toxicity including sleep disturbance, weight gain, hypertension, gastritis, behavioral change, osteoporosis, adrenal insufficiency, immune suppression, and steroid myopathy. For these reasons, long-term steroids are avoided when possible.

IVIG is another well-established first-line treatment and is used when a rapid platelet response is desired, most often in the setting of active bleeding. Dosing is 0.8–1 g/kg ×1 in children and 2 g/kg divided in either 2, 4, or 5 days in adults. A systematic review of ten randomized controlled trials comparing corticosteroids with IVIG in pediatrics concluded that children treated with IVIG were more likely to achieve a platelet count >20,000/microL after 48 hours of therapy than those treated with prednisone [21]. As emphasized previously, treatment goals should be control of bleeding, not achievement of a particular platelet count. Use of IVIG was compared to observation in childhood ITP, and IVIG was not associated with a reduced risk of chronic ITP. Reactions to IVIG are common and include a spectrum from mild headache, chills, and flushing to aseptic meningitis, anaphylaxis, thromboembolic events, and hemolysis. Serious reactions occur in 2–6% of patients [22]. Risk correlates with dose and rate of infusion and can be reduce with premedication with acetaminophen and diphenhydramine.

Anti-Rh (D) binds to the Rh (D) antigen on red blood cells which leads immune-mediated clearance of the red cells, which serve as "decoys" for the Fc receptor on reticuloendothelial cells. Anti-D immunoglobulin may be used a select population of patients who are Rh+, have a negative direct antiglobulin test, and have not undergone splenectomy. This strategy has been shown to be as effective as IVIG in children with newly diagnosed ITP [23, 24]. Anti-D, however, is associated with increased side effects that can include fatal intravascular hemolysis in about 1 in 1000 patients [25, 26].

Adjunct therapies may be used in addition to the above therapies depending on the source of bleeding. In the case of the adolescent female, attention must be paid to prevent heavy menstrual bleeding (HMB). Fibrinolytics may be used to manage mucosal bleeding, including gastrointestinal bleeding or HMB, but are strictly contraindicated for hematuria. Hormonal therapy should also be employed if the patient is experiencing HMB.

75–90% of patients respond to first-line therapies [4]. The average time to platelet response to IVIG is 1–4 days, and time to response to glucocorticoids is 2–14 days [27]. Once platelet counts have normalized and have remained stable for 2–6 months, the risk of recurrence in children is <5% [28] but is higher in adolescents and adults. Relapsed disease and chronic ITP will be discussed later in the chapter, but the rate of relapse and chronic ITP is higher in adolescents than in children. Poor response to first-line therapy should prompt providers to investigate other etiologies of thrombocytopenia including bone marrow failure, malignancy, and infections.

Treatment Strategies: Second Line

Second-line therapies are indicated for patients with thrombocytopenia lasting more than 3–6 months or those with symptoms or bleeding risk that is not controlled with first-line therapy. These treatment options include rituximab, thrombopoietin receptor agonists, and splenectomy.

Rituximab is a monoclonal antibody targeting CD20 that depletes B cells to suppress production of antibodies. It is considered second line in treatment of pediatric ITP but first line in treatment of adult ITP. Accepted standard dosing is 375 mg/m2 ×4 doses. The safety and efficacy of rituximab in children and adolescent chronic ITP

were assessed in a prospective study of 36 patients ages 2.6–18.3 years. These patients were treated with standard dose rituximab, and 11 of the 36 patients achieved a platelet count above 50,000/microL [29]. Eight of these 11 responders maintained a platelet count over 150,000/microL without further treatment 1 year later [30]. Another study had similar response rates in 15 of 24 patients with 9 patients having long-term complete response (platelet count >150,000/microL) [31]. Rituximab was well tolerated in all of these trials with a rate of serum sickness around 5%. In the treatment of adult patients, the use of rituximab with dexamethasone in previously untreated adults with ITP had a higher sustained response rate at 6 months, defined as a platelet count >50,000/microL, than those treated with dexamethasone alone (63% vs 36%). Additionally, dexamethasone and rituximab therapy was used as an effective salvage therapy in 56% of those patients who did not respond to dexamethasone monotherapy [32].

Thrombopoietin (TPO) is a hormone produced by the liver which regulates platelet production by binding and activating TPO receptors on the megakaryocyte surface. Two TPO-R agonists are currently approved by the FDA for treatment of chronic or refractory ITP, romiplostim and eltrombopag. Thrombopoietin receptor agonists have dramatically changed the treatment of ITP. Recent studies of these agents have demonstrated both safety and efficacy in adults and children when compared to placebo. Notably, a meta-analysis of six randomized controlled trials showed significantly improved platelet counts (RR 3.42; 95% CI 2.51–4.65) and decreased incidence of bleeding (RR 0.74; 95% CI 0.66–0.83) in adults [33]. The EXTEND trial followed adult patients with chronic ITP on TPO-agonists and showed an overall response rate of 85% with a median platelet count increasing to >50,000/mm3 by 2 weeks and remaining increased for the duration of the study [34]. A meta-analysis of five randomized controlled pediatric trials including 261 patients confirmed the safety and efficacy over placebo [35]. Major side effects of TPO agonists are mild grade 1–2 headache, nasopharyngitis, fatigue, and VTE [36].

Splenectomy is a last resort, used in patients whose disease is refractory to medical management. Splenectomy carries significant risks including infection, thrombosis, pulmonary hypertension, and postoperative complications. Vaccinations against encapsulated organisms should be given prior to surgery, including pneumococcus, meningococcus, and *Haemophilus influenzae*. In the adolescent population, a high rate of spontaneous remission suggests that if possible, splenectomy should be delayed for at least 12 months unless the patient has severe and unresponsive disease [37].

Relapsed Disease and Chronic ITP

One-third of adult patients who initially respond to first-line therapies develop recurrent severe thrombocytopenia [4]. If the patient had a good response to first-line therapy, the same therapy may be given again. The rate of chronic ITP is about 10–21% in children, and the rate of chronic ITP is higher in adolescents than in younger children [2–4, 37, 38]. By comparison the incidence of chronic ITP in adults (age >18) is 23.6%. Factors associated with an increased risk of chronic ITP are older age, less severe thrombocytopenia at diagnosis, insidious onset of symptoms, lack of associated infection, and lack of mucosal bleeding at diagnosis [2, 14, 15, 39–41]. We are limited by lack of data specific to the adolescent population, but the 2011 ASH guidelines recommend that the management of adolescents should follow the usual management of children with ITP [11].

Special Populations: Pregnancy

The incidence of ITP in pregnancy is 1–10 in 10,000 [42] and requires treatment in about 30% of cases [43]. Bleeding complications are rare, but women with ITP prior to pregnancy have a higher incidence of fetal loss and low birth weight for gestational age than those without a history of ITP prior to pregnancy [44]. The goal of treatment is to maintain the maternal platelet count above 30,000/microL until 36-week gestation or near delivery. Platelets should be monitored every 2–4 weeks depending on the stability of the platelet counts. Asymptomatic patients with a platelet count >30,000/microL should be monitored carefully but do not require treatment until near delivery. Symptomatic patients, or those with a platelet count <30,000/microL, should receive either IVIG or corticosteroids, which have been shown to have similar efficacy [4, 11, 45]. Patients who are refractory to therapy can be treated with combination therapy of IVIG and corticosteroids. Refractory ITP can be treated with splenectomy, preferably in the second trimester [46]. Most other agents used to treat refractory ITP are not safe in pregnancy, including Danazol, Vinca alkaloids, and cyclophosphamide [42].

ITP is not an indication for caesarian delivery. The optimal platelet count for delivery is 75,000/microL, but 50,000/microL is generally safe for an uncomplicated delivery or caesarian section. The platelet threshold for safe neuraxial anesthesia is not known, and practice varies considerably from institution to institution. Generally, the platelet goal at our center is 75,000–80,000/microL in these patients.

Fetal intracranial hemorrhage has been reported in 0–1.5% of cases of maternal ITP. There is poor correlation between maternal and fetal platelet counts [47]. A neonatal platelet count should be obtained at delivery to determine the need for neonatal treatment of ITP.

Summary

ITP in adolescents is similar to ITP in adults and children in terms of diagnosis and presentation. The clinical course is a hybrid, with more patients requiring therapy, and many patients eventually achieving remission. Therapy is guided by bleeding symptoms, rather than absolute platelet counts, but also by prophylaxis against bleeding, given the increased physical activity in this age group. Careful attention should be paid to females with heavy menstrual bleeding. Lastly, the psychosocial aspects of care for patients in this vulnerable age group must be considered, with attention to aspects of independence and shared decision making.

References

1. Kühne T, Imbach P, Bolton-Maggs PHB, Berchtold W, Blanchette V, Buchanan GR. Newly diagnosed idiopathic thrombocytopenic purpura in childhood: an observational study. Lancet. 2001;358(9299):2122–5. https://doi.org/10.1016/S0140-6736(01)07219-1.

2. Rosthøj S, Hedlund-Treutiger I, Rajantie J, et al. Duration and morbidity of newly diagnosed idiopathic. Most. 2003;143(3):302–7. http://www.ncbi.nlm.nih.gov/pubmed/14517509.

3. Kühne T, Buchanan GR, Zimmerman S, et al. A prospective comparative study of 2540 infants and children with newly diagnosed idiopathic thrombocytopenic purpura (ITP) from the intercontinental childhood ITP study group. J Pediatr. 2003;143(5):605–8. https://doi.org/10.1067/S0022-3476(03)00535-3.

4. Rodeghiero F, Stasi R, Gernsheimer T, et al. Standardization of terminology, definitions and outcome criteria in immune thrombocytopenic purpura of adults and children: report from an international working group. Blood. 2009;113(11):2386–93. https://doi.org/10.1182/blood-2008-07-162503.

5. Zufferey A, Kapur R, Semple J. Pathogenesis and therapeutic mechanisms in immune thrombocytopenia (ITP). J Clin Med. 2017;6(2):16. https://doi.org/10.3390/jcm6020016.

6. Olsson B, Andersson PO, Jernås M, et al. T-cell-mediated cytotoxicity toward platelets in chronic idiopathic thrombocytopenic purpura. Nat Med. 2003;9(9):1123–4. https://doi.org/10.1038/nm921.

7. Khodadi E, Asnafi AA, Shahrabi S, Shahjahani M, Saki N. Bone marrow niche in immune thrombocytopenia: a focus on megakaryopoiesis. Ann Hematol. 2016;95(11):1765–76. https://doi.org/10.1007/s00277-016-2703-1.

8. Terrell DR, Beebe LA, Neas BR, Vesely SK, Segal JB, George JN. Prevalence of primary immune thrombocytopenia in Oklahoma. Am J Hematol. 2012;87(9):848–52. https://doi.org/10.1002/ajh.23262.

9. Frederiksen H, Schmidt K. The incidence of idiopathic thrombocytopenic purpura in adults increases with age. Blood. 1999;94(3):909–13.

10. Neylon AJ, Saunders PWG, Howard MR, Proctor SJ, Taylor PRA. Clinically significant newly presenting autoimmune thrombocytopenic purpura in adults: a prospective study of a population-based cohort of 245 patients. Br J Haematol. 2003;122(6):966–74. https://doi.org/10.1046/j.1365-2141.2003.04547.x.

11. Neunert C, Lim W, Crowther M, Cohen A, Solberg L, Crowther MA. The American Society of Hematology 2011 evidence-based practice guideline for immune thrombocytopenia. Blood. 2011;117(16):4190–207. https://doi.org/10.1182/blood-2010-08-302984.

12. Oncology PH, George JN, Cohen AR, Blanchette VS. Self-reported initial management of childhood idiopathic thrombocytopenic purpura: results of a survey of members of the American Society of Pediatric Hematology/Oncology, 2001. J Pediatr. 2003;25(2):130–3.

13. Heitink-Pollé KMJ, Uiterwaal CSPM, Porcelijn L, et al. Intravenous immunoglobulin vs observation in childhood immune thrombocytopenia: a randomized controlled trial. Blood. 2018;132(9):883–91. https://doi.org/10.1182/blood-2018-02-830844.

14. Glanz J, France E, Xu S, Hayes T, Hambidge S. A population-based, multisite cohort study of the predictors of chronic idiopathic thrombocytopenic purpura in children. Pediatrics. 2008;121(3):10–5. https://doi.org/10.1542/peds.2007-1129.

15. Revel-Vilk S, Yacobovich J, Frank S, et al. Age and duration of bleeding symptoms at diagnosis best predict resolution of childhood immune thrombocytopenia at 3, 6, and 12 months. J Pediatr. 2013;163(5):1335–9. https://doi.org/10.1016/j.jpeds.2013.06.018.

16. Cohen YC, Djuibegovic B, Shamai-Lubovitz O, Mozes B. The bleeding risk and natural history of idiopathic thrombocytopenic purpura in patients with persistent low platelet counts. Arch Intern Med. 2000;160(11):1630–8. https://doi.org/10.1001/archinte.160.11.1630.

17. Kühne T, Berchtold W, Michaels LA, et al. Newly diagnosed immune thrombocytopenia in children and adults: a comparative prospective observational registry of the intercontinental cooperative immune thrombocytopenia study group. Haematologica. 2011;96(12):1831–7. https://doi.org/10.3324/haematol.2011.050799.

18. Neunert C, Noroozi N, Norman G, et al. Severe bleeding events in adults and children with primary immune thrombocytopenia: a systematic review. J Thromb Haemost. 2015;13(3):457–64. https://doi.org/10.1111/jth.12813.

19. Neunert CE, Buchanan GR, Imbach P, et al. Severe hemorrhage in children with newly diagnosed immune thrombocytopenic purpura. Blood. 2008;112(10):4003–8. https://doi.org/10.1182/blood-2008-03-138487.

20. Wei Y, Ji XB, Wang YW, Wang JX, et al. High-dose dexamethasone vs prednisone for treatment of adult immune thrombocytopenia: a prospective multicenter randomized trial. Blood. 2016;127(3):296–302. https://doi.org/10.1182/blood-2015-07-659656.

21. Blanchette VS, Luke B, Andrew M, et al. A prospective, randomized trial of high-dose intravenous immune globulin G therapy, oral prednisone therapy, and no therapy in childhood acute immune thrombocytopenic purpura. J Pediatr. 1993;123(6):989–95. https://doi.org/10.1016/S0022-3476(05)80400-7.

22. Perez EE, Orange JS, Bonilla F, et al. Update on the use of immunoglobulin in human disease: a review of evidence. J Allergy Clin Immunol. 2017;139(3):S1–S46. https://doi.org/10.1016/j.jaci.2016.09.023.

23. Son DW, Jeon IS, Yang SW, Cho SH. A single dose of anti-D immunoglobulin raises platelet count

as efficiently as intravenous immunoglobulin in newly diagnosed immune thrombocytopenic purpura in korean children. J Pediatr Hematol Oncol. 2008;30(8):598–601. https://doi.org/10.1097/MPH.0b013e31817541ba.

24. Tarantino MD, Madden RM, Fennewald DL, Patel CC, Bertolone SJ. Treatment of childhood acute immune thrombocytopenic purpura with anti- D immune globulin or pooled immune globulin. J Pediatr. 1999;134(1):21–6. https://doi.org/10.1016/S0022-3476(99)70367-7.

25. Alioglu B, Avci Z, Ozyurek E, Ozbek N. Anti-D immunoglobulin-induced prolonged intravascular hemolysis and neutropenia. J Pediatr Hematol Oncol. 2007;29(9):636–9. https://doi.org/10.1097/MPH.0b013e318142ac5f.

26. Gaines AR. Disseminated intravascular coagulation associated with acute hemoglobinemia or hemoglobinuria following Rho(D) immune globulin intravenous administration for immune thrombocytopenic purpura. Blood. 2005;106(5):1532–7. https://doi.org/10.1182/blood-2004-11-4303.

27. Beck CE, et al. Corticosteroids Versus Intravenous Immune Globulin for the Treatment of Acute Immune Thrombocytopenic Purpura in Children: A Systemic Review and Meta-Analysis of Randomized Controlled Trials. The Journal of Pediatrics. 2005;147(4):521–27.

28. Gebauer E, Vijatov G. Idiopathic thrombocytopenic purpura in children. Med Pregl. 1998;51(3–4):127–34.

29. Bennett CM, Rogers ZR, Kinnamon DD, et al. Brief report Prospective phase 1/2 study of rituximab in childhood and adolescent chronic immune thrombocytopenic purpura. Blood. 2019;107(7):2639–43. https://doi.org/10.1182/blood-2005-08-3518.A.

30. Bennett CM, Rogers ZR, Kinnamon DD, et al. Chronic immune thrombocytopenic purpura Brief report Prospective phase 1/2 study of rituximab in childhood and adolescent chronic immune thrombocytopenic purpura. Child A Glob J Child Res. 2011;107(7):2639–42. https://doi.org/10.1182/blood-2005-08-3518.

31. Wang J, Wiley JM, Luddy R, Greenberg J, Feuerstein MA, Bussel JB. Chronic immune thrombocytopenic purpura in children: assessment of rituximab treatment. J Pediatr. 2005;146(2):217–21. https://doi.org/10.1016/j.jpeds.2004.09.004.

32. Zaja F, Baccarani M, Mazza P, Bocchia M, Gugliotta L, Zaccaria A, Vianelli N, Defina M, Tieghi A, Amadori S, Campagna S. Dexamethasone plus rituximab yields higher sustained response rates than dexamethasone monotherapy in adults with primary immune thrombocytopenia. Blood. 2010;115(14):2755–62. https://doi.org/10.1182/blood-2009-07-229815. LK - http://sfx.library.uu.nl/utrecht?sid=EMBASE&issn=00064971&id=doi:10.1182%2Fblood-2009-07-229815&atitle=Dexamethasone+plus+rituximab+yields+higher+sustained+response+rates+than+dexamethasone+monotherapy+in+adults+with+primary+immune+thrombocytopenia&stitle=Blood&title=Blood&volume=115&issue=14&spage=2755&epage=2762&aulast=Zaja&aufirst=Francesco&auinit=F.&aufull=Za

ja+F.&coden=BLOOA&isbn=&pages=2755-2762&date=2010&auinit1=F&auinitm=

33. Elgebaly AS, El Ashal G, Elfil M, Menshawy A. Tolerability and efficacy of eltrombopag in chronic immune thrombocytopenia: meta-analysis of randomized controlled trials. Clin Appl Thromb. 2017;23(8):928–37. https://doi.org/10.1177/1076029616663849.

34. Saleh MN, Bussel JB, Cheng G, et al. Safety and efficacy of eltrombopag for treatment of chronic immune thrombocytopenia: results of the long-term, open-label EXTEND study. Blood. 2013;121(3):537–45. https://doi.org/10.1182/blood-2012-04-425512.

35. Guo JC, Zheng Y, Chen HT, et al. Efficacy and safety of thrombopoietin receptor agonists in children with chronic immune thrombocytopenia: a metaanalysis. Oncotarget. 2018;9(6):7112–25. https://doi.org/10.18632/oncotarget.23487.

36. Ghanima W, Cooper N, Rodeghiero F, Godeau B, Bussel JB. Thrombopoietin receptor agonists: ten years later. Haematologica. 2019;104(6):1112–23. https://doi.org/10.3324/haematol.2018.212845.

37. Imbach P, Kühne T, Müller D, et al. Childhood ITP: 12 months follow-up data from the prospective registry I of the Intercontinental Childhood ITP Study Group (ICIS). Pediatr Blood Cancer. 2006;46(3):351–6. https://doi.org/10.1002/pbc.20453.

38. Zeller B, Rajantie J, Hedlund-Treutiger I, et al. Childhood idiopathic thrombocytopenic purpura in the Nordic countries: epidemiology and predictors of chronic disease. Acta Paediatr Int J Paediatr. 2005;94(2):178–84. https://doi.org/10.1080/08035250410025294.

39. Ahmed S, Siddiqui AK, Shahid RK, Kimpo M, Sison CP, Hoffman MA. Prognostic variables in newly diagnosed childhood immune thrombocytopenia. Am J Hematol. 2004;77(4):358–62. https://doi.org/10.1002/ajh.20205.

40. Bruin M, Bierings M, Uiterwaal C, et al. Platelet count, previous infection and FCGR2B genotype predict development of chronic disease in newly diagnosed idiopathic thrombocytopenia in childhood: results of a prospective study. Br J Haematol. 2004;127(5):561–7. https://doi.org/10.1111/j.1365-2141.2004.05235.x.

41. Bennett CM, Neunert C, Grace RF, et al. Predictors of remission in children with newly diagnosed immune thrombocytopenia: data from the Intercontinental Cooperative ITP Study Group Registry II participants. Pediatr Blood Cancer. 2018;65(1):1–7. https://doi.org/10.1002/pbc.26736.

42. Silver RM, Richard L. Thrombocytopenia in pregnancy. Gynecology. 1999;67:117–28.

43. Webert KE, Mittal R, Sigouin C, et al. A retrospective 11-year analysis of obstetric patients with idiopathic thrombocytopenic purpura a retrospective 11-year analysis of obstetric patients with idiopathic thrombocytopenic purpura. Blood. 2011;102(13):4306–11. https://doi.org/10.1182/blood-2002-10-3317.

44. Al-Jama FE, Rahman J, Al-Suleiman SA, Rahman MS. Outcome of pregnancy in women with idiopathic

thrombocytopenic purpura. Aust New Zeal J Obstet Gynaecol. 1998;38(4):410–3. https://doi.org/10.1111/j.1479-828X.1998.tb03099.x.

45. Nicolescu A, Vladareanu AM, Voican I, Onisai M, Vladareanu R. Therapeutic options for immune thrombocytopenia (ITP) during pregnancy. Maedica (Buchar). 2013;8(2):182–8. http://www.ncbi.nlm.nih.gov/pubmed/24371483%0A. http://www.pubmedcentral.nih.gov/articlerender.fcgi?artid=PMC3865128.

46. Anglin BV, Rutherford C, Ramus R, Lieser M, Jones DB. Immune thrombocytopenic purpura during pregnancy: laparoscopic treatment. JSLS. 2001;5(1):63–7.

47. Sainio S, Kekomäki R, Riikonen S, Teramo K. Maternal thrombocytopenai at term: a population-based study. Acta Obstet Gynecol Scand. 2000;79(9):744–9. https://doi.org/10.1034/j.1600-0412.2000.079009744.x.

Autoimmune Hemolytic Anemia in Adolescent Females

Taylor Olmsted Kim and James B. Bussel

Introduction

Autoimmune hemolytic anemia (AIHA) is characterized by immune dysregulation leading to autoantibodies directed against endogenous red cell antigens, resulting in premature erythrocyte destruction and anemia. It is a rare disorder affecting 0.2 per 10^5 children annually. AIHA has a slight male predominance and a median age of presentation of 3.8 years [1, 2]. The exact incidence in adolescents has not been reported; however, adolescents who develop AIHA are more likely to have chronically relapsing disease that is often secondary to a systemic immune abnormality [3].

AIHA can be categorized by the type of autoantibodies binding red cells or by the presence or absence and type of an underlying disorder. Young children most commonly have idiopathic disease, often following a viral infection. In contrast, the adolescent population more commonly has secondary causes and AIHA, and other immune cytopenias may often be the presenting feature of a systemic immunodeficiency or systemic autoimmune disease.

Initial Diagnostic Testing

Direct Antiglobulin Test

To diagnose autoimmune-mediated hemolysis, two components are required: proof of ongoing hemolysis and serologic evidence of an autoantibody targeting a red cell antigen. The direct antiglobulin test (DAT), formerly the Coombs test, is the most important and specific test in the diagnosis of AIHA [4]. The DAT detects autoantibodies bound to a patient's red blood cells which potentially lead to red cell destruction.

A reagent containing polyspecific antibodies against human globulin (IgG) is applied to washed patient red blood cells. If the red cells have been coated with IgG antibody in vivo, they will agglutinate on exposure to antihuman globulin antibodies which typically bind the heavy chain of the IgG molecule, constituting a positive result. The degree of DAT positivity is subjectively defined by the degree of agglutination from 0 to 4+ [5]. The strength of DAT positivity roughly correlates to degree of hemolysis;

T. O. Kim (✉)
Baylor College of Medicine, Department of Pediatrics, Houston, TX, USA

Texas Children's Hematology Center, Houston, TX, USA
e-mail: teolmste@txch.org

J. B. Bussel
Weill Cornell Medicine, Department of Pediatrics, New York, NY, USA

Weill Cornell Medicine, Internal Medicine, New York, NY, USA

Weill Cornell Medicine, Obstetrics and Gynecology, New York, NY, USA

© Springer Nature Switzerland AG 2020
L. V. Srivaths (ed.), *Hematology in the Adolescent Female*,
https://doi.org/10.1007/978-3-030-48446-0_22

however, the potency of antibody-antigen reaction can be a confounding factor which may be impacted by characteristics of the antigen or the specific antibody [6] (see Fig. 22.1).

If the polyspecific DAT is positive, additional testing is performed using specific antiglobulins to distinguish IgG from C3d-coated red blood cells (see Fig. 22.1).

Limitations of DAT Testing

While the DAT remains an essential component in diagnosing AIHA, the test has several limitations. DAT testing may be falsely negative if clinically relevant antibody titers are below the limits of detection or due to errors in specimen handling or the functioning of reagents [7]. Additionally, the standard DAT only tests for IgG and C3 antibodies. Rarely, AIHA can be caused by other antibody types such as IgA [8]. Specialized centers can test additional antibodies and can be helpful when the clinical picture is consistent with AIHA but the DAT is negative. False positives can result from technical errors such as over-centrifugation, clotted specimens, delayed test interpretation, or improper handling of reagents.

In normal healthy populations, a positive DAT is found in approximately 1 in 1000 to 1 in 14,000 donors. The incidence of a positive result in absence of hemolysis is even higher in hospitalized patients, up to 15% [7]. Therefore, a positive DAT must be interpreted in conjunction with the clinical presentation, as a positive DAT does not diagnose AIHA in the absence of hemolysis.

Warm Autoimmune Hemolytic Anemia

The most common type of AIHA in adolescents is warm AIHA (W-AIHA), comprising 75–90% of all cases [9, 10]. W-AIHA occurs when polyclonal IgG autoantibodies are formed and directed against protein or glycoprotein complexes on the red cell surface. These antibodies bind red cells optimally at body temperature (37 °C). Once erythrocytes in circulation are coated with autoantibodies, upon passage through the spleen, they are bound by Fc receptors on splenic macrophages. Red cells may be fully phagocytosed or, more commonly, are partially engulfed and digested. This results in spherocytic cells with decreased surface-area-to-volume ratio. Abnormal microcytic spherocytes are then trapped and destroyed on a subsequent passage through the blood vessels of the reticuloendothelial system [11].

Presentation W-AIHA may present with severe, acute onset of hemolytic anemia, though some patients are minimally affected with slower onset of symptoms. Symptoms include fatigue, pallor, dyspnea, dizziness, and jaundice. Jaundice may be prominent initially and give way to pallor. In severe cases or those with comorbidities, patients can manifest evidence of heart failure.

Anemia is variable depending on disease acuity, but is often severe. It is impacted by the degree of compensatory erythropoiesis. Typically, the reticulocyte percentage is elevated greater than 3%; however, if early in disease presentation, reticulocytosis may be absent [12, 13]. It is important in assessing the degree of compensatory erythrocyte production to correct the reticulocyte count for the absolute number of red cells. Specifically, in a very anemic patient, a relatively high reticulocyte percentage may be misleading in that the absolute number of reticulocytes may be relatively low. In the setting of brisk reticulocytosis or red cell clumping, there is often an elevated mean corpuscular volume.

Laboratory evidence of active hemolysis includes elevated total bilirubin, indirect bilirubin, and lactic dehydrogenase (LDH) levels. Haptoglobin levels are decreased in the great majority of affected adolescents; if there is detectable haptoglobin on testing, the diagnosis should be reconsidered [14]. Peripheral smear typically demonstrates anemia, poikilocytosis, anisocytosis, and polychromasia; spherocytes are present in the setting of warm AIHA [13] (see Fig. 22.2a).

In primary W-AIHA, the DAT is commonly positive for bound IgG and negative for bound C3-d. When IgG binding is robust and IgG

Direct Antiglobulin Test (DAT)

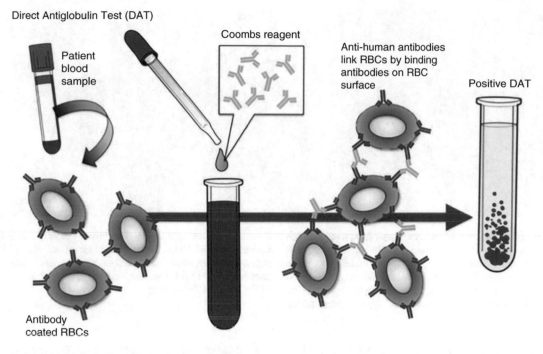

Indirect Antiglobulin Test (Screen)

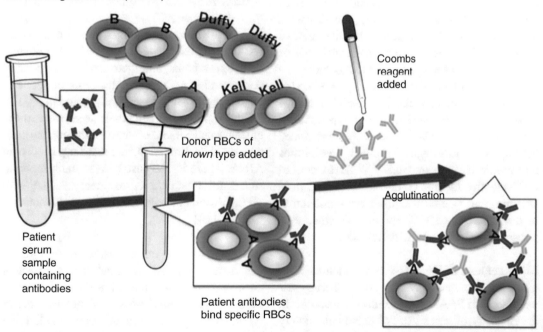

Fig. 22.1 *Direct antiglobulin test (DAT)*: antibody-coated erythrocytes in the patient's blood are bound by Coombs reagent resulting in agglutination. A positive test is graded based on the degree of agglutination. *Indirect antiglobulin test*: in this test, a patient's serum is incu-bated with donor erythrocytes with known antigenic characteristics. Following incubation, the DAT is performed to identify the red blood cell antigen types bound by antibody (agglutinated). (Figure printed with permissions from Taylor Kim)

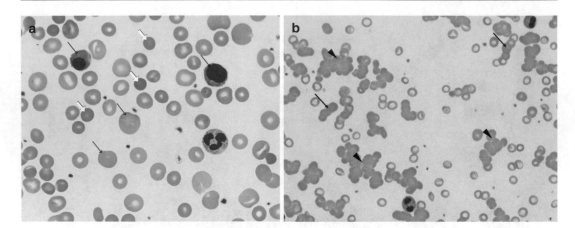

Fig. 22.2 (a) Peripheral blood smear from a patient with warm AIHA. White arrows indicate spherocytes that result from partial engulfment of the red cell by splenic macrophages. Black arrows mark nucleated red blood cells, and red arrows indicated reticulocytes, both markers of compensatory hematopoiesis. (Image courtesy of Dr. Amanda Grimes). (b) Peripheral blood smear from a patient with cold AIHA. Triangles indicate red cell clumping, and arrows mark areas of rouleaux formation that results from the IgM pentamer binding. (Image courtesy of Dr. M. Tarek Elghetany)

molecules come in close proximity to each other, complement fixation can occur, leading to positive C3-d testing. Generally, the driver of hemolysis can be determined by the relative strength of IgG and C3. In approximately 5% of cases, the DAT is negative despite a clinical picture consistent with AIHA. This may be related to a low-affinity or low-titer IgG, IgA, or monomeric IgM antibodies [15]. In our experience, a frequent cause of DAT-negative "autoimmune" hemolysis is misdiagnosis. Other possibilities that mimic the presentation of W-AIHA but are DAT-negative include GI or other bleeding, thalassemia, paroxysmal nocturnal hemoglobinuria, or a red cell enzyme defect such as glucose-6-phosphate dehydrogenase deficiency.

Management of W-AIHA Is Confirmed Steroids are the mainstay of upfront therapy for patients with W-AIHA and induce a response in the majority of cases [2]. For hemodynamically unstable patients, IV methylprednisolone should be started at 30 mg/kg/day divided every 12–24 hours. Once a patient is hemodynamically stable, hemoglobin maintained without transfusions, and reticulocytosis ceased, patients may be transitioned to oral steroids (prednisone or prednisolone) at 1–2 mg/kg/day. Once stable on oral dosing for 2–3 weeks, steroids can be tapered. A French study has suggested that the steroid taper should be prolonged to 6 months since those who taper longer than 6 months are less likely to relapse [2, 16]. This is one potential treatment schema, and there are a wide range of dosing and tapering schedules reported, none of which have been extensively validated [17]. While high-dose dexamethasone is used in the upfront management of immune thrombocytopenia, there is limited data regarding its use in AIHA. There is one case series which reported successful treatment of refractory AIHA with 40 mg dexamethasone for 4 days per month for 6 cycles [18].

If patients are unresponsive to steroids or experience a relapse, rituximab is effective with an overall response rate of 80% or more [2]. Some suggest rituximab should not be used in ALPS patients and perhaps other underlying immune deficiency due to risk for lasting hypogammaglobulinemia.

Unlike in treatment of ITP, IVIG has been shown to be clearly less effective in AIHA [9]. If used, higher doses may be required [19].

Splenectomy is used for steroid and rituximab refractory W-AIHA in adults but is typically avoided in children. This paradigm needs to be reconsidered in adolescents who have humoral immunity. If splenectomy is performed, patients require immunization against encapsulated organisms and possibly institution of antibiotic prophylaxis; if there is any suspicion of immune deficiency, it is prudent to ascertain response to vaccination before proceeding. Finally, in addition to the risk of sepsis with polysaccharide-encapsulated organisms, infection with intracellular organisms (e.g., malaria, dengue virus, and babesia), the increased risks of both thrombosis and pulmonary hypertension should be considered [2].

Cold Agglutinin Disease

Cold agglutinin disease or cold AIHA (C-AIHA) is rare in the pediatric population even in adolescents. It is seen most often in elderly adults. Cold agglutinin disease is caused by IgM pentamers, which upon binding trigger complement activation. These erythrocytes undergo complement-mediated lysis within the vasculature [15].

Presentation Most cases of C-AIHA develop 1–2 weeks following an infection, although the infection may often remain unidentified. The most commonly implicated organism is *Mycoplasma pneumoniae*. Other common inciting infections include influenza, cytomegalovirus, and varicella infection [15]. Epstein-Barr virus infectious mononucleosis is of particular relevance for adolescents with the peak incidence in patients ages 15–24 [20].

Cold agglutinins themselves are common, and develops in over 60% of those with mononucleosis, but hemolysis is rare or is very mild given the optimal binding temperatures (4 °C and 22 °C) are well below temperatures patients are normally exposed to and typically IgM antibodies do not bind red cells at 37 °C. Hemolysis may flare when the patient is cold or become apparent only in areas where the blood is cooled as it travels away from the body core. This presents with

acrocyanosis of the digits, nose and ears and/or livedo reticularis [21].

Laboratory features include nonspecific signs of hemolysis with several distinctions unique to C-AIHA. The DAT may reveal complement only on red cells. Other features include hemoglobinuria caused by intravascular hemolysis, hypocomplementemia, as well as red cell clumping and rouleaux formation on peripheral smear (see Fig. 22.2b). Red cell agglutination on peripheral smear may falsely overestimate anemia and dramatically increase mean corpuscular volume on automated cell counters [22].

Management Because C-AIHA is typically milder, symptomatic management is appropriate for many patients. This includes keeping the patient warm and warming any blood products or fluids prescribed [9]. Recently used treatments have consisted of immunosuppression including rituximab and oral agents such as azathioprine and chlorambucil. Investigational agents with promise include inhibitors of complement. Treatments such as steroids, IVIG, and even splenectomy are ineffective. For severely affected patients, a single 1–2-volume plasmapheresis can be used to quickly remove circulating IgM antibodies. In some adult patients, rituximab is used; however, its use is not common in pediatric cases, largely due to the rarity of cases [9]. In an emergency, eculizumab could be considered [23].

Paroxysmal Cold Hemoglobinuria (PCH)

PCH is caused by Donath-Landsteiner antibodies. At cold temperatures, these antibodies fix complement, and then upon rewarming, complement is amplified resulting in intravascular hemolysis [22].

Presentation PCH is atypical in adolescents with a median age of presentation of 5 years old [24]. It occurs following a viral illness with hemoglobinuria as a prominent feature [25]. Other symptoms are consistent with cold agglutinin disease.

Management Though acute episodes may be severe, PCH is self-limited and resolves after days to weeks typically. Steroids may be used if initial symptoms are severe.

Secondary Causes of AIHA

Drug-Induced AIHA

Drug-induced AIHA (D-AIHA) has been reported in association with approximately 125 different drugs. Cephalosporins are the most commonly implicated class of drugs. Other common causative agents include piperacillin, β-lactamase inhibitors, and platinum-containing medications [26].

D-AIHA occurs by several different mechanisms. First is drug-independent autoantibody formation, seen with the classical description of α-methyldopa-related AIHA. The drug alters proteins on the red cell surface which are subsequently identified as foreign. Alternatively, hemolysis can be induced in a drug-dependent mechanism via haptenization. The drug itself is not antigenic but when bound to proteins on the erythrocyte becomes immunogenic. Finally, first-generation cephalosporins and β-lactamase inhibitors may induce changes to the red cell surface proteins such that they are bound in a nonspecific fashion by plasma proteins. Erythrocytes are then opsonized and destroyed by the reticuloendothelial system [15, 26].

Diagnosis may be difficult given the unavailability of sites that perform specific testing of drug-induced hemolysis. Antibody-mediated hemolysis in the setting of a known-causative medication is sufficient for diagnosis. If testing is undertaken and a drug *metabolite* is the culprit, a test system in which the parent compound is added to patient serum and erythrocytes will be negative.

Posttransplant Cytopenias

Autoimmune cytopenias may develop following solid organ and hematopoietic stem cell transplantation and are associated with increased morbidity and mortality [27]. AIHA is more common than ITP, occurring in ~1.37% posttransplant patients [28]. While the underlying cause of posttransplant cytopenias is incompletely understood, it is often attributed to alterations in T-cell immunity driven by calcineurin inhibitors or, in the case of HSCT, abnormal autoreactive clones repopulating the marrow due to relative deficiency of regulatory T cells [29]. Initial management involves decreasing the dose of tacrolimus or cyclosporine or switching immune suppressants (especially tacrolimus to cyclosporine, in our experience). Other causes of autoimmune cytopenias include viral infections, graft-versus-host disease, or delayed immune reconstitution [29].

Evans Syndrome

Adolescent Population Adolescent AIHA is more likely to be chronic and secondary to an underlying disorder. Adolescents have a variable response to therapy and a more unfavorable mortality rate [30]. This patient group is also more likely to have Evans syndrome (ES).

ES is defined as having two autoimmune cytopenias, which may present simultaneously or more often sequentially [31]. ES commonly presents with AIHA and immune thrombocytopenia (ITP) [32]. There may be autoimmune neutropenia instead of AIHA or ITP. ITP can present with an autoantibody against red cells identified by a positive DAT in the absence of hemolysis. The latter is usually not considered ES, but is monitored closely in case hemolysis develops. When autoimmune hemolysis develops in a patient with ITP, the platelet count may increase, dramatically confirming the limited ability of the spleen to phagocytize particles and its preference for antibody-coated red cells over antibody-coated platelets [33].

Chronic refractory AIHA in isolation or in conjunction with another cytopenia as in the case of ES is evaluated and managed similarly. While ES is a clinical diagnosis, increasingly the underlying genetic or molecular defect in these patients can be identified and may guide management in certain cases.

Laboratory Workup for Secondary AIHA

In the case of refractory, chronic autoimmune hemolytic anemia, or multilineage autoimmune cytopenias or ones with suggestive findings in history or examination, further evaluation for an underlying autoimmune, rheumatologic, immunodeficiency or lymphoproliferative disorder is indicated. Table 22.1 indicates recommended testing for this subset of patients [9].

Chronic Infections Chronic infections including cytomegalovirus (CMV), Epstein-Barr virus (EBV), *Helicobacter pylori* (*H. pylori*), hepatitis C virus (HCV), and human immunodeficiency virus (HIV) are associated with development of autoimmune cytopenias. These infections may present with an isolated DAT+ AIHA, but testing should be pursued if there are additional (subtle)

Table 22.1 Recommended evaluation in the setting of refractory cytopenias

Laboratory testing	Diagnoses considered
Flow cytometry for double-negative T cells (ideally four color flow) TCRα/β+CD3+CD4−CD8−	ALPS, other rare immunodeficiencies
ANA	SLE or other systemic autoimmune disease
Antiphospholipid antibodies	APS SLE
Quantitative immunoglobulins ± Specific antibodies (e.g., pneumococcal titers)	CVID, XLA Specific antibody deficiency Selective IgA deficiency IgG subclass deficiency SCID
Lymphocyte subsets	SCID, DiGeorge syndrome

ALPS autoimmune lymphoproliferative syndrome, *ANA* antinuclear antibody, *SLE* systemic lupus erythematosus, *CVID* common variable immunodeficiency, *XLA* X-linked agammaglobulinemia, *APS* antiphospholipid antibody syndrome, *SCID* severe combined immunodeficiency

suggestive symptoms such as atypical lymphocytes, lymphadenopathy, hepatosplenomegaly, and transaminitis or if the patient has risk factors for infection [9, 34].

Malignancy-Related AIHA Autoimmune cytopenias are known to develop in patients with malignancies, most commonly leukemias or lymphomas. W-AIHA may be associated with chronic lymphocytic leukemia (CLL), non-Hodgkin lymphoma (NHL), or Hodgkin lymphoma (HL). Cold agglutinin disease is associated with solid tumors, CLL, macroglobulinemia, and premalignant monoclonal gammopathy of undetermined significance (MGUS) [15]. The great majority of patients affected by these conditions occur in older adults. However, adolescents with NHL and HL do infrequently develop AIHA (and ITP). Specific treatment is uncertain but treatment of the underlying condition is sufficient in most cases.

Lymphoproliferative   Disorders Lymphoproliferative disorders such as ALPS, Castleman disease, and Rosai-Dorfman disease may cause AIHA. ALPS is characterized by chronic lymphoproliferation in the absence of overt malignancy or infection. Classically, affected patients initially develop neck adenopathy and then pronounced hepatosplenomegaly. Patients with ALPS frequently experience chronic multilineage cytopenias. ALPS patients are at risk for hematologic malignancies including leukemias and lymphomas. Distinguishing ALPS from lymphoma/leukemia may be very difficult [35].

ALPS is a genetic disorder in which well over 80% of cases are caused by autosomal dominant germline mutations in *FAS (CD95)*. Other patients may have inherited defects in genes encoding the *FAS* ligand or several caspase genes [36–40]. Collectively, these defects lead to disruption of the *FAS* apoptotic pathway. This results in persistence and proliferation of abnormal lymphocytes that would normally undergo apoptosis and thus leads to persistent autoimmunity [41].

It is important to identify underlying ALPS syndrome because this is one of the secondary

Table 22.2 Diagnostic criteria for autoimmune lymphoproliferative syndrome

Required features	*Primary* accessory criteria	*Secondary* accessory criteria
1. Nonmalignant, noninfectious lymphadenopathy or splenomegaly for >6 months 2. Elevated CD3+TCRαβ+CD4−CD8− (double-negative) T cells in the setting of normal lymphocyte counts	1. Defective lymphocyte apoptosis 2. Somatic or germline pathogenic mutation in *FAS, FASLG,* or *CASP10* genes	1. Elevated plasma-soluble FASL levels (>200 pg/mL) *or* elevated plasma IL-10 (>20 pg/mL) *or* plasma elevated vitamin B12 (>1500 ng/L) OR elevated plasma IL-18 (>500 pg/mL) 2. Immunohistologic findings consistent with ALPS as determined by an experienced hematopathologist 3. Autoimmune cytopenias *and* elevated immunoglobulin G 4. Family history of nonmalignant and noninfectious lymphoproliferation

diagnoses that dictates specific therapy. Diagnostic criteria for ALPS are shown in Table 22.2 [35]. A definitive diagnosis necessitates both required features and at least one *primary* accessory criterion. A probable diagnosis needs both required features and at least one *secondary* accessory criterion.

First-line therapy for ALPS is sirolimus, an mTOR inhibitor [9, 42]. Mycophenolate mofetil was the standard treatment previously and is still an acceptable alternative. Rituximab and splenectomy are both used in refractory AIHA but are relatively contraindicated in ALPS. ALPS patients treated with rituximab may not recover their B-cell population, resulting in the need for chronic IVIG supplementation. Splenectomized ALPS patients are at a significantly increased risk for pneumococcal sepsis [9]. IVIG is typically not effective for ALPS patients and is used only for IgG supplementation (if required).

Immunodeficiency Syndromes DiGeorge syndrome, IgA deficiency, SCID, and most commonly CVID all may have AIHA as a component of the constellation of their symptoms.

CVID Autoimmune cytopenias occur in 11–18% of those with CVID [43]. Of those, up to 5.5–7% have AIHA [43]. Ultimately, up to 25% of CVID patients develop autoimmune disease including ITP, AIHA, autoimmune neutropenia, and/or ES during the course of illness [43]. CVID patients with autoimmune cytopenias are more likely to have disease affecting the liver, GI tract, and lungs [43]. Some CVID cases present as evaluation for leukemia or lymphoma due to cytopenias with lymphoid hyperplasia, granuloma, and/or splenomegaly.

The diagnosis of CVID is made on the basis of hypogammaglobulinemia and poor response vaccines. Other symptoms of immunodeficiency include increased susceptibility to infection, autoimmunity, lung disease, and/or polyclonal lymphoproliferation [44]. Unlike ALPS, there are many genetic abnormalities shown to cause complex CVID, although these are only identified in approximately 1/3 cases. Some patients have primarily hypogammaglobulinemia, and others have a complex condition with multiple features.

Mutations in *ICOS, CD19, BAFF-R,* and *TNFRSF13B* [encodes transmembrane activator and CAML interactor (TACI)] are associated with up to 15% of CVID cases; TACI deficiency comprises as many as 10% of CVID cases [45]. TACI is expressed on peripheral B cells and plays a role immunoglobulin switching [45].

Treatment for CVID involves immunoglobulin replacement and standard therapies for concurrent autoimmune cytopenias. Rituximab is particularly effective for ITP and AIHA but mandates monthly SQ or IVIG for IgG replacement, likely for life.

Adolescent Population: CVID is typically diagnosed between ages 20 and 45 years but occurs in adolescents [46]. CVID does not have a gender predilection; however, females may be more likely to experience autoimmune or rheumatologic disorders [46].

Systemic Autoimmunity AIHA is frequently associated with autoimmune disease, most commonly systemic lupus erythematosus (SLE). Other systemic disorders associated with autoimmune cytopenias include antiphospholipid antibody syndrome, Sjögren's disease, or Hashimoto's thyroiditis [41]. An estimated 50% of SLE patients present with an isolated hematologic abnormality including immune thrombocytopenia (ITP), AIHA, or a combination of ITP and AIHA [47].

Adolescent Population Adolescents are more likely than school-aged children to have an underlying systemic autoimmune disorder driving AIHA [30]. SLE has a much higher prevalence in females [48]. Adolescent patients with AIHA, especially females, warrant further investigation for the presence of systemic autoimmunity. An antinuclear antibody titer with reflex to specific antibodies (e.g., anti-dsDNA, anti-Sm, and anti-RNP) is a reasonable initial screening test for SLE. Complement C3 and C4 levels may be helpful. There is no standard cut-off for ANA positivity; however, in our experience, a titer of ≥1:160 should be considered a true positive. Lower titers are less specific and should be interpreted in context of the clinical scenario. A negative ANA does not rule out underlying autoimmunity [49]. There may be substantial time from initial presentation with autoantibodies to the diagnosis of SLE [50]. Because the risk is so high, the adolescent female patient with relapsing AIHA should undergo serial screening for SLE.

Identifying AIHA caused by SLE is important for diagnostic purposes but also can aid in predicting clinical course. Childhood SLE has a more severe phenotype necessitating the use of aggressive immune suppression [51]. The AIHA generally comes under control with appropriate treatment of the underlying autoimmune disorder.

Novel Molecular Diagnoses Increasingly, novel genetic alterations are being identified as the causative lesion in ES and AIHA, as preliminarily described under CVID. Lipopolysaccharide-responsive and beige-like anchor (LRBA) protein deficiency [52–54], activated phosphoinositide 3-kinase δ (PI3KD) syndrome [55, 56], cytotoxic T-lymphocyte-associated protein 4 (CTLA-4) haploinsufficiency [57, 58], and signal transducer and activator of transcription (STAT) 1 and 3 gain-of-function mutations [59], among other disorders, lead to selection of autoreactive T cells and loss of tolerance along with hypogammaglobulinemia. Autoimmune cytopenias are often a feature of all of these disorders; however, typically other symptoms are present as well. Identification of these disorders is particularly important given the fact that, in some cases, targeted therapies are available.

CTLA-4 Haploinsufficiency and LRBA Deficiency Via regulation of a co-stimulatory molecule, CD28, CTLA-4 impacts activation and proliferation of T cells [60]. CTLA-4 haploinsufficiency patients experience lymphoproliferation, recurrent infections, hypogammaglobulinemia, and lymphocytic infiltration of the lungs, intestines, kidneys, reticuloendothelial system, and central nervous system [61, 62]. LRBA regulates CTLA-4 intracellular vesicle trafficking. Patients with homozygous or compound heterozygous LRBA mutations develop autoimmunity and enteritis [41]. With a common molecular effect, both CTLA-4 haploinsufficiency and LRBA deficiency can be treated with a CTLA-4 fusion protein, abatacept, designed to restore CTLA-4 function [63].

Adolescent Population The median age of onset for CTLA-4 haploinsufficiency is 11 years old. The mean age of diagnosis of LRBA deficiency is 13 years; however, patients may have symptoms in early childhood or in later adulthood [54].

PI3KD Syndrome Activated PI3K-delta syndrome results from a gain-of-function mutation in the catalytic subunit of PI(3)K, which is thought to play a role in innate immunity via activation of the mTOR pathway. PI3K may also promote development of effector T cells through Akt phosphorylation [41]. The majority of patients present with recurrent respiratory tract infections with lymphadenopathy and hepatosplenomegaly. AIHA and multilineage cytopenias have been reported [56]. M-TOR inhibitors especially sirolimus have been used to treat PI3KD syndrome. Lenisolib (CDZ173) is a selective inhibitor of PI3KD and is currently being studied in a clinical trial (#NCT02435173) [64].

Adolescent Population The average age on onset of symptoms is approximately 1–7 years old but may occur in adolescents [56].

STAT1 and STAT3 Gain of Function STAT1 gain of function results in hyperresponsiveness to IFN-γ, while STAT3 gain of function causes impaired apoptosis [41]. Both these disorders present in young children and, however, can be considered in adolescents. Clinically, STAT1 gain-of-function mutations are characterized by chronic mucocutaneous candidiasis and other skin infections as well as autoimmune disorders including cytopenias; iron deficiency may also cause anemia [65]. STAT3 gain of function is characterized by autoimmune cytopenias, lymphoproliferation, and multi-organ disease including enteritis, endocrinopathies, and pulmonary and renal manifestations [66]. Targeted therapies for STAT1 gain of function include ruxolitinib, which inhibits JAK1/JAK 2, an upstream IFN-γ receptor. Tocilizumab, an IL-6 inhibitor, and ABT-737, a Bcl-2 inhibitor, have been used to repress the downstream effects of excess STAT3 signaling [22].

Other Autoimmune Lymphoproliferative Diseases Ras-associated autoimmune leukoproliferative disorder (RALD) presents similarly to ALPS including elevated double-negative T-cell populations, but does not meet diagnostic criteria for ALPS. It is caused by NRAS and KRAS mutations leading to abnormal augmentation of RAF/MEK/ErK signaling. This condition is reported in school-age to adolescent patients [67–69]. Dianzani autoimmune lymphoproliferative disease (DALD) also presents with symptoms of ALPS, and defective *FAS*-mediated apoptosis, but lacks elevated double-negative T cells. Among seven DALD patients, the age of symptom onset ranged from 4 months to 13 years

[70]. Both disorders frequently require broad immunosuppression, but targeted therapies also exist [22].

Many additional disorders may feature AIHA as a part of the symptomatology including immunodysregulation, polyendocrinopathy and enteropathy, X-linked (IPEX) syndrome, or CD25 deficiency; this presents most commonly in younger children [62].

Genotypes do not correlate consistently with specific phenotypes. Thus, genetic workup is best performed by screening a panel of candidate genes or by whole-exome sequencing rather than assuming which defect is most likely.

Management of Refractory Disease

Given its low incidence and common occurrence secondary to underlying defects, upfront therapies for AIHA have not been compared formally in the pediatric or adolescent populations. However, steroids and then rituximab are widely accepted and have been used for decades as upfront management. When patients fail these standard therapies, management of AIHA becomes variable. There is a paucity of formal trials establishing the best second- and third-line treatments for AIHA.

There is increasing emphasis on genetic diagnosis which may help identify targeted treatments, assumed to be optimal. As more cases are accumulated, the initial diagnostic workup may increasingly involve genomic sequencing to better distinguish cases and clarify the pathophysiology. Furthermore, these cytopenias are often only one part of difficult complex diagnoses.

The selection of treatments should be individualized, involve discussion with the patient and parents, and consider cost, route of administration, efficacy, and side effects. Additionally, individual physician or treatment center experience may have a substantial impact on treatments selected. Some therapies are used as a temporizing measures with the goal of rapidly controlling acute severe anemia. Such temporizing agents commonly include a high-dose steroid burst with or without IVIG, but these treatments are not optimal for long-term management.

For difficult refractory cases, physicians may use a combination of treatments. Information on the effectiveness of combination treatments is limited. General principles are to select the most effective treatments in addition to ones with different, complementary mechanisms and without overlapping toxicities. A treatment which on its own is ineffective may be a useful component of a combination plan. Erythropoietin and thrombopoietin agonists have not demonstrated benefit in treating AIHA.

Treatment for Adolescents Rituximab is often the optimal next treatment given certain exceptions. The majority of third-line agents can be used to treat adolescent females with AIHA, with

some considerations unique to this age group. For patients of childbearing age, it is important for families to be aware which potential treatments can be teratogenic or need to be used cautiously in adolescent females who may be planning pregnancy (see Table 22.3). For example, high-dose cyclophosphamide can negatively impact fertility. In this age group, certain cosmetic side effects including gingival hyperplasia or hair growth associated with calcineurin inhibitors [71] or acne and weight gain related to corticosteroids are particularly distressing for many patients. Furthermore, as with patients of any age, the use of rituximab limits the ability to vaccinate for at least 4–6 months. AIHA itself leads to more than 2.5 times greater risk for venous thromboembolism versus those without AIHA [72]. Along with other factors, concomitant oral contraceptive use may exacerbate this risk.

Table 22.3 Potential therapies for AIHA are listed alphabetically including the route of administration, side effects, relevant considerations for the adolescent female population, as well as safety of use in the case of pregnancy

Treatment	Route	Flares or chronic use	Role in therapy	Important side effects	Issues in the adolescent female	Pregnancy considerations
Alemtuzumab	IV, SC	Chronic	Third line	Significant long-lasting immune suppression may rarely cause severe ITP	None	Fetal B- and T-lymphodepletion Contraception recommended during therapy to 6 months after last dose [73]
Antithymocyte globulin (rarely used)	IV	Chronic	Third line	Significant immune suppression, serum sickness, infusion reactions	None	Adverse events reported in animal studies [73]
Calcineurin inhibitors	PO	Chronic	Third line	Nephrotoxic, electrolyte abnormalities, risk of PML drug-level monitoring required	Cosmetic side effects: gingival hyperplasia, acne, hair growth	Low risk in human studies [73]
Corticosteroids	PO, IV	Flares, chronic	First or second line	Weight gain, mood changes, hypertension, hyperglycemia, loss of bone mineral density, cataracts, and many others	Weight gain, loss of bone density, acne, DVT risk for those also taking estrogen	Potential increased risk for oral clefts and decreased birth weight when used in first trimester [73] generally considered safe in pregnancy [73] Variability in transplacental passage

(continued)

Table 22.3 (continued)

Treatment	Route	Flares or chronic use	Role in therapy	Important side effects	Issues in the adolescent female	Pregnancy considerations
Cyclophosphamide	PO	Chronic	Third line	Myelosuppression, GI toxicity, increased risk MDS/AML, PML, bladder fibrosis	Infertility, amenorrhea, hair loss	Teratogenic, avoid pregnancy for up to 1 year after completing medication course [73]
Danazol	PO	Chronic	Third line	Androgenic effects, blood lipid changes, hepatotoxicity, intracranial hypertension	Mild androgenic effects: menstrual irregularities (may be useful in patients with heavy menses), weight gain, breast atrophy, vaginal dryness, hirsutism, acne	Contraindicated. Risk for androgenic effects to female fetus [73]
IVIG	IV	Flares, chronic	First line	Headache, aseptic meningitis, nausea, vomiting (thrombosis, renal toxicity, and hemolysis all reduced by changes in preparation)	None	Safe for use during pregnancy [73]
Methotrexate	PO	Chronic	Third line	Dose-dependent myelosuppression, hepatic and renal toxicity	None	Contraindicated in other autoimmune disorders including psoriasis and rheumatoid arthritis risk for fetal death and congenital defects [73]
Mycophenolate mofetil	PO, IV	Chronic	Second or third line	Diarrhea, neutropenia, risk for PML	May lessen effectiveness of birth control	Black box warning: associated with first trimester pregnancy loss and congenital malformations pregnancy test required prior to and during treatment [73]
Plasmapheresis	IV	Flares	First-line (CAH only)	Central line insertion, hypotension, hypocalcemia primarily used for non-IgG-mediated disease (single apheresis); if used for IgG-mediated disease needs 2–3 days to take effect	None	Low risk for morbidity to patient or fetus [74]

Table 22.3 (continued)

Treatment	Route	Flares or chronic use	Role in therapy	Important side effects	Issues in the adolescent female	Pregnancy considerations
Purine analogues	PO	Chronic	Third line	Dose-dependent myelosuppression, genetic polymorphisms impact metabolism, rare hepatotoxicity PML risk (azathioprine)	None	Case reports of fetal loss during the first trimester (mercaptopurine) Thioguanine and azathioprine are contraindicated per manufacturer but have been used safely for autoimmune cytopenias and azathioprine extensively in renal transplantation [73, 75]
Rituximab	IV (recently anti-CD20s can be given SQ)	Flares, chronic	Second line	First infusion-related reactions, serum sickness. PML risk. Risk of prolonged hypogammaglobulinemia (especially ALPS or with high-dose dexamethasone), neutropenia, activation of hepatitis B	None	Risk for B-cell depletion in newborn for up to 6 months [73]
Sirolimus	PO	Chronic	First-line (ALPS), third line	Requires monitoring: drug Levels, liver enzymes, lipids	None	Limited data: only case reports of safe pregnancy with sirolimus use in posttransplant patients [73]
Splenectomy	N/A	Chronic	Second or third line	Requires surgical procedure. Risk of encapsulated organisms, sepsis, DVT, pulmonary hypertension contraindicated in ALPS	Confirm fully vaccinated including all five strains of *N. meningitis* may require vaccine titers	If required (very rarely) recommended for second trimester only
Vincristine/Vinblastine	IV	Chronic	Third line	Neuropathy, foot drop, pancreatitis, extravasation risk	None	Teratogenic, risk for fetal loss [73]

Very limited data regarding incidence or course of affected newborns

Conclusion

Autoimmune hemolytic anemia encompasses a broad spectrum of disorders, some primary idiopathic and many secondary to infections, immunodeficiency, neoplasia, medication-induced, or rheumatologic conditions. The adolescent female patient with AIHA should be managed similarly to other patients, with increased suspicion for systemic autoimmune disorders, such as SLE, that commonly develop in female patients. Adolescent females can generally be managed with standard therapies with special attention to the side effect profile of each medication including potential effects if taken during pregnancy. Adolescent males would be managed similarly, but with lower likelihood of systemic autoimmune disorders and higher likelihood of X-linked diseases.

References

1. Aladjidi N, Leverger G, Leblanc T, et al. New insights into childhood autoimmune hemolytic anemia: a French national observational study of 265 children. Haematologica. 2011;96(5):655–63.
2. Zanella A, Barcellini W. Treatment of autoimmune hemolytic anemias. Haematologica. 2014;99(10):1547–54.
3. Habibi B, Homberg JC, Schaison G, Salmon C. Autoimmune hemolytic anemia in children. A review of 80 cases. Am J Med. 1974;56(1):61–9.
4. Coombs RR, Mourant AE, Race RR. A new test for the detection of weak and incomplete Rh agglutinins. Br J Exp Pathol. 1945;26:255–66.
5. Quist E, Koepsell S. Autoimmune hemolytic anemia and red blood cell autoantibodies. Arch Pathol Lab Med. 2015;139(11):1455–8.
6. Kaplan M, Hammerman C, Vreman HJ, Wong RJ, Stevenson DK. Direct antiglobulin titer strength and hyperbilirubinemia. Pediatrics. 2014;134(5):e1340–4.
7. Zantek ND, Koepsell SA, Tharp DR Jr, Cohn CS. The direct antiglobulin test: a critical step in the evaluation of hemolysis. Am J Hematol. 2012;87(7):707–9.
8. McGann PT, McDade J, Mortier NA, Combs MR, Ware RE. IgA-mediated autoimmune hemolytic anemia in an infant. Pediatr Blood Cancer. 2011;56(5):837–9.
9. Teachey DT, Lambert MP. Diagnosis and management of autoimmune cytopenias in childhood. Pediatr Clin N Am. 2013;60(6):1489–511.
10. Bass GF, Tuscano ET, Tuscano JM. Diagnosis and classification of autoimmune hemolytic anemia. Autoimmun Rev. 2014;13(4-5):560–4.
11. Ravetch JV. Fc receptors. Curr Opin Immunol. 1997;9(1):121–5.
12. Liesveld JL, Rowe JM, Lichtman MA. Variability of the erythropoietic response in autoimmune hemolytic anemia: analysis of 109 cases. Blood. 1987;69(3):820–6.
13. Liebman HA, Weitz IC. Autoimmune hemolytic anemia. Med Clin North Am. 2017;101(2):351–9.
14. Marchand A, Galen RS, Van Lente F. The predictive value of serum haptoglobin in hemolytic disease. JAMA. 1980;243(19):1909–11.
15. Qasim S. Background, presentation and pathophysiology of autommune hemolytic anemia. In: Despotovic JM, editor. Immune hematology, vol. 1. Cham, Switzerland: Springer International Publishing AG; 2018.
16. Dussadee K, Taka O, Thedsawad A, Wanachiwanawin W. Incidence and risk factors of relapses in idiopathic autoimmune hemolytic anemia. J Med Assoc Thai. 2010;93(Suppl 1):S165–70.
17. Kalfa TA. Warm antibody autoimmune hemolytic anemia. Hematology Am Soc Hematol Educ Program. 2016;2016(1):690–7.
18. Meyer O, Stahl D, Beckhove P, Huhn D, Salama A. Pulsed high-dose dexamethasone in chronic autoimmune haemolytic anaemia of warm type. Br J Haematol. 1997;98(4):860–2.
19. Bussel JB, Cunningham-Rundles C, Abraham C. Intravenous treatment of autoimmune hemolytic anemia with very high dose gammaglobulin. Vox Sang. 1986;51(4):264–9.
20. Heath CW Jr, Brodsky AL, Potolsky AI. Infectious mononucleosis in a general population. Am J Epidemiol. 1972;95(1):46–52.
21. Packman CH. The clinical pictures of autoimmune hemolytic anemia. Transfus Med Hemother. 2015;42(5):317–24.
22. Kim TO, Despotovic JM. Primary and secondary immune cytopenias: evaluation and treatment approach in children. Hematol Oncol Clin North Am. 2019;33(3):489–506.
23. Roth A, Bommer M, Huttmann A, et al. Eculizumab in cold agglutinin disease (DECADE): an open-label, prospective, bicentric, nonrandomized phase 2 trial. Blood Adv. 2018;2(19):2543–9.
24. Petz LD. Cold antibody autoimmune hemolytic anemias. Blood Rev. 2008;22(1):1–15.
25. Heddle NM. Acute paroxysmal cold hemoglobinuria. Transfus Med Rev. 1989;3(3):219–29.
26. Garratty G. Immune hemolytic anemia associated with drug therapy. Blood Rev. 2010;24(4-5):143–50.
27. Sanz J, Arriaga F, Montesinos P, et al. Autoimmune hemolytic anemia following allogeneic hematopoietic stem cell transplantation in adult patients. Bone Marrow Transplant. 2007;39(9):555–61.
28. Neunert CE, Despotovic JM. Autoimmune hemolytic anemia and immune thrombocytopenia following hematopoietic stem cell transplant: a critical review of the literature. Pediatr Blood Cancer. 2019;66(4):e27569.

29. Park JA, Lee HH, Kwon HS, Baik CR, Song SA, Lee JN. Sirolimus for refractory autoimmune hemolytic anemia after allogeneic hematopoietic stem cell transplantation: a case report and literature review of the treatment of post-transplant autoimmune hemolytic anemia. Transfus Med Rev. 2016;30(1):6–14.

30. Heisel MA, Ortega JA. Factors influencing prognosis in childhood autoimmune hemolytic anemia. Am J Pediatr Hematol Oncol. 1983;5(2):147–52.

31. Omar Niss REW. Treatment of autoimmune hemolytic anemia. In: Despotovic JM, editor. Immune hematology, vol. 1. Cham, Switzerland: Springer International Publishing AG; 2018.

32. Norton A, Roberts I. Management of Evans syndrome. Br J Haematol. 2006;132(2):125–37.

33. Scaradavou A, Bussel J. Evans syndrome. Results of a pilot study utilizing a multiagent treatment protocol. J Pediatr Hematol Oncol. 1995;17(4):290–5.

34. Miano M. How I manage Evans syndrome and AIHA cases in children. Br J Haematol. 2016;172(4):524–34.

35. Oliveira JB, Bleesing JJ, Dianzani U, et al. Revised diagnostic criteria and classification for the autoimmune lymphoproliferative syndrome (ALPS): report from the 2009 NIH International Workshop. Blood. 2010;116(14):e35–40.

36. Holzelova E, Vonarbourg C, Stolzenberg MC, et al. Autoimmune lymphoproliferative syndrome with somatic Fas mutations. N Engl J Med. 2004;351(14):1409–18.

37. Del-Rey M, Ruiz-Contreras J, Bosque A, et al. A homozygous Fas ligand gene mutation in a patient causes a new type of autoimmune lymphoproliferative syndrome. Blood. 2006;108(4):1306–12.

38. Wang J, Zheng L, Lobito A, et al. Inherited human caspase 10 mutations underlie defective lymphocyte and dendritic cell apoptosis in autoimmune lymphoproliferative syndrome type II. Cell. 1999;98(1):47–58.

39. Chun HJ, Zheng L, Ahmad M, et al. Pleiotropic defects in lymphocyte activation caused by caspase-8 mutations lead to human immunodeficiency. Nature. 2002;419(6905):395–9.

40. Dowdell KC, Niemela JE, Price S, et al. Somatic FAS mutations are common in patients with genetically undefined autoimmune lymphoproliferative syndrome. Blood. 2010;115(25):5164–9.

41. Grimes AB. Evans syndrome: background, clinical presentation, pathophysiology, and management. In: Despotovic JM, editor. Immune hematology, vol. 1. Cham, Switzerland: Springer International Publishing AG; 2018.

42. Bride KL, Vincent T, Smith-Whitley K, et al. Sirolimus is effective in relapsed/refractory autoimmune cytopenias: results of a prospective multi-institutional trial. Blood. 2016;127(1):17–28.

43. Feuille EJ, Anooshiravani N, Sullivan KE, Fuleihan RL, Cunningham-Rundles C. Autoimmune cytopenias and associated conditions in CVID: a report from the USIDNET registry. J Clin Immunol. 2018;38(1):28–34.

44. Ameratunga R, Brewerton M, Slade C, et al. Comparison of diagnostic criteria for common variable immunodeficiency disorder. Front Immunol. 2014;5:415.

45. Poodt AE, Driessen GJ, de Klein A, van Dongen JJ, van der Burg M, de Vries E. TACI mutations and disease susceptibility in patients with common variable immunodeficiency. Clin Exp Immunol. 2009;156(1):35–9.

46. Cunningham-Rundles C. Common variable immune deficiency: dissection of the variable. Immunol Rev. 2019;287(1):145–61.

47. Zhang L, Wu X, Wang L, et al. Clinical features of systemic lupus erythematosus patients complicated with Evans syndrome: a case-control, Single Center Study. Medicine. 2016;95(15):e3279.

48. Rees F, Doherty M, Grainge MJ, Lanyon P, Zhang W. The worldwide incidence and prevalence of systemic lupus erythematosus: a systematic review of epidemiological studies. Rheumatology. 2017;56(11):1945–61.

49. Leuchten N, Hoyer A, Brinks R, et al. Performance of antinuclear antibodies for classifying systemic lupus erythematosus: a systematic literature review and meta-regression of diagnostic data. Arthritis Care Res. 2018;70(3):428–38.

50. Arbuckle MR, McClain MT, Rubertone MV, et al. Development of autoantibodies before the clinical onset of systemic lupus erythematosus. N Engl J Med. 2003;349(16):1526–33.

51. Sassi RH, Hendler JV, Piccoli GF, et al. Age of onset influences on clinical and laboratory profile of patients with systemic lupus erythematosus. Clin Rheumatol. 2017;36(1):89–95.

52. Lopez-Herrera G, Tampella G, Pan-Hammarstrom Q, et al. Deleterious mutations in LRBA are associated with a syndrome of immune deficiency and autoimmunity. Am J Hum Genet. 2012;90(6):986–1001.

53. Kostel Bal S, Haskologlu S, Serwas NK, et al. Multiple presentations of LRBA deficiency: a single-center experience. J Clin Immunol. 2017;37(8):790–800.

54. Gamez-Diaz L, August D, Stepensky P, et al. The extended phenotype of LPS-responsive beige-like anchor protein (LRBA) deficiency. J Allergy Clin Immunol. 2016;137(1):223–30.

55. Lucas CL, Kuehn HS, Zhao F, et al. Dominant-activating germline mutations in the gene encoding the PI(3)K catalytic subunit p110delta result in T cell senescence and human immunodeficiency. Nat Immunol. 2014;15(1):88–97.

56. Coulter TI, Chandra A, Bacon CM, et al. Clinical spectrum and features of activated phosphoinositide 3-kinase delta syndrome: a large patient cohort study. J Allergy Clin Immunol. 2017;139(2):597–606 e594.

57. Kuehn HS, Ouyang W, Lo B, et al. Immune dysregulation in human subjects with heterozygous germline mutations in CTLA4. Science. 2014;345(6204):1623–7.

58. Kucuk ZY, Charbonnier LM, McMasters RL, Chatila T, Bleesing JJ. CTLA-4 haploinsufficiency in a patient with an autoimmune lymphoproliferative disorder. J Allergy Clin Immunol. 2017;140(3):862–864 e864.

59. Consonni F, Dotta L, Todaro F, Vairo D, Badolato R. Signal transducer and activator of transcription gain-of-function primary immunodeficiency/immunodysregulation disorders. Curr Opin Pediatr. 2017;29(6):711–7.
60. Besnard C, Levy E, Aladjidi N, et al. Pediatric-onset Evans syndrome: heterogeneous presentation and high frequency of monogenic disorders including LRBA and CTLA4 mutations. Clin Immunol. 2018;188:52–7.
61. Schubert D, Bode C, Kenefeck R, et al. Autosomal dominant immune dysregulation syndrome in humans with CTLA4 mutations. Nat Med. 2014;20(12):1410–6.
62. Mitsuiki N, Schwab C, Grimbacher B. What did we learn from CTLA-4 insufficiency on the human immune system? Immunol Rev. 2019;287(1): 33–49.
63. Verma N, Burns SO, Walker LSK, Sansom DM. Immune deficiency and autoimmunity in patients with CTLA-4 (CD152) mutations. Clin Exp Immunol. 2017;190(1):1–7.
64. Rao VK, Webster S, Dalm V, et al. Effective "activated PI3Kdelta syndrome"-targeted therapy with the PI3Kdelta inhibitor leniolisib. Blood. 2017;130(21):2307–16.
65. Toubiana J, Okada S, Hiller J, et al. Heterozygous STAT1 gain-of-function mutations underlie an unexpectedly broad clinical phenotype. Blood. 2016;127(25):3154–64.
66. Fabre A, Marchal S, Barlogis V, et al. Clinical aspects of STAT3 gain-of-function germline mutations: a systematic review. J Allergy Clin Immunol Pract. 2019;7(6):1958–1969.e9.
67. Levy-Mendelovich S, Lev A, Rechavi E, et al. T and B cell clonal expansion in Ras-associated lymphoproliferative disease (RALD) as revealed by next-generation sequencing. Clin Exp Immunol. 2017;189(3):310–7.
68. Niemela JE, Lu L, Fleisher TA, et al. Somatic KRAS mutations associated with a human nonmalignant syndrome of autoimmunity and abnormal leukocyte homeostasis. Blood. 2011;117(10):2883–6.
69. Toyoda H, Deguchi T, Iwamoto S, et al. Weekly rituximab followed by monthly rituximab treatment for autoimmune disease associated with RAS-associated autoimmune leukoproliferative disease. J Pediatr Hematol Oncol. 2018;40(8):e516–8.
70. Dianzani U, Bragardo M, DiFranco D, et al. Deficiency of the Fas apoptosis pathway without Fas gene mutations in pediatric patients with autoimmunity/lymphoproliferation. Blood. 1997;89(8):2871–9.
71. Hardinger K, Magee CC. Pharmacology of cyclosporine and tacrolimus. In: Kam A, editor. Waltham: UpToDate; 2019.
72. Ungprasert P, Tanratana P, Srivali N. Autoimmune hemolytic anemia and venous thromboembolism: a systematic review and meta-analysis. Thromb Res. 2015;136(5):1013–7.
73. Online L. Lexi-Drugs Online. Hudson: Wolters Kluwer Clinical Drug Information, Inc.; 2013. Accessed 5 Sept 2019.
74. Watson WJ, Katz VL, Bowes WA Jr. Plasmapheresis during pregnancy. Obstet Gynecol. 1990;76(3 Pt 1):451–7.
75. Neunert C, Lim W, Crowther M, et al. The American Society of Hematology 2011 evidence-based practice guideline for immune thrombocytopenia. Blood. 2011;117(16):4190–207.

Evans Syndrome in the Adolescent Female

23

Amanda B. Grimes and Vicky R. Breakey

Introduction

Evans syndrome (ES) is defined as the presence of autoimmune cytopenias affecting two or more blood cell lines, either simultaneously or sequentially, in a single individual. Most often, this refers to the combination of autoimmune hemolytic anemia (AIHA) and immune thrombocytopenia (ITP), but can include autoimmune neutropenia (AIN) as well. The etiology of ES has historically been attributed to pathologic autoantibody production against the blood cells, with the true underlying etiology remaining unknown. However, recent advances in our understanding of this complex disorder have revealed frequent association with more well-described underlying disorders of immune regulation. Nevertheless, "idiopathic" ES still precedes the diagnosis of an underlying autoimmune disorder or immunodeficiency in the majority of cases [1–3]. Improved insight into the pathology behind ES over the recent years highlights the importance of thorough investigation for underlying immune dysregulation disorders when applying this "diagnosis of exclusion," especially among adolescent females, who are known to be at higher risk for the development of systemic autoimmune disease. This chapter will review the clinical features, pathophysiology, diagnosis, and management of ES in adolescent females.

Clinical Features

In both children and adults, the largest series of ES patients to date have shown AIHA and ITP to occur at initial presentation about half of the time (~48% of children and 55% of adults) [4–6]. However, many patients ultimately diagnosed with ES will present initially with only one autoimmune cytopenia – ITP first in ~29% and AIHA first in ~24% of children and 16% of adults [4–6]. AIN is present in 20% of children [5] and ~15% of adults with ES [6]. Clinically, patients with ES will present with symptoms related to the autoimmune cytopenia(s) of which their syndrome is comprised (i.e., symptomatic anemia, jaundice, and evidence of hemolysis in AIHA, or petechiae, bruising, and bleeding in ITP). Heavy menstrual bleeding is often a presenting feature of ITP in adolescent females; and may therefore present with associated anemia as well. Therefore, care must be taken to differentiate whether this associated anemia is secondary to acute blood loss (with or without iron deficiency) or secondary to an autoimmune hemolytic process which may present concomitantly with ITP, making a diagnosis of ES (see Fig. 23.1). Importantly, as opposed to

A. B. Grimes (✉)
Baylor College of Medicine, Texas Children's Cancer and Hematology Centers, Houston, TX, USA
e-mail: abgrimes@txch.org

V. R. Breakey
McMaster University, Division of Pediatric Hematology/Oncology, Hamilton, ON, Canada

© Springer Nature Switzerland AG 2020
L. V. Srivaths (ed.), *Hematology in the Adolescent Female*,
https://doi.org/10.1007/978-3-030-48446-0_23

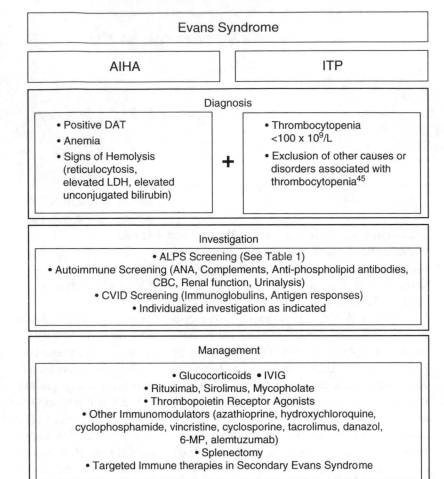

AIHA: Autoimmune Hemolytic Anemia, ITP: Immune Thrombocytopenia, DAT: Direct
Antiglobulin Test, LDH: Lactate Dehydrogenase, ALPS: Autoimmune Lymphoproliferative
Syndrome, ANA: Antinuclear Antibodies, CBC: Complete Blood Count, CVID: Common
Variable Immunodeficiency, IVIG: Intravenous Immunoglobulin, 6-MP: 6-Mercaptopurine

the often spontaneously resolving and non-recur-
ring single-lineage autoimmune cytopenias, the
ITP and AIHA presenting in ES are often associated with a chronic, relapsing, and treatment-
refractory disease course [5, 7–9] – especially ES
which is determined to be secondary to an underlying disorder of immune regulation [5, 10].
Notably, mortality among patients with ES is
reported to be as high as 10% in children [4, 5]
and as high as 24% in adults [6] – a mortality rate
which is significantly increased above that seen
among patients with ITP, AIHA, or AIN alone.

Although ES is traditionally known as an "idiopathic" condition, well-defined immune disorders
are now being identified as the etiology of disease

in ~50% of ES cases [1, 6]. The most commonly
identified diseases driving ES are autoimmune
lymphoproliferative syndrome (ALPS) [11, 12],
common variable immunodeficiency (CVID) [1,
4, 6, 13], and systemic autoimmune disease, most
often systemic lupus erythematosus (SLE) [1, 5,
6]. With improving diagnostic capabilities, including increased access to genetic testing, it is
expected that inherited immunologic diseases
responsible for driving the autoimmunity of ES
will be increasingly identified, including monogenic disorders such as cytotoxic T-lymphocyte
antigen-4 (CTLA-4) haploinsufficiency and
lipopolysaccharide-responsive and beige-like
anchor (LRBA) protein deficiency [2, 3, 14].

ES which is driven by ALPS is clinically defined by defective lymphocyte apoptosis resulting in chronic nonmalignant noninfectious lymphoproliferation and elevated double-negative T (DNT) cells. Following the characterization of ALPS during the 1990s [15–18], Teachey and colleagues first reported the association of ALPS with idiopathic ES, finding diagnostic evidence of underlying ALPS in 50% of idiopathic ES patients followed at their institution over a 5-year period [11]. A follow-up multi-institutional study in 2010 confirmed prior findings, with 21 of 45 pediatric ES patients (47%) meeting diagnostic criteria for ALPS [12]. In order to streamline ongoing investigations within the field, revised diagnostic criteria and classification for ALPS were released following the NIH international workshop in 2009, with hopes of standardizing the diagnosis of ALPS and modernizing the classification to rely less heavily on outdated and cumbersome testing techniques such as Fas-mediated apoptosis assays and more heavily on the highly sensitive and specific DNT cell testing, as well as the newer mutation-specific variations of disease [19]. These diagnostic criteria are outlined in Table 23.1.

Autoimmune cytopenias may also be a presenting manifestation of systemic autoimmune disease, particularly in adolescent females; and systemic autoimmunity is in fact diagnosed in ~8% of pediatric ES patients [1, 5] and 21% of adult ES patients [6]. SLE is the most common autoimmune disease diagnosed in patients with ES [5, 6], but other primary autoimmune diseases may be associated with ES as well, including Hashimoto's thyroiditis, type 1 diabetes [1], antiphospholipid antibody syndrome, and Sjögren syndrome [6]. At a minimum, however, ES patients should be screened for SLE [10]. See Table 23.2 for the classification criteria defining SLE [20–22].

CVID, much like ES, is a heterogeneous and phenotypically variable disorder, depending on underlying immune pathology, but unified by its most prominent feature, hypogammaglobulinemia. Consensus criteria for the diagnosis of CVID are outlined in Table 23.3 [23]. The incidence of CVID among pediatric ES patients is reported at ~10% on average [1, 4], although some smaller series report CVID incidence up to 83% in pediatric ES patients [13]. Conversely, the prevalence of autoimmune cytopenias in CVID is ~10–20% [24–27], with one large series of 990 CVID patients specifically reporting ES in 3.8% of patients [27] and a smaller series of 326 CVID patients corroborating these findings, with a 3.4% incidence of ES reported [24]. The defining features of CVID – hypogammaglobulinemia and impaired antibody responses [28] – provide clear rationale for the infectious complications common to this condition. However, as immunoglobulin replacement therapy has become stan-

Table 23.1 Diagnostic criteria for ALPS [19]

Required criteria		Accessory criteria
Definitive ALPS diagnosis: Both required criteria plus a primary accessory criteria		
Probable ALPS diagnosis: Both required criteria plus a secondary accessory criteria		
Chronic nonmalignant, noninfectious lymphoproliferation (lymphadenopathy or splenomegaly)	*Primary*	Defective lymphocyte apoptosis
		Somatic or germline pathogenic mutation in *FAS*, *FASL*, or *CASP10*
	Secondary	Elevated plasma biomarkers: sFASL (>200 pg/ml) or vitamin B12 (>1500 ng/L) or IL-10 (>20 pg/ml) or IL-18 (>500 pg/ml)
Elevated peripheral blood DNT cells[a] (≥1.5% of total lymphocytes or ≥2.5% of CD3+ lymphocytes)		Immunohistological findings consistent with ALPS
		Autoimmune cytopenias and polyclonal hypergammaglobulinemia
		Family history of ALPS or nonmalignant/noninfectious lymphoproliferation (+/− autoimmunity)

sFASL soluble FAS ligand, *IL-10* Interleukin-10, *IL-18* Interleukin-18
[a]DNT cells: CD3+TCRαβ+CD4−CD8− Double negative T cells

Table 23.2 Classification criteria[a] for the diagnosis of SLE [20–22]

American College of Rheumatology (ACR) Criteria [20, 21]	Systemic Lupus International Collaborating Clinics (SLICC) Criteria [22]	
(SLE diagnosis is made *when 4 of 11 criteria* are met[b])	(SLE diagnosis is made when *4 of 17 criteria* are met, including at least 1 clinical and 1 immunologic criterion[b]; *OR biopsy-proven lupus nephritis* with ANA or anti-dsDNA)	
Malar rash	*Clinical criteria*	*Acute cutaneous lupus*
Photosensitivity		*Chronic cutaneous lupus*
Discoid rash		*Nonscarring alopecia*
Oral ulcers		*Oral or nasal ulcers*
Arthritis		*Joint disease* (synovitis OR tenderness and a.m. stiffness)
Serositis (pleuritic or pericardial)		*Serositis* (pleuritic or pericardial)
Renal disorder (proteinuria OR cellular casts)		*Renal involvement* (proteinuria OR red blood cell casts)
Neurologic disorder (seizures OR psychosis)		*Neurologic involvement* (seizures, psychosis, myelitis, neuropathy, and others)
Hematologic disorder (hemolytic anemia OR leukopenia OR lymphopenia OR thrombocytopenia)		*Hemolytic anemia*
		Leukopenia OR *lymphopenia*
		Thrombocytopenia
ANA (elevated antinuclear antibody titer)	*Immunologic criteria*	*ANA* (elevated antinuclear antibody titer)
Immunologic disorders (anti-DNA antibody OR anti-Smith antibody OR positive antiphospholipid antibody [anticardiolipin IgG or IgM antibodies] OR lupus anticoagulant OR false-positive serologic test for syphilis)		*Anti-dsDNA* (anti-double-stranded DNA) antibody
		Anti-Sm (anti-Smith) antibody
		Antiphospholipid antibody positivity (lupus anticoagulant, anticardiolipin antibody, anti-beta 2-glycoprotein antibody, or false positive test for rapid plasma reagin)
		Low complement (C3, C4, OR CH50)
		Direct Coombs test positivity

[a]Classification criteria are summarized here, but full definitions of individual criterion should be referenced in the original publications delineating SLE classification criteria [20–22]
[b]Criteria need not be present concurrently, but are cumulative over any interval of observation

dard practice, infectious complications have been surpassed by the autoimmune and lymphoproliferative complications of disease. Interestingly, these autoimmune, lymphoproliferative, and granulomatous complications occur at a significantly increased rate among CVID patients with autoimmune cytopenias (69.4%) compared to those without autoimmune cytopenias (43.5%) [27]. This shared phenotype of autoimmunity and lymphoproliferative complications among this subset of CVID patients suggests a common underlying immunopathology in many cases. Importantly, the autoimmune cytopenias appear to precede the diagnosis of CVID more than 50%

of the time; and, therefore, one should maintain a high level of clinical suspicion for possible development of CVID in adolescent females diagnosed with ES.

Pathophysiology

The pathophysiology in ES is largely attributed to that of its individual components: ITP, AIHA, and/or AIN, which are described in more detail within their respective chapters of this book. Traditionally, autoimmune cytopenias in ES have been ascribed to aberrant autoantibody produc-

Table 23.3 Consensus definition of CVID [23]

Required criteria:
Low IgG (according to age-adjusted laboratory reference range, measured twice, >3 weeks apart)
Low IgA or IgM as well (some experts *require low IgA* to define CVID)
Impairment of T-dependent or T-independent antigen response (if IgG >100 mg/dL)
Exclusion of other causes of hypogammaglobulinemia (drug-induced, single gene and other immune defects, chromosomal anomalies, infectious diseases, malignancy, other systemic disorders, and immunodeficiency caused by excessive loss of immunoglobulins [nephrosis, severe burns, lymphangiectasia, protein-losing enteropathy])
Characteristic clinical manifestations:
Infection
Autoimmunity
Lymphoproliferation
Occasionally Asymptomatic (especially in familial cases)
Genetic investigations:
Not generally required for diagnosis, especially in patients with infections alone; however, for those with immune dysregulation, autoimmunity, malignancy, or other complications, molecular genetic diagnosis should be considered, as monogenic disorders may be amenable to specific therapies

IgG Immunoglobulin G, *IgA* Immunoglobulin A, *IgM* Immunoglobulin M

tion and the cascade of downstream events that follows, with more recent delineation of the role of cell-mediated immunity in the pathogenesis of disease as well. However, ES is unique in that unifying immune pathology driving the multilineage autoimmune cytopenias in ES is being identified with rapidly increasing frequency [1–3, 6, 11, 12, 14]. This allows for better understanding of the true mechanisms of pathogenesis, in not only cases of secondary ES but also in idiopathic ES presenting with similar clinical features. For example, ALPS is a syndrome in which lymphocyte homeostasis is disrupted due to mutations affecting the *FAS* apoptotic pathway, resulting in aberrant lymphocyte survival, chronic lymphoproliferation, dysregulated immune tolerance, and autoimmunity [10, 11, 29, 30]. Fas expressed on the surface of activated B and T lymphocytes and Fas ligand expressed on activated T lymphocytes normally interact to trigger activation of the intracellular caspase cascade, leading to cellular

apoptosis [10]. This apoptotic pathway typically functions to downregulate the immune response by eliminating excess activated and autoreactive lymphocytes, but is rendered dysfunctional via mutations in *FAS* (60–70%), *FASL* (<1%), and *CASP10* genes (2–3%) in patients with ALPS [29]. This results in the persistence of TCRα/β⁺CD3⁺CD4⁻CD8⁻ double-negative T (DNT) cells characteristic of this condition, as well as the characteristic clinical phenotype of chronic lymphoproliferation and autoimmunity.

In contrast to ALPS, CVID is thought to be the result of multiple genetic, environmental, and immunologic factors, as monogenic drivers of disease have been identified in only ~2% of cases [23, 31]. The immune dysregulation in CVID is classically thought to result from impaired B cell maturation [14]; but there are many complex immune mechanisms at play in the pathology of this diverse and multifaceted disease. B lymphocyte development remains key to the pathology of disease however, as impaired B cell maturation may result in altered B cell receptor signaling pathways, ultimately resulting in failure of central tolerance checkpoints. When central tolerance induction fails, autoreactive B cells normally selected for receptor editing or blocked development will evade detection and escape to the periphery unchecked [32, 33]. Decreased levels of isotype-switched memory B cells, suggesting defective germinal center development [34], and greater preservation of IgM production, suggesting potential defects in T cell involvement in immunoglobulin switching [25], have been associated with the development of autoimmunity in CVID as well.

In systemic autoimmune diseases such as SLE, autoimmunity is clearly the prominent feature, and the occurrence of autoimmune cytopenias is so common that they are often included in the diagnostic criteria of disease [20–22]. However, these autoimmune cytopenias may be an initial presentation of disease and therefore considered idiopathic until the underlying autoimmune disease is ultimately diagnosed. Among patients with SLE complicated by ES, for example, ~50% may be diagnosed with hematologic abnormalities (i.e., AIHA and/or ITP) months to years before developing full-blown clinical manifestations of SLE [35]. One of the most prominent and unifying pathologic features of systemic autoimmunity is the failure to induce lymphocyte tolerance. Defective apoptosis in immature B cells, unbalanced pro-survival signals (such as those provided by B cell activating factor [BAFF]), and altered B cell receptor signaling are all cited as contributing to the failure of central and peripheral B cell tolerance induction in systemic autoimmunity [32, 33, 36]. Defective T cell tolerance may result from the failure to generate regulatory T cells, or to anergize immature T cells which express autoreactive T cell receptors [33]. In SLE specifically, humoral autoimmunity is largely implicated in the generation of autoimmune cytopenias, with immunological changes including increased plasma cell precursors [37], expansion of CD19^{hi}CD21$^{lo/neg}$ B cells [37] which appear to be anergic but express germline autoreactive antibodies [38], and several hematologic-specific autoantibodies unique to SLE complicated by ES [39]. Additionally, the complement deficiency which is well-described in SLE [14], most notably involving C4, is significantly more pronounced in patients with ITP related to SLE [40] and ES related to SLE [35] as compared to patients with "primary" ITP or ES, or SLE not complicated by autoimmune cytopenias [35].

In addition to these more well-defined entities, several ALPS-like syndromes and ALPS-CVID overlap syndromes have been described, in which clinical phenotypes including multilineage autoimmune cytopenias that may be initially identified as ES indicate similar underlying immune dysregulation. These include RAS-associated autoimmune leukoproliferative disease (RALD), associated with somatic mutations in the *NRAS* or *KRAS* genes [19, 41, 42]; Dianzani autoimmune lymphoproliferative disease (DALD), in which an associated gene mutation has not yet been identified; and classes in which lymphoproliferation and immunodeficiency, rather than autoimmunity, are more prominent features, such as caspase-8 deficiency state (CEDS) [43, 44] and X-linked lymphoproliferative syndrome type 1 (XLP1) [19]. Furthermore, with next-generation

and ever-advancing sequencing techniques in today's genomic landscape, novel monogenic disorders of immune regulation including CTLA-4 haploinsufficiency and LRBA deficiency are being identified and better understood all the time [2, 3].

Diagnosis

When an adolescent female presents with anemia, thrombocytopenia, and/or neutropenia, the etiology of cytopenias must first be defined. In the case of thrombocytopenia, platelet size variance including large and giant platelets, with elevated immature platelet fraction, and no other etiology of thrombocytopenia is consistent with a diagnosis of ITP [45], while autoimmune hemolytic anemia is confirmed by positive direct antiglobulin test (DAT) with evidence of hemolysis, including reticulocytosis, elevated lactate dehydrogenase (LDH), and unconjugated bilirubin levels. See Fig. 23.1 for diagnostic and management algorithm. Once multilineage autoimmune cytopenias are confirmed, and a diagnosis of ES is made, patients should be screened for underlying immune dysregulation disorders as indicated. Given the noted well-established associations, adolescents should be screened for ALPS, CVID, and SLE at a minimum (see Tables 23.1, 23.2, and 23.3), while screening in some adolescents should also be expanded to include infectious etiologies such as human immunodeficiency virus (HIV) and hepatitis C virus (HCV), in addition to malignancies, as leukemias and lymphomas are reported in ~10% of adults with ES [6, 10]. Beyond these routine recommendations, however, investigation should be conducted as clinically indicated, given the wide array of clinical entities capable of driving ES, including infections, drugs, vaccinations, immunodeficiencies (combined immunodeficiencies, DiGeorge syndrome, selective IgA deficiency), autoimmune diseases, lymphoproliferative diseases, hemophagocytic disorders, malignancies, and other disorders of immune dysregulation, both well-established and novel (CTLA-4 haploinsufficiency, LRBA deficiency, activated phosphoinositide 3-kinase delta [PI3KD] syndrome, and others) [9] .Given the rapidly increasing identification rate of monogenic drivers of ES [2, 3], genetic investigations should be pursued if feasible.

Management

ES is managed in accordance with the particular autoimmune cytopenias and accompanying symptoms with which a patient presents. However, ES does tend to be a more refractory and chronic disease, often less responsive to frontline therapies used in the single-lineage autoimmune cytopenias ITP, AIHA, and AIN [7–10, 46, 47]. Furthermore, ES which is secondary to an underlying disorder of immune dysregulation such as ALPS, warrants a management strategy targeting the primary immune pathology, as well as consideration of the potential toxicities associated with certain treatment options in the setting of underlying systemic immune dysregulation.

Frontline management of ES does not differ from that of frontline ITP or AIHA management presenting alone, with the goal of controlling acute symptoms of bleeding or anemia, generally with corticosteroids, or with intravenous immunoglobulin (IVIG) or anti-D immune globulin in the case of ITP. Children [9] and adults [6] with ES achieve at least partial response to corticosteroid therapy ~80% of the time. These response rates appear to be maintained with repeat steroid courses for relapsed autoimmune cytopenias; however, the chronic relapsing course of autoimmune cytopenias in ES, not to mention longer treatment duration requirements in ES, necessitates consideration of alternate treatment strategies in order to avoid prolonged corticosteroid therapy and accompanying side effects, both short and long term [48]. Similarly, the majority of ES patients who respond to frontline ITP-directed therapies will have short-lived responses, may lose response to these therapies more quickly on repeat treatments [8], and will more than likely have persistent and/or relapsing disease, necessitating second-line therapies [9].

There are many "secondary" immunomodulating treatment options from which to choose, including azathioprine, cyclosporine, 6-mercaptopurine (6-MP) or 6-thioguanine (6-TG), hydroxychloroquine, vincristine, cyclophosphamide, tacrolimus, danazol, splenectomy, alemtuzumab (anti-CD52 antibody), mycophenolate mofetil (MMF), rituximab (anti-CD20 antibody), rapamycin (sirolimus), and more recently thrombopoietin receptor agonists (TPO-RAs) eltrombopag and romiplostim, among others [49–52]; but current advances in the understanding of ES have helped to narrow treatment strategies in the recent years (see Fig. 23.1).

Primary Evans Syndrome

For primary ES, with no well-defined underlying disorder of immune dysregulation, the most well-studied and efficacious second-line therapies include rituximab, sirolimus, MMF, and other immunomodulatory agents – with an aim toward targeting the global immune dysregulation of ES.

Rituximab, an anti-CD20 antibody which causes rapid and targeted B cell depletion, given weekly for 4 weeks at a dose of 375 mg/m^2 results in a 75 80% initial response rate in children [53, 54] and adults [6] with ES, with a long-term relapse-free response rate ~60% in adults followed for 1–3.5 years [6] and a relapse-free response rate in children varying from 65% [53] down to 36% in those children followed for 6 years [54]. Interestingly, the complete response (CR) rate was significantly higher in children with AIHA alone treated with rituximab (74%) compared to those with ES treated with rituximab (46%); and 6-year relapse-free survival for children with ES treated with rituximab was significantly lower (36%) than that for children with AIHA alone (53%) [54]. As with all monoclonal antibodies, rituximab carries a risk of infusion reaction. However, infusion reactions are generally mild, with grade 3 or 4 reactions occurring <1–9% of the time [55]. Other concerns related to the use of rituximab include prolonged hypogammaglobulinemia and infection risk following therapy. This is of particular concern in patients with known underlying ALPS, CVID, or other immunodeficiencies (see section "Special Considerations for Secondary Evans Syndrome"), but should also be used with appropriate caution and counseling in all ES patients, given that some underlying disorders may take years to evolve.

Sirolimus is a mammalian target of rapamycin (mTOR) inhibitor, blocking the response of T and B lymphocyte activation by cytokines, which prevents cell cycle progression and proliferation [56]. In addition to its attenuation of lymphoproliferation and autoimmunity, sirolimus may also have anti-malignancy potential [57]. Sirolimus is generally initiated at a dose of 2–2.5 mg/m² per day (maximum initial dose of 4 mg per day), titrating to a goal serum trough level between 5 and 15 ng/mL. The most common adverse effects associated with sirolimus therapy in ES patients were grade 1–2 mucositis and elevations of triglyceride and cholesterol levels, with rarer events including hypertension, headache, acne, sun sensitivity, and exacerbation of gastroesophageal reflux, with an overall good safety and tolerability profile [47].

MMF inactivates inosine monophosphate, a key enzyme in purine synthesis, inhibiting proliferation of T and B lymphocytes, and has been proven very effective in the treatment of ES, resulting in ~80% response rate in all patients with ES [58]. MMF is typically prescribed at 600 mg/m² twice daily. Importantly, the response seen with MMF is generally sustainable, allowing for the avoidance of less desirable treatment strategies or prolonged steroid exposure in many ES patients [46, 58, 59]. MMF is well-tolerated in general, although the most common treatment-limiting toxicities are cytopenias (leukopenia, neutropenia, anemia) and GI toxicities (diarrhea, abdominal pain, and transaminitis). Notably, however, MMF does not induce lymphocyte death, while sirolimus has been shown to reduce DNT cells and result in markedly reduced lymphoproliferation.

In the case of chronic or refractory ITP not controlled with systemic immunomodulation, TPO-RAs eltrombopag and romiplostim may be used, although ideal therapeutic options in the setting of ES are directed at the underlying immunopathology. Both eltrombopag [51, 60–63] and romiplostim [52, 64, 65] have shown excellent efficacy in the treatment of chronic and/or refractory ITP, with response rates ~80%, decreased bleeding events, improved health-related quality of life, and favorable adverse event profiles. However, patients receiving TPO-RA therapy should still be closely monitored for development of adverse events, including thrombosis (with both agents), transaminitis, and potential cataract formation (with eltrombopag), and development of neutralizing antibodies (with romiplostim). Investigations regarding potential immunomodulatory properties of these TPO-RAs are currently ongoing.

Special Considerations for Secondary Evans Syndrome

Evans syndrome which is identified to be secondary to ALPS, an ALPS-related disorder, CVID, systemic autoimmune disease, or another disorder of immune dysregulation, requires careful strategization when considering treatment options. For example, while rituximab is generally an excellent treatment option for patients with refractory autoimmune cytopenias in ES, the response rate in patients with ALPS is 58%, as compared to a response rate of 76% in patients with primary ES [46, 53]. Furthermore, the risk of clinically significant hypogammaglobulinemia following rituximab therapy may be disproportionately high in patients with underlying immunodeficiency, including those with ALPS, given that a subset of ALPS patients are predisposed to develop CVID [66]. In one series, complications among ALPS patients treated with rituximab for refractory autoimmune cytopenias included prolonged hypogammaglobulinemia, prolonged impairment and/or absence of antibody responses, and prolonged neutropenia [46]. Therefore, rituximab therapy should generally be avoided in patients with ALPS. Similarly, splenectomy should be avoided in patients with ALPS, as responses in this population are generally short-lived, and post-splenectomy toxicities are significantly more pronounced [46, 67–69]. More than 70% of patients with ES related to ALPS will ultimately relapse following splenectomy [69], with median time to relapse of ~1 month in one series, but potentially occurring up to several years following splenectomy [8, 69]. More importantly, severe invasive bacterial infections are noted in up to 50% of splenectomized ALPS patients, with higher risk related to a younger age at the time of splenectomy, overall resulting in a bacteremia-related mortality rate ranging from 12% to 22% in splenectomized ALPS patients [67–69].

On the other hand, responses to MMF are even better in patients with ALPS-related ES than those obtained in patients with primary ES [58], with 92% sustained response rate documented in ALPS patients treated with MMF for refractory autoimmune cytopenias [46, 59]. Additionally, Teachey and colleagues recently demonstrated that the mTOR inhibitor sirolimus is an effective and safe treatment for autoimmune cytopenias in highly refractory ES patients. Moreover, this medication is effective when used alone, thereby sparing the effects of additional steroid therapy. Significantly, the treatment effect was better among ES patients treated with sirolimus than among those with single-lineage autoimmune cytopenias, with particularly excellent activity in ALPS [47]. The cohort of ALPS patients had rapid response in autoimmune cytopenias, durable CR, improvement in lymphoproliferative symptoms, and disappearance of DNT cell populations (with sparing of other lymphocyte populations) as well [47, 50]. Given these findings, sirolimus is now considered as an earlier treatment option in ALPS patients who require chronic therapy [47].

Even as ES therapies are evolving toward more mechanistically driven approaches however (such as targeting lymphocyte dysregulation with MMF and sirolimus in ALPS), and away from the broader empiric immunosuppressive approaches, work remains ongoing toward further honing more targeted approaches to therapy. Some of the novel monogenic disorders now being described provide good examples for targeted therapeutic possibilities. For example, in CTLA-4 haploinsufficiency and LRBA deficiency, the immunoglobulin-CTLA4 fusion protein abatacept can help to restore the immunoregulatory activity of CTLA-4 [70, 71]; mTOR inhibition [72] and the newer selective PI3Kδ inhibitor leniolisib [73] have shown promising effects in PI3KD syndrome; JAK1/2 inhibitors (ruxolitinib) have effected positive results in signal transducer and activator of transcription (STAT)1 gain of function disease [74]; and the small molecule Bcl-2 inhibitor, ABT-737, has demonstrated reversal of the constitutive activation effects of STAT3 gain of function [75]. These are a collection of examples in which targeted therapies may result in improved outcomes for patients with secondary ES in the future.

An ancillary consideration in the management of ES pertains to the increased risk for secondary malignancy and the need for careful surveillance in this population of patients. Although the increased risk for lymphoma in ALPS is not definitively established [29], most data suggest ~5–10% risk for secondary lymphomas in ALPS patients [10]. Additionally, CVID patients carry a higher risk of developing lymphomas as well [23, 31], most commonly non-Hodgkin's B cell lymphomas, particularly when CVID is complicated by lymphoproliferation [25].

ES therapy must be individualized, as some patients may need chronic therapy for recalcitrant symptomatic disease, while some patients may require only intermittent therapy for occasional symptomatic disease flares [10, 49]. In general, invasive therapies such as splenectomy, and certainly hematopoietic stem cell transplant, should be reserved for multi-treatment-refractory and severely symptomatic ES patients.

Conclusion

ES is a descriptive diagnosis, defining a condition in which two or more autoimmune cytopenias are diagnosed, either simultaneously or sequentially. The disease course is generally more chronic, severe, and treatment-refractory in ES than in isolated autoimmune cytopenias, likely due to the complex underlying immune dysregulation. Immunopathology in ES can generally be ascribed to a disturbance in lymphocyte development or function, such that the immune balance is tipped toward autoreactivity. The genetic and biological drivers of immune dysregulation are now being increasingly identified; but at least 50% of ES cases are "idiopathic," indicating the need for thorough clinical investigation of underlying causes, especially in adolescent females, who are more likely to have secondary ES and to therefore require individualized treatment strategies.

References

1. Al Ghaithi I, Wright NAM, Breakey VR, Cox K, Warias A, Wong T, O'Connell C, Price V. Combined autoimmune cytopenias presenting in childhood. Pediatr Blood Cancer. 2016;63:292–8.
2. Besnard C, Levy E, Aladjidi N, Stolzenberg MC, Magerus-Chatinet A, Alibeu O, Nitschke P, Blanche S, Hermine O, Jeziorski E, Landman-Parker J, Leverger G, Mahlaoui N, Michel G, Pellier I, Suarez F, Thuret I, de Saint-Basile G, Picard C, Fischer A, Neven B, Rieux-Laucat F, Quartier P, Members of the French reference center for pediatric autoimmune cytopenias (CEREVANCE). Pediatric-onset Evans syndrome: heterogeneous presentation and high frequency of monogenic disorders including LRBA and CTLA4 mutations. Clin Immunol. 2018;188:52–7.
3. Hadjadj J, Aladjidi N, Fernandes H, Leverger G, Magerus-Chatinet A, Mazerolles F, Stolzenberg MC, Jacques S, Picard C, Rosain J, Fourrage C, Hanein S, Zarharte M, Pasquet M, Abou Chahla W, Barlogis V, Bertrand Y, Pellier I, Colomb Bottollier E, Fouyssac F, Blouin P, Thomas C, Cheikh N, Dore E, Pondarre C, Plantaz D, Jeziorski E, Millot F, Garcelon N, Ducassou S, Perel Y, Leblanc T, Neven B, Fischer A, Rieux-Laucat F, Members of the French Reference Center for Pediatric Autoimmune Cytopenias (CEREVANCE). Pediatric Evans syndrome is associated with a high frequency of potentially damaging variants in immune genes. Blood. 2019;134(1):9–21.
4. Aladjidi N, Leverger G, Leblanc T, Quitterie Picat M, Michel G, Bertrand Y, Bader-Meunier B, Robert A, Nelken B, Gandemer V, Savel H, Stephan JL, Fouyssac F, Jeanpetit J, Thomas C, Rohrlich P, Baruchel A, Fischer A, Chêne G, Perel Y, for the Centre de Référence National des Cytopénies Autoimmunes de l'Enfant (CEREVANCE). New insights into childhood autoimmune hemolytic anemia: a French national observational study of 2f children. Haematologica. 2011;96(5):655–63.
5. Aladjidi N, Fernandes H, Leblanc T, Vareliette A, Rieux-Laucat F, Bertrand Y, Chambost H, Pasquet M, Mazinque F, Guitton C, Pellier I, Roqueplan-
Bellmann F, Armari-Alla C, Thomas C, Marie-Cardine A, Lejars O, Fouyssac F, Bayart S, Lutz P, Piquet C, Jeziorski E, Rohrlich P, Lemoine P, Bodet D, Paillard C, Couillault G, Millot F, Fischer A, Pérel Y, Leverger G. Evans syndrome in children: long-term outcome in a prospective French national observational cohort. Front Pediatr. 2015;3:79.
6. Michel M, Chanet V, Dechartres A, Morin AS, Piette JC, Cirasino L, Emilia G, Zaja F, Ruggeri M, Andrès E, Bierling P, Godeau B, Rodeghiero F. The spectrum of Evans syndrome in adults: new insight into the disease based on the analysis of 68 cases. Blood. 2009;114(15):3167–72.
7. Wang WC. Evans syndrome in childhood: pathophysiology, clinical course, and treatment. Am J Pediatr Hematol Oncol. 1988;10(4):330–8.
8. Mathew P, Chen G, Wang W. Evans syndrome: results of a national survey. J Pediatr Hematol Oncol. 1997;19(5):433–7.
9. Miano M. How I manage Evans syndrome and AIHA cases in children. Br J Haematol. 2016;172:524–34.
10. Teachey DT, Lambert MP. Diagnosis and management of autoimmune cytopenias in childhood. Pediatr Clin N Am. 2013;60(6):1489–511.
11. Teachey DT, Manno CS, Axsom KM, Andrews T, Choi JK, Greenbaum BH, McMann JM, Sullivan KE, Travis SF, Grupp SA. Unmasking Evans syndrome: T-cell phenotype and apoptotic response reveal autoimmune lymphoproliferative syndrome (ALPS). Blood. 2005;105(6):2443–8.
12. Seif AE, Manno CS, Sheen C, Grupp SA, Teachey DT. Identifying autoimmune lymphoproliferative syndrome in children with Evans syndrome: a multi-institutional study. Blood. 2010;115(11):2142–5.
13. Savaşan S, Warrier I, Buck S, Kaplan J, Ravindranath Y. Increased lymphocyte Fas expression and high incidence of common variable immunodeficiency disorder in childhood Evans' syndrome. Clin Immunol. 2007;125(3):224–9.
14. Seidel MG. Autoimmune and other cytopenias in primary immunodeficiencies: pathomechanisms, novel differential diagnoses, and treatment. Blood. 2014;124(15):2337–44.
15. Watanabe-Fukunaga R, Brannan CI, Copeland NG, Jenkins NA, Nagata S. Lymphoproliferative disorder in mice explained by defects in Fas antigen that mediates apoptosis. Nature. 1992;356(6367):314–7.
16. Fisher GH, Rosenberg FJ, Straus SE, Dale JK, Middleton LA, Lin AY, Strober W, Lenardo MJ, Puck JM. Dominant interfering Fas gene mutations impair apoptosis in a human autoimmune lymphoproliferative syndrome. Cell. 1995;81(6):935–46.
17. Drappa J, Vaishnaw AK, Sullivan KE, Chu JL, Elkon KB. Fas gene mutations in the Canale-Smith syndrome, an inherited lymphoproliferative disorder associated with autoimmunity. N Engl J Med. 1996;335(22):1643–9.
18. Sneller MC, Wang J, Dale JK, Strober W, Middleton LA, Choi Y, Fleisher TA, Lim MS, Jaffe ES, Puck JM, Lenardo MJ, Straus SE. Clinical, immunologic, and

genetic features of an autoimmune lymphoproliferative syndrome associated with abnormal lymphocyte apoptosis. Blood. 1997;89(4):1341–8.

19. Oliveira JB, Bleesing JJ, Dianzani U, Fleisher TA, Jaffe ES, Lenardo MJ, Rieux-Laucat F, Siegel RM, Su HC, Teachey DT, Rao VK. Revised diagnostic criteria and classification for the autoimmune lymphoproliferative syndrome (ALPS): report from the 2009 NIH International Workshop. Blood. 2010;116(14):e35–40.

20. Tan EM, Cohen AS, Fries JF, Masi AT, McShane DJ, Rothfield NF, Schaller JG, Talal N, Winchester RJ. The 1982 revised criteria for the classification of systemic lupus erythematosus. Arthritis Rheum. 1982;25:1271.

21. Hochberg MC. Updating the American College of Rheumatology revised criteria for the classification of systemic lupus erythematosus (letter). Arthritis Rheum. 1997;40:1725.

22. Petri M, Orbai AM, Alarcón GS, Gordon C, Merrill JT, Fortin PR, Bruce IN, Isenberg D, Wallace DJ, Nived O, Sturfelt G, Ramsey-Goldman R, Bae SC, Hanly JG, Sanchez-Guerrero J, Clarke A, Aranow C, Manzi S, Urowitz M, Gladman D, Kalunian K, Costner M, Werth VP, Zoma A, Bernatsky S, Ruiz-Irastorza G, Khamashta MA, Jacobsen S, Buyon JP, Maddison P, Dooley MA, van Vollenhoven RF, Ginzler E, Stoll T, Peschken C, Jorizzo JL, Callen JP, Lim SS, Fessler BJ, Inanc M, Kamen DL, Rahman A, Steinsson K, Franks AG Jr, Sigler L, Hameed S, Fang H, Pham N, Brey R, Weisman MH, McGwin G Jr, Magder LS. Derivation and validation of the Systemic Lupus International Collaborating Clinics classification criteria for systemic lupus erythematosus. Arthritis Rheum. 2012;64:2677.

23. Bonilla FA, Barlan I, Chapel H, Costa-Carvalho BT, Cunningham-Rundles C, de la Morena MT, Espinosa-Rosales FJ, Hammarstrom L, Nonoyama S, Quinti I, Routes JM, Tang ML, Warnatz K. International Consensus Document (ICON): common variable immunodeficiency disorders. J Allergy Clin Immunol Pract. 2016;4(1):38–59.

24. Wang J, Cunningham-Rundles C. Treatment and outcome of autoimmune hematologic disease in common variable immunodeficiency (CVID). J Autoimmun. 2005;25(1):57–62.

25. Chapel H, Lucas M, Lee M, Bjorkander J, Webster D, Grimbacher B, Fieschi C, Thon V, Abedi MR, Hammarstrom L. Common variable immunodeficiency disorders: division into distinct clinical phenotypes. Blood. 2008;112(2):277–86.

26. Gathmann B, Mahlaoui N, Ceredih L, Gerard E, Oksenhendler K, Warnatz I, et al. European Society for Immunodeficiencies Registry Working. Clinical picture and treatment of 2212 patients with common variable immunodeficiency. J Allergy Clin Immunol. 2014;134:116–26.

27. Feuille EJ, Anooshiravani N, Sullivan KE, Fuleihan RL, Cunningham-Rundles C. Autoimmune cytopenias and associated conditions in CVID: a report from the USIDNET registry. J Clin Immunol. 2018;38(1):28–34.

28. Ameratunga R, Brewerton M, Slade C, Jordan A, Gillis D, Steele R, Koopmans W, Woon ST. Comparison of diagnostic criteria for common variable immunodeficiency disorder. Front Immunol. 2014;5:415.

29. Teachey D. New advances in the diagnosis and treatment of autoimmune lymphoproliferative syndrome. Curr Opin Pediatr. 2012;24:1–8.

30. Straus SE, Sneller M, Lenardo MJ, Puck JM, Strober W. An inherited disorder of lymphocyte apoptosis: the autoimmune lymphoproliferative syndrome. Ann Intern Med. 1999;130:591–601.

31. Maglione PJ. Autoimmune and lymphoproliferative complications of common variable immunodeficiency. Curr Allergy Asthma Rep. 2016;16(3):19.

32. Meffre E. The establishment of early B cell tolerance in humans: lessons from primary immunodeficiency diseases. Ann N Y Acad Sci. 2011;1246:1–10.

33. von Boehmer H, Melchers F. Checkpoints in lymphocyte development and autoimmune disease. Nat Immunol. 2010;11(1):14–20.

34. Wehr C, Kivioja T, Schmitt C, Ferry B, Witte T, Eren F, Vlkova M, Hernandez M, Detkova D, Bos PR, Poerksen G, von Bernuth H, Baumann U, Goldacker S, Gutenberger S, Schlesier M, Bergeron-van der Cruyssen F, Le Garff M, Debré P, Jacobs R, Jones J, Bateman E, Litzman J, van Hagen PM, Plebani A, Schmidt RE, Thon V, Quinti I, Espanol T, Webster AD, Chapel H, Vihinen M, Oksenhendler E, Peter HH, Warnatz K. The EUROclass trial: defining subgroups in common variable immunodeficiency. Blood. 2008;111(1):77–85.

35. Zhang L, Wu X, Wang L, Li J, Chen H, Zhao Y, Zheng W. Clinical features of systemic lupus erythematosus patients complicated with Evans syndrome: a case-control, single center study. Medicine (Baltimore). 2016;95(15):e3279.

36. Newman K, Owlia MB, El-Hemaidi I, Akhtari M. Management of immune cytopenias in patients with systemic lupus erythematosus – old and new. Autoimmun Rev. 2013;12(7):784–91.

37. Warnatz K, Wehr C, Dräger R, Schmidt S, Eibel H, Schlesier M, Peter HH. Expansion of CD19(hi) CD21(lo/neg) B cells in common variable immunodeficiency (CVID) patients with autoimmune cytopenia. Immunobiology. 2002;206(5):502–13.

38. Isnardi I, Ng YS, Menard L, Meyers G, Saadoun D, Srdanovic I, Samuels J, Berman J, Buckner JH, Cunningham-Rundles C, Meffre E. Complement receptor 2/CD21- human naïve B cells contain mostly autoreactive unresponsive clones. Blood. 2010;115(24):5026–36.

39. Nakamura M, Tanaka Y, Satoh T, Kawai M, Hirakata M, Kaburaki J, Kawakami Y, Ikeda Y, Kuwana M. Autoantibody to CD40 ligand in systemic lupus erythematosus: association with thrombocytopenia but not thromboembolism. Rheumatology (Oxford). 2006;45(2):150–6.

40. Liu Y, Chen S, Sun Y, Lin Q, Liao X, Zhang J, Luo J, Qian H, Duan L, Shi G. Clinical characteristics of immune thrombocytopenia associated with autoimmune disease: a retrospective study. Medicine (Baltimore). 2016;95(50):e5565.

41. Oliveira JB, Bidère N, Niemela JE, Zheng L, Sakai K, Nix CP, Danner RL, Barb J, Munson PJ, Puck JM, Dale J, Straus SE, Fleisher TA, Lenardo MJ. NRAS mutation causes a human autoimmune lymphoproliferative syndrome. Proc Natl Acad Sci U S A. 2007;104(21):8953–8.

42. Niemela J, Lu L, Fleisher TA, Davis J, Caminha I, Natter M, Beer LA, Dowdell KC, Pittaluga S, Raffeld M, Rao VK, Oliveira JB. Somatic KRAS mutations associated with a human nonmalignant syndrome of autoimmunity and abnormal leukocyte homeostasis. Blood. 2011;117:2883–6.

43. Campagnoli MF, Garbarini L, Quarello P, Garelli E, Carando A, Baravalle V, Doria A, Biava A, Chiocchetti A, Rosolen A, Dufour C, Dianzani U, Ramenghi U. The broad spectrum of autoimmune lymphoproliferative disease: molecular bases, clinical features and long-term follow-up in 31 patients. Haematologica. 2006;91(4):538–41.

44. Chun HJ, Zheng I, Ahmad M, Wang J, Speirs CK, Siegel RM, Dale JK, Puck J, Davis J, Hall CG, Skoda-Smith S, Atkinson TP, Straus SE, Lenardo MJ. Pleiotropic defects in lymphocyte activation caused by caspase-8 mutations lead to human immunodeficiency. Nature. 2002;419(6905):395–9.

45. Neunert C, Lim W, Crowther M, Cohen A, Solberg L Jr, Crowther MA, American Society of Hematology. The American Society of Hematology 2011 evidence-based practice guideline for immune thrombocytopenia. Blood. 2011;117(16):4190–207.

46. Rao VK, Oliveira JB. How I treat autoimmune lymphoproliferative syndrome. Blood. 2011;118(22):5741–51.

47. Bride KL, Vincent T, Smith-Whitley K, Lambert MP, Bleesing JJ, Seif AE, Manno CS, Casper J, Grupp SA, Teachey DT. Sirolimus is effective in relapsed/refractory autoimmune cytopenias: results of a prospective multi-institutional trial. Blood. 2016;127(1):17–28.

48. Fan J, He H, Zhao W, Wang Y, Lu J, Li J, Li J, Xiao P, Lu Y, Chai Y, Hu S. Clinical features and treatment outcomes of childhood autoimmune hemolytic anemia: a retrospective analysis of 68 cases. J Pediatr Hematol Oncol. 2016;38(2):e50–5.

49. Norton A, Roberts I. Management of Evans syndrome. Br J Haematol. 2005;132:125–37.

50. Teachey DT, Greiner R, Seif A, Attiyeh E, Bleesing J, Choi J, Manno C, Rappaport E, Schwabe D, Sheen C, Sullivan KE, Zhuang H, Wechsler DS, Grupp SA. Treatment with sirolimus results in complete responses in patients with autoimmune lymphoproliferative syndrome. Br J Haematol. 2009;145(1):101–6.

51. Bussel JB, Cheng G, Saleh MN, et al. Eltrombopag for the treatment of chronic idiopathic thrombocytopenic purpura. N Engl J Med. 2007;357:2237–47.

52. Kuter DJ, Bussel JB, Lyons RM, et al. Efficacy of romiplostim in patients with chronic immune thrombocytopenic purpura: a double-blind randomised controlled trial. Lancet. 2008;371:395–403.

53. Bader-Meunier B, Aladjidi N, Bellmann F, Monpoux F, Nelken B, Robert A, Armari-Alla C, Picard C, Ledeist F, Munzer M, Yacouben K, Bertrand Y, Pariente A, Chaussé A, Perel Y, Leverger G. Rituximab therapy for childhood Evans syndrome. Haematologica. 2007;92(12):1691–4.

54. Ducassou S, Leverger G, Fernandes H, Chambost H, Bertrand Y, Armari-Alla C, Nelken B, Monpoux F, Guitton C, Leblanc T, Fisher A, Lejars O, Jeziorski E, Fouissac F, Lutz P, Pasquet M, Pellier I, Piquet C, Vic P, Bayart S, Marie-Cardine A, Michel M, Perel Y, Aladjidi N. Benefits of rituximab as a second-line treatment for autoimmune haemolytic anaemia in children: a prospective French cohort study. Br J Haematol. 2017;177(5):751–8.

55. Genentech Inc. Rituxan (rituximab) package insert. South San Francisco: Genentech Inc; 2013.

56. Kelly PA, Gruber SA, Behbod F, Kahan BD. Sirolimus, a new, potent immunosuppressive agent. Pharmacotherapy. 1997;17(6):1148.

57. Euvrard S, Morelon E, Rostaing L, Goffin E, Brocard A, Tromme I, Broeders N, del Marmol V, Chatelet V, Dompmartin A, Kessler M, Serra AL, Hofbauer GF, Pouteil-Noble C, Campistol JM, Kanitakis J, Roux AS, Decullier E, Dantal J, TUMORAPA Study Group. Sirolimus and secondary skin-cancer prevention in kidney transplantation. N Engl J Med. 2012;367(4):329.

58. Miano M, Ramenghi U, Russo G, Rubert L, Barone A, Tucci F, Farruggia P, Petrone A, Mondino A, Lo Valvo L, Crescenzio N, Bellia F, Olivieri I, Palmisani E, Caviglia I, Dufour C, Fioredda F. Mycophenolate mofetil for the treatment of children with immune thrombocytopenia and Evans syndrome. A retrospective data review from the Italian Association of Paediatric Haematology/Oncology. Br J Haematol. 2016;175(3):490–5.

59. Rao VK, Dugan F, Dale JK, Davis J, Tretler J, Hurley JK, Fleisher T, Puck J, Straus SE. Use of mycophenolate mofetil for chronic, refractory immune cytopenias in children with autoimmune lymphoproliferative syndrome. Br J Haematol. 2005;129(4):534–8.

60. Bussel JB, Provan D, Shamsi T, et al. Effect of Eltrombopag on platelet counts and bleeding during treatment of chronic idiopathic thrombocytopenic purpura: a randomised, double-blind, placebo-controlled trial. Lancet. 2009;373:641–8.

61. Cheng G, Saleh MN, Marcher C, et al. Eltrombopag for management of chronic immune thrombocytopenia (RAISE): a 6-month, randomised, phase 3 study. Lancet. 2011;377:393–402.

62. Bussel JB, Saleh MN, Vasey SY, et al. Repeated short-term use of eltrombopag in patients with chronic immune thrombocytopenia (ITP). Br J Haematol. 2013;160:538–46.

63. Saleh MN, Bussel JB, Cheng G, et al. Safety and efficacy of eltrombopag for treatment of chronic immune
thrombocytopenia: results of the long-term, open-
label EXTEND study. Blood. 2013;121:537–45.
64. Kuter DJ, Rummel M, Boccia R, et al. Romiplostim
or standard of care in patients with immune thrombocytopenia. N Engl J Med. 2010;363(20):1889–99.
65. Rodeghiero F, Stasi R, Giagounidis A, et al. Long-term
safety and tolerability of romiplostim in patients with
primary immune thrombocytopenia: a pooled analysis
of 13 clinical trials. Eur J Haematol. 2013;91:423–36.
66. Teachey DT, Seif AE, Grupp SA. Advances in the
management and understanding of autoimmune lymphoproliferative syndrome (ALPS). Br J Haematol.
2010;148:205–16.
67. Neven B, Magerus-Chatinet A, Florkin B, Gobert D,
Lambotte O, De Somer L, Lanzarotti N, Stolzenberg
MC, Bader-Meunier B, Aladjidi N, Chantrain C,
Bertrand Y, Jeziorski E, Leverger G, Michel G,
Suarez F, Oksenhendler E, Hermine O, Blanche S,
Picard C, Fischer A, Rieux-Laucat F. A survey of
90 patients with autoimmune lymphoproliferative
syndrome related to TNFRSF6 mutation. Blood.
2011;118(18):4798–807.
68. Neven B, Bruneau J, Stolzenberg MC, Meyts
I, Magerus-Chatinet A, Moens L, Lanzarotti N,
Weller S, Amiranoff D, Florkin B, Bader-Meunier
B, Leverger G, Ferster A, Chantrain C, Blanche S,
Picard C, Molina TJ, Brousse N, Durandy A, Rizzi
M, Bossuyt X, Fischer A, Rieux-Laucat F. Defective
anti-polysaccharide response and splenic marginal
zone disorganization in ALPS patients. Blood.
2014;124(10):1597–609.
69. Price S, Shaw PA, Seitz A, Joshi G, Davis J, Niemela
JE, Perkins K, Nornung RL, Folio L, Rosenberg PS,
Puck JM, Hsu AP, Lo B, Pittaluga S, Jaffe ES, Fleisher
TA, Rao VK, Lenardo MJ. Natural history of autoim-
mune lymphoproliferative syndrome associated with
FAS gene mutations. Blood. 2014;123(13):1989–99.
70. Lo B, Zhang K, Lu W, Zheng L, Zhang Q,
Kanellopoulou C, Zhang Y, Liu Z, Fritz JM, Marsh
R, Husami A, Kissell D, Nortman S, Chaturvedi V,
Haines H, Young LR, Mo J, Filipovich AH, Bleesing
JJ, Mustillo P, Stephens M, Rueda CM, Chougnet CA,
Hoebe K, McElwee J, Hughes JD, Karakoc-Aydiner
E, Matthews HF, Price S, Su HC, Rao VK, Lenardo

MJ, Jordan MB. Autoimmune Disease. Patients with
LRBA deficiency show CTLA4 loss and immune dysregulation responsive to abatacept therapy. Science.
2015;349(6246):436–40.
71. Lee S, Moon JS, Lee CR, Kim HE, Baek SM,
Hwang S, Kang GH, Seo JK, Shin CH, Kang HJ,
Ko JS, Park SG, Choi M. Abatacept alleviates severe
autoimmune symptoms in a patient carrying a de
novo variant in CTLA-4. J Allergy Clin Immunol.
2016;137(1):327–30.
72. Lucas CL, Kuehn HS, Zhao F, Niemela JE, Deenick
EK, Palendira U, Avery DT, Moens L, Cannons
JL, Biancalana M, Stoddard J, Ouyang W, Frucht
DM, Rao VK, Atkinson TP, Agharahimi A, Hussey
AA, Folio LR, Olivier KN, Fleisher TA, Pittaluga
S, Holland SM, Cohen JI, Oliveira JB, Tangye SG,
Schwartzberg PL, Lenardo MJ, Uzel G. Dominant-
activating germline mutations in the gene encod-
ing the PI(3)K catalytic subunit p110δ result in T
cell senescence and human immunodeficiency. Nat
Immunol. 2014;15(1):88–97.
73. Rao VK, Webster S, Dalm VASH, Sedivá A, van
Hagen PM, Holland S, Rosensweig SD, Christ AD,
Sloth B, Cabanski M, Joshi AD, de Buck S, Doucet
J, Guerini D, Kalis C, Pylvaenaeinen I, Soldermann
N, Kashyap A, Uzel G, Lenardo MJ, Patel DD,
Lucas CL, Burkhart C. Effective 'Activated PI3Kδ
Syndrome'-targeted therapy with the PI3Kδ inhibitor
leniolisib. Blood. 2017;130(21):2307–16.
74. Weinacht KG, Charbonnier LM, Alrogi F, Plant A,
Qiao Q, Wu H, Ma C, Torgerson TR, Rosenzweig
SD, Fleisher TA, Notarangelo LD, Hanson IC, Forbes
LR, Chatila TA. Ruxolitinib reverses dysregulated
T helper cell responses and controls autoimmunity
caused by a novel signal transducer and activator of
transcription 1 (STAT1) gain-of-function mutation. J
Allergy Clin Immunol. 2017;139(5):1629–40.
75. Nabhani S, Schipp C, Miskin H, Levin C, Postovsky
S, Dujovny T, Koren A, Harlev D, Bis AM, Auer F,
Keller B, Warnatz K, Gombert M, Ginzel S, Borkhardt
A, Stepensky P, Fischer U. STAT3 gain-of-function
mutations associated with autoimmune lymphoproliferative syndrome like disease deregulate lymphocyte
apoptosis and can be targeted by BH3 mimetic com-
pounds. Clin Immunol. 2017;181:32–42.

Antiphospholipid Syndrome

Neha Bhasin, Christine Knoll, and Leslie M. Skeith

Introduction

Antiphospholipid syndrome (APS) is a multisystem autoimmune disorder that is an important cause of venous and arterial thromboembolism and pregnancy-related morbidity [1]. Among all adult patients with thrombosis, APS is often diagnosed in patients at a younger age [2]. Antiphospholipid syndrome can be classified as a primary condition (primary APS) or in the presence of other systemic autoimmune diseases (secondary APS) [3]. The most common autoimmune condition that is associated with secondary APS is systemic lupus erythematosus (SLE) [2, 4].

While APS in adults has been relatively well characterized, there are few studies describing pediatric APS and even fewer studies describing primary pediatric APS. The true prevalence of primary pediatric APS is not known, and there is little information about the influence of age,

comorbidities, clinical manifestations, or outcomes in pediatric APS. We currently use the same classification criteria for both adult and pediatric APS, although obstetric morbidity may be less applicable in a pediatric population [2, 4, 5]. In this chapter, pediatric APS will be reviewed including the definition, pathophysiology, clinical manifestations, laboratory manifestations, and differential diagnosis and management.

Definition

Antiphospholipid syndrome is an acquired thrombotic disorder characterized by venous, arterial, small-vessel thromboembolism, or obstetric morbidity in the presence of persistently positive antiphospholipid (aPL) antibodies. The revised Sapporo criteria is a consensus-based diagnostic criteria that was originally developed for research purposes and requires at least one clinical criterion and one laboratory criterion to be met [1, 6, 7].

Clinical criteria for APS:

1. *Thrombosis:* One or more clinical episodes of venous, arterial, or small-vessel thrombosis, in any tissue or organ. For histopathologic confirmation, thrombosis should be present without significant vessel wall inflammation.

N. Bhasin
Department of Pediatrics, University of Arizona, Tucson, AZ, USA

C. Knoll
Department of Child Health, Phoenix Children's Hospital, Phoenix, AZ, USA

L. M. Skeith (✉)
Department of Medicine, University of Calgary, Calgary, Alberta, Canada

© Springer Nature Switzerland AG 2020
L. V. Srivaths (ed.), *Hematology in the Adolescent Female*,
https://doi.org/10.1007/978-3-030-48446-0_24

2. *Obstetric morbidity:*
   (a) One or more unexplained deaths of a morphologically normal fetus at or beyond the 10th week of gestation
   (b) One or more premature births of a morphologically normal neonate before the 34th week of gestation because of eclampsia or severe preeclampsia defined according to standard definitions, or recognized features of placental insufficiency
   (c) Three or more unexplained consecutive spontaneous abortions before the 10th week of gestation, with maternal anatomic or hormonal abnormalities and paternal and maternal chromosomal causes excluded

Laboratory criteria for APS:

Laboratory criteria for APS include the following laboratory tests, detected on two or more occasions at least 12 weeks apart:

(a) Lupus anticoagulant (LAC) present in plasma, detected according to the guidelines of the International Society on Thrombosis and Haemostasis [8]
(b) Anticardiolipin antibody (aCL) of IgG and/or IgM isotype in serum or plasma, present in medium or high titer (>40 GPL or MPL, or >99th percentile), measured by a standardized ELISA
(c) Anti-β2-glycoprotein I (aβ2GPI) antibody of IgG and/or IgM isotype in serum or plasma (in titer greater than the 99th percentile), measured by a standardized ELISA

Catastrophic APS (CAPS) is a rare and severe form of APS, usually presenting with small-vessel thrombosis with microangiopathic hemolytic anemia and thrombocytopenia [9, 10]. Catastrophic APS is fatal in over 40% of cases [11]. Diagnosis is based on clinical involvement of at least three organ systems over a short period of time with histopathologic evidence of microvascular occlusive disease and presence of aPL [12–14]. A recent clinical practice guideline on the diagnosis and management of CAPS recommended using the Preliminary Criteria for Classification of CAPS as described below, and recommended not delaying empiric treatment in patients with suspected CAPS [15].

The preliminary criteria for classification of CAPS:

1. Evidence of involvement of three or more organs, systems, and/or tissues
2. Development of manifestations simultaneously or in less than a week
3. Confirmation by histopathology of small-vessel occlusion in at least one organ or tissue
4. Laboratory confirmation of the presence of antiphospholipid antibodies

Definite CAPS:
All four criteria
Probable CAPS:

- All four criteria, except for only two organs, systems, and/or tissues involved
- All four criteria, except for the absence of laboratory confirmation at least 6 weeks apart because of the early death of a patient never tested for aPL before the CAPS
- 1, 2, and 4
- 1, 3, and 4 and the development of a third event in more than a week but less than a month, despite anticoagulation

Pathophysiology

The mechanisms by which APS causes thrombotic and obstetrical complications are not fully understood. There is a heterogeneous group of antibodies directed against phospholipids and phospholipid-binding proteins, which can be both diagnostic and pathogenic [16]. The pathogenesis of APS is largely thought to be related to aPLs that bind to phospholipid-binding proteins, such as aβ2GPI. Antibodies that bind to phospholipid directly, such as aCL, have also been shown to be pathogenic in mice models [17]. There are other aPLs that are not part of the revised revised Sapporo criteria, such as anti-phosphatidylserine and prothrombin (anti-PS/PT), anti-phosphatidylinositol, and antibodies against domain 1 of aβ2GP, I that continue to be a focus of ongoing research.

Although aβ2GPI is thought to be one of the primary antibodies in APS, its inhibition does not directly have thrombotic effects as evidenced by the lack of a thrombotic phenotype in β2GPI-deficient individuals. Multiple pathogenic mechanisms of APS have been proposed including inhibition of the natural anticoagulant and fibrinolytic systems; activation of endothelial cells, platelets, and monocytes; procoagulant effects of extracellular vesicles; and complement activation and disruption of the anticoagulant annexin A5 shield on cellular surfaces [11]. Some studies suggest that a direct activity of aPL may be involved in the development of non-thrombotic manifestations and pregnancy morbidity. In particular, aPL can directly bind to trophoblast cells causing direct cellular injury, reduction of the secretion of human chorionic gonadotropin, and abnormalities in placentation [18].

Antiphospholipid antibodies can induce activation of platelets, which increase expression of glycoprotein IIb-IIIa, synthesis of thromboxane A2, and secretion of platelet factor-4, a chemokine with procoagulant and pro-thrombotic effects. Moreover, aPL may interfere with proteins implicated in the coagulation cascade such as prothrombin, factor X, protein C, protein S, and plasmin, thus affecting the balance between procoagulant and anticoagulant factors and hampering fibrinolysis [19].

It is unclear why high aPL titers may persist for years in asymptomatic patients. One proposed theory is a "two-hit" model, where APS represents a condition necessary but not sufficient to induce thrombosis. The "two-hit model" proposes that aPL increase the risk of thrombotic events ("first hit") but thrombus formation takes place only if another procoagulant or inflammatory condition occurs ("second hit"), such as surgery, trauma pregnancy, or infection [19].

Over the past two decades, complement activation has emerged as an attractive target for mechanistic and therapeutic investigations with studies showing complement activation in aPL-mediated thrombosis and obstetrical complications. The complement system, consisting of over 50 plasma proteins involved in innate host defense, is organized into the classical, lectin, and alternative pathway. These pathways converge at the level of complement component C3 and the terminal complement pathway that leads to generation of C5a, a potent pro-inflammatory molecule, and C5b-9 (the membrane attack complex). Anti- β2GPI antibodies are associated with complement activation, and the complement and coagulation pathways are closely linked. There is complement activation in murine models of aPL-induced thrombosis and fetal loss and early evidence of complement activation in patients with APS [11].

Studies have demonstrated that aPL-induced complement activation may lead to neutrophil expression of tissue factor (TF) mediated through the C5a receptor, leading to expression of procoagulant activity (Fig. 24.1) [11, 20]. C5a also induces TF expression on monocytes and endothelial cells. In addition, deposition of C5b-9 on the endothelial surface leads to secretion of high-molecular-weight multimers of von Willebrand factor, expression of P-selectin, and plasma membrane vesiculation that exposes a catalytic surface for the prothrombinase complex. Complement activation can also contribute to depressed fibrinolysis, a recognized thrombogenic mechanism in APS.

A minority of patients (1%) with aPL develop CAPS, manifesting as small-vessel thrombosis in three or more organs within the span of a week in the absence of small-vessel inflammation on histopathologic examination. The pathophysiology of CAPS is not clearly defined; however, some researchers hypothesize that a precipitating factor, such as surgery, pregnancy, or infection, may cause an acute endothelial injury, which initiates a cycle of cytokine overproduction and systemic inflammatory response leading to microangiopathy and small-vessel thrombosis [21]. Recently, rare mutations in complement regulatory genes have been identified in patients who develop CAPS [22]. Increased serum C5b-9 has been detected in patients with CAPS, with case reports of clinical and laboratory improvement after treatment with eculizumab, a complement inhibitor. Further research is still needed before these therapies become widespread practice.

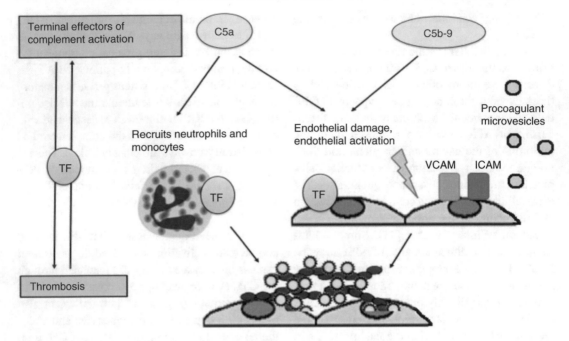

Fig. 24.1 Procoagulant effects of complement activation

Activation of complement leads to generation of C5a and C5b, which combines with other terminal complement components to form the membrane attack complex. C5a is an anaphylatoxin that recruits neutrophils and leads to expression of tissue factor on neutrophils, monocytes, and endothelial cells, which is associated with procoagulant activity. Deposition of the membrane attack complex on the endothelium leads to endothelial injury and procoagulant changes including expression of adhesion molecules, secretion of von Willebrand factor, and release of procoagulant microvesicles [11].

Clinical Manifestations

Pediatric APS is rare with the true incidence unknown, as most reports of pediatric APS are based on small cohort and registry studies [23–25]. Similar to APS in adults, there is a female predominance in pediatric APS [26]. In the largest international pediatric registry of 121 children, APS was found to be slightly more predominant among girls than boys (1.2:1). The mean age of APS onset has been reported as 11.5

(±4.6) years in one study and 12.9 years in another small cohort study [27]. In contrast, in a predominantly adult prospective cohort of 1000 APS patients, the mean age of symptom onset was 34 ± 13 years (range 0–81 years) [28]. An additional series of 50 children with APS reported that females outnumbered males (31 vs. 19) with the age of onset of 102 years (range 8 months to 16 years) [1].

Antiphospholipid syndrome should be suspected in patients that have unexplained venous or arterial thrombotic events or obstetric morbidity, particularly if they have a systemic autoimmune disorder. Systemic lupus erythematosus and lupus-like conditions account for the majority of cases in small case series [26]. Other autoimmune causes include juvenile idiopathic arthritis, Henoch-Schonlein purpura, Behcet disease, hemolytic-uremic syndrome, juvenile dermatomyositis, and rheumatic fever [27]. Primary APS presents in younger children and has a higher incidence of arterial thrombosis compared to secondary APS, which presents in older children and has a higher incidence of venous thrombosis [1]. Some children who present with primary APS may later develop SLE [27].

Positive aPL occurs in the highest percentage in pediatric SLE compared to other autoimmune diseases [29, 30]. The risk of thrombosis with positive aPLs may be as low as <1% with isolated aPL and up to 5% per year and 35% at 10 years for individuals with triple-positive antibodies (positive LAC, aCL, and B2GP1) [31–33].

Thrombosis can occur in any organ system, and arterial, venous, and small-vessel thrombosis, and multiple thrombotic events can occur in the same patient. In a large prospective cohort of largely adult patients, the most frequent venous thrombotic events were deep vein thrombosis (DVT), pulmonary embolism (PE), and cerebral vein thrombosis [28]. The most common arterial thrombotic events were ischemic stroke and transient ischemic attacks. Other arterial thrombotic sites include coronary, hepatic, mesenteric, renal, retinal, and peripheral arteries. Other less common thrombotic complications include upper extremity DVT, splanchnic vein thrombosis including Budd-Chiari syndrome, renal vein thrombosis, or retinal vein occlusion. Adrenal infarcts are thought to be secondary to adrenal vein thrombosis. While not part of the revised Sapporo criteria, superficial vein thrombosis, pulmonary hypertension due to recurrent/chronic pulmonary embolism, and diffuse pulmonary hemorrhage due to microthrombosis are possible in APS [3].

The Ped-APS Registry is an international registry and is the largest collection of pediatric patients with APS. In this registry, there are 121 children from 24 centers in which data was collected [27]. Only patients with thrombosis who fulfilled the revised Sapporo criteria were included in the registry. Of the thrombotic events in this registry, 60% of patients presented with venous thrombosis, 32% with arterial thrombosis, 6% with small-vessel thrombosis, and 2% with mixed arterial and venous thrombosis. The most common initial thrombotic event was lower extremity DVT ($n = 49$), ischemic stroke ($n = 31$), and cerebral sinus vein thrombosis ($n = 8$).

In a Mexican cohort of 32 children with APS evaluated retrospectively, 19 patients (59%) had SLE, 12 (38%) had primary APS, and 1 (3%) had immune thrombocytopenic purpura. Thrombotic events in this study included 14 patients (44%) with small-vessel thrombosis, 10 (31%) with venous thrombosis, and 8 (25%) with arterial thrombosis. Interestingly, the most common presentation was digital ischemia ($n = 14$), followed by lower extremity DVT ($n = 10$) [26].

In another retrospective study of 28 children, there were 12 patients (43%) with venous thrombosis and 11 (40%) with arterial thrombosis. The most common initial manifestations were DVT (32.1%) and stroke (25%). None had both venous and arterial thromboses. Two female patients were diagnosed with APS and thrombosis during the onset of SLE [34].

In a case series cohort of 50 pediatric APS patients, all patients had at least one thrombotic event: venous thrombosis in 35 patients and arterial thrombosis in 22 patients; 7 patients had both arterial and venous thromboses [5]. Interestingly, arterial thrombosis was more common in the younger (<10 years old) population (63% vs. 28%) [1].

Obstetrical complications include recurrent early pregnancy loss (<10 weeks gestation), late fetal loss, or placenta-mediated pregnancy complications such as early-onset (<34 weeks gestation) or severe preeclampsia or placental insufficiency [35]. Little information has been published in the obstetric morbidity among adolescent females with APS.

Non-thrombotic complications of APS include hematologic manifestations including thrombocytopenia, cardiac valve disease, nephropathy, skin manifestations including livedo reticularis, and neurologic complications including transverse myelitis. Non-criteria manifestations that may be more prevalent in the pediatric setting include Raynaud's phenomenon, autoimmune cytopenias, epilepsy, migraine headache, and chorea. While rare, renal thrombotic microangiopathy has been described in a pediatric population. Many of these potential complications are also seen in SLE and other autoimmune disorders, so this can be challenging to diagnosis [36, 37].

In the Ped-APS Registry, the most common "non-criteria" manifestations were hematological (39%), skin disorders (25%), and non-thrombotic neurological disorders (16%) [27]. In the retrospective study of 28 children, 5 patients presented with non-thrombotic manifestations, including thrombocytopenia, hemolytic anemia, epilepsy, and chorea with livedo reticularis. The most common initial non-criteria manifestations were thrombocytopenia (17.9%) and hemolytic anemia (10.7%). Chorea was observed in two patients at the time of presentation. Epilepsy, pseudotumor cerebri, migraine, livedo reticularis, Raynaud's phenomenon, TIA, and visual disturbances attributable to retinal artery emboli from mitral valve vegetation were each present in a single patient [3, 34].

Laboratory Manifestations

In comparison to adults, there have been differences reported in laboratory features of pediatric patients. Studies have shown higher rate of LAC and IgM aCL in pediatric patients compared to adults, with a comparable prevalence of IgG aCL and aβ2GPI antibodies [27, 38]. Similar to adults, the specificity of aCL and aβ2GPI ELISA tests for aPL-related clinical events increases with higher titers of these antibodies.

In a single-center study aimed to evaluate the frequency of aPL positivity associated with other risk factors and outcomes in children, 16 out of 138 (11.6%) children with thrombosis displayed positive aPL, 11 out of 16 with positive aPL (68.8%) had more than 1 pro-thrombotic risk factor other than circulating aPL, and 5 out of the 16 with positive aPL (31.3%) had no additional risk factors. Ten (62.5%) had arterial thrombosis, five had (31.3%) venous thrombosis, and one (6.3%) had purpura fulminans [3, 39].

Pediatric Catastrophic APS

As previously defined, CAPS is a rare and severe form of APS that represents less than 1% of all patients with APS and has also been described in children [12–14]. The international CAPS Registry of the European Forum on aPL reported 45 pediatric cases. The clinical and laboratory features, treatments, and outcomes

were not significantly different in children compared to adults. There was a higher prevalence of infection as a triggering factor in pediatric CAPS (60.9% vs. 26.8%) compared to adults. The majority of pediatric patients (68.9%) had primary APS and 28.9% had SLE. Peripheral vessel thrombosis was more prevalent in pediatric patients compared to adults (52.2% vs. 34.3%). In addition, CAPS was the first manifestation of APS more frequently in pediatric patients compared to adults (86.6% vs. 45.2%), but pediatric patients showed a tendency of lower mortality probably considering their relative vascular health, although the difference was not statistically significant (26.1 vs. 40.2%; odds ratio, 1.9; 95% confidence interval, 0.96–3.79) [15, 40].

Neonatal APS

While rare, neonatal APS does occur. It is defined as thrombosis that occurs during the first 28 days of an infant's life, which is most likely secondary to transplacental passage of maternal aPL. In general, neonates represent the largest childhood group that develop thrombotic events. Neonates potentially have a higher thrombotic risk due to decreased thrombin-plasminogen; decreased coagulation factors; decreased platelet aggregation (confirmed increased or decreased aggregation); decreased protein C, protein S, antithrombin III; and relative vitamin K deficiency. Babies born to mothers with APS have detectable aCL that decrease over time and are eventually resolved by 6 months of age. Antiphospholipid antibodies have transplacental passage rates of about 30%; however, thrombosis in infants born to mothers with APS is rare [41]. The thrombotic events seen in this age group are usually arterial and often stroke like lesions, suggestive of intrauterine thromboembolism originating from the placenta. Most have other risk factors including preeclampsia, intrauterine growth restriction, asphyxia, sepsis, arterial or venous catheter, and congenital thrombophilia [16, 41–47]. There are rare cases of de novo neonatal APS. This is defined as thrombosis and positive aPL in babies and negative assays in the mothers. Most cases were found to have additional thrombosis risk factors [46, 47].

Differential Diagnosis

Several infectious agents may induce transient aPL positivity, but these infectious agents may also act as an inflammatory second hit in APS pathogenesis [27, 48]. These include parvovirus B19, cytomegalovirus, varicella-zoster virus, HIV, streptococcal and staphylococcal infections, mycoplasma pneumonia, and gram-negative bacteria. Lupus anticoagulant positivity was detected in 84% of a pediatric series during a screening before adenotonsillectomy, which is a selected group with recurrent sinus, tonsillar, and upper respiratory tract infections [27]. Varicella zoster virus was found in pediatric cases with cerebrovascular disease in association with purpura fulminans after chickenpox infection linked to the presence of LAC and acquired protein S deficiency [48]. The presence of LAC has also been described in Lemierre syndrome, commonly associated with an anaerobic gram-negative bacillus, *Fusobacterium necrophorum* [49]. Only a few cases of thrombosis have been reported in young children with postinfectious LAC without an underlying autoimmune disease. LAC is transiently present in most children, and there is no associated thrombosis. Vaccination-induced aPL may also occur in children either because of the infectious or the adjuvant components. The majority of these postinfectious aPL are immunologically different than the true autoimmune ones since they do not require β2GPI for their binding [50].

APS is just one of many potential causes of thrombosis in the pediatric population. While awaiting confirmation of APS with repeat aPL at least 12 weeks apart, other possible causes should be considered and potentially pursued depending on the clinical scenario. Inherited thrombophilia testing may be warranted in some cases. Inherited thrombophilias include factor V Leiden mutation, prothrombin gene mutation, antithrombin III deficiency, protein S deficiency, or protein C deficiency. Other pro-thrombotic states include trauma, surgery, malignancy, inflammatory conditions such as inflammatory bowel disease, protein-losing states such as nephrotic syndrome and protein-losing enteropathy, and drugs such as estrogen and steroids. Primary hematologic disorders such as sickle cell anemia, essential thrombocythemia, or paroxysmal nocturnal hemoglobinuria may be considered depending if other findings are present such as anemia, hemolysis, or other cytopenias.

Management

The management of APS has been in continuous evolution over several decades. Different factors such as the aPL profile (type, number, and titer of aPL antibodies), clinical manifestations, and the presence of additional cardiovascular risk factors may affect future risk of thrombosis and the associated treatment. The 2019 European League Against Rheumatism (EULAR) Task Force guidelines focus on design tailored treatment strategies taking into account individual risk assessments based on available evidence for adult patients with APS [21].

Minimizing additional risk factors in patients with APS or persistently positive aPL is recommended. In adolescents, hormone contraceptives should be avoided if possible. Hormone therapy that appears safe, even without anticoagulation, is the progesterone-only intrauterine device or the Micronor progesterone-only pill. Management of any additional vascular risk factors (e.g., hypercholesterolemia, hypertension, diabetes, obesity, smoking) is recommended in patients with APS with or without prior thrombosis. Thromboprophylaxis during high-risk situations (surgery, postpartum, long-lasting immobilization) is recommended.

Primary Prevention

Primary prophylaxis with low-dose aspirin (75–100 mg daily) for patients with asymptomatic aPL is debated. While controversial, there may be of possible benefit if existing cardiovascular risk factors or autoimmune disease is present based on existing limited data.

In patients with aPL associated with SLE, hydroxychloroquine (HCQ) is commonly prescribed. In addition to benefits to SLE, HCQ has shown antithrombotic mechanisms based on platelet inhibition, reduction of aPL-β2GPI complexes binding to phospholipid surfaces, and reduction of aPL titers and their procoagulant effect [51]. There is little evidence to use HCQ for primary thromboprophylaxis in the absence of a secondary autoimmune disease.

Secondary prevention

After treatment of an initial venous or arterial thrombotic event for 3–6 months, long-term anticoagulation is typically recommended given the high risk of thrombotic recurrence. Initial treatment is often therapeutic-dose low-molecular-weight heparin (LMWH) or unfractionated heparin, bridged to a vitamin K antagonist (e.g., warfarin) with an INR target between 2 and 3. If unfractionated heparin is used, monitoring with anti-Xa levels or a PTT-insensitive assay may be needed in patients with a positive LAC to ensure adequate anticoagulation.

In the pediatric population where warfarin monitoring with blood work may be a challenge, continuing daily LMWH injections may be an option but has been less well studied.

Randomized trials have evaluated high-intensity warfarin (INR 3–4) in adult patients with past thrombosis compared to standard-intensity warfarin (INR 2–3), and there was no difference in recurrent thrombosis with a potentially higher bleeding rate [52, 53]. Based on observational data, some experts argue for more aggressive treatment in patients at high risk of recurrent stroke such as with the addition of an antiplatelet agent or high-intensity warfarin.

Recent studies have shown the efficacy and safety of direct oral anticoagulants (DOACs) in a general pediatric population with venous thromboembolism [54]. However, caution is needed in patients with APS. Two randomized controlled trials in the adult population have shown an increased thrombotic risk with rivaroxaban, compared to warfarin.

The TRAPS (Trial on Rivaroxaban in AntiPhospholipid Syndrome) was a multicenter, randomized, controlled, open-label, non-inferiority trial comparing rivaroxaban 20 mg daily versus standard-intensity warfarin among high-risk adult APS patients with triple positivity (positive for LAC, aCL, and aβ2GPI) and thrombosis. After randomizing 59 patients to the rivaroxaban arm and 61 patients to the warfarin arm, the study was terminated early because there were significantly more events in the rivaroxaban group; thromboembolic events and major bleeding occurred in 12% and 7% in the rivaroxaban arm compared with 0% and 3% in the warfarin arm, respectively [55]. The thromboembolic events in the rivaroxaban arm were all arterial events with ischemic stroke and myocardial infarctions, including in patients with only a history of VTE.

The second published randomized controlled, open-label, non-inferiority trial compared rivaroxaban 20 mg daily versus warfarin among adult APS patients with a positive LAC or moderate-high titer [56] aCL or aβ2GPI IgG. Non-inferiority was not met; there were more thromboembolic events in the rivaroxaban arm (11.6% versus 6.3%), which included CAPS and predominantly arterial events [55].

Based on the available evidence from the adult population, DOACs should be avoided in pediatric patients with confirmed APS. Trials are ongoing that will provide additional evidence for these patients.

Refractory of Refractory Thrombosis

There are varying practices for the management of refractory thrombosis and may include increasing the dose of LMWH and the addition of an antiplatelet to anticoagulation or high-intensity warfarin (INR 3–4). Additional therapies may include the addition of a statin or HCQ in refractory cases [56].

Pregnancy Management

For *pregnancy* management in women with APS, the objectives are to improve both maternal and fetal-neonatal outcomes. Preconception planning with a multidisciplinary team of providers is needed to optimize the management of APS and concomitant autoimmune diseases like SLE, with close monitoring throughout pregnancy of the patient and the fetus.

Pregnant patients with past venous or arterial thrombosis who are on anticoagulation should receive therapeutic dose of LMWH throughout their pregnancy, as they are at a higher risk of recurrent thrombosis. After pregnancy confirmation, patient should discontinue warfarin and switch to LMWH (with or without aspirin) because warfarin has a known teratogenicity in pregnancy. In the absence of a history of thrombosis, the role of prophylactic-dose LMWH during pregnancy *to prevent thrombosis* is less certain. Based on a review of all randomized trials of patients with positive aPL, there were no thrombotic events during pregnancy among patients who were on the aspirin/placebo arms of the randomized trials [57].

Daily low-molecular-weight heparin injections throughout pregnancy may also be used to *prevent future pregnancy loss*. For patients with persistently positive aPL and pregnancy loss that meets the definition of the revised Sapporo criteria, prophylactic-dose LMWH and aspirin throughout pregnancy is recommended in the 2019 EULAR guidelines and is common practice. This is surprisingly based on limited and mixed evidence with earlier positive randomized or quasi-randomized trials, and two more recent negative randomized trials [58–62]. Despite use of LMWH/aspirin during pregnancy, the reported live birth rates of recently published cohort studies are still lower than the general population.

For those who do not meet the clinical definition of obstetrical APS (e.g., two early pregnancy losses) or have other placenta-mediated pregnancy complications, the role of LMWH is even less certain. There has been one small randomized trial published in women who had a previous early delivery for preeclampsia and/or a small-for-gestational age infant <34 weeks gestation, which showed no difference in reduction of early-onset preeclampsia among patients with positive aPLs who received LMWH versus no LMWH in pregnancy [63]. In the 2019 EULAR guidelines, either aspirin alone or LMWH/aspirin is recommended based on patient-specific risk factors and patient preference. Aspirin is recommended during pregnancy for preeclampsia prevention among patients at risk of preeclampsia, primarily based on non-APS data [64].

If patients with APS are on therapeutic-dose LMWH, then stopping 24 hours prior to induction of labor is often needed. If patients are on prophylactic-dose LMWH, this can often be stopped at least 12 hours before delivery, but may be stopped earlier if the indication is to prevent early pregnancy loss.

Postpartum, patients with APS who have had past thrombosis should transition from LMWH back to warfarin; both LMWH and VKA such as warfarin are safe in breast-feeding. For patients with APS without past thrombosis, there may be a role for LMWH thromboprophylaxis for 6 weeks postpartum, particularly if there is a high-titer or multiple positive antibodies or concomitant autoimmune disease.

Catastrophic APS Management

Catastrophic APS (CAPS) is treated aggressively with a combination of full-dose anticoagulation with unfractionated, high-dose corticosteroids, plasma exchange, and/or intravenous immunoglobulins based on recent clinical practice guideline recommendations [65]. For patients with refractory CAPS, rituximab, an anti-CD20 chimeric monoclonal antibody, has been used. Eculizumab, a humanized monoclonal antibody against complement protein C5, is a promising future therapy for CAPS that requires further study [9].

Management of Non-criteria Manifestations

Thrombocytopenia and autoimmune hemolytic anemia (AIHA) related to APS are usually mild and generally do not require any active therapeutic intervention. First-line treatment of immune thrombocytopenia is corticosteroids, with intravenous immunoglobulins as an alternative. In case of symptomatic or severe hemolytic anemia, corticosteroids are the first-line treatment, similar to autoimmune hemolytic anemia without aPL present. Immunosuppressive therapy or rituximab may be used in cases of immune-mediated cytopenias that are refractory to steroids.

Generally, no treatment is required for valve abnormalities associated with APS, but full anticoagulation therapy is recommended if emboli or thrombi are demonstrated. Of note, only a minority of patients will develop severe valve damage, thus needing surgical replacement with a mechanical valve or bioprosthesis.

The treatment of neurological manifestations associated with aPL but not meeting the revised Sapporo classification criteria (such as chorea, myelitis, and multiple sclerosis-like disease) may include corticosteroids and/or immunosuppressive agents. There is limited evidence for anticoagulation in these cases. Chorea can be managed with a symptomatic treatment based on anti-dopaminergic drugs or dopamine-depleting agents.

Patients with aPL-associated nephropathy should be treated with antiplatelet agent or anticoagulant, together with a strict control of arterial hypertension and proteinuria with angiotensin-converting enzyme inhibitors and/or angiotensin-receptor blockers. In case of concomitant lupus nephritis, introduction of immunosuppressive therapy is necessary.

References

1. Meroni PL, Argolini LM, Pontikaki I. What is known about pediatric antiphospholipid syndrome? Expert Rev Hematol. 2016;9(10):977–85.
2. Levine JS, Branch DW, Rauch J. The antiphospholipid syndrome. N Engl J Med. 2002;346(10):752–63.
3. Cervera R, Piette JC, Font J, et al. Antiphospholipid syndrome: clinical and immunologic manifestations and patterns of disease expression in a cohort of 1,000 patients. Arthritis Rheum. 2002;46(4):1019–27.
4. Shoenfeld Y. Systemic antiphospholipid syndrome. Lupus. 2003;12(7):497–8.
5. Ravelli A, Martini A. Antiphospholipid antibody syndrome in pediatric patients. Rheum Dis Clin N Am. 1997;23(3):657–76.
6. Lackner KJ, Peetz D, von Landenberg P. Revision of the Sapporo criteria for the antiphospholipid syndrome-- coming to grips with evidence and Thomas Bayes? Thromb Haemost. 2006;95(6):917–9.
7. Miyakis S, Lockshin MD, Atsumi T, et al. International consensus statement on an update of the classification criteria for definite antiphospholipid syndrome (APS). J Thromb Haemost. 2006;4(2):295–306.
8. Devreese KM, Pierangeli SS, de Laat B, et al. Testing for antiphospholipid antibodies with solid phase assays: guidance from the SSC of the ISTH. J Thromb Haemost. 2014;12(5):792–5.
9. Legault K, Schunemann H, Hillis C, et al. McMaster RARE-Bestpractices clinical practice guideline on diagnosis and management of the catastrophic antiphospholipid syndrome. J Thromb Haemost. 2018;16(8):1656–64.
10. Legault KJ, Ugarte A, Crowther MA, Ruiz-Irastorza G. Prevention of recurrent thrombosis in antiphospholipid syndrome: different from the general population? Curr Rheumatol Rep. 2016;18(5):26.
11. Chaturvedi S, Brodsky RA, McCrae KR. Complement in the pathophysiology of the antiphospholipid syndrome. Front Immunol. 2019;10:449.
12. Erkan D, Espinosa G, Cervera R. Catastrophic antiphospholipid syndrome: updated diagnostic algorithms. Autoimmun Rev. 2010;10(2):74–9.
13. Asherson RA. The catastrophic antiphospholipid syndrome. J Rheumatol. 1992;19(4):508–12.
14. Cervera R. CAPS Registry. Lupus. 2012;21(7):755–7.
15. Aguiar CL, Erkan D. Catastrophic antiphospholipid syndrome: how to diagnose a rare but highly fatal disease. Ther Adv Musculoskelet Dis. 2013;5(6):305–14.
16. Meroni PL, Borghi MO, Raschi E, Tedesco F. Pathogenesis of antiphospholipid syndrome: understanding the antibodies. Nat Rev Rheumatol. 2011;7(6):330–9.
17. Manukyan D, Muller-Calleja N, Jackel S, et al. Cofactor-independent human antiphospholipid antibodies induce venous thrombosis in mice. J Thromb Haemost. 2016;14(5):1011–20.
18. Di Simone N, Raschi E, Testoni C, et al. Pathogenic role of anti-beta 2-glycoprotein I antibodies in antiphospholipid associated fetal loss: characterisation of beta 2-glycoprotein I binding to trophoblast cells and functional effects of anti-beta 2-glycoprotein I antibodies in vitro. Ann Rheum Dis. 2005;64(3):462–7.
19. Negrini S, Pappalardo F, Murdaca G, Indiveri F, Puppo F. The antiphospholipid syndrome: from pathophysiology to treatment. Clin Exp Med. 2017;17(3):257–67.
20. Ritis K, Doumas M, Mastellos D, et al. A novel C5a receptor-tissue factor cross-talk in neutrophils links

innate immunity to coagulation pathways. J Immunol. 2006;177(7):4794–802.

21. Uthman I, Noureldine MHA, Ruiz-Irastorza G, Khamashta M. Management of antiphospholipid syndrome. Ann Rheum Dis. 2019;78(2):155–61.

22. Chaturvedi S, Braunstein EM, Yuan X, et al. Rare germline mutations in complement regulatory genes make the antiphospholipid syndrome catastrophic. Blood. 2019;134(Supplement_1):4.

23. Garcia-Carrasco M, Galarza C, Gomez-Ponce M, et al. Antiphospholipid syndrome in Latin American patients: clinical and immunologic characteristics and comparison with European patients. Lupus. 2007;16(5):366–73.

24. Avcin T, Silverman ED. Antiphospholipid antibodies in pediatric systemic lupus erythematosus and the antiphospholipid syndrome. Lupus. 2007;16(8):627–33.

25. Gomez-Puerta JA, Martin H, Amigo MC, et al. Long-term follow-up in 128 patients with primary antiphospholipid syndrome: do they develop lupus? Medicine (Baltimore). 2005;84(4):225–30.

26. Zamora-Ustaran A, Escarcega-Alarcon RO, Garcia-Carrasco M, et al. Antiphospholipid syndrome in Mexican children. Isr Med Assoc J. 2012;14(5):286–9.

27. Avcin T, Cimaz R, Silverman ED, et al. Pediatric antiphospholipid syndrome: clinical and immunologic features of 121 patients in an international registry. Pediatrics. 2008;122(5):e1100–7.

28. Cervera R, Boffa MC, Khamashta MA, Hughes GR. The euro-phospholipid project: epidemiology of the antiphospholipid syndrome in Europe. Lupus. 2009;18(10):889–93.

29. de Laat B, Derksen RH, Urbanus RT, de Groot PG. IgG antibodies that recognize epitope Gly40-Arg43 in domain I of beta 2 glycoprotein I cause LAC, and their presence correlates strongly with thrombosis. Blood. 2005;105(4):1540–5.

30. Giron-Gonzalez JA, Garcia del Rio E, Rodriguez C, Rodriguez-Martorell J, Serrano A. Antiphospholipid syndrome and asymptomatic carriers of antiphospholipid antibody: prospective analysis of 404 individuals. J Rheumatol. 2004;31(8):1560–7.

31. Mustonen P, Lehtonen KV, Javela K, Puurunen M. Persistent antiphospholipid antibody (aPL) in asymptomatic carriers as a risk factor for future thrombotic events: a nationwide prospective study. Lupus. 2014;23(14):1468–76.

32. Pengo V, Testa S, Martinelli I, et al. Incidence of a first thromboembolic event in carriers of isolated lupus anticoagulant. Thromb Res. 2015;135(1):46–9.

33. Pengo V, Ruffatti A, Legnani C, et al. Incidence of a first thromboembolic event in asymptomatic carriers of high-risk antiphospholipid antibody profile: a multicenter prospective study. Blood. 2011;118(17):4714–8.

34. Berkun Y, Padeh S, Barash J, et al. Antiphospholipid syndrome and recurrent thrombosis in children. Arthritis Rheum. 2006;55(6):850–5.

35. Schreiber K, Hunt BJ. Managing antiphospholipid syndrome in pregnancy. Thromb Res. 2019;181(Suppl 1):S41–6.

36. George D, Erkan D. Antiphospholipid syndrome. Prog Cardiovasc Dis. 2009;52(2):115–25.

37. Ravelli A, Martini A. Antiphospholipid syndrome. Pediatr Clin N Am. 2005;52(2):469–91, vi.

38. Hunt BJ. Pediatric antiphospholipid antibodies and antiphospholipid syndrome. Semin Thromb Hemost. 2008;34(3):274–81.

39. Tavil B, Ozyurek E, Gumruk F, Cetin M, Gurgey A. Antiphospholipid antibodies in Turkish children with thrombosis. Blood Coagul Fibrinolysis. 2007;18(4):347–52.

40. Berman H, Rodriguez-Pinto I, Cervera R, et al. Pediatric catastrophic antiphospholipid syndrome: descriptive analysis of 45 patients from the "CAPS Registry". Autoimmun Rev. 2014;13(2):157–62.

41. Thornburg C, Pipe S. Neonatal thromboembolic emergencies. Semin Fetal Neonatal Med. 2006;11(3):198–206.

42. Boffa MC, Lachassinne E. Infant perinatal thrombosis and antiphospholipid antibodies: a review. Lupus. 2007;16(8):634–41.

43. Peixoto MV, de Carvalho JF, Rodrigues CE. Clinical, laboratory, and therapeutic analyses of 21 patients with neonatal thrombosis and antiphospholipid antibodies: a literature review. J Immunol Res. 2014;2014:672603.

44. Boffa MC, Aurousseau MH, Lachassinne E, et al. European register of babies born to mothers with antiphospholipid syndrome. Lupus. 2004;13(9):713–7.

45. Mekinian A, Lachassinne E, Nicaise-Roland P, et al. European registry of babies born to mothers with antiphospholipid syndrome. Ann Rheum Dis. 2013;72(2):217–22.

46. Schmidt B, Andrew M. Neonatal thrombosis: report of a prospective Canadian and international registry. Pediatrics. 1995;96(5 Pt 1):939–43.

47. Mekinian A, Carbillon L, Nicaise-Roland P, et al. Mothers' antiphospholipid antibodies during pregnancy and the relation to offspring outcome. Clin Exp Rheumatol. 2014;32(3):446.

48. Hernandez-Molina G, Espericueta-Arriola G, Cabral AR. The role of lupus anticoagulant and triple marker positivity as risk factors for rethrombosis in patients with primary antiphospholipid syndrome. Clin Exp Rheumatol. 2013;31(3):382–8.

49. Goldenberg NA, Knapp-Clevenger R, Hays T, Manco-Johnson MJ. Lemierre's and Lemierre's-like syndromes in children: survival and thromboembolic outcomes. Pediatrics. 2005;116(4):e543–8.

50. Shoenfeld Y, Blank M, Cervera R, Font J, Raschi E, Meroni PL. Infectious origin of the antiphospholipid syndrome. Ann Rheum Dis. 2006;65(1):2–6.

51. Belizna C. Hydroxychloroquine as an anti-thrombotic in antiphospholipid syndrome. Autoimmun Rev. 2015;14(4):358–62.

52. Crowther MA, Ginsberg JS, Julian J, et al. A comparison of two intensities of warfarin for the prevention of recurrent thrombosis in patients with the antiphospholipid antibody syndrome. N Engl J Med. 2003;349(12):1133–8.

53. Finazzi G, Marchioli R, Brancaccio V, et al. A randomized clinical trial of high-intensity warfarin vs. conventional antithrombotic therapy for the prevention of recurrent thrombosis in patients with the antiphospholipid syndrome (WAPS). J Thromb Haemost. 2005;3(5):848–53.

54. von Vajna E, Alam R, So TY. Current clinical trials on the use of direct oral anticoagulants in the pediatric population. Cardiol Ther. 2016;5(1):19–41.

55. Ordi-Ros J, Saez-Comet L, Perez-Conesa M, et al. Rivaroxaban versus vitamin K antagonist in antiphospholipid syndrome: a randomized noninferiority trial. Ann Intern Med. 2019;171(10):685–94.

56. Garcia D, Erkan D. Diagnosis and Management of the Antiphospholipid Syndrome. N Engl J Med. 2018;378(21):2010–21.

57. Skeith L. Anticoagulating patients with high-risk acquired thrombophilias. Blood. 2018;132(21):2219–29.

58. Kutteh WH. Antiphospholipid antibody-associated recurrent pregnancy loss: treatment with heparin and low-dose aspirin is superior to low-dose aspirin alone. Am J Obstet Gynecol. 1996;174(5):1584–9.

59. Rai R, Cohen H, Dave M, Regan L. Randomised controlled trial of aspirin and aspirin plus heparin in pregnant women with recurrent miscarriage associated with phospholipid antibodies (or antiphospholipid antibodies). BMJ. 1997;314(7076):253–7.

60. Goel N, Tuli A, Choudhry R. The role of aspirin versus aspirin and heparin in cases of recurrent abortions with raised anticardiolipin antibodies. Med Sci Monit. 2006;12(3):CR132–6.

61. Laskin CA, Spitzer KA, Clark CA, et al. Low molecular weight heparin and aspirin for recurrent pregnancy loss: results from the randomized, controlled HepASA trial. J Rheumatol. 2009;36(2):279–87.

62. Farquharson RG, Quenby S, Greaves M. Antiphospholipid syndrome in pregnancy: a randomized, controlled trial of treatment. Obstet Gynecol. 2002;100(3):408–13.

63. van Hoorn ME, Hague WM, van Pampus MG, Bezemer D, de Vries JI, Investigators F. Low-molecular-weight heparin and aspirin in the prevention of recurrent early-onset pre-eclampsia in women with antiphospholipid antibodies: the FRUIT-RCT. Eur J Obstet Gynecol Reprod Biol. 2016;197:168–73.

64. Rolnik DL, Wright D, Poon LCY, et al. ASPRE trial: performance of screening for preterm pre-eclampsia. Ultrasound Obstet Gynecol. 2017;50(4):492–5.

65. Erkan D. Therapeutic and prognostic considerations in catastrophic antiphospholipid syndrome. Autoimmun Rev. 2006;6(2):98–103.

Thrombotic Microangiopathy in the Adolescent Female

25

Clay T. Cohen, Tammuella Chrisentery Singleton, and Sarah E. Sartain

Adolescent and young adult females have menstrual cycles that can be associated with menorrhagia, anemia, fatigue, and headaches. While understanding these common occurrences, it is important to note the possibility of a rare but life-threatening disorder with similar, yet progressive symptoms. Bleeding is accompanied by thrombocytopenia, microangiopathic hemolytic anemia (MAHA), and organ dysfunction which are defining features consistent with a group of disorders known as thrombotic microangiopathy (TMA). The family of TMA that affect children and adolescents typically include thrombotic thrombocytopenic purpura (TTP), hemolytic uremic syndrome (HUS) caused by Shiga toxin-producing *Escherichia coli* (STEC), and complement-, metabolism-,and drug-mediated TMA [1]. Additionally, there are several "TMA-like" disorders that can present similarly to TMA, including disseminated intravascular coagulation (DIC), *h*emolysis, *e*levated *l*iver enzymes, and *l*ow *p*latelets of pregnancy (HELLP syndrome), and severe hypertension (Table 25.1).

C. T. Cohen (✉) · S. E. Sartain
Department of Pediatrics, Section of Hematology-Oncology, Baylor College of Medicine, Texas Children's Hospital, Houston, TX, USA
e-mail: ctcohen@texaschildrens.org

T. C. Singleton
Pediatric Hematology, Mississippi Center for Advanced Medicine, Madison, MS, USA

The MAHA and platelet consumption associated with TMA contributes to organ dysfunction resulting from microvascular thrombosis and endothelial damage [2]. Although these conditions have similar clinical presentations, the underlying pathophysiology is different. TTP is a rare disease, with the first instance reported in the literature by Moschocowitz in an adolescent female [3]. TTP results from a severe deficiency of the von Willebrand factor (VWF)-cleaving protease ADAMTS13 (a disintegrin and metalloproteinase with a thrombospondin type 1 motif, member 13) [2, 4]. This severe deficiency results in an accumulation of ultra-large VWF multimers that causes platelet aggregation in the microvasculature [1, 4–7]. The deficiency of ADAMTS13 activity can be acquired, due to anti-ADAMTS13 autoantibodies or congenital (Upshaw-Schulman syndrome). Acquired TTP is a relatively rare disorder, with an annual estimated incidence of 1/250,000. It is estimated that only 5% of patients with TTP present with the congenital form, amounting to 2.2 cases per million per year [8]. However, among certain groups, congenital TTP may be more common than expected. For example, in pregnant women, congenital TTP may represent 25% of all TTP cases, and this precipitating factor would certainly include the adolescent and young adult female.

An unexpected presentation of TTP in the adolescent female can result in a delayed diagnosis with catastrophic outcomes if the signs and symptoms of the disorder are not recognized. A

© Springer Nature Switzerland AG 2020
L. V. Srivaths (ed.), *Hematology in the Adolescent Female*,
https://doi.org/10.1007/978-3-030-48446-0_25

Table 25.1 Thrombotic microangiopathy syndromes in the adolescent female

TMA disorder	Pathophysiology	Key findings	Treatment
TTP	Deficiency or inhibitor to ADAMTS13	Microangiopathic hemolytic anemia, thrombocytopenia, ADAMTS13 activity<10% Lack of coagulation abnormalities, mild kidney dysfunction (if present), +/− neurological changes	Acquired TTP: plasma exchange, glucocorticoids, +/− rituximab or other immunosuppressive agent Congenital TTP: plasma infusion
Complement-mediated TMA	Uncontrolled activation of the alternative complement pathway (increased formation and activity of the C5b-9 complex)	Acute kidney injury, hypertension No evidence of ADAMTS13 deficiency, or Shiga toxin-producing infection	Complement blockade: eculizumab Plasma exchange or infusion
ST-HUS	Infection with a Shiga toxin-producing organism	Abdominal pain, diarrhea (often bloody) Acute kidney injury	Supportive care
Metabolism-mediated TMA	Disorder of cobalamin metabolism	Elevated homocysteine and methylmalonic acid levels Neurologic sequelae, often presents in infancy	Hydroxocobalamin supplementation
Drug-mediated TMA	Drug-mediated immune reaction or toxic cellular injury	Kidney dysfunction and hypertension often with sudden onset following exposure to the offending agent	Stop offending drug Supportive care
Coagulation-mediated TMA	Genetic mutations in thrombomodulin, plasminogen, or diacylglycerol kinase ε	Acute kidney injury, often presenting in infancy	Plasma exchange/infusion Anti-complement therapy
HELLP syndrome	Unclear, may be severe form of preeclampsia or due to complement dysregulation	Hemolysis, elevated liver proteins, and low platelets Often presents in the third trimester of pregnancy	Delivery of the fetus with associated pregnancy-related supportive care

TTP thrombotic thrombocytopenic purpura, *TMA* thrombotic microangiopathy, *ST-HUS* Shiga toxin-mediated hemolytic uremic syndrome

familiarity with primary TMA syndromes and other TMA-mimicking systemic disorders could prevent a delay in diagnosis and facilitate lifesaving intervention. Distinguishing among the different types of TMA disorders can be diagnostically difficult; however, subsequent management decisions depend upon the confirmation of the etiology of the TMA to determine the appropriate therapy [9, 10].

Diagnostic Considerations in TMA

TTP

TTP is one of the hematological emergencies with a high mortality rate and often rapid clinical progression that must be considered when approaching a patient with suspected TMA. Classically, TTP has been described by a pentad of clinical signs and symptoms: thrombocytopenia, MAHA, neurological abnormalities, renal dysfunction, and fever. In clinical practice, however, TTP rarely presents with all of the findings of the pentad [11]. The combination of thrombocytopenia (frequently below 20,000 cells/μL), MAHA (presence of schistocytes on the peripheral smear), and an elevated lactate dehydrogenase (LDH) is sufficient to suspect TTP [1, 10, 12]. Patients with acute onset TTP often have vague, nonspecific symptoms and may present critically ill, appearing only mildly affected, or anywhere in-between. The cause of TTP is a marked reduction of the VWF multimer-cleaving protease, ADAMTS13. Decreased ADAMTS13 activity results in erythrocyte fragmentation due to increased platelet adhesion to unprocessed, ultra-large VWF multimers in the microcirculation [1]. TTP is usually caused by an acquired inhibitory antibody to ADAMTS13 and less commonly secondary to a congenital deficiency of ADAMTS13 [13]. It is important to note that women with hereditary TTP may have their first presentation of the disease during pregnancy [14, 15]. Mutational analysis in pregnancy has been previously evaluated, and a predominance of the exon 24 missense mutation c.3178C > T in a homozygous and compound heterozygous form was noted [16]. Knowledge of genetic mutations may help with early detection and early intervention in patients presenting with congenital TTP as adolescents or young adults [16–19]. This association with pregnancy and delayed onset of symptoms in women may also be related to phenotypic variability that can be seen even within families [13, 17, 19, 20].

In a case of suspected TTP, the diagnosis is confirmed by noting a severe deficiency of ADAMTS13 activity (<10%) [21]. However, ADAMTS13 activity assays are often not readily available, and treatment should begin prior to confirmation of the diagnosis if there is a high index of suspicion for TTP. In addition to MAHA and thrombocytopenia, additional laboratory evaluation will note normal coagulation studies (D-dimers, prothrombin time [PT], partial thromboplastin time [PTT], and fibrinogen levels), negative Coombs testing, and often reticulocytosis and elevated indirect bilirubin.

Complement-Mediated TMA

Complement-mediated TMA, including atypical HUS and TMA occurring after bone marrow or solid tumor transplantation, is caused by uncontrolled activation of the alternative complement pathway leading to acute kidney injury and failure. The underlying defect is an inherited or acquired over production of complement components or inhibition of complement regulatory proteins, resulting in increased C3 hydrolysis, and ultimately formation of the C5b-9 terminal complement (or membrane-attack) complex [22–26]. This increase in complement activity leads to

cellular injury, platelet and neutrophil activation, endothelial cell injury, and glomerular capillary and arteriole thrombi development, resulting in acute kidney injury and hypertension [27, 28]. While most laboratories do not offer diagnostic laboratory tests, the diagnosis of complement-mediated TMA can be confirmed through complement genetic studies (including testing the following genes: *CFH, CD46, CFI, C3, CFB, THBD, CFHR1, CFHR5,* and *DGKE1*) [29]. Additional laboratory investigation that may be helpful includes complement studies, including complement protein levels (C3, C4, complement factor [F]B), complement regulatory protein levels (FH, FI), and complement split products (soluble C5b-9) [29]. Diagnostic criteria include kidney dysfunction (elevated creatinine), MAHA, thrombocytopenia, an ADAMTS13 activity >10% (excluding TTP), and negative stool tests for Shiga toxin-producing infection (excluding STEC-HUS) [30].

STEC-HUS

STEC-HUS often presents with bloody diarrhea in addition to renal dysfunction. As opposed to complement-mediated TMA, the cause is glomerular endothelial cell injury secondary to the Shiga exotoxin following infection with a Shiga toxin-producing organism. The most common age of presentation of STEC-HUS is between 1 and 5 years of age and less likely to occur during the adolescent time period [31].

Drug-Mediated TMA

Drug-mediated TMA can occur secondary to an immunologic reaction or to a toxic dose-related reaction [13]. Quinine was the first drug found to induce TMA through the development of platelet-reactive antibodies and endothelial cell activation [32]. Clinical relapses may occur following cessation of the offending agent upon re-exposure. Many drugs used with solid organ and allogenic bone marrow transplant have also been implicated in episodes of TMA, including sirolimus, cyclosporine, etoposide, cytarabine, and mitomycin [33–35]. Intravenous injection of the oral long-acting opioid oxymorphone hydrochloride has recently been associated with a toxic, dose-dependent drug-mediated TMA [36, 37]. Presentation of drug-mediated TMA is often sudden, with acute kidney injury developing within hours of exposure to the offending drug [13].

Other TMA Disorders

Additional causes of TMA include metabolism-mediated and coagulation-mediated TMA. In both classes TMA is caused by a hereditary defect and tends to present early in life (often the first year of life) though later presentation is possible. Metabolism-mediated TMA involves disorders of cobalamin (vitamin B-12) metabolism [38]. Coagulation-mediated TMAs are caused by genetic abnormalities in diacylglycerol kinase ε (DGKE), protein kinase C, or thrombomodulin [39, 40]. HELLP syndrome (*h*emolysis, *e*levated *l*iver enzymes, and *l*ow *p*latelets) is a TMA that occurs during pregnancy.

TMA-Mimicking Disorders

There are additional TMA-mimicking disorders that should also be considered when approaching an adolescent patient with possible TMA. DIC will present with the combination of thrombocytopenia and MAHA, though will also have coagulation abnormalities (abnormal PT, PTT, D-dimer, and fibrinogen) in the setting of a systemic illness. Thrombocytopenia and anemia (with the presence of schistocytes in some cases) can occur in the pregnancy-related condition preeclampsia. Severe hypertension can also cause a TMA-like picture.

Non-TMA Disorders to Consider

Evans syndrome, immune cytopenias affecting at least two cell lines, may occur in the setting of a systemic rheumatologic disorder (systemic lupus erythematosus [SLE]) or in isolation. Anemia

and thrombocytopenia alongside reticulocytosis and an increased immature platelet fraction (indicating active replacement of the destroyed red blood cells and platelets) are typically seen. Schistocytes should not be seen in the peripheral smear of an Evans syndrome patient. A number of different infections may present with MAHA and should also be considered and ruled out; these include human immunodeficiency virus (HIV) and cytomegalovirus as well as systemic bacterial infections.

Initial Evaluation

When presented with an adolescent patient with anemia and thrombocytopenia, timely evaluation and a systematic approach are necessary to avoid the consequences of delayed diagnosis and treatment. Confirmation of schistocytes on the peripheral smear will indicate that the anemia is secondary to a microangiopathy. A review of all medications (including over the counter and illicit drugs) is important to ensure there is not the presence of TMA-associated drugs. A pregnancy test will rule out TMA-mimicking diagnoses (preeclampsia and HELLP syndrome) if negative. In addition to a complete blood count (CBC), the laboratory evaluation should also include coagulation studies (D-dimer, PT, PTT, and fibrinogen levels). An abnormal coagulation profile in the setting of an acutely ill patient will differentiate DIC from TTP (as TTP should have a normal coagulation profile). A chemistry panel is important to check creatinine and possible electrolyte abnormalities in the setting of kidney dysfunction. If necessary, additional labs to confirm intravascular hemolysis may be helpful, including decreased haptoglobin and increased plasma hemoglobin. Direct antiglobulin, or Coombs, testing will be negative in TMA syndromes. Homocysteine, methylmalonic acid, and vitamin B-12 levels should be obtained to rule out severe vitamin B-12 deficiency as the cause of TMA. If other signs and symptoms are present that may indicate a systemic rheumatological condition (joint pain, rashes, etc.), it may be helpful to obtain serologic testing for SLE and other autoimmune diseases. Considering serologic testing is especially important prior to the initiation of plasma exchange in the setting of possible TTP. Blood cultures and infection specific testing (HIV as an example) should be obtained in patients with possible systemic infections. Stool cultures and Shiga toxin testing should also be obtained in the presence of bloody diarrhea to rule out STEC-HUS. Head imaging is warranted with neurological changes due to the risk of intracranial hemorrhage and infarction in the setting of TMA syndromes, acute kidney injury, and hypertension.

While the above evaluation is important, if there is suspicion for TTP (which should be present in the setting of MAHA, thrombocytopenia, and an elevated LDH), clinical evaluation should not delay the initiation of therapy for TTP. Though a deficiency of ADAMTS13 (<10%) is necessary to confirm the diagnosis of TTP, initiation of treatment for presumed TTP should not wait on the laboratory results.

Management of Thrombotic Microangiopathy

TMA is a serious condition that should be treated promptly to reverse the microangiopathic process and halt end-organ damage. Distinguishing among the different types of TMA can be diagnostically challenging, often leading to treatment delays. Initial management decisions should be based upon whether there is a high suspicion for TTP or complement-mediated TMA, as therapies differ between these distinct TMA syndromes.

TTP

Because of the high risk of sudden decompensation, the adolescent female with presumed TTP should be treated immediately, without waiting for diagnostic testing to result [41]. While plasma infusion is the most appropriate therapy for congenital TTP, plasma exchange is the preferred treatment for acquired TTP, as it replenishes ADAMTS13 and removes the anti-ADAMTS13 autoantibodies and ultra-large VWF multimers. High-dose corticosteroids should be simultaneously initiated to inhibit antibody production for a more sustained response [42, 43]. It is also critical to eliminate or treat the offending cause, such as drugs, infection, or other autoimmune process. Plasma exchange should occur daily until the platelet count has normalized (>150,000/mm3 for at least 1 day), LDH has decreased to normal levels, hemoglobin has begun to rise, and ADAMTS13 levels have risen above 10% [44, 45]. The duration of plasma exchange varies greatly, with most studies reporting a treatment duration of 7–20 days [12, 46].

Patients with a more severe course, or those with multiple exacerbations or relapses, may benefit from stronger immunosuppression [47]. Rituximab, an anti-CD20 monoclonal antibody, is an immunosuppressive agent considered a standard second-line therapy for antibody-mediated TTP. Recent studies evaluating rituximab as a first-line agent in combination with plasma exchange, or as prophylaxis against relapse, have been promising [43, 48, 49]. The drug is especially efficacious in patients with evidence of TTP and underlying systemic autoimmunity [50] and, therefore, must be considered in the adolescent female patient.

A variety of other immunosuppressive agents have been trialed in the treatment of TTP, including vincristine, cyclophosphamide, azathioprine, cyclosporine A, intravenous immunoglobulin, mycophenolate mofetil, and bortezomib. Results of these case reports and retrospective reviews are varied [51–54]. Splenectomy has been performed as a measure to prevent TTP relapse with some success [55], but is not routinely recommended because of the complications and infection risk with which it is associated.

Decisions on the most appropriate treatment regimen for a particular patient can be challenging, given the number and different therapies available. The adolescent female poses an even greater challenge because, depending on age, this population could be considered for adult-based treatment regimens. In adult TTP, the PLASMIC score is a tool that can be used to quantify the likelihood of TTP by assigning points for a number of clinical features [56, 57]. Patients who are deemed intermediate- to high-risk (scores of 5–7) should likely begin more intensive treatment regimens with glucocorticoids and rituximab in addition to plasma exchange.

Complement-Mediated TMA

Because immediately available confirmatory tests for complement-mediated TMA are lacking, the decision to treat TMA with anti-complement therapy should be based on a presumptive clinical diagnosis. Therapy should be initiated rapidly, within 24–48 hours of presentation, in order to halt the irreversible renal injury observed.

Treatment of the complement-mediated TMAs involves complement blockade, plasma exchange or infusion, and/or supportive measures. Complement blockade is achieved with the humanized monoclonal antibody to C5, eculizumab. This agent blocks C5 cleavage by the C5 convertase of the alternative complement pathway, thereby preventing the production of the terminal complement components C5a and the membrane-attack complex C5b-9 [58]. Eculizumab is administered as an intravenous infusion in weekly doses, usually up to 4 weeks, followed by a maintenance regimen consisting of every-other-week dosing, which may continue for months, or even indefinitely, depending on the cause of the TMA [59–61]. The eculizumab dose or schedule should be altered to achieve complete complement suppression, measured by CH50 assay [62, 63]. There is risk for life-threatening meningococcal infections with eculizumab treatment, and, therefore, patients should receive vaccinations for *Neisseria meningitidis*, *S. pneumoniae*, and *Haemophilus influenza* type b prior to treatment.

The annual cost of eculizumab therapy is estimated to be greater than $400,000 [64], and, thus, its use may be prohibitive in the treatment of complement-mediated TMA. In this case, plasma therapy is a reasonable intervention, although only about one-half of patients with complement-mediated TMA will respond [65, 66]. Plasma exchange is likely more efficacious than plasma

infusion as it will function to remove unwanted complement activation products and antibodies against complement proteins, in addition to replacing any deficient complement components. Patients with complement-mediated TMA caused by antibodies against complement factor H may benefit from immune suppression in addition to plasma exchange or eculizumab [67, 68].

Supportive care for complement-mediated TMA includes red blood cell and platelet transfusion, correction of electrolyte abnormalities, and, in cases of severe renal disease, dialysis [69].

TMA Syndromes and TMA-Mimicking Disorders

Management of STEC-HUS is primarily based on supportive care, but in cases where there is severe central nervous system involvement, plasma therapy and/or anti-complement therapy may be trialed. Treatment of drug-induced TMA is discontinuation of the offending drug, while treatment of metabolism-mediated TMA is by administration of high-dose hydroxocobalamin. Coagulation-mediated TMAs are often treated with plasma exchange or with anti-complement therapy. Management of DIC is achieved by treating the underlying cause of the DIC. Patients with SLE who also present with MAHA, thrombocytopenia, nephritis, and TMA on kidney biopsy are best managed by the treatment of the SLE rather than with TTP-specific treatment. Finally, hypertension-related TMA is managed with anti-hypertensive therapy, while HELLP syndrome is ultimately treated by delivery of the fetus.

Outcomes of Thrombotic Microangiopathy

TTP

TTP is a life-threatening condition with high morbidity and mortality. The mortality rate in untreated TTP approaches 90% [14] but with treatment is approximately 10–20% [12]. A high percentage of patients with acquired TTP eventually develop other underlying autoimmune diseases, including SLE and anti-phospholipid antibody syndrome [11, 70, 71]. A thorough screening for signs and symptoms of autoimmunity should be performed, and development of symptoms should be monitored over time. Relapses occur in 20–65% of TTP patients [72–74]. Relapse rates are high in patients presenting with severe ADAMTS13 deficiency (<10%) and can be common in patients with an underlying autoimmune disorder [11, 47, 72, 73]. Relapses are most common in the year following the initial TTP episode [72]. TTP survivors can develop varying degrees of neuropsychological deficits, including problems with memory, cognition, concentration, and depression, which can severely affect quality of life [75].

Complement-Mediated TMA

Mortality rates in complement-mediated TMA approach 20–25% [63, 65, 76, 77]. In those that survive, renal injury can be devastating, with many patients progressing to chronic kidney disease or even end stage renal disease (ESRD) requiring renal transplantation. In complement-mediated TMA specifically, mortality is higher in children than adults (6.7% versus 0.8% at 1 year), but adults have a higher likelihood of progressing to ESRD than children (46% versus 16%) at initial presentation [78]. Prognosis in complement-mediated TMA is dependent on genotype, with variability in the clinical course and outcome depending on the affected complement component.

New Therapies on the Horizon for Thrombotic Microangiopathy

An emerging therapy for TTP is recombinant ADAMTS13 [79, 80], which is currently in Phase 3 trials. This product was developed as a replacement product for use in congenital TTP but may have potential use in acquired TTP as well.

Another therapy that has recently shown efficacy in a small group of patients is the factor concentrate Koate-DVI, which is a FVIII/VWF biologic product indicated for FVIII replacement therapy in hemophilia A. This product has higher concentrations of ADAMTS13 than other plasma-derived concentrates and currently available plasma. A cohort of eight congenital TTP patients have been successfully treated for varying periods with this agent [81]. While it requires more study, this factor shows promise as a potential agent that can be used in an outpatient setting to prevent or treat acute exacerbations of TTP.

Most recently, a Phase 3 trial of caplacizumab, an anti-VWF humanized immunoglobulin fragment that functions by inhibiting the interaction between VWF and platelets, has shown promise as a potential therapy for acquired TTP. In this study, treatment with caplacizumab was associated with (1) a faster normalization of platelet count; (2) a lower incidence of TTP-related death, recurrence of TTP, or a thromboembolic event during the treatment period; and (3) a lower rate of recurrence of TTP during the trial than the placebo [82]. Caplacizumab efficacy and safety have not been evaluated in the pediatric or adolescent population, but in the adult population, it is often considered in patients with severe features of TTP, such as neurologic abnormalities, who warrant more aggressive initial therapy. Adolescent females approaching adult age may be candidates for this therapeutic agent.

There has been a recent effort to develop complement-blocking agents that target the alternative complement pathway amplification loop, which is a major driving force behind complement activation in the complement-mediated TMAs. Agents targeting complement components C3, FB, FD, and properdin are under different stages of development [83]. These agents provide an upstream inhibition of complement prior to current complement-blocking agent, eculizumab, and may have more impact on terminal complement pathway inhibition.

In conclusion, TMAs are a group of disorders that have life-threatening consequences if not recognized and treated in a timely manner. Adolescent women are a unique population, and clinicians caring for them should be aware of the

TMA syndromes, and disorders closely mimicking TMA, to avoid damaging delays in diagnosis and treatment.

References

1. Moake JL. Thrombotic microangiopathies. N Engl J Med. 2002;347(8):589–600.
2. Furlan M, Robles R, Solenthaler M, Wassmer M, Sandoz P, Lammle B. Deficient activity of von Willebrand factor-cleaving protease in chronic relapsing thrombotic thrombocytopenic purpura. Blood. 1997;89(9):3097–103.
3. Moschcowitz E. Hyaline thrombosis of the terminal arterioles and capillaries: a hitherto undescribed disease. Proc N Y Pathol Soc. 1924;24:21–4.
4. Furlan M, Lammle B. Aetiology and pathogenesis of thrombotic thrombocytopenic purpura and haemolytic uraemic syndrome: the role of von Willebrand factor-cleaving protease. Best Pract Res Clin Haematol. 2001;14(2):437–54.
5. Furlan M, Robles R, Galbusera M, Remuzzi G, Kyrle PA, Brenner B, et al. von Willebrand factor-cleaving protease in thrombotic thrombocytopenic purpura and the hemolytic-uremic syndrome. N Engl J Med. 1998;339(22):1578–84.
6. Tsai HM, Lian EC. Antibodies to von Willebrand factor-cleaving protease in acute thrombotic thrombocytopenic purpura. N Engl J Med. 1998;339(22):1585–94.
7. Fujimura Y, Matsumoto M, Isonishi A, Yagi H, Kokame K, Soejima K, et al. Natural history of Upshaw-Schulman syndrome based on ADAMTS13 gene analysis in Japan. J Thromb Haemost. 2011;9 Suppl 1:283–301.
8. Levy GG, Nichols WC, Lian EC, Foroud T, McClintick JN, McGee BM, et al. Mutations in a member of the ADAMTS gene family cause thrombotic thrombocytopenic purpura. Nature. 2001;413(6855):488–94.
9. George JN. Congenital thrombotic thrombocytopenic purpura: lessons for recognition and management of rare syndromes. Pediatr Blood Cancer. 2008;50(5):947–8.
10. Scully M, Hunt BJ, Benjamin S, Liesner R, Rose P, Peyvandi F, et al. Guidelines on the diagnosis and management of thrombotic thrombocytopenic purpura and other thrombotic microangiopathies. Br J Haematol. 2012;158(3):323–35.
11. George JN. How I treat patients with thrombotic thrombocytopenic purpura: 2010. Blood. 2010;116(20):4060–9.
12. Rock GA, Shumak KH, Buskard NA, Blanchette VS, Kelton JG, Nair RC, et al. Comparison of plasma exchange with plasma infusion in the treatment of thrombotic thrombocytopenic purpura. Canadian Apheresis Study Group. N Engl J Med. 1991;325(6):393–7.
13. George JN, Nester CM. Syndromes of thrombotic microangiopathy. N Engl J Med. 2014;371(7):654–66.
14. Moatti-Cohen M, Garrec C, Wolf M, Boisseau P, Galicier L, Azoulay E, et al. Unexpected frequency of Upshaw-Schulman syndrome in pregnancy-onset thrombotic thrombocytopenic purpura. Blood. 2012;119(24):5888–97.
15. von Auer C, von Krogh AS, Kremer Hovinga JA, Lammle B. Current insights into thrombotic microangiopathies: thrombotic thrombocytopenic purpura and pregnancy. Thromb Res. 2015;135 Suppl 1:S30–3.
16. Scully M, Thomas M, Underwood M, Watson H, Langley K, Camilleri RS, et al. Thrombotic thrombocytopenic purpura and pregnancy: presentation, management, and subsequent pregnancy outcomes. Blood. 2014;124(2):211–9.
17. Epperla N, Hemauer K, Friedman KD, George JN, Foy P. Congenital thrombotic thrombocytopenic purpura related to a novel mutation in ADAMTS13 gene and management during pregnancy. Am J Hematol. 2016;91(6):644–6.
18. von Krogh AS, Quist-Paulsen P, Waage A, Langseth OO, Thorstensen K, Brudevold R, et al. High prevalence of hereditary thrombotic thrombocytopenic purpura in central Norway: from clinical observation to evidence. J Thromb Haemost. 2016;14(1):73–82.
19. Fuchs WE, George JN, Dotin LN, Sears DA. Thrombotic thrombocytopenic purpura. Occurrence two years apart during late pregnancy in two sisters. JAMA. 1976;235(19):2126–7.
20. George JN, Charania RS. Evaluation of patients with microangiopathic hemolytic anemia and thrombocytopenia. Semin Thromb Hemost. 2013;39(2):153–60.
21. George JN. Measuring ADAMTS13 activity in patients with suspected thrombotic thrombocytopenic purpura: when, how, and why? Transfusion. 2015;55(1):11–3.
22. Fremeaux-Bacchi V, Dragon-Durey MA, Blouin J, Vigneau C, Kuypers D, Boudailliez B, et al. Complement factor I: a susceptibility gene for atypical haemolytic uraemic syndrome. J Med Genet. 2004;41(6):e84.
23. Richards A, Kemp EJ, Liszewski MK, Goodship JA, Lampe AK, Decorte R, et al. Mutations in human complement regulator, membrane cofactor protein (CD46), predispose to development of familial hemolytic uremic syndrome. Proc Natl Acad Sci U S A. 2003;100(22):12966–71.
24. Goicoechea de Jorge E, Harris CL, Esparza-Gordillo J, Carreras L, Arranz EA, Garrido CA, et al. Gain-of-function mutations in complement factor B are associated with atypical hemolytic uremic syndrome. Proc Natl Acad Sci U S A. 2007;104(1):240–5.
25. Ying L, Katz Y, Schlesinger M, Carmi R, Shalev H, Haider N, et al. Complement factor H gene mutation associated with autosomal recessive atypical hemolytic uremic syndrome. Am J Hum Genet. 1999;65(6):1538–46.
26. Dragon-Durey MA, Loirat C, Cloarec S, Macher MA, Blouin J, Nivet H, et al. Anti-Factor H autoantibodies

associated with atypical hemolytic uremic syndrome. J Am Soc Nephrol. 2005;16(2):555–63.

27. Sperati CJ, Moliterno AR. Thrombotic microangiopathy: focus on atypical hemolytic uremic syndrome. Hematol Oncol Clin North Am. 2015;29(3):541–59.

28. Greenbaum LA. Atypical hemolytic uremic syndrome. Adv Pediatr. 2014;61(1):335–56.

29. Goodship TH, Cook HT, Fakhouri F, Fervenza FC, Fremeaux-Bacchi V, Kavanagh D, et al. Atypical hemolytic uremic syndrome and C3 glomerulopathy: conclusions from a "Kidney Disease: Improving Global Outcomes" (KDIGO) Controversies Conference. Kidney Int. 2017;91(3):539–51.

30. Legendre CM, Licht C, Muus P, Greenbaum LA, Babu S, Bedrosian C, et al. Terminal complement inhibitor eculizumab in atypical hemolytic-uremic syndrome. N Engl J Med. 2013;368(23):2169–81.

31. Fakhouri F, Zuber J, Fremeaux-Bacchi V, Loirat C. Haemolytic uraemic syndrome. Lancet (London, England). 2017;390(10095):681–96.

32. Gottschall JL, Neahring B, McFarland JG, Wu GG, Weitekamp LA, Aster RH. Quinine-induced immune thrombocytopenia with hemolytic uremic syndrome: clinical and serological findings in nine patients and review of literature. Am J Hematol. 1994;47(4):283–9.

33. Sartelet H, Toupance O, Lorenzato M, Fadel F, Noel LH, Lagonotte E, et al. Sirolimus-induced thrombotic microangiopathy is associated with decreased expression of vascular endothelial growth factor in kidneys. Am J Transplant. 2005;5(10):2441–7.

34. Rabadi SJ, Khandekar JD, Miller HJ. Mitomycin-induced hemolytic uremic syndrome: case presentation and review of literature. Cancer Treat Rep. 1982;66(5):1244–7.

35. Moake JL, Byrnes JJ. Thrombotic microangiopathies associated with drugs and bone marrow transplantation. Hematol Oncol Clin North Am. 1996;10(2):485–97.

36. Ambruzs JM, Serrell PB, Rahim N, Larsen CP. Thrombotic microangiopathy and acute kidney injury associated with intravenous abuse of an oral extended-release formulation of oxymorphone hydrochloride: kidney biopsy findings and report of 3 cases. Am J Kidney Dis. 2014;63(6):1022–6.

37. Lammle B. Opana ER-induced thrombotic microangiopathy. Blood. 2017;129(7):808–9.

38. Koenig JC, Rutsch F, Bockmeyer C, Baumgartner M, Beck BB, Kranz B, et al. Nephrotic syndrome and thrombotic microangiopathy caused by cobalamin C deficiency. Pediatr Nephrol (Berlin, Germany). 2015;30(7):1203–6.

39. Lemaire M, Fremeaux-Bacchi V, Schaefer F, Choi M, Tang WH, Le Quintrec M, et al. Recessive mutations in DGKE cause atypical hemolytic-uremic syndrome. Nat Genet. 2013;45(5):531–6.

40. Delvaeye M, Noris M, De Vriese A, Esmon CT, Esmon NL, Ferrell G, et al. Thrombomodulin mutations in atypical hemolytic-uremic syndrome. N Engl J Med. 2009;361(4):345–57.

41. Ridolfi RL, Bell WR. Thrombotic thrombocytopenic purpura. Report of 25 cases and review of the literature. Medicine (Baltimore). 1981;60(6):413–28.

42. George JN. Clinical practice. Thrombotic thrombocytopenic purpura. N Engl J Med. 2006;354(18):1927–35.

43. Scully M, Goodship T. How I treat thrombotic thrombocytopenic purpura and atypical haemolytic uraemic syndrome. Br J Haematol. 2014;164(6):759–66.

44. Allford SL, Hunt BJ, Rose P, Machin SJ. Guidelines on the diagnosis and management of the thrombotic microangiopathic haemolytic anaemias. Br J Haematol. 2003;120(4):556–73.

45. Wu N, Liu J, Yang S, Kellett ET, Cataland SR, Li H, et al. Diagnostic and prognostic values of ADAMTS13 activity measured during daily plasma exchange therapy in patients with acquired thrombotic thrombocytopenic purpura. Transfusion. 2015;55(1):18–24.

46. Fontana S, Kremer Hovinga JA, Studt JD, Alberio L, Lammle B, Taleghani BM. Plasma therapy in thrombotic thrombocytopenic purpura: review of the literature and the Bern experience in a subgroup of patients with severe acquired ADAMTS-13 deficiency. Semin Hematol. 2004;41(1):48–59.

47. Sadler JE, Moake JL, Miyata T, George JN. Recent advances in thrombotic thrombocytopenic purpura. Hematology Am Soc Hematol Educ Program. 2004:407–23.

48. Bresin E, Gastoldi S, Daina E, Belotti D, Pogliani E, Perseghin P, et al. Rituximab as pre-emptive treatment in patients with thrombotic thrombocytopenic purpura and evidence of anti-ADAMTS13 autoantibodies. Thromb Haemost. 2009;101(2):233–8.

49. Scully M, McDonald V, Cavenagh J, Hunt BJ, Longair I, Cohen H, et al. A phase 2 study of the safety and efficacy of rituximab with plasma exchange in acute acquired thrombotic thrombocytopenic purpura. Blood. 2011;118(7):1746–53.

50. Boye J, Elter T, Engert A. An overview of the current clinical use of the anti-CD20 monoclonal antibody rituximab. Ann Oncol. 2003;14(4):520–35.

51. Tsai HM. Current concepts in thrombotic thrombocytopenic purpura. Annu Rev Med. 2006;57:419–36.

52. Ahmad HN, Thomas-Dewing RR, Hunt BJ. Mycophenolate mofetil in a case of relapsed, refractory thrombotic thrombocytopenic purpura. Eur J Haematol. 2007;78(5):449–52.

53. Shortt J, Oh DH, Opat SS. ADAMTS13 antibody depletion by bortezomib in thrombotic thrombocytopenic purpura. N Engl J Med. 2013;368(1):90–2.

54. Eskazan AE. Bortezomib therapy in patients with relapsed/refractory acquired thrombotic thrombocytopenic purpura. Ann Hematol. 2016;95(11):1751–6.

55. Fontana S, Kremer Hovinga JA, Lammle B, Mansouri TB. Treatment of thrombotic thrombocytopenic purpura. Vox Sang. 2006;90(4):245–54.

56. Jamme M, Rondeau E. The PLASMIC score for thrombotic thrombocytopenic purpura. Lancet Haemat. 2017;4(4):e148–e9.

57. Bendapudi PK, Hurwitz S, Fry A, Marques MB, Waldo SW, Li A, et al. Derivation and external validation of the PLASMIC score for rapid assessment of adults with thrombotic microangiopathies: a cohort study. Lancet Haematol. 2017;4(4):e157–e64.

58. Cofiell R, Kukreja A, Bedard K, Yan Y, Mickle AP, Ogawa M, et al. Eculizumab reduces complement activation, inflammation, endothelial damage, thrombosis, and renal injury markers in aHUS. Blood. 2015;125(21):3253–62.

59. Olson SR, Lu E, Sulpizio E, Shatzel JJ, Rueda JF, DeLoughery TG. When to stop eculizumab in complement-mediated thrombotic microangiopathies. Am J Nephrol. 2018;48(2):96–107.

60. Ardissino G, Testa S, Possenti I, Tel F, Paglialonga F, Salardi S, et al. Discontinuation of eculizumab maintenance treatment for atypical hemolytic uremic syndrome: a report of 10 cases. Am J Kidney Dis. 2014;64(4):633–7.

61. Schoettler M, Lehmann L, Li A, Ma C, Duncan C. Thrombotic microangiopathy following pediatric autologous hematopoietic cell transplantation: a report of significant end-organ dysfunction in eculizumab-treated survivors. Biol Blood Marrow Transplant. 2019;25(5):e163–e8.

62. Ardissino G, Tel F, Sgarbanti M, Cresseri D, Giussani A, Griffini S, et al. Complement functional tests for monitoring eculizumab treatment in patients with atypical hemolytic uremic syndrome: an update. Pediatr Nephrol (Berlin, Germany). 2018;33(3):457–61.

63. Jodele S, Fukuda T, Vinks A, Mizuno K, Laskin BL, Goebel J, et al. Eculizumab therapy in children with severe hematopoietic stem cell transplantation-associated thrombotic microangiopathy. Biol Blood Marrow Transplant. 2014;20(4):518–25.

64. Parker C. Eculizumab for paroxysmal nocturnal haemoglobinuria. Lancet (London, England). 2009;373(9665):759–67.

65. Noris M, Caprioli J, Bresin E, Mossali C, Pianetti G, Gamba S, et al. Relative role of genetic complement abnormalities in sporadic and familial aHUS and their impact on clinical phenotype. Clin J Am Soc Nephrol. 2010;5(10):1844–59.

66. Jodele S, Laskin BL, Goebel J, Khoury JC, Pinkard SL, Carey PM, et al. Does early initiation of therapeutic plasma exchange improve outcome in pediatric stem cell transplant-associated thrombotic microangiopathy? Transfusion. 2013;53(3):661–7.

67. Boyer O, Balzamo E, Charbit M, Biebuyck-Gouge N, Salomon R, Dragon-Durey MA, et al. Pulse cyclophosphamide therapy and clinical remission in atypical hemolytic uremic syndrome with anti-complement factor H autoantibodies. Am J Kidney Dis. 2010;55(5):923–7.

68. Sana G, Dragon-Durey MA, Charbit M, Bouchireb K, Rousset-Rouviere C, Berard E, et al. Long-term remission of atypical HUS with anti-factor H antibodies after cyclophosphamide pulses. Pediatr Nephrol (Berlin, Germany). 2014;29(1):75–83.

69. Loirat C, Fakhouri F, Ariceta G, Besbas N, Bitzan M, Bjerre A, et al. An international consensus approach to the management of atypical hemolytic uremic syndrome in children. Pediatr Nephrol (Berlin, Germany). 2016;31(1):15–39.

70. Porta C, Caporali R, Montecucco C. Thrombotic thrombocytopenic purpura and autoimmunity: a tale of shadows and suspects. Haematologica. 1999;84(3):260–9.

71. Muscal E, Edwards RM, Kearney DL, Hicks JM, Myones BL, Teruya J. Thrombotic microangiopathic hemolytic anemia with reduction of ADAMTS13 activity: initial manifestation of childhood-onset systemic lupus erythematosus. Am J Clin Pathol. 2011;135(3):406–16.

72. Kremer Hovinga JA, Vesely SK, Terrell DR, Lammle B, George JN. Survival and relapse in patients with thrombotic thrombocytopenic purpura. Blood. 2010;115(8):1500–11; quiz 662.

73. Vesely SK, George JN, Lammle B, Studt JD, Alberio L, El-Harake MA, et al. ADAMTS13 activity in thrombotic thrombocytopenic purpura-hemolytic uremic syndrome: relation to presenting features and clinical outcomes in a prospective cohort of 142 patients. Blood. 2003;102(1):60–8.

74. Sadler JE. Pathophysiology of thrombotic thrombocytopenic purpura. Blood. 2017;130(10):1181–8.

75. Lewis QF, Lanneau MS, Mathias SD, Terrell DR, Vesely SK, George JN. Long-term deficits in health-related quality of life after recovery from thrombotic thrombocytopenic purpura. Transfusion. 2009;49(1):118–24.

76. Loirat C, Fremeaux-Bacchi V. Atypical hemolytic uremic syndrome. Orphanet J Rare Dis. 2011;6:60.

77. Uderzo C, Bonanomi S, Busca A, Renoldi M, Ferrari P, Iacobelli M, et al. Risk factors and severe outcome in thrombotic microangiopathy after allogeneic hematopoietic stem cell transplantation. Transplantation. 2006;82(5):638–44.

78. Fremeaux-Bacchi V, Fakhouri F, Garnier A, Bienaime F, Dragon-Durey MA, Ngo S, et al. Genetics and outcome of atypical hemolytic uremic syndrome: a nationwide French series comparing children and adults. Clin J Am Soc Nephrol. 2013;8(4):554–62.

79. Sayani FA, Abrams CS. How I treat refractory thrombotic thrombocytopenic purpura. Blood. 2015;125(25):3860–7.

80. Schiviz A, Wuersch K, Piskernik C, Dietrich B, Hoellriegl W, Rottensteiner H, et al. A new mouse model mimicking thrombotic thrombocytopenic purpura: correction of symptoms by recombinant human ADAMTS13. Blood. 2012;119(25):6128–35.

81. Aledort LM, Singleton TC, Ulsh PJ. Treatment of congenital thrombotic thrombocytopenia Purpura: a new paradigm. J Pediatr Hematol Oncol. 2017;39(7):524–7.

82. Scully M, Cataland SR, Peyvandi F, Coppo P, Knobl P, Kremer Hovinga JA, et al. Caplacizumab treatment for acquired thrombotic thrombocytopenic Purpura. N Engl J Med. 2019;380(4):335–46.

83. Harris CL, Pouw RB, Kavanagh D, Sun R, Ricklin D. Developments in anti-complement therapy; from disease to clinical trial. Mol Immunol. 2018;102:89–119.

Part VI

Bone Marrow Failure Disorders in the Adolescent Female

Bone Marrow Failure Disorders in the Adolescent Female

Ghadir S. Sasa and Adrianna Vlachos

Hematopoiesis and Bone Marrow Failure Mechanisms

Hematopoiesis is the process of blood cell formation. It is a complex and delicate process that starts from hematopoietic pluripotent stem cells, cells that are characterized by their unique ability for both self-renewal and differentiation. Committed progenitor cells are next in the hierarchy, display more limited ability for self-renewal, and undergo several steps of differentiation and maturation, ultimately leading to the production of an adequate number of mature peripheral blood cells. This process is under significant regulation by several factors such as chemokines, cytokines, growth factors, and the bone marrow microenvironment, all of which are essential in complete function of the bone marrow cells. A full review of hematopoiesis is beyond the scope of this chapter, and readers are directed to reviewing other didactic resources [1–3].

Bone marrow failure is a term used to describe the group of disorders whereby the process of hematopoiesis has been impaired enough to affect the sufficient production of mature peripheral blood leukocytes, erythrocytes, and/or platelets. Mechanistically, several models have been proposed to result in impaired hematopoiesis [4] as follows:

1. An external injury is incurred, such as exposure of the bone marrow to irradiation or medications that halt the proliferation of stem cells. An example of this mechanism is the transient pancytopenia that occurs after a course of chemotherapy is administered to a patient with cancer.
2. The hematopoietic stem cells themselves are abnormal and unable to proliferate properly and/or undergo premature apoptosis. Inherited bone marrow failure syndromes (IBMFS) are such disorders that display flawed survival ability.
3. The immune system attacks the hematopoietic stem cells, resulting in exhaustion of the proliferative capacity of remaining cells.
4. Abnormalities in bone marrow microenvironment, which in turn inhibit hematopoiesis.

It is noteworthy that these mechanisms are not all mutually exclusive, as a patient with

G. S. Sasa (✉)
Department of Pediatrics, Section of Hematology-Oncology, Baylor College of Medicine,
Houston, TX, USA
e-mail: gssasa@texaschildrens.org

A. Vlachos
Zucker School of Medicine at Hofstra/Northwell, Division of Hematology/Oncology and Stem Cell Transplantation, Cohen Children's Medical Center, New Hyde Park, NY, USA

Feinstein Institutes for Medical Research, Manhasset, NY, USA

© Springer Nature Switzerland AG 2020
L. V. Srivaths (ed.), *Hematology in the Adolescent Female*,
https://doi.org/10.1007/978-3-030-48446-0_26

genetically abnormal cells might accrue further injury at time of exposure to marrow suppressive medications, for example.

Clinical Evaluation of the Adolescent Female with Bone Marrow Failure

Patients with bone marrow failure usually present with symptoms related to the cytopenia(s), such as easy bruising, bleeding, fatigue, or evidence of infection, depending on the affected blood cell line. Occasionally, they might be asymptomatic of their cytopenia(s), yet abnormalities in blood counts are uncovered during medical evaluation of other conditions.

Upon presentation of an adolescent with single, bi-, or pancytopenia, a careful evaluation through comprehensive medical history, physical examination, and laboratory testing are required to first discern whether the etiology of the defect is due to impaired production of blood cells or due to increased destruction and then to discern whether the cause is inherited vs acquired (Table 26.1). Destructive causes (e.g., immune cytopenias) are not the focus of this chapter and therefore will not be discussed here. Once destructive causes are excluded, the decision to the exact timing of bone marrow evaluation through aspiration and biopsy with correlative cytogenetic testing is individualized based on the severity and extent of cytopenias. However, it is prudent to proceed with prompt examination in those with severe single cytopenia and in those with bi- or pancytopenia, as earlier diagnosis of bone marrow failure aids in proper administration of directed therapy and supportive care. Bone marrow examination allows assessment of cellularity and morphology of cells and excludes the presence of hematologic malignancy, myelodysplastic syndrome, or infiltrative disorders. Cytogenetics is important again to uncover presence of clones. Genetic testing through next-generation sequencing, deletion analysis, and whole exome sequencing is increasingly and more readily being used as an adjunct to all the above to confirm and better define various inherited conditions leading to, or associated with, cytopenias. Certain molecular tests are key to screen for some inherited marrow failure disorders, such as chromosome breakage testing for Fanconi anemia or measurement of telomere lengths to evaluate for a telomere biology disorder/dyskeratosis congenita.

The importance of distinguishing between inherited and acquired causes is very important for two main reasons:

1. Treatment options are considerably different between inherited and acquired causes, as is described in depth in the following sections. Briefly, while immunosuppression might improve blood counts in a patient with idiopathic aplastic anemia, it is unlikely to result in any response in a patient with an inherited marrow failure syndrome. Additionally, while stem cell transplant might be curative of all causes of severe marrow failure, knowledge of an inherited cause would require adjustments to the stem cell transplant conditioning regimen. Transplant may require the use of reduced intensity regimens and, importantly, is vital in donor selection, for instance.

2. When a genetic/inherited cause is diagnosed, counseling and genetic testing of siblings and parents are recommended, both for reasons of choosing an unaffected marrow donor and extending medical care, therapy, and surveillance to affected family members, as needed. For the adolescent female, knowledge of risk of transmittal to offspring is important for her to know, as she ages and considers having her own children.

In conclusion, the evaluation of an adolescent female with bone marrow failure ought to be detailed and comprehensive, as ramifications of the correct diagnosis are immense to the patient and extend even beyond her to her family. This group is unique in that medical providers might oversee the possibility of an inherited cause, yet absolutely should consider and evaluate for one.

Table 26.1 Clinical and laboratory evaluation of adolescent females presenting with blood cytopenia(s), key points of consideration

Elements of evaluation	Specific evaluations	Significance of evaluation
Patient's personal history	Symptoms related to cytopenia	Establishes effect and extent of cytopenia
	Onset of symptoms	May help distinguish between inherited and acquired causes
	Environmental exposures to toxins (e.g., benzene, ionizing radiation)	May establish cause of cytopenia and may reverse with removal from exposure
	Medications	May explain cytopenia and improve with withdrawal from use
	Illicit drug use	May explain cytopenia or impact choices for treatment
	Past history of congenital abnormalities	Some abnormalities are associated with IBMFS
	Past history of growth or developmental delay	May help distinguish between inherited and acquired causes
Patient's family history	History of autoimmunity	May help point toward acquired rather than inherited causes
	History of cytopenia(s)	Favors inherited rather than acquired causes
	History of early onset or specific malignancies (e.g., MDS or HNSCC)	Favors inherited causes
	History of early graying, lung or liver failure	May indicate TBD/DC
Patient's physical examination	Growth parameters	Short stature may be associated with IBMFS; eating disorders might be an acquired and possibly reversible cause of marrow failure [111]
	Limb abnormalities	Changes could be associated to an IBMFS such as FA or DBA
	Skin and nail abnormalities (may be subtle)	Nail dystrophy, oral leukoplakia, or skin hyperpigmentation might provide diagnosis of TBD/DC; café au lait is seen in patients with FA
Basic laboratory evaluation	Complete blood count with differential	Establishes extent and severity of cytopenia(s); red cell macrocytosis might indicate inherited rather than acquired cause
	Basic metabolic panel	Assesses overall well-being of patient
	Liver function tests	Hepatitis might be associated with AA; presence of liver dysfunction may change treatment choice
	Pregnancy test	Pregnancy has been associated with onset or relapse of AA [112]; may also result in worsening anemia in DBA [75]
	Viral serology testing	May establish cause of cytopenia; baseline evaluation pre-blood transfusions; important to know as treatment options are considered (e.g., CMV status in patients who might need HSCT)
Molecular testing	FLAER-based PNH testing in patients with bi- or pancytopenia	Might be more associated with idiopathic AA rather than an IBMFS [113]
	Chromosome breakage testing	Establishes diagnosis of FA
	Telomere length testing using flow-FISH	Aids in diagnosis of TBD/DC

(continued)

Table 26.1 (continued)

Elements of evaluation	Specific evaluations	Significance of evaluation
Genetic testing	Sanger sequencing of individual genes of interest or, when a specific inherited disease is considered, gene panels of implicated genes. Whole exome sequencing to be considered when index of suspicion high for an inherited cause	May confirm a genetic/inherited cause of cytopenia; important for choosing an unaffected sibling donor for patients with IBMFS
Pathology	Bone marrow aspiration with flow cytometry	Helps assess morphology and maturation of cells; excludes malignancy
	Bone marrow biopsy	Assesses cellularity of the bone marrow; assesses for fibrosis
	Cytogenetics	Evaluates for hematologic clones

Abbreviations: *AA*, aplastic anemia, CMV cytomegalovirus, *DBA* Diamond-Blackfan anemia, *FA* Fanconi anemia, *FLAER* fluorescent aerolysin, *HSCT* hematopoietic stem cell transplantation, *IBMFS* inherited bone marrow failure syndrome, *PNH* paroxysmal nocturnal hemoglobinuria, *TBD/DC* telomere biology disorder/dyskeratosis congenita

Genetic Disorders Leading to Bone Marrow Failure

Fanconi Anemia (FA)

Fanconi anemia (FA) is a genetic disorder associated with variable congenital abnormalities, predisposition to bone marrow failure, as well as malignancy [5, 6]. The pathophysiology stems from chromosomal instability due to defects in proteins essential to DNA repair [7, 8]. Table 26.2 details modes of inheritance and genes implicated in FA, all of which comprise a pathway that repairs and removes DNA interstrand crosslinks, thereby allowing proper DNA replication and gene transcription [8]. The genes are grouped according to their function in the DNA repair pathway as upstream genes (FANCA, B, C, E, F, G, L, M, and T), ID2 complex (FANCD2 and I), and downstream genes (FANCD1, J, N, O, P, Q, R, S, U, V, and W) [9]. The upstream protein products combine to form the FA core complex upon DNA damage, which monoubiquitinates the ID2 complex, which in turn activates the downstream gene protein products, resulting in DNA repair [7, 8]. Chromosome breakage testing establishes the diagnosis of FA, where lymphoblastoid cell lines created from a proband display increased chromosomal breakage and radial ray forms when cells are exposed to diepoxybutane and mitomycin C [10]. Complementation analysis by somatic cell methods and next-generation

sequencing looking for variants in genes involved in FA confirm the diagnosis and detail the genotype [11, 12].

FA is usually diagnosed in the first decade of life at the median age of 7 years, yet it has also been diagnosed in patients as young as newborn and in those older than 50 years [13]. FA is suspected in patients who present with single cytopenias, pancytopenia, or in those with red cell macrocytosis with or without anemia and with a high fetal hemoglobin [14–16]. Physical abnormalities are found in 75% of patients with FA, most commonly in the form of abnormal skin pigmentation, short stature, and upper extremity malformations [6, 17]. On occasion, malignancies such as myelodysplastic syndrome or squamous cell carcinoma of the head and neck in young adults prompt the diagnosis of FA [17].

From a hematologic standpoint, the severity of the marrow failure state guides consideration of the treatment route [14]. For example, periodic monitoring of blood counts and marrow cellularity might be sufficient in mild marrow failure, whereas more high-risk treatment as detailed below would be needed for patients in the moderate to severe marrow failure groups. The cytopenias described in the severity scale (Table 26.3; [18]) have to be persistent and otherwise unexplained. In addition to supportive care with blood transfusions when needed and iron chelation if a patient is needing chronic red cell transfusions, options for treatment of the FA-associated marrow failure include using:

Table 26.2 Modes of inheritance of inherited marrow failure disorders and genes involved[a]

Disease	Genes involved in autosomal recessive disease	Genes involved in autosomal dominant disease	Genes involved in X-linked recessive disease
FA	*FANCA, FANCC, FANCD1/BRCA2, FANCD2, FANCE, FANCF, FANCG, FANCI, FANCJ/BRIP1, FANCL, FANCM, FANCN/PALB2, FANCO/RAD51C, FANCP/SLX4, FANCQ/ERCC4/XPF, FANCR/RAD51, FANCS/BRCA1, FANCT/UBE2T, FANCU/XRCC2, FANCV/REV7, and FANCW/RFWD3*	*FANCR/RAD51*	*FANCB*
TBD/ DC	*TERT, NOP10, NHP2, PARN, WRAP53, ACD, STN1, CTC1, RTEL1, POT1*	*TERT, TERC, NAF1, PARN, ACD, RTEL1, TINF2*	*DKC1*
SDS	*SBDS, EFL1, DNAJC21*	*SRP54*	
DBA		*RPL5, RPL11, RPL35a, RPS10, RPS24, RPS17, RPL15, RPS28, RPS29, RPS7, RPS15, RPS27a, RPS27, RPL9, RPL18, RPL26, RPL27, RPL31*	*TSR2, GATA1*

[a]Data collated from several reviews [18, 27, 61, 114]
Abbreviations: *DBA* Diamond-Blackfan anemia, *FA* Fanconi anemia, *SDS* Shwachman-Diamond Syndrome, *TBD/DC* telomere biology disorders/dyskeratosis congenita

Table 26.3 Severity of bone marrow failure in Fanconi anemia [18]

	Mild	Moderate	Severe
Absolute neutrophil count (ANC)	<1500/mm³	<1000/mm³	<500/mm³
Platelet count	150,000–50,000/mm³	<50,000/mm³	<30,000/mm³
Hemoglobin level	≥8 g/dL	<8 g/dL	<8 g/dL

1. Androgens which may improve anemia and/or thrombocytopenia and, less so, neutropenia in 50–60% of treated patients [19, 20]. This improvement might be transient. Adverse effects observed and monitored for include virilization, accelerated growth spurt with premature closure of epiphyses, hypertension, and liver toxicity such as transaminitis, cholestatic jaundice, or hepatic adenoma development [20]. Of important note, use of androgens would not prevent development of MDS or AML [19, 20].

2. Growth factors such as granulocyte colony-stimulating factor (GCSF) have been used in scenarios where patients have severe neutropenia along with a bacterial infection and usually only as a bridge to stem cell transplantation. Continued monitoring of the bone marrow for development of dysplasia or leukemia is warranted with prolonged use of GCSF [18].

3. Hematopoietic stem cell transplantation (HSCT): Hematopoietic stem cell transplantation remains the curative option for FA-associated marrow failure but is a high-risk procedure given the inherent increased sensitivity that FA patients have to chemotherapy and irradiation. Conditioning regimens have been modified to reduce toxicities experienced by FA patients and improve survival, and the current recommendations are to use reduced intensity, fludarabine-based conditioning. Guidelines for HSCT timing and type are beyond the scope of this chapter, and readers are directed to review the consensus guidelines established by the Fanconi Anemia Research Foundation in 2014 (See https://www.fanconi.org/explore/clinical-care-guidelines) and other reviews [14, 18]. It is impor-

tant to note that while HSCT cures the marrow failure state, it increases the risk of FA complications in other systems, and patients continue to warrant surveillance for organ dysfunctions as well as malignancy development [13, 21, 22].

The risk for malignancy development has come from analyses of data from several FA patient cohorts, which have compared the number of patients with certain cancers to the expected number in the database from the SEER (Surveillance, Epidemiology, and End Results) [23–26]. The information showed an overall risk of any cancer of 20- to 50-fold, solid tumors 20- to 40-fold, acute myelogenous leukemia 300- to 800-fold, head and neck squamous cell carcinoma (HNSCC) 200- to 800-fold, esophageal cancer 1300- to 6000-fold, vulvar cancer 500- to 4000-fold, and myelodysplastic syndrome more than 5000-fold [13, 23–26]. Patients with FA are at a very high risk of developing malignancies and develop them at an earlier age. Use of HSCT further increases the risk of HNSCC and gynecologic SCC, as well as non-melanoma skin cancers [5, 13].

For the adolescent female with FA-associated marrow failure, full discussion of the risks involved in each treatment modality is of paramount importance, e.g., some of the adverse effects of androgen use might not be desirable and the patient may opt to pursue HSCT instead. Alternatively, the patient might have undergone HSCT as a younger child and would need to receive education on the need for additional surveillance of the endocrine dysfunction or malignancy screening. Additionally, the hematologist often serves as the primary care provider for a patient with FA, and it is important that patients be referred to gynecologists and endocrinologists as they approach their teenage years. Issues such as delayed menarche, irregular menstruation, and excessive bleeding due to concurrent thrombocytopenia are a few examples of issue that might arise in FA adolescent female.

Telomere Biology Disorders/ Dyskeratosis Congenita

Telomere biology disorders/dyskeratosis congenita (TBD/DC) are a heterogeneous group of disorders that affect multiple systems [27, 28]. The classical form includes a mucocutaneous triad of oral leukoplakia, lacy hyperpigmented skin changes, and dystrophic nails and includes a significant predisposition to marrow failure and cancer [27, 28]. Nonhematologic features are multiple and include strictures of lacrimal ducts, esophagus, or urethra; gastrointestinal enteropathies; abnormal teeth; early gray hair; and early hair loss [27, 28].

Over the last two decades, our understanding of the pathophysiology of TBD/DC has dramatically evolved due to improved understanding of telomeres and their role in human disease [27, 29]. Telomeres are specialized nucleoprotein structures at the end of eukaryotic chromosomes which protect chromosome ends, serve to solve the "end replication" problem, and are essential for maintenance of genetic stability [29]. In humans, telomeres consist of tandem repeats of TTAGGG nucleotides and a multi-protein complex called shelterin which protects telomere ends from DNA damage response [29, 30]. The normal length of telomeres is maintained through the enzyme telomerase reverse transcriptase (encoded by *TERT*), its RNA component (encoded by *TERC*), along with the function of several other proteins [27, 29, 31]. TBD/DC occurs when maintenance of normal telomere lengths is altered to where very short telomeres are observed, which in turn, results in cellular apoptosis or senescence [27, 32]. Genetic mutations in 14 genes affecting all components of the nucleoprotein complex have been observed in patients with TBD/DC, with significant variability in inheritance patterns as noted in Table 26.2 [27].

Bone marrow failure due to premature hematopoietic stem cell exhaustion is a prominent presentation of TBD/DC, where at least a single cytopenia rate of up to 80% by the age of 30 years has been observed [28, 33]. Patients may develop a single cytopenia (frequently thrombocytopenia

[33]) before progressing to pancytopenia or later evolve into myelodysplastic syndrome [27].

Classic TBD/DC should be considered in patients with [27]:

1. All three mucocutaneous changes described above, which are often subtle findings.
2. Any one mucocutaneous change in combination with bone marrow failure and two other physical features consistent with TBD/DC.
3. Bone marrow failure, myelodysplastic syndrome, and/or pulmonary fibrosis associated with previously described pathogenic germline mutation in a TBD-associated gene.
4. Two or more features seen in TBD/DC associated with telomere length below the first percentile for age.

The testing of average telomere lengths involves flow cytometry with fluorescent in situ hybridization of telomeres in leukocyte subsets [34–36]. Using this method, measured telomere lengths of less than the first percentile in three of six of the lymphocyte subsets are both highly sensitive and specific for TBD/DC diagnosis [35, 36]. Use of this testing is widely being incorporated in assessing patients, not only with evidence of bone marrow failure and myelodysplastic syndrome but also in adults found with pulmonary fibrosis, unexplained liver disease, or early onset head and neck squamous cell carcinomas. Once a patient is identified to have very short telomeres, genetic testing further confirms the diagnosis and aids in genetic counseling being offered to affected families [27].

The management of the TBD/DC-associated marrow failure closely parallels that of patients with FA-associated marrow failure, as described above, with the following notable differences:

1. Androgens may result in response rates in 70–80% of patients, but close attention is needed to ensure safety with close monitoring for liver toxicity [37].
2. GCSF should not be used concurrently with androgens due to two reported cases of splenic peliosis and rupture [38].

3. HSCT remains the only curative option. Similar to HSCT for FA, initial studies utilizing myeloablative regimens had extremely high mortality rates due to organ toxicity, particularly of the lungs, and endothelial injury [39]. The introduction of reduced intensity, fludarabine-based conditioning regimens has improved survival rates to about 65% [40], and more recent studies are studying whether elimination of DNA alkylating agents and radiation would reduce short- and long-term complications seen in TBD/DC patients post-transplant (Clinical trials.gov NCT01659606).

Patients with TBD/DC, similar to FA, have high risks of malignancies (fourfold increase) when compared to unaffected individuals. The types of cancers seen are head and neck (~70-fold), anogenital SCC (~50-fold), MDS (~500-fold), and AML (~70-fold) [5].

The adolescent female diagnosed with TBD/DC would need care to be delivered in a center that is familiar with all manifestations of TBD/DC. The same concepts described above for FA regarding discussion of treatment options of bone marrow failure apply. As hematologists often serve as providers of comprehensive care for TBD/DC, special care needs to be given to issues such as bone health and pulmonary and liver function. Care of a TBD/DC patient post-HSCT is also unique, and efforts have been made to delineate the surveillance and follow-up of this rare patient population [22].

Shwachman-Diamond Syndrome

Shwachman-Diamond Syndrome (SDS) is a disorder characterized by exocrine pancreatic insufficiency resulting in fat malabsorption, bone marrow dysfunction, and variable skeletal abnormalities [13, 41]. Patients have a high propensity to progress to myelodysplastic syndrome (MDS) and acute myelogenous leukemia (AML) [41, 42].

Most patients with SDS are diagnosed in early childhood, although some may present in later childhood or even as adults, with the bone marrow failure component with or without mild pancreatic insufficiency [43, 44]. Diagnosing SDS has evolved over time and is reviewed in the draft consensus guidelines for diagnosis and treatment of SDS [44]. The clinical diagnosis briefly requires both of the following criteria [44]:

1. Evidence of pancreatic exocrine dysfunction, typically by testing for pancreatic enzymes (amylase, lipase, trypsinogen) and evaluating for evidence of fat malabsorption. Exclusion of other known causes of pancreatic insufficiency (e.g., cystic fibrosis, Pearson syndrome) is warranted.
2. Presence of hematological changes as described below, with exclusion of other known causes of bone marrow failure, such as FA.

Molecular diagnosis of SDS is established by presence of pathogenic biallelic mutations in *SBDS*, which is found in up to 90% of patients with SDS [41, 45]. In a small number of patients, newer genes implicated to result in disorders very similar to SDS are *DNAJC21* [46], *EFL1* [47], and *SRP54* [48] (Table 26.2). SDS is a disorder of ribosomal function, where the protein product of *SBDS* gene cooperates with elongation factor-like GTPase 1 (EFL1) to catalyze release of the ribosome anti-association factor eIF6 and activate translation [49].

Failure to thrive due to pancreatic exocrine deficiency is often the presenting symptom in children with SDS, usually within the first year of life [44]. The fat malabsorption is treated with pancreatic enzymes taken with meals and snacks [41, 50]. Often improvement in pancreatic function is seen, and patients may not require enzyme therapy during adolescence and adulthood [41]. Patients have presented with bone marrow failure/MDS/AML without significant failure to thrive or pancreatic dysfunction.

From a hematological standpoint, nearly all patients with SDS have neutropenia of variable severity, which might be intermittent or persistent [44, 51]. In addition to the quantitative defect, neutrophils have been reported to have defects in migration or chemotaxis [52–54]. Other less commonly observed cytopenias include normo- or macrocytic anemia with high fetal hemoglobin, which again might be intermittent and of fluctuating severity and mild-moderate thrombocytopenia [44, 51]. A smaller number of patients have been reported with pancytopenia [55]. Bone marrow biopsies most often have hypocellularity with left shift in granulopoiesis, and fluctuating mild dysplasia is commonly observed [44, 51]. Persistent or progressive dysplasia is concerning for malignant transformation into MDS/AML. It is important to note that patients with SDS are prone to development of cytogenetic clones, most commonly del (20) (q11) and isochromosome 7q i(7)(q10) and that mere presence of such clones does not portend evolution of MDS/AML [44, 56–58].

Use of granulocyte colony-stimulating factor (GCSF) is considered for recurrent invasive bacterial and/or fungal infection due to severe neutropenia, with the goal to use the lowest dose possible to prevent infections rather than achieve normal hematological parameters [44]. Often doses may be given a few times a week and not needed daily [44]. Allogeneic HSCT remains a curative option but is being reserved for patients who have severe cytopenias or MDS/AML [41, 44], as its application is associated with increased transplant-related toxicities, particularly of the heart, lung, and liver [59]. Use of reduced intensity regimens in more recent years has improved outcome, but further larger studies are needed to confirm safety of wider application [60].

Diamond-Blackfan Anemia

Diamond-Blackfan anemia (DBA) is a clinically and genetically heterogeneous disorder, hematologically characterized by inherited red cell aplasia. Physical anomalies, including craniofacial defects, thumb deformities, and short stature, occur in about 50% of patients. Through studies conducted by the DBA Registry and the National Cancer Institute, DBA patients have been found to have a fivefold increased risk of cancer, where the most common cancers observed are MDS/AML, colon carcinoma, osteosarcoma, and genitourinary cancers [5, 61–63].

A consensus clinical diagnosis for classic DBA states that individuals with this disorder present within the first year of life and have normochromic, macrocytic anemia, reticulocytopenia, limited cytopenias of other lineages, and a visible paucity of erythroid precursor cells in the bone marrow [64]. Elevated erythrocyte adenosine deaminase (eADA) activity is observed in over 75–90% of cases [61]. About 10% of patients present later in childhood or adolescence, or even in adulthood, with macrocytic anemia and are found to have a hypocellular bone marrow with a paucity of red cell precursors.

DBA is a ribosomopathy, as 21 genes that either code for ribosomal subunits or indirectly alter ribosomal biogenesis have been reported to result in disease. About 25% of mutations affect *RPS19* ([61]. The ribosomal gene mutations in DBA reported to date have all been heterozygous and include missense, nonsense, frameshift, and splice site mutations as well as large deletions [43, 61]. Genetic testing can currently provide a diagnosis in over 70% of cases [61, 65].

Regarding management of persistent and transfusion-dependent anemia, the majority of patients respond to glucocorticoids, with up to 80% achieving some improvement in erythropoiesis [66]. The exact mechanism by which glucocorticoids resolves the defect in erythropoiesis has been under investigation for quite some time. Evidence has shown that there is nonspecific anti-apoptotic effect on erythroid progenitors at the colony-forming unit-erythroid/proerythroblast progenitor interface [66]. In the mouse model Flygare et al. demonstrated increased red cell production through self-renewal of the burst-forming unit-erythroid [66–68]. Up to 20% of patients are able to enter into a state of remission by age 25 years, some of which might be spontaneous and not necessarily related to treatment with glucocorticoids [66]. Long-term administration of glucocorticoids, however, can be deleterious and has been reported to result in impaired bone health, hypertension, diabetes mellitus, and cataract formation, among other adverse effects in patients with DBA [69, 70]. Therefore, it is advisable to maintain patients on the lowest dose of glucocor-

ticoids that allows for an adequate hemoglobin response [71].

Chronic red cell transfusions are needed in those patients whose erythroid defect is refractory to glucocorticoids, along with need for iron chelation to minimize the secondary effects of iron overload. Allogeneic SCT should be considered early in such patients, particularly if an unaffected matched sibling donor is available, as improved survival was noted when matched sibling donor SCT was implemented in patients younger than 9 years [71]. The role of unrelated donor SCT and exact timing of SCT consideration remains unclear and requires further larger studies, though use of treosulfan-based conditioning is showing promising results [60].

There are several considerations regarding DBA in the adolescent female. First, continued surveillance for adverse effects of chronic steroid use or iron overload is warranted, including involvement of subspecialists such as endocrinologists and gynecologists who are familiar with this disorder when possible, as some clinical observational studies suggest that females with DBA have an increased incidence of delayed puberty, irregular menstrual cycles, and decreased fertility [72–74]. Second, counseling is needed regarding the risk for malignancies as the onset of such malignancies may occur during adolescent or early adulthood years [62, 63] and the adolescent needs to report symptoms, such as extremity swelling, abdominal discomfort, and rectal bleeding, to allow for early diagnosis and treatment. Thirdly, recurrence of anemia after being in a remission or stable state on glucocorticoid therapy can occur and has been reported during puberty and pregnancy. During puberty, increases in the glucocorticoid doses may be necessary. However, if the dose increases over the maximum maintenance dose of 0.5 mg/kg/day, the patient may require transfusion therapy. Pregnancy in patients with DBA is considered high risk as it is associated with complications to the mother, fetus, or both [64, 75]. Transfusions are often needed in the patient with DBA to keep the hemoglobin >10 gm/dL while she is pregnant. Estrogen-containing oral contraceptives can disrupt the steady state of a non-transfused female with DBA. Progesterone-containing products have been better tolerated (personal observation). Lastly, genetic counseling about the autosomal dominant inheritance of this disorder and the 50% chance of an offspring being affected should be provided to the adolescent female as she enters young adulthood.

Acquired Causes of Bone Marrow Failure

Idiopathic Severe Aplastic Anemia (SAA)

In the adolescent female who presents with significant pancytopenia or bicytopenia, a major consideration is to elucidate whether the marrow failure state is genetic in nature or acquired. Inherited bone marrow failure disorders must be thoroughly considered and evaluated for, as described in the previous sections. Once an inherited cause has been eliminated, idiopathic severe aplastic anemia (SAA) might be the diagnosis, if the following diagnostic criteria are met, as set by Camitta [76]:

1. Bone marrow hypocellularity, with less than 25% hematopoietic cells
2. Two of the three peripheral blood cytopenias: absolute neutrophil count (ANC) less than 500/uL, platelet count less than 20,000/uL, and anemia with low absolute reticulocyte count of <60,000/uL

When ANC is less than 200/uL, very severe aplastic anemia is diagnosed.

Pathophysiology of SAA

Idiopathic SAA is believed to be the result of an immune attack, primarily by activated, oligoclonal cytotoxic T cells, which produce cytokines that cause apoptosis of the hematopoietic stem and progenitor cells through the Fas/Fas ligand pathway [77, 78]. The exact antigens that activate cytotoxic T cells remain unclear.

Supportive Care for SAA

The high risk of bacterial and fungal infections constitutes a major cause of mortality cause in SAA [79–82], and immediate evaluation of fever with judicious use of empiric antibiotics is warranted. Fungal infections, especially *Aspergillus* spp., should be evaluated in the patient with prolonged or recurrent unexplained fever [79–82]. The use of prophylactic antibiotics is variable across centers, except for use of prophylaxis for *Pneumocystis jirovecii* [83]. Another supportive care measure is the use of packed red cell and platelet transfusions to maintain adequate cardiopulmonary function and prevent bleeding, respectively. Blood products should be irradiated to prevent transfusion-associated graft vs host disease and to prevent allo-sensitization of patients [84].

Due to risk of significant bleeding with menstruation in severe thrombocytopenia, platelet transfusions might be needed more frequently during menstruation or menstrual suppression using oral contraception, or leuprolide may need to be instituted [85].

Iron overload may develop over time in patients who receive multiple red cell transfusions, and monitoring should occur so that iron chelation can be appropriately started. Serum ferritin is a crude marker of iron overload; however, when serum ferritin level is more than 1000 ug/L, liver and cardiac iron concentration should be checked with an MRI T2*or ferriscan. Chelation agents used vary between centers and are individually based, depending on anticipated toxicities with the available agents (e.g., deferiprone might be avoided due to risk of agranulocytosis; deferasirox might cause nephrotoxicity in those on cyclosporine) [86].

Definitive Therapies for SAA

SAA is a life-threatening disorder, and prompt institution of definitive therapy is paramount in the outcome of treated patients [87]. The two major pillars of definitive therapy for SAA are immunosuppressive therapy (IST) and hematopoietic stem cell transplantation (HSCT) [85].

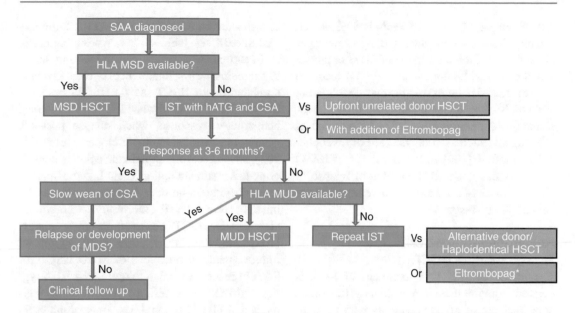

Fig. 26.1 Schematic treatment algorithm for SAA in children. Grey boxes indicate insufficient information to recommend treatment and need for additional studies. Abbreviations CSA Cyclosporine A, hATG horse antithymocyte globulin, HLA human leukocyte antigen, HSCT hematopoietic stem cell transplantation, SAA idiopathic severe aplastic anemia, IST immunosuppressive therapy, MDS myclodysplastic syndrome, MSD matched sibling donor, MUD matched unrelated donor. *Use of eltrombopag is not recommended for patients with MDS

The decision-making of which treatment to apply highly depends on the availability of a matching donor and is detailed in Fig. 26.1 and discussed below.

Immunosuppressive Therapy (IST)

The current standard of care for patients with SAA who lack a matched sibling donor is to receive immunosuppression with horse anti-thymocyte globulin (hATG) and cyclosporine A (CSA), which in combination have been effective in decreasing the activated cytotoxic T cells and dampening the ongoing marrow destruction [78, 85]. Due to the need for hematopoietic stem cells to recover hematopoiesis, response to treatment is generally assessed several months after initiation of IST and is measured by improvement of peripheral blood counts, and not by evaluation of the marrow cellularity [88]. Definitions of hematologic response differ between studies, but a refractory state is agreed on as continuing to meet criteria for SAA 6 months after initiation of IST. Complete response is achieved when blood counts return to normal or at least when the ANC

increases to >1000/uL, hemoglobin is >10 gm/dL, and platelets are >100,000/uL without transfusions [85, 88]. Partial response is when peripheral cytopenias improve above the criteria for the SAA diagnosis but less than complete response. Several studies of the efficacy of IST with hATG and CSA have resulted in hematologic recovery in 60–70% of cases [89–93]. Specific to the adolescent group, Dufour et al. reported 3-year overall survival of 90% in patients who received IST alone [94].

Several postulations have been made regarding SAA that is refractory to IST, including misdiagnosis of a genetic etiology of the marrow failure or hypoplastic MDS, neither of which is responsive to immunosuppression. Alternatively, the immune mechanism causing marrow failure may not be susceptible to hATG/CSA. Lastly, the degree of hematopoietic destruction at time of IST treatment could be extensive to where recovery of remaining cells is minimal [95].

Aside from refractory SAA, the two other concerns with IST as the treatment option are the risks of relapse and clonal evolution [90, 96]. The rate of relapse of SAA at 5 years is 33%, which can be delayed, but not prevented, by a slow taper of CSA [97]. Clonal evolution of MDS or paroxysmal nocturnal hemoglobinuria (PNH) occurs in 15% of treated patients over the decade following IST [78, 88, 98]. It is important to note that intensification of immunosuppression by addition of other agents such as sirolimus [99] or mycophenolate mofetil [100] to the backbone of hATG and CSA has not decreased rates of relapse or clonal evolution, nor has it improved the rates of hematopoietic response.

Hematopoietic Stem Cell Transplantation (HSCT)

The utility of HSCT in treatment of SAA is derived from the need to replace a dysfunctional bone marrow of affected patients with hematopoietic stem cells derived from healthy donors, thereby restoring normal hematopoiesis. This treatment requires administration of conditioning regimens, which, in SAA patients, would mostly focus on immunosuppression of the host to allow engraftment of donor cells to occur. HSCT is associated with several short- and long-term risks that are beyond the scope of this chapter but briefly include graft failure, graft-vs-host disease (GvHD), infectious complications, and organ injury.

When an adolescent with SAA has an available HLA-matched sibling donor, hematopoietic stem cell transplantation (HSCT) should be the treatment of choice as it has been shown to be curative and the young age of transplanted patients is one of the factors associated with improved overall survival [101]. The European Group for Blood and Marrow Transplantation (EBMT) reviewed results of 940 matched sibling donor transplants of SAA, and overall survival was 84% in patients younger than 20 years, and a similar 3-year overall survival of 86% was found in a study of 537 adolescents, including 227 females [101]. Results from the Center for International Blood and Marrow Transplant Research (CIBMTR) showed a slightly higher overall survival of 90% in the 1013 patients younger than 18 years transplanted between 2006 and 2016 (D'Souza A, Fretham C. Current Uses and Outcomes of Hematopoietic Cell Transplantation (HCT): CIBMTR Summary Slides, 2018. Available at https://www.cibmtr.org).

In patients who lack a matched sibling donor, IST remains the first treatment of choice. Matched unrelated donor HSCT (MUD HSCT) has been historically considered when IST fails to mount a hematologic response, when relapse post-IST occurs, or when hematologic clones evolve [95, 102]. Several reasons explain the delay in considering this treatment option, including the time lag to identifying an unrelated donor, as well as the inherent risks of GvHD, morbidity, and mortality after MUD HSCT observed in early reports [102]. However, there have been significant improvements in outcomes of MUD HSCT for SAA in recent years due to optimized HLA typing and the use of different conditioning regimens and GvHD prophylaxis. Bacigalupo et al. compared the outcomes of MUD HSCT to matched sibling donor HSCT and found that the outcome of the former was not statistically inferior, although there was greater risk of acute and chronic GvHD [101]. They additionally found that the use of peripheral stem cells is the strongest negative predictor of survival, followed by an interval of diagnosis to transplant of 180 days or more, older patients (>20 years), not using ATG in the conditioning regimen, and positive cytomegalovirus in either patient or donor [101]. A different study evaluating outcomes of the adolescent age group, specifically, also concluded that early transplant and use of bone marrow cells rather than peripheral stem cells were associated with improved outcome [94]. Furthermore, use of upfront MUD HSCT in about 30 children, including 8 adolescents, had excellent outcomes equaling survival of matched sibling donor HSCT, while at the same time showing decreased survival in those receiving MUD HSCT post-IST failure [103]. These results have prompted reconsideration of the treatment approach to include the possibility of MUD HSCT earlier in the course of SAA, if a donor is identifiable in a timely manner. Further larger studies are in progress to compare efficacy of upfront MUD HSCT to IST (ClinicalTrials.gov NCT02845596).

It is noteworthy that advances have also been made in alternative donor transplants for SAA, including successful use of haploidentical donor bone marrow cells followed by post-transplant cyclophosphamide for GvHD prophylaxis and graft rejection prevention [104]. Larger studies are being conducted to evaluate outcome of such alternative transplants, and it remains a second line treatment option at this point (ClinicalTrials. gov NCT02918292).

Considerations of Choice Between IST and HSCT

Matched sibling HSCT is preferred over IST as it restores hematopoiesis more rapidly, thereby reducing the risks of potentially life-threatening bacterial and fungal infections seen with prolonged neutropenia, and minimizes exposure to blood products with all the risks associated with transfusions over time, such as iron overload. It is also preferred as it would effectively eliminate the risks of later clonal evolution into MDS or PNH. However, these benefits need to be weighed against the potential for transplant-associated complications.

On the other hand, patients who receive and respond to IST have minimal to no long-term toxicity, and in most centers, institution of treatment does not require time delays. The downfalls include possible refractoriness to treatment with high potential of infections in the interim, as well as the need for long-term follow-up for onset of relapse and clonal evolution.

As is described above, there is a recent shift in paradigm of treatment choices to include earlier consideration of MUD HSCT when possible [103, 105], but more studies are needed to compare the treatment modalities more comprehensively. Due to the complexity of decision-making, it is highly recommended that patients with SAA are cared for by centers that are specialized in evaluation and care delivery to this unique population.

Alternative Treatments

The addition of hematopoietic-stimulating factors such as granulocyte-stimulating growth factor [106–108] and recombinant erythropoietin did not augment responses seen with IST [108]. However, the use of eltrombopag, a thrombopoietin mimetic, in 43 patients with refractory SAA,

induced a durable hematologic response in 40% of patients in at least one blood lineage, while 8 patients developed clones [109]. A larger study of 88 adult patients who received eltrombopag at different time points of IST initiation showed an improved and quicker onset of response when eltrombopag was started at time of IST initiation [110]. Similar studies in children and adolescents are ongoing in both the upfront as well as the refractory and relapsed SAA settings (ClinicalTrials.gov NCT03025698).

References

1. Mills SE, editor. Histology for pathologists. Philadelphia, PA: Lippincott Williams & Wilkins; 2012.
2. DeVita, Hellman, and Rosenberg's Cancer: Principles & Practice of Oncology. 2015.
3. Sieff CA, G.Q.D, Zon LI. Anatomy and physiology of hematopoiesis. In: Orkin SH, Fisher DE, Ginsburg D, Look AT, Lux SE, Nathan DG, editors. Nathan and Oski's hematology and oncology of infancy and childhood. Philadelphia, PA: Saunders, Elsevier; 2015. p. 3–51. e21.
4. Akiko Shimamura DAW. Acquired aplastic anemia and pure red cell aplasia. In: Orkin SH, Fisher DE, Ginsburg D, Look AT, Lux SE, Nathan DG, editors. Nathan and Oski's hematology and oncology of infancy and childhood. Philadelphia, PA: Elsevier; 2015. p. 161–81.
5. Alter BP, et al. Cancer in the National Cancer Institute inherited bone marrow failure syndrome cohort after fifteen years of follow-up. Haematologica. 2018;103(1):30–9.
6. Shimamura A, Alter BP. Pathophysiology and management of inherited bone marrow failure syndromes. Blood Rev. 2010;24(3):101–22.
7. Wang AT, Smogorzewska A. SnapShot: Fanconi anemia and associated proteins. Cell. 2015;160(1–2):354–354 e1.
8. Rodriguez A, D'Andrea A. Fanconi anemia pathway. Curr Biol. 2017;27(18):R986–8.
9. Fiesco-Roa MO, et al. Genotype-phenotype associations in Fanconi anemia: a literature review. Blood Rev. 2019;37:100589.
10. Auerbach AD. Diagnosis of Fanconi anemia by diepoxybutane analysisz. Curr Protoc Hum Genet. 2015;85:8 7 1–8 7 17.
11. Ameziane N, et al. Genetic subtyping of Fanconi anemia by comprehensive mutation screening. Hum Mutat. 2008;29(1):159–66.
12. Ameziane N, et al. Diagnosis of fanconi anemia: mutation analysis by next-generation sequencing. Anemia. 2012;2012:132856.

13. Alter BP. Inherited bone marrow failure syndromes: considerations pre- and posttransplant. Hematology Am Soc Hematol Educ Program. 2017;2017(1):88–95.

14. Dufour C. How I manage patients with Fanconi anaemia. Br J Haematol. 2017;178(1):32–47.

15. Butturini A, et al. Hematologic abnormalities in Fanconi anemia: an International Fanconi Anemia Registry study. Blood. 1994;84(5):1650–5.

16. Kutler DI, et al. A 20-year perspective on the International Fanconi Anemia Registry (IFAR). Blood. 2003;101(4):1249–56.

17. Auerbach AD. Fanconi anemia and its diagnosis. Mutat Res. 2009;668(1–2):4–10.

18. Mehta PA, Tolar J. Fanconi Anemia. 2002 Feb 14 [Updated 2018 Mar 8]. In: Adam MP, Ardinger HH, Pagon RA, et al., editors. GeneReviews® [Internet]. Seattle (WA): University of Washington, Seattle; 1993–2020. Available from: https://www.ncbi.nlm.nih.gov/books/NBK1401/.

19. Scheckenbach K, et al. Treatment of the bone marrow failure in Fanconi anemia patients with danazol. Blood Cells Mol Dis. 2012;48(2):128–31.

20. Paustian L, et al. Androgen therapy in Fanconi anemia: a retrospective analysis of 30 years in Germany. Pediatr Hematol Oncol. 2016;33(1):5–12.

21. Dietz AC, et al. Current knowledge and priorities for future research in late effects after hematopoietic cell transplantation for inherited bone marrow failure syndromes: consensus statement from the second pediatric blood and marrow transplant consortium international conference on late effects after pediatric hematopoietic cell transplantation. Biol Blood Marrow Transplant. 2017;23(5):726–35.

22. Dietz AC, et al. Late effects screening guidelines after hematopoietic cell transplantation for inherited bone marrow failure syndromes: consensus statement from the second pediatric blood and marrow transplant consortium international conference on late effects after pediatric HCT. Biol Blood Marrow Transplant. 2017;23(9):1422–8.

23. Alter BP, et al. Malignancies and survival patterns in the National Cancer Institute inherited bone marrow failure syndromes cohort study. Br J Haematol. 2010;150(2):179–88.

24. Rosenberg PS, Greene MH, Alter BP. Cancer incidence in persons with Fanconi anemia. Blood. 2003;101(3):822–6.

25. Rosenberg PS, Alter BP, Ebell W. Cancer risks in Fanconi anemia: findings from the German Fanconi Anemia Registry. Haematologica. 2008;93(4):511–7.

26. Tamary H, et al. Frequency and natural history of inherited bone marrow failure syndromes: the Israeli Inherited Bone Marrow Failure Registry. Haematologica. 2010;95(8):1300–7.

27. Niewisch MR, Savage SA. An update on the biology and management of dyskeratosis congenita and related telomere biology disorders. Expert Rev Hematol. 2019;12(12):1037–52.

28. Dokal I. Dyskeratosis congenita in all its forms. Br J Haematol. 2000;110(4):768–79.

29. Bertuch AA. The molecular genetics of the telomere biology disorders. RNA Biol. 2016;13(8):696–706.

30. de Lange T. Shelterin-mediated telomere protection. Annu Rev Genet. 2018;52:223–47.

31. Schmidt JC, Cech TR. Human telomerase: biogenesis, trafficking, recruitment, and activation. Genes Dev. 2015;29(11):1095–105.

32. Harley CB, Futcher AB, Greider CW. Telomeres shorten during ageing of human fibroblasts. Nature. 1990;345(6274):458–60.

33. Dokal I. Dyskeratosis congenita. Hematology Am Soc Hematol Educ Program. 2011;2011:480–6.

34. Gutierrez-Rodrigues F, et al. Direct comparison of flow-FISH and qPCR as diagnostic tests for telomere length measurement in humans. PLoS One. 2014;9(11):e113747.

35. Alter BP, et al. Telomere length is associated with disease severity and declines with age in dyskeratosis congenita. Haematologica. 2012;97(3):353–9.

36. Alter BP, et al. Very short telomere length by flow fluorescence in situ hybridization identifies patients with dyskeratosis congenita. Blood. 2007;110(5):1439–47.

37. Khincha PP, et al. Response to androgen therapy in patients with dyskeratosis congenita. Br J Haematol. 2014;165(3):349–57.

38. Giri N, et al. Splenic peliosis and rupture in patients with dyskeratosis congenita on androgens and granulocyte colony-stimulating factor. Br J Haematol. 2007;138(6):815–7.

39. de la Fuente J, Dokal I. Dyskeratosis congenita: advances in the understanding of the telomerase defect and the role of stem cell transplantation. Pediatr Transplant. 2007;11(6):584–94.

40. Gadalla SM, et al. Outcomes of allogeneic hematopoietic cell transplantation in patients with dyskeratosis congenita. Biol Blood Marrow Transplant. 2013;19(8):1238–43.

41. Nelson AS, Myers KC. Diagnosis, treatment, and molecular pathology of Shwachman-Diamond syndrome. Hematol Oncol Clin North Am. 2018;32(4):687–700.

42. Alter BP. Inherited bone marrow failure syndromes: considerations pre- and posttransplant. Blood. 2017;130(21):2257–64.

43. Wilson DB, et al. Inherited bone marrow failure syndromes in adolescents and young adults. Ann Med. 2014;46(6):353–63.

44. Dror Y, et al. Draft consensus guidelines for diagnosis and treatment of Shwachman-Diamond syndrome. Ann N Y Acad Sci. 2011;1242:40–55.

45. Boocock GR, et al. Mutations in SBDS are associated with Shwachman-Diamond syndrome. Nat Genet. 2003;33(1):97–101.

46. Dhanraj S, et al. Biallelic mutations in DNAJC21 cause Shwachman-Diamond syndrome. Blood. 2017;129(11):1557–62.

47. Stepensky P, et al. Mutations in EFL1, an SBDS partner, are associated with infantile pancytopenia, exocrine pancreatic insufficiency and skeletal anomalies in a Shwachman-Diamond like syndrome. J Med Genet. 2017;54(8):558–66.

48. Carapito R, et al. Mutations in signal recognition particle SRP54 cause syndromic neutropenia with Shwachman-Diamond-like features. J Clin Invest. 2017;127(11):4090–103.

49. Tan S, et al. EFL1 mutations impair eIF6 release to cause Shwachman-Diamond syndrome. Blood. 2019;134(3):277–90.

50. Mack DR, et al. Shwachman syndrome: exocrine pancreatic dysfunction and variable phenotypic expression. Gastroenterology. 1996;111(6):1593–602.

51. Hashmi SK, et al. Comparative analysis of Shwachman-Diamond syndrome to other inherited bone marrow failure syndromes and genotype-phenotype correlation. Clin Genet. 2011;79(5):448–58.

52. Rothbaum RJ, Williams DA, Daugherty CC. Unusual surface distribution of concanavalin A reflects a cytoskeletal defect in neutrophils in Shwachman's syndrome. Lancet. 1982;2(8302):800–1.

53. Orelio C, et al. Altered intracellular localization and mobility of SBDS protein upon mutation in Shwachman-Diamond syndrome. PLoS One. 2011;6(6):e20727.

54. Stepanovic V, et al. The chemotaxis defect of Shwachman-Diamond syndrome leukocytes. Cell Motil Cytoskeleton. 2004;57(3):158–74.

55. Donadieu J, et al. Classification of and risk factors for hematologic complications in a French national cohort of 102 patients with Shwachman-Diamond syndrome. Haematologica. 2012;97(9):1312–9.

56. Dror Y, et al. Clonal evolution in marrows of patients with Shwachman-Diamond syndrome: a prospective 5-year follow-up study. Exp Hematol. 2002;30(7):659–69.

57. Smith A, et al. Intermittent 20q- and consistent i(7q) in a patient with Shwachman-Diamond syndrome. Pediatr Hematol Oncol. 2002;19(7):525–8.

58. Valli R, et al. Shwachman-Diamond syndrome with clonal interstitial deletion of the long arm of chromosome 20 in bone marrow: haematological features, prognosis and genomic instability. Br J Haematol. 2019;184(6):974–81.

59. Donadieu J, et al. Hematopoietic stem cell transplantation for Shwachman-Diamond syndrome: experience of the French neutropenia registry. Bone Marrow Transplant. 2005;36(9):787–92.

60. Burroughs LM, et al. Allogeneic hematopoietic cell transplantation using treosulfan-based conditioning for treatment of marrow failure disorders. Biol Blood Marrow Transplant. 2017;23(10):1669–77.

61. Da Costa L, Narla A, Mohandas N. An update on the pathogenesis and diagnosis of Diamond-Blackfan anemia. F1000Res. 2018;7

62. Vlachos A, et al. Incidence of neoplasia in Diamond Blackfan anemia: a report from the Diamond Blackfan Anemia Registry. Blood. 2012;119(16):3815–9.

63. Vlachos A, et al. Increased risk of colon cancer and osteogenic sarcoma in Diamond-Blackfan anemia. Blood. 2018;132(20):2205–8.

64. Vlachos A, et al. Diagnosing and treating Diamond Blackfan anaemia: results of an international clinical consensus conference. Br J Haematol. 2008;142(6):859–76.

65. Ulirsch JC, et al. The genetic landscape of Diamond-Blackfan anemia. Am J Hum Genet. 2018;103(6):930–47.

66. Narla A, Vlachos A, Nathan DG. Diamond Blackfan anemia treatment: past, present, and future. Semin Hematol. 2011;48(2):117–23.

67. Sjogren SE, et al. Glucocorticoids improve erythroid progenitor maintenance and dampen Trp53 response in a mouse model of Diamond-Blackfan anaemia. Br J Haematol. 2015;171(4):517–29.

68. Flygare J, et al. HIF1alpha synergizes with glucocorticoids to promote BFU-E progenitor self-renewal. Blood. 2011;117(12):3435–44.

69. Lipton JM, et al. Improving clinical care and elucidating the pathophysiology of Diamond Blackfan anemia: an update from the Diamond Blackfan Anemia Registry. Pediatr Blood Cancer. 2006;46(5):558–64.

70. Willig TN, et al. Identification of new prognosis factors from the clinical and epidemiologic analysis of a registry of 229 Diamond-Blackfan anemia patients. DBA group of Societe d'Hematologie et d'Immunologie Pediatrique (SHIP), Gesellshaft fur Padiatrische Onkologie und Hamatologie (GPOH), and the European Society for Pediatric Hematology and Immunology (ESPHI). Pediatr Res. 1999;46(5):553–61.

71. Vlachos A, Muir E. How I treat Diamond-Blackfan anemia. Blood. 2010;116(19):3715–23.

72. Tufano AM, et al. Deleterious consequences of Diamond Blackfan anemia on reproductive health and pregnancy outcomes: a report from the Diamond Blackfan Anemia Registry (DBAR). Blood. 2014;124(21):4399.

73. Lahoti A, et al. Endocrine dysfunction in Diamond-Blackfan Anemia (DBA): a report from the DBA Registry (DBAR). Pediatr Blood Cancer. 2016;63(2):306–12.

74. Bartels M, Bierings M. How I manage children with Diamond-Blackfan anaemia. Br J Haematol. 2019;184(2):123–33.

75. Faivre L, et al. High-risk pregnancies in Diamond-Blackfan anemia: a survey of 64 pregnancies from the French and German registries. Haematologica. 2006;91(4):530–3.

76. Camitta BM, Storb R, Thomas ED. Aplastic anemia (second of two parts): pathogenesis, diagnosis, treatment, and prognosis. N Engl J Med. 1982;306(12):712–8.

77. Young NS. Current concepts in the pathophysiology and treatment of aplastic anemia. Hematology Am Soc Hematol Educ Program. 2013;2013:76–81.
78. Young NS. Aplastic Anemia. N Engl J Med. 2018;379(17):1643–56.
79. Weinberger M, et al. Patterns of infection in patients with aplastic anemia and the emergence of Aspergillus as a major cause of death. Medicine (Baltimore). 1992;71(1):24–43.
80. Torres HA, et al. Infections in patients with aplastic anemia: experience at a tertiary care cancer center. Cancer. 2003;98(1):86–93.
81. Valdez JM, et al. Decreased infection-related mortality and improved survival in severe aplastic anemia in the past two decades. Clin Infect Dis. 2011;52(6):726–35.
82. Quarello P, et al. Epidemiology of infections in children with acquired aplastic anaemia: a retrospective multicenter study in Italy. Eur J Haematol. 2012;88(6):526–34.
83. Williams DA, et al. Diagnosis and treatment of pediatric acquired aplastic anemia (AAA): an initial survey of the North American Pediatric Aplastic Anemia Consortium (NAPAAC). Pediatr Blood Cancer. 2014;61(5):869–74.
84. Marsh J, et al. Should irradiated blood products be given routinely to all patients with aplastic anaemia undergoing immunosuppressive therapy with antithymocyte globulin (ATG)? A survey from the European Group for Blood and Marrow Transplantation Severe Aplastic Anaemia Working Party. Br J Haematol. 2010; 150(3):377–9.
85. DeZern AE, Guinan EC. Aplastic anemia in adolescents and young adults. Acta Haematol. 2014;132(3–4):331–9.
86. Marsh JC, Kulasekararaj AG. Management of the refractory aplastic anemia patient: what are the options? Blood. 2013;122(22):3561–7.
87. Locasciulli A, et al. Outcome of patients with acquired aplastic anemia given first line bone marrow transplantation or immunosuppressive treatment in the last decade: a report from the European Group for Blood and Marrow Transplantation (EBMT). Haematologica. 2007;92(1):11–8.
88. Scheinberg P, Young NS. How I treat acquired aplastic anemia. Blood. 2012;120(6):1185–96.
89. Frickhofen N, et al. Antithymocyte globulin with or without cyclosporin a: 11-year follow-up of a randomized trial comparing treatments of aplastic anemia. Blood. 2003;101(4):1236–42.
90. Rosenfeld S, et al. Antithymocyte globulin and cyclosporine for severe aplastic anemia: association between hematologic response and long-term outcome. JAMA. 2003;289(9):1130–5.
91. Fuhrer M, et al. Immunosuppressive therapy for aplastic anemia in children: a more severe disease predicts better survival. Blood. 2005;106(6):2102–4.
92. Fuhrer M, et al. Relapse and clonal disease in children with aplastic anemia (AA) after immunosuppressive therapy (IST): the SAA 94 experience. German/Austrian Pediatric Aplastic Anemia Working Group. Klin Padiatr. 1998;210(4):173–9.
93. Scheinberg P, et al. Long-term outcome of pediatric patients with severe aplastic anemia treated with antithymocyte globulin and cyclosporine. J Pediatr. 2008;153(6):814–9.
94. Dufour C, et al. Outcome of aplastic anemia in adolescence: a survey of the Severe Aplastic Anemia Working Party of the European Group for Blood and Marrow Transplantation. Haematologica. 2014;99(10):1574–81.
95. Marsh JC, Kulasekararaj AG. Management of the refractory aplastic anemia patient: what are the options? Hematology Am Soc Hematol Educ Program. 2013;2013:87–94.
96. Rogers ZR, et al. Immunosuppressive therapy for pediatric aplastic anemia: a North American Pediatric Aplastic Anemia Consortium study. Haematologica. 2019;104(10):1974–83.
97. Scheinberg P, et al. Prolonged cyclosporine administration after antithymocyte globulin delays but does not prevent relapse in severe aplastic anemia. Am J Hematol. 2014;89(6):571–4.
98. Maciejewski JP, Selleri C. Evolution of clonal cytogenetic abnormalities in aplastic anemia. Leuk Lymphoma. 2004;45(3):433–40.
99. Scheinberg P, et al. Treatment of severe aplastic anemia with a combination of horse antithymocyte globulin and cyclosporine, with or without sirolimus: a prospective randomized study. Haematologica. 2009;94(3):348–54.
100. Scheinberg P, et al. Treatment of severe aplastic anemia with combined immunosuppression: antithymocyte globulin, ciclosporin and mycophenolate mofetil. Br J Haematol. 2006;133(6):606–11.
101. Bacigalupo A, et al. Current outcome of HLA identical sibling versus unrelated donor transplants in severe aplastic anemia: an EBMT analysis. Haematologica. 2015;100(5):696–702.
102. Davies JK, Guinan EC. An update on the management of severe idiopathic aplastic anaemia in children. Br J Haematol. 2007;136(4):549–64.
103. Dufour C, et al. Similar outcome of upfront-unrelated and matched sibling stem cell transplantation in idiopathic paediatric aplastic anaemia. A study on behalf of the UK Paediatric BMT Working Party, Paediatric Diseases Working Party and Severe Aplastic Anaemia Working Party of EBMT. Br J Haematol. 2015;171(4):585–94.
104. DeZern AE, Brodsky RA. Haploidentical donor bone marrow transplantation for severe aplastic anemia. Hematol Oncol Clin North Am. 2018;32(4):629–42.
105. Georges GE, Doney K, Storb R. Severe aplastic anemia: allogeneic bone marrow transplantation as first-line treatment. Blood Adv. 2018;2(15):2020–8.

106. Gluckman E, et al. Results and follow-up of a phase III randomized study of recombinant human-granulocyte stimulating factor as support for immunosuppressive therapy in patients with severe aplastic anaemia. Br J Haematol. 2002;119(4):1075–82.

107. Tichelli A, et al. A randomized controlled study in patients with newly diagnosed severe aplastic anemia receiving antithymocyte globulin (ATG), cyclosporine, with or without G-CSF: a study of the SAA Working Party of the European Group for Blood and Marrow Transplantation. Blood. 2011;117(17):4434–41.

108. Marsh JC, Ganser A, Stadler M. Hematopoietic growth factors in the treatment of acquired bone marrow failure states. Semin Hematol. 2007;44(3):138–47.

109. Olnes MJ, et al. Eltrombopag and improved hematopoiesis in refractory aplastic anemia. N Engl J Med. 2012;367(1):11–9.

110. Townsley DM, et al. Eltrombopag added to standard immunosuppression for aplastic anemia. N Engl J Med. 2017;376(16):1540–50.

111. Takeshima M, et al. Anorexia nervosa-associated pancytopenia mimicking idiopathic aplastic anemia: a case report. BMC Psychiatry. 2018;18(1):150.

112. McGowan KE, et al. Aplastic anaemia in pregnancy – a single centre, North American series. Br J Haematol. 2019;184(3):436–9.

113. DeZern AE, et al. Detection of paroxysmal nocturnal hemoglobinuria clones to exclude inherited bone marrow failure syndromes. Eur J Haematol. 2014;92(6):467–70.

114. Nelson A, Myers K. Shwachman-Diamond Syndrome. 2008 Jul 17 [Updated 2018 Oct 18]. In: Adam MP, Ardinger HH, Pagon RA, et al., editors. GeneReviews® [Internet]. Seattle (WA): University of Washington, Seattle; 1993–2020. Available from: https://www.ncbi.nlm.nih.gov/books/NBK1756/.

Part VII

Blood Disorders in the Pregnant Adolescent

Adolescent Pregnancy Complicated by Thrombosis

Candice M. Dersch and Peter A. Kouides

Introduction

Pregnancy in adolescence has significant physical, psychological, social, and economic impact on the lives of young women. Each year, more than 21 million girls aged 15–19 and two million under age 15 become pregnant in developing countries [1]. Pregnancy occurs in approximately 25% of adolescents worldwide and 13% of adolescents in the United States [2].

Adolescent pregnancy is associated with increased maternal and fetal risk. Adverse outcomes include preterm labor and delivery, low birthweight infants, pregnancy-related infections, preeclampsia and eclampsia [3]. Worldwide, pregnancy and complications related to childbirth remain the number one cause of death for adolescent girls aged 15–19 years [4]. The risk of maternal mortality is highest for adolescent girls under 15 years old, and complications in pregnancy and childbirth are higher among adolescent girls age 10–19 years when compared to women age 20–24 [4, 5].

In 2014, an analysis by the World Health Organization identified hemorrhage to be the leading cause of maternal death in developing countries, followed by venous thromboembolic events [5]. In the United States, venous thromboembolism (VTE) accounts for 9.2% of all maternal deaths [6]. Women and girls with hematologic disorders are at increased risk for pregnancy-related complications, including thrombosis and bleeding. Care of pregnant adolescents with hematologic disorders should employ a multidisciplinary approach, including maternal fetal medicine specialists, hematologists, obstetricians, anesthesiologists, transfusion medicine specialists, and other care providers as needed.

Venous Thromboembolism in Pregnancy

Background and Physiology

Adolescent girls are known to have a lower absolute risk of thromboembolism than non-pregnant adult women. However, risk of VTE has been shown to be higher in adolescent girls than in the general pediatric population [7]. Intuitively, this is related to increases in endogenous estrogen as well as use of exogenous estrogen. The risk of adolescent VTE in girls peaks at 15–18 years of age, and use of exogenous estrogen is most highly correlated with VTE risk in this age group [7]. The

C. M. Dersch (✉)
Tuft University School of Medicine, Maine Medical Center, Portland, ME, USA
e-mail: derscc@mmc.org

P. A. Kouides
University of Rochester School of Medicine and Dentistry, Rochester Regional Health, Rochester, NY, USA

© Springer Nature Switzerland AG 2020
L. V. Srivaths (ed.), *Hematology in the Adolescent Female*,
https://doi.org/10.1007/978-3-030-48446-0_27

rate of VTE in adolescents is increasing, likely due to the increased prevalence of risk factors for VTE in this population [8]. Similar to adults, additional risk factors for thrombosis may be present in pregnant adolescents, including obesity, smoking, and decreased mobility [9]. Non-pregnant adolescents with VTE are more likely to have two or more risk factors for VTE [10], and this compounding of risk is likely present in pregnant adolescents as well, although there are no studies to date to demonstrate this. Thus, we must rely on recommendations for studies in pregnant adults to guide our evaluation and management of VTE in pregnant adolescents.

In pregnancy, physiologic, hormonal, and anatomic changes lead to a transient hypercoagulable state that results in an increased risk of thromboembolic events. Although this may confer a survival benefit by decreasing the risk of postpartum hemorrhage, it also results in a five to tenfold increase in the risk of thromboembolism during pregnancy and in the postpartum period [11]. The increase in risk starts as early as 6 weeks of pregnancy, but is greatest in the third trimester and the 6 weeks following delivery. The transient hypercoagulable state in pregnancy largely results from increases in estradiol and progesterone. More specifically, hormonal changes increase factor levels of fibrinogen (factor I), VII, VIII, X, Von Willebrand factor, and plasminogen activator inhibitors 1 and 2. There is also a hormone mediated reduction in the natural anticoagulant activity of protein C and S. These changes all contribute to the increased risk of VTE in pregnancy and up to 12 weeks postpartum.

Physiologic and anatomic changes also contribute to the elevated risk of VTE. Progesterone mediated venous stasis is exacerbated by compression of the vena cava and pelvic veins by the enlarged uterus, specifically on the left side, similar to May-Thurner syndrome, and play a role in increased risk of VTE [12]. Risk factors specifically identified in adolescents with VTE include inherited thrombophilia, infection, recent surgery, and immobility, among others [7]. Pregnancy-related conditions such as preeclampsia, infection and multiple gestation further increase the risk of VTE [13]. Furthermore, paradoxically, the risk of postpartum VTE increases in the setting of postpartum hemorrhage [14].

As noted above, all women with an inherited thrombophilia are at increased risk of thrombosis in pregnancy. Thrombophilia is present in 20–50% of women who develop VTE in pregnancy or in the postpartum period [15]. Therefore, evaluation of thrombosis in pregnancy for women of any age usually includes evaluation for inherited thrombophilia, as the subsequent finding of an inherited thrombophilic defect would be of value if the patient has female family members that may also be at risk for thrombotic events while on combined hormonal contraception or in pregnancy. Absolute risk for VTE in patients with defined genetic thrombophilia is outlined in Table 27.1 below.

Table 27.1 Risk of VTE in pregnant women with various thrombophilias

Thrombophilia	Asymptomatic carriers	Positive family history of VTE	Personal history of VTE
	Estimated absolute risk of VTE events per 1000 patients[a]		
Factor V Leiden (heterozygous)	8	15	100
Factor II G20210A (heterozygous)	6	15	>100
Factor V Leiden (homozygous)	34	70	170
Factor II G20210A (homozygous)	26	70	>170
Antithrombin deficiency	4	20	400
Protein C deficiency	4	20	40–170
Protein S deficiency	3	20	0–220

Sources: Robertson L et al. Br J Haematol. 2006;132(2):171–196; Bates SM et al. Chest. 2012;141(2)(suppl):e691S-e736S; American College of Obstetricians and Gynecologists Women's Health Care Physicians. Obstet Gynecol. 2018;132(1):e18–e34. Refs. [15–17]
Reprinted with permission from Rybstein and DeSancho [45]
[a]Assuming a baseline risk of 1 VTE event per 1000 pregnant patients without a known thrombophilia. *VTE* venous thromboembolism

Diagnosis of VTE in Pregnancy

Approximately 80% of thrombotic events in pregnancy are venous, with approximately 75–80% of these being deep vein thrombosis (DVT). The remaining 20–25% are pulmonary emboli (PE), which constitute the majority of postpartum VTE [13]. Diagnosing VTE in pregnancy can be challenging due to anatomic and physiologic changes, as well as concern for limiting radiation exposure to the developing fetus.

Deep vein thrombosis is the most commonly assessed form of VTE in pregnancy. Similar to non-pregnant women, more than 80% of pregnant women with a DVT present with complaints of pain and swelling in the calf [16]. However, the specificity for leg symptoms is poor in pregnancy. Only 10% of pregnant women presenting with symptoms suspicious for DVT are ultimately confirmed as VTE, which is much lower than the 25% in the non-pregnant population [17]. Compression ultrasonography of the proximal veins is the recommended initial diagnostic imaging modality for suspected DVT. More proximal iliac vein Doppler ultrasonography or magnetic resonance imaging (MRI) may be needed to rule out iliac vein thrombosis if lower extremity ultrasound is negative and suspicion remains high for DVT [18].

In non-pregnant patients, several validated models use D-dimer to calculate risk of VTE and aid in clinical decision-making [19]. D-dimer levels in pregnancy are higher and increase with each trimester, making interpretation of D-dimer challenging in this population. Studies have been done to establish normative values for D-dimer in each trimester of pregnancy [20]. Risk assessment models utilizing D-dimer for clinical decision-making during evaluation of VTE, especially PE, in pregnancy have been investigated and may be of value [21, 22], but there is no single model currently recommended by major organizations issuing guidelines [23].

Evaluation for PE is challenging in pregnancy. Typical symptoms of PE, including shortness of breath and tachycardia, occur frequently and can be normal in pregnancy. Pregnant women are at increased risk for PE, and untreated PE can have catastrophic effects for the mother and fetus; therefore suspicion for PE in pregnancy must remain high. Similar to the lower sensitivity for DVT screening in pregnancy, studies have shown the prevalence of PE for women screened in pregnancy to be much lower than in non-pregnant women [24]. For symptomatic patients, the American Thoracic Society recommends chest radiography (CXR) as the initial imaging procedure for evaluation of PE in pregnancy. Chest radiography should be performed unless clinical signs or symptoms of DVT are also present, in which case lower extremity compression ultrasonography should be performed [25]. If the CXR is normal and suspicion for PE remains high, a ventilation/perfusion scan (V/Q) should be considered next for the pregnant adolescent. Radiation exposure to the maternal chest is a concern for future breast and lung cancer, and exposure is higher from a single CTA than a single V/Q. Although there is still debate on the recommended next imaging modality for adult pregnant women, the increased concern for radiation exposure to adolescent breast and lung tissue due to both organ sensitivity and longer life expectancy makes V/Q preferable in this scenario [26]. However, if V/Q is not available, or if the CXR is abnormal, CTA is recommended [25].

Fetal risk from radiation exposure is a frequent concern when imaging is indicated in pregnancy. Fetal radiation exposure from a CTA remains lower than a V/Q. Patients can be reassured that radiation exposure from CXR, V/Q, and CTA combined remains 100–200 times lower than the dose associated with significant risk of fetal anomalies. Potential fetal and maternal risks must also be weighed against the mortality risk of 20–30% for an untreated maternal PE [27].

Management of VTE in Pregnancy

Anticoagulation is recommended following the diagnosis of VTE in pregnancy, and treatment should not be delayed due to pregnancy. There is currently lack of data to suggest adolescents should be treated differently from their adult counterparts. Therefore, recommended treatment for pregnancy will be reviewed here.

Low-molecular-weight heparin (LMWH) and subcutaneous unfractionated heparin (SUH) are the mainstays of therapy for VTE in pregnancy. Neither LMWH nor SUH crosses the placenta, and numerous studies have demonstrated their safety in pregnancy. Alternatives, including vitamin K antagonists, are generally avoided in pregnancy. Their use is limited to high-risk patients, such as those with mechanical heart valves. Vitamin K antagonists are known teratogens, being most deleterious at 6–12 weeks of gestation. They should therefore be avoided not only in early pregnancy but also in adolescents at high risk of unplanned pregnancy. Direct oral anticoagulants (DOACs) cross the placenta, and data regarding their safety in pregnancy is extremely limited. Thus, DOACs should be avoided in pregnancy.

Low-molecular-weight heparin is preferred to SUH for anticoagulation in pregnancy for several reasons. Unfractionated heparin has a higher risk of heparin-induced thrombocytopenia (HIT). Although HIT is uncommon in pregnancy, the exact frequency is unknown. The risk of HIT is higher if patients are first treated with SUH and transitioned to LMWH. A platelet count 4–7 days following initiation of LMWH or SUH should be drawn to assess for the presence of HIT. Risk of heparin-induced osteoporosis has also been evaluated in pregnant patients and is likely less when LMWH is used [28]. Local sensitivity reactions including erythema, itching, and pain are quite common with both LMWH and SUH. Unless a severe type 1 sensitivity reaction is suspected, switching from one LMWH to another is recommended. Approximately one-third of patients who are switched from one LMWH to another because of a skin reaction will have a recurrent skin reaction. Switching to fondaparinux is recommended in these patients. Although fondaparinux does cross the placenta, umbilical anti-Xa levels are subtherapeutic in the fetus, at one-tenth of the maternal level. Even at this level, fondaparinux must be stopped prior to delivery to allow for safe maternal neuraxial analgesia and fetal delivery. Additionally, safety data for use of fondaparinux in the first trimester are lacking [29].

LMWH is also preferred to SUH in adolescent pregnancy because administration is less frequent, and more frequent dosing may lower medication compliance in adolescent patients [30]. Additionally, SUH produces a less predictable therapeutic response than LMWH in pregnancy. While studies do not conclusively support routine Xa monitoring in pregnant women requiring full-dose anticoagulation, periodic Xa monitoring is reasonable in the obese patient, since Xa levels fall by 25% in the third trimester as the blood volume rises. Monitoring is also reasonable if renal function is reduced [31, 32].

For patients with newly diagnosed VTE in pregnancy, full anticoagulation is recommended through 6 weeks postpartum. Management of anticoagulation during labor and immediately following delivery require careful consideration, and a multidisciplinary approach is recommended to optimize care. Treatment dose LMWH can be safely used until 24 hours before planned delivery, while prophylactic doses can be continued until 12 hours before delivery [33]. Patients with VTE earlier in pregnancy can be transitioned to SUH 3–4 weeks prior to estimated delivery. The shorter half-life of SUH can allow for more flexibility in management while awaiting spontaneous labor. Although randomized clinical trial data are lacking, most experts advise a planned induction of labor if VTE occurred in the 8 weeks prior to delivery. Hospital admission and transition to intravenous SUH prior to delivery are appropriate if the VTE occurred in the 4 weeks prior to delivery. For VTE occurring less than 2 weeks before delivery, a retrievable filter can be considered [34].

Spinal hematoma after regional anesthesia placement in anticoagulated pregnant women is uncommon, but the exact incidence remains unknown. To minimize risk, neuraxial anesthesia should not be placed before 24 h from last dose therapeutic dose of LMWH or 12 h from last prophylactic dose [13].

Low-molecular-weight heparin and SUH in prophylactic and therapeutic doses can be safely reinitiated postpartum. Timing is dependent on individual patient risk of VTE versus postpartum hemorrhage [35]. To avoid an increased risk of postpartum bleeding, anticoagulation can be restarted 4–6 h following a vaginal delivery or 6–12 h following cesarean delivery [13]. Anticoagulation can be considered up to 12 weeks postpartum as the increased risk of VTE is known to persist through 12 weeks post-delivery [36].

VTE Prophylaxis in Pregnancy

Antepartum prophylaxis for pregnant women at risk for VTE is more controversial, and no studies evaluating risk in adolescent pregnancy are currently available. Current standard of care is application of recommendations for adult pregnancy. A complete individualized risk assessment including presence of known genetic or acquired thrombophilia, personal and family history of prior VTE, maternal obesity, and other factors for VTE must be considered. Although the level of acceptable VTE risk without prophylaxis will differ between patients, a risk of 3% or greater was determined by consensus opinion to be an acceptable point at which prophylaxis can be considered [37]. A summary of the recommendations for thromboprophylaxis in pregnancies complicated by inherited thrombophilia is summarized in Table 27.2 below. As with any

Table 27.2 Recommended thromboprophylaxis for pregnancies complicated by inherited thrombophilias[a]

Clinical scenario	Antepartum management	Postpartum management
Low-risk thrombophilia[b] without previous VTE	Surveillance without anticoagulation therapy	Surveillance without anticoagulation therapy or postpartum prophylactic anticoagulation therapy if the patient has additional risks factors[c]
Low-risk thrombophilia[b] with a family history (first-degree relative) of VTE	Surveillance without anticoagulation therapy or prophylactic LMWH/UFH	Postpartum prophylactic anticoagulation therapy or intermediate-dose LMWH/UFH
Low-risk thrombophilia[b] with a single previous episode of VTE—not receiving long-term anticoagulation therapy	Prophylactic or intermediate-dose LMWH/UFH	Postpartum prophylactic anticoagulation therapy or intermediate-dose LMWH/UFH
High-risk thrombophilia[d] without previous VTE	Prophylactic or intermediate-dose LMWH/UFH	Postpartum prophylactic anticoagulation therapy or intermediate-dose LMWH/UFH

Table 27.2 (continued)

Clinical scenario	Antepartum management	Postpartum management
High-risk thrombophilia[d] with a single previous episode of VTE or an affected first-degree relative—not receiving long-term anticoagulation therapy	Prophylactic, intermediate-dose, or adjusted-dose LMWH/UFH	Postpartum prophylactic anticoagulation therapy, or intermediate or adjusted-dose LMWH/UFH for 6 weeks (therapy level should be equal to the selected antepartum treatment)
Thrombophilia with two or more episodes of VTE—not receiving long-term anticoagulation therapy	Intermediate-dose or adjusted-dose LMWH/UFH	Postpartum anticoagulation therapy with intermediate-dose or adjusted-dose LMWH/UFH for 6 weeks (therapy level should be equal to the selected antepartum treatment)
Thrombophilia with two or more episodes of VTE—receiving long-term anticoagulation therapy	Adjusted-dose LMWH/UFH	Resumption of long-term anticoagulation therapy. Oral anticoagulants may be considered postpartum based upon planned duration of therapy, lactation, and patient preference

Reprinted with permission from inherited thrombophilias in pregnancy. ACOG Practice Bulletin No. 197 [37]
Abbreviations: *LMWH* low-molecular-weight heparin, *UFH* unfractionated heparin, *VTE* venous thromboembolism
[a]Postpartum treatment levels should be equal to antepartum treatment
[b]Low-risk thrombophilia: factor V Leiden heterozygous; prothrombin G20210A heterozygous; protein C or protein S deficiency
[c]First-degree relative with a history of a thrombotic episode or other major thrombotic risk factors (e.g., obesity, prolonged immobility, cesarean delivery)
[d]High-risk thrombophilias include factor V Leiden homozygosity, prothrombin gene G20210A mutation homozygosity, heterozygosity for factor V Leiden and prothrombin G20210A mutation, or antithrombin deficiency

treatment, risk of VTE prophylaxis must be balanced against risk of withholding treatment. Both LMWH and SUH can be used for VTE prophylaxis in pregnancy.

Other VTE in Pregnancy

More than 99% of VTE in pregnancy is DVT or PE, but ovarian vein thrombosis (OVT) and cerebral vein thrombosis (CVT) are worth discussing because they have both been described in adolescent pregnancy. Ovarian vein thrombosis is an uncommon complication of pregnancy. Incidence is estimated from 1/600 to 1/2000 deliveries. Cases of OVT in postpartum adolescents have been reported [38]. Cesarean delivery is a known risk factor for OVT, and patients with OVT most often present with pelvic pain and fever. Therapeutic anticoagulation therapy is recommended when symptomatic OVT is diagnosed. Antibiotics are recommended if infection is also suspected.

Cerebral vein thrombosis (CVT) is an uncommon event, with an incidence of 7/1000000 in the general population. Pregnancy is a known risk factor for CVT, and the risk of CVT in pregnancy is 11.6/100000 deliveries [39, 40]. Cerebral vein thrombosis has also been reported in pregnant and postpartum adolescents [41]. Presence of an inherited thrombophilia is a risk factor for CVT, with 20% or more of patients diagnosed with an inherited thrombophilia during evaluation [42]. Being overweight or obese has also been shown to be a risk factor for CVT in pediatric and adolescent populations, but the effect pregnancy-related weight gain is unknown [43]. The most common symptoms of CVT are headache and seizure, making differentiation from eclampsia difficult in pregnancy. Magnetic resonance imaging with venography is the preferred diagnostic imaging modality. Therapeutic anticoagulation with LMWH is recommended following diagnosis. In some patients, thrombolytic therapy or surgical thrombectomy are indicated. Recurrence risk is low in subsequent pregnancies [44].

References

1. Blum RW, Gates WH. United Nations Population Fund. Girlhood, not motherhood: preventing adolescent pregnancy. UNFPA; 2015. https://unfpa.org/sites/default/files/pub-pdf/Girlhood_not_motherhood_final_web.pdf. Accessed 23 Sept 2019.
2. Leftwich HK, Alves MV. Adolescent pregnancy. Pediatric Clin N Am. 2017;64:381–8.
3. WHO. Global health estimates 2015: deaths by cause, age, sex, by country and by region, 2000–2015. Geneva: WHO; 2016 http://wwwwhoint/healthinfo/global_burden_disease/en/. Accessed 24 Sept 2019.
4. Ganchimeg T, Ota E, Morisaki N, Laopaiboon M, Lumbiganon P, Zhang J, et al. Pregnancy and childbirth outcomes among adolescent mothers: a World Health Organization multicountry study. BJOG. 2014;121(Suppl 1):40–8.
5. Say L, Chou D, Gemmill A, Tunçalp Ö, Moller AB, Daniels J, et al. Global causes of maternal death: a WHO systematic analysis. Lancet Glob Health. 2014;2:e323–33.
6. Centers for Disease Control and Prevention. Pregnancy mortality surveillance system. Aug 7, 2018. https://www.cdc.gov/reproductivehealth/maternalinfanthealth/pmss.html. Accessed 23 Sept 2019.
7. Tuckuviene R, Christensen A, Helgestad J, Johnsen SP, Kristensen SR. Pediatric venous and arterial noncerebral thromboembolism in Denmark: A nationwide population-based study. J Pediatr. 2011;159:663–9.
8. Srivaths L, Dietrich JE. Prothrombotic risk factors and preventive strategies in adolescent venous thromboembolism. Clin Appl Thromb Hemost. 2016;22:512–9.
9. Macklon NS, Greer IA. Venous thromboembolic disease in obstetrics and gynaecology: the Scottish experience. Scott Med J. 1996;41:83–6.
10. Ishola T, Kirk SE, Guffey D, Voigt K, Shah MD, Srivaths L. Risk factors and co-morbidities in adolescent thromboembolism are different than those in younger children. Thromb Res. 2016;141:178–82.
11. Pomp ER, Lenselink AM, Rosendaal FR, Doggen CJ. Pregnancy, the postpartum period and prothrombotic defects: risk of venous thrombosis in the MEGA study. J Thromb Haemost. 2008;6:632–7.
12. Gordon MC. Maternal physiology. In: Gabbe SG, Niebyl JR, Leigh Simpson J, Landon MB, Galan HL, Jauniaux ERM, Driscott DA, Verghella V, Grobman WA, editors. Obstetrics: normal and problem pregnancies. 7th ed. Philadelphia: PA Saunders; 2017. p. 38–63.
13. American College of Obstetricians and Gynecologists. Practice Bulletin No. 196: Thromboembolism in pregnancy. Obstet Gynecol. 2018;132:e1–e17.
14. Bourjeily G, Paidas M, Khalil H, Rosene-Montella K, Rodger M. Pulmonary embolism in pregnancy. Lanced. 2010;375:500–12.

15. James AH. Venous thromboembolism in pregnancy. Arterioscler Thromb Vasc Biol. 2009;29:326–31.
16. James AH, Tapson VF, Goldhaber SZ. Thrombosis during pregnancy and the postpartum period. Am J Obstet Gynecol. 2005;193:216–9.
17. Ginsberg JS, Greer I, Hirsh J. Use of antithrombotic agents during pregnancy. Chest. 2001;119:122S–31S.
18. Bates SM, Greer IA, Middeldorp S, Veenstra DL, Prabulos AM, Vandvik PO. VTE, thrombophilia, antithrombotic therapy, and pregnancy: Antithrombotic Therapy and Prevention of Thrombosis, 9th ed: American College of Chest Physicians Evidence-Based Clinical Practice Guidelines. Chest. 2012;141(2 Supple);e691S–e736S.
19. Wicki J, Perneger TV, Junod AF, Bounameaux H, Perrier A. Assessing clinical probability of pulmonary embolism in the emergency ward: a simple score. Arch Intern Med. 2001;161:92–7.
20. Gutiérrez García I, Pérez Cañadas P, Martínez Uriarte J, García Izquierdo O, Angeles Jódar Pérez M, García de Guadiana Romualdo L. D-dimer during pregnancy: establishing trimester-specific reference intervals. Scand J Clin Lab Invest. 2018;78:439–42.
21. Righini M, Robert-Ebadi H, Elias A, Sanchez O, Le Moigne E, Schmidt J, et al. Diagnosis of pulmonary embolism during pregnancy: A Multicenter Prospective Management Outcome Study. Ann Intern Med. 2018;169:766–73.
22. van der Pol LM, Tromeur C, Bistervels IM, Ni Ainle F, van Bemmel T, Bertoletti L, et al. Pregnancy-Adapted YEARS algorithm for diagnosis of suspected pulmonary embolism. N Engl J Med. 2019;380:1139–49.
23. Parilla BV, Fournogerakis R, Archer A, Sulo S, Laurent L, Lee P, et al. Diagnosing pulmonary embolism in pregnancy: Are biomarkers and clinical predictive models useful? AJP Rep. 2016;6:e160–4.
24. Kline JA, Richardson DM, Than MP, Penaloza A, Roy PM. Systematic review and meta-analysis of pregnant patients investigated for suspected pulmonary embolism in the emergency department. Acad Emerg Med. 2014;21:949–59.
25. Revel MP, Cohen S, Sanchez O, Collignon MA, Thiam R, Redheuil A, et al. Pulmonary embolism during pregnancy: diagnosis with lung scintigraphy or CT angiography? Radiology. 2011;258:590–8.
26. American College of Radiology ACR Appropriateness Criteria Suspected Pulmonary Embolism, Revised 2016:1–14.
27. Kouides P, Paidas M. Chapter 3: Consultative Hematology II: women's health issues. In: Cuker A, Altman JK, Gerda AT, Wun T, editors. American Society of hematology self-assessment program. Washington, DC: ASH Publications; 2019. p. 78–9.
28. Le Templier G, Rodger MA. Heparin-induced osteoporosis and pregnancy. Curr Opin Pulm Med. 2008;14:403–7.
29. DeCarolis S, di Pasquo E, Rossi E, Del Sordo G, Buonomo A, Schiavino D, et al. Fondaparinux in pregnancy: Could it be a safe option? A review of the literature. Thromb Res. 2015;135(6):1049–51.
30. Taddeo D, Egedy M, Frappier JY. Adherence to treatment in adolescents. Paediatri Child Health. 2008;13:19–24.
31. Bates SM, Rajasekhar A, Middeldorp S, McLintock C, Rodger MA, James AH, et al. American Society of Hematology 2018 Guidelines for management of venous thromboembolism: venous thromboembolism in the context of pregnancy. Blood Adv. 2018;2:3317–59.
32. Royal College of Obstetricians and Gynaecologists. Green-top Guideline No. 37b. Thromboembolic disease in pregnancy and the puerperium: acute management. April 2015. https://www.rcog.org.uk/globalassets/documents/guidelines/gtg-37b.pdf. Accessed 13 Oct 2019.
33. D'Alton ME, Friedman AM, Smiley RM, Montgomery DM, Paidas MJ, D'Oria R, et al. National partnership for maternal safety: consensus bundle on venous thromboembolism. Obstet Gynecol. 2016;128:688–98.
34. Crosby DA, Ryan K, McEniff N, Dicker P, Regan C, Lynch C, et al. Retrievable inferior vena cava filters in pregnancy: risk versus benefit? Eur J Obstet Gynecol Reprod Biol. 2018;222:25–30.
35. Bates SM, Middeldorp S, Rodger M, James AH, Greer I. Guidance for the treatment and prevention of obstetric-associated venous thromboembolism. J Thromb Thrombolysis. 2016;41:92–128.
36. Kamel H, Navi BB, Sriram N, Hovscpian DA, Devereux RB, Elkind MS. Risk of a thrombotic event after the 6-week postpartum period. N Engl J Med. 2014;370:1307–15.
37. American College of Obstetricians and Gynecologists. Practice Bulletin No.197. Inherited Thrombophilias in pregnancy. Obstet Gynecol. 2018;132:e18–34.
38. Arkadopoulos N, Dellaportas D, Yiallourou A, Koureas A, Voros D. Ovarian vein thrombosis mimicking acute abdomen: a case report and literature review. World J Emerg Surg. 2011;6:45.
39. Dangal G, Thapa LB. Cerebral venous sinus thrombosis presenting in pregnancy and puerperium. BMJ Case Rep. 2009;2009:bcr0620092045. https://doi.org/10.1136/bcr.06.2009.2045.
40. Lanska DJ, Kryscio RJ. Risk factors for peripartum and postpartum stroke and intracranial venous thrombosis. Stroke. 2000;31:1274–82.
41. Imai WK, Everhart FR Jr, Sanders JM Jr. Cerebral venous sinus thrombosis: Report of a case and review of the literature. Pediatrics. 1982;70:965–70.
42. Ahmad A. Genetics of cerebral vein thrombosis. J Pak Med Assoc. 2006;56(11):488–90.

43. Pearson V, Ruzas C, Krebs N, Goldenberg N, Manco-Johnson M, Bernard T. Overweight and obesity are increased in childhood-onst cerebrovascular disease. J Child Neurol. 2013;28(4):517–9.

44. Mehraein S, Ortwein H, Busch M, Weih M, Einhäupl K, Masuhr F. Risk of recurrence of cerebral venous and sinus thrombosis during subsequent pregnancy and puerperium. J Neurol Neurosurg Psychiatry. 2003;74:814–6.

45. Rybstein M, DeSancho MT. Risk factors for and clinical management of venous thromboembolism during pregnancy. Clin Adv Hematol Oncol.2019;17(7):396–404.

Bleeding Disorders in Pregnancy

Maissa Janbain and Peter A. Kouides

Background

Management of bleeding in pregnant adolescents is challenging, as adolescents are in general more likely to terminate a pregnancy than adult women, and if they carry a pregnancy, they are more likely to deliver prematurely. In one case control study, adolescents were not found to be at increased risk of obstetrical complications including postpartum hemorrhage when compared to adult women [1]. However, the risk of bleeding remains significant for women with an existing bleeding disorder, when compared to women with no existing bleeding disease, especially delayed postpartum hemorrhage occurring 2–3 weeks after delivery [2, 3]. There are limited data on the prevalence of bleeding disorders in adolescents. The most common bleeding disorder is von Willebrand disease, a quantitative or qualitative deficiency of von Willebrand protein. Hemophilia carriership is another risk factor for bleeding; this is particularly true for hemophilia A carriers who have a level <60% through pregnancy with emerging data that even carriers with "normalized" levels may bleed postpartum [4–6].

Platelet defects, acquired or inherited, are very common cause of bleeding in adolescents, especially mild cases, raising awareness to consider them in all adolescents presenting with menorrhagia [7]. Finally other clotting factor deficiencies encoded by genes on chromosomes other than X chromosomes affect women and men equally, with earlier and more evident presentation in adolescent girls because of menstruation.

Diagnosis of a Suspected Bleeding Disorder in a Pregnant Adolescent

Not every adolescent with bleeding disorder will be identified prior to pregnancy as they may not have experienced challenges such as wisdom tooth extraction and increased menstrual flow might be considered normal in their families. Therefore, it is recommended to screen for bleeding disorders during their first obstetrical visit if there is a personal (manifest by an increased bleeding score) [8] or family bleeding history, taking into consideration the normal physiologic increase in factor levels (specifically FVIII and von Willebrand factor (VWF) levels) that occur with advancing pregnancy. History should include questions assessing for menorrhagia, anemia, personal and family history of bleeding symptoms per a bleeding assessment tool [8]. Physical exam should assess for petechiae, ecchymosis, and epistaxis. In one study, a positive bleeding history by

M. Janbain (✉)
Tulane School of Medicine, New Orleans, LA, USA
e-mail: mjanbain@tulane.edu

P. A. Kouides
University of Rochester School of Medicine and Dentistry, Rochester Regional Health, Rochester, NY, USA

© Springer Nature Switzerland AG 2020
L. V. Srivaths (ed.), *Hematology in the Adolescent Female*,
https://doi.org/10.1007/978-3-030-48446-0_28

itself has a sensitivity of 82% for detecting an inherited bleeding disorder in the setting of heavy menses [9]. As FVIII increases during pregnancy, it is recommended to perform genetic mutation analysis if levels are within the normal range and an affected individual is available for testing or their mutation is known.

Management of Pregnancy and Childbirth in Adolescents with Bleeding Disorder

The challenge remains in the two thirds of pregnancies that are unplanned, especially if the adolescent has not yet been diagnosed or counseled about her bleeding disorder. In the case of hemophilia carriership, genetic counseling should be offered, and prenatal diagnostic options should be discussed including chorionic villus sampling, amniocentesis, and fetal sex determination.

There does not appear to be an increased risk of miscarriage in women with bleeding disorders except in the case of congenital fibrinogen deficiency and congenital FXIII deficiency. Replacement therapy is required during pregnancy, to maintain levels of fibrinogen above 100 mg/dL and FXIII trough levels above 3 IU/dL.

The majority of hemophilia carriers and pregnant women with type 1 VWD or low VWF do not require replacement therapy nor DDAVP as levels of FVIII and VWF are expected to increase during pregnancy >100%, associated with an improvement in bleeding symptoms. But in women with non-DDAVP responsive VWD, i.e., severe type 1 (<30% VWF) or type 2 or 3, at the time of delivery, historically the target level for replacement was 50% or higher, but recent studies strongly suggest undertreatment resulting in increased blood loss, so postpartum replacement ideally should aim for VWF levels >~100 IU/dL (i.e., closer to levels that are observed in normal pregnant women) [6, 10–12]. It is possible that the undertreatment is in part also because the dosing is not weight-based, that is, taking into consideration the increased plasma volume peripartum. Treatment should be for 3–5 days in the case of a vaginal delivery and 5–7 days for a cesarean section (CS) [13]. Table 28.1 includes specific factor replacement therapies in different bleeding disorders and the desired target levels.

Patients should be co-managed by their obstetrician and a hematologist during their pregnancy and the postpartum period. Invasive fetal monitoring procedures should be avoided if the fetus might be potentially affected with a moderate to severe bleeding disorder. Delivery method should be the least traumatic, avoiding forceps and vacuum extraction. Some obstetricians prefer planning cesarean delivery ahead of time, as the outcome of non-operative vaginal delivery cannot be predicted or guaranteed [14, 15].

In the hemophilia carrier expecting an affected infant, the risk of intracranial hemorrhage is 2.5% compared to 0.06% in the general population (odds ratio 44-fold), and the risk of extracranial hemorrhage is 3.7% compared with 0.47% (odds ratio eightfold). The majority of cases were due to instrumentation (vacuum extraction or forceps). Nonetheless, although not proven conclusively due to lack of randomized data, cesarean delivery is recommended over vaginal delivery to reduce that risk. In high-risk infants, the critical issue is the availability of a multidisciplinary team in an obstetric unit with facilities for high-risk deliveries. Of course, the problem is that many carriers are not diagnosed until after delivery, and even in those who are known carriers, an affected infant may not be anticipated if they are not properly counseled. It should be recognized that preconception counseling with genotyping is currently available, as well as pre-and postimplantation options, including preimplantation genetic diagnosis and postimplantation fetal DNA sex determination, chorionic villus sampling, and amniocentesis [16].

Factor levels should be checked during third trimester of pregnancy. Central neuraxial anesthesia is safe in type 1 VWD and hemophilia A after achieving a VWF level of 50%. But regarding type 2 and 3 VWD, the 2017 Royal College of Obstetricians and Gynaecologists guidelines advise "that neuraxial anesthesia be avoided unless VWF activity is more than 50% and the hemostatic defect has been corrected; this may be

Table 28.1 Specific factor replacement in inherited bleeding disorders peripartum

Factor deficiency	Patients' factor level (normal)	Desired level	Recommendation
VWD type 1	<50%	>100%	VWF concentrate 40–60 IU/kg, then 20–40 IU/kg q 12 h, then daily 3–5 days if vaginal delivery, 5–7 days if cesarean
VWD types 2, 3	<50%	>100%	VWF concentrate 60–80 IU/kg, then 40–60 IU/kg q 12 h, then daily 3–5 days if vaginal delivery, 5–7 days if cesarean
FI (fibrinogen)	<0.5 g/L	1–1.5 g/L × 3 days	Pregnancy prophylaxis: fibrinogen concentrate 50–100 mg/kg twice a week to maintain level at >1 g/L (more during labor) × 3 days. Cryoprecipitate 15–20 mL/kg, SD-FFP 15–30 mL/kg. TXA 15–20 mg/kg IV, then 1 g po tid.
FII	<20% (50–150%)	20–40%	PCC 20–40 U/kg, then PCC 10–20 IU/kg q 48 h to maintain levels for it least 3 days
FV	<20% (50–150%)	20–40%	FFP 15–30 ml/kg, later FFP 10 ml/kg q 12 h for at least 3 days. For severe bleeding or cesarean, give platelet transfusion (FV + VIII give DDAVP,FFP).
FVII	<20% (50–150%)	>40%	rFVIIa 15–30 µg/kg q 4–6 h for at least 3–5 days
FVIII, FIX	<50% (50–150%)	>100%	FVIII earner: FVIII concentrate 20–40 IU/kg: FIX carrier: 40–50 IU/kg
FX	<30% (50–150%)	>40%	PDFX concentrate 1500 U (18.8–25 U/kg), PCC 10–20 U/kg qd × 3 days, FFP
FXI	<15–20% (70–150%)	>30–40%	If bleeding phenotype or prior h/o PPH-FXI concentrate 15–20 U/kg if available: FFP, TXA alone at 1 g qtg. rFVIIa for inhibitors
FXIII	<30% (70–150%)	>20%	Pd-FXIII 20–40 U/kg × 1, rFXIII-A 35 U/kg, cryoprecipitate, FFP

Adapted from Pavord S et al., BJOC, 2017;124;e193–e263. It should be recognized that these represent expert opinion recommendations, and treatment duration and intensity are based on not only the factor level but historical assessment of the bleeding phenotype

DDAVP 1-desamino-8D-arginine vasopressin, *FFP* fresh frozen plasma, *PCC* prothrombin complex concentrate, *PDFX* plasma-derived FX, *PdFXIII* plasma-derived FXIIII, *PPH-FXI* postpartum hemorrhage-FXI concentrate, *rFXIII-A* recombinant FXIII, *SD-FFP* solvent detergent fresh frozen plasma, *TXA* tranexamic acid, *VWD* von Willebrand disease, *VWF* von Willebrand factor

difficult to achieve in type 2 and central neuraxial anesthesia should not be given in cases of type 3." In type 2 N, central neuraxial anesthesia is safe if the FVIII level is replaced to >50% [13].

In addition to factor replacement therapy peripartum as previously mentioned, antifibrinolytics (aminocaproic acid and tranexamic acid) can be considered as adjunctive therapy to improve hemostasis in these patients particularly in those with past history of postpartum hemorrhage or a high bleeding score >10 or severe factor deficiency or severe type 1 VWD or type 2 VWD or type 3 VWD, as intuitively the risk of postpartum hemorrhage exceeds 20% [17]. The recommended dose of tranexamic acid is 1gm intravenous every 6 hours as long as the bleeding continues. Close monitoring after delivery is cru-

cial as women with inherited bleeding disorders have significantly longer postpartum bleeding, especially delayed bleeding that occurs between 24 hours and 6 weeks postpartum [18]. In general, women with von Willebrand disease were found to bleed on average for at least 15 days postpartum [19]; therefore frequent contact with their provider is requested [20]. This is due to the rapid decline in their hemostatic factors back to their baseline levels, usually low in these women depending on the type of their inherited bleeding disease. Primary postpartum hemorrhage (PPH) that occurs immediately after delivery is defined as an estimated blood loss of >500 ml for vaginal delivery or >1000 ml for cesarean deliveries. This latter type of PPH is mainly due to uterine atony, retained placental products, and genital tract trauma, and this is true for all women with and without bleeding disorders. The risk factors for uterine atony are mainly prolonged induced labor, especially in third stage of labor. Management of women with bleeding disorders should aggressively aim to reduce this stage of labor with prophylactic use of uterotonics to improve muscle contractility. In addition, genital and perineal trauma should be minimized as much as possible, as one patient series had shown increased perineal hematoma in women with inherited bleeding disorders [21].

References

1. Al-Ramahi M, Saleh S. Outcome of adolescent pregnancy at a university hospital in Jordan. Arch Gynecol Obstet. 2006;273(4):207–10.
2. James AH, Jamison MG. Bleeding events and other complications during pregnancy and childbirth in women with von Willebrand disease. J Thromb Haemost. 2007;5(6):1165–9.
3. James AH. More than menorrhagia: a review of the obstetric and gynaecological manifestations of bleeding disorders. Haemophilia. 2005;11(4):295–307.
4. Paroskie A, Gailani D, DeBaun MR, Sidonio RF Jr. A cross-sectional study of bleeding phenotype in haemophilia A carriers. Br J Haematol. 2015;170(2):223–8.
5. Plug I, Mauser-Bunschoten EP, Brocker-Vriends AH, van Amstel HK, van der Bom JG, van Diemen-Homan JE, et al. Bleeding in carriers of hemophilia. Blood. 2006;108(1):52–6.
6. Stoof SC, van Steenbergen HW, Zwagemaker A, Sanders YV, Cannegieter SC, Duvekot JJ, et al. Primary postpartum haemorrhage in women with von Willebrand disease or carriership of haemophilia despite specialised care: a retrospective survey. Haemophilia. 2015;21(4):505–12.
7. James AH, Lukes AS, Brancazio LR, Thames E, Ortel TL. Use of a new platelet function analyzer to detect von Willebrand disease in women with menorrhagia. Am J Obstet Gynecol. 2004;191(2):449–55.
8. Elbatarny M, Mollah S, Grabell J, Bae S, Deforest M, Tuttle A, et al. Normal range of bleeding scores for the ISTH-BAT: adult and pediatric data from the merging project. Haemophilia. 2014;20(6):831–5.
9. Philipp CS, Faiz A, Dowling NF, Beckman M, Owens S, Ayers C, et al. Development of a screening tool for identifying women with menorrhagia for hemostatic evaluation. Am J Obstet Gynecol. 2008;198(2):163.e1–8.
10. Kouides PA. Preventing postpartum haemorrhage-when guidelines fall short. Haemophilia. 2015;21(4):502–4.
11. James AH, Konkle BA, Kouides P, Ragni MV, Thames B, Gupta S, et al. Postpartum von Willebrand factor levels in women with and without von Willebrand disease and implications for prophylaxis. Haemophilia. 2015;21(1):81–7.
12. Lavin M, Aguila S, Dalton N, Nolan M, Byrne M, Ryan K, et al. Significant gynecological bleeding in women with low von Willebrand factor levels. Blood Adv. 2018;2(14):1784–91.
13. Management of Inherited Bleeding Disorders in Pregnancy: Green-top Guideline No. 71 (joint with UKHCDO). BJOG. 2017;124(8):e193–e263.
14. Lee CA, Chi C, Pavord SR, Bolton-Maggs PH, Pollard D, Hinchcliffe-Wood A, et al. The obstetric and gynaecological management of women with inherited bleeding disorders–review with guidelines produced by a taskforce of UK Haemophilia Centre Doctors' Organization. Haemophilia. 2006;12(4):301–36.
15. Nichols WL, Hultin MB, James AH, Manco-Johnson MJ, Montgomery RR, Ortel TL, et al. von Willebrand disease (VWD): evidence-based diagnosis and management guidelines, the National Heart, Lung, and Blood Institute (NHLBI) Expert Panel report (USA). Haemophilia. 2008;14(2):171–232.
16. James AH, Hoots K. The optimal mode of delivery for the haemophilia carrier expecting an affected infant is caesarean delivery. Haemophilia. 2010;16(3):420–4.
17. Kouides PA. Antifibrinolytic therapy for preventing VWD-related postpartum hemorrhage: indications and limitations. Blood Adv. 2017;1(11):699–702.
18. Castaman G, James PD. Pregnancy and delivery in women with von Willebrand disease. Eur J Haematol. 2019;103(2):73–9.
19. Roque H, Funai E, Lockwood CJ. von Willebrand disease and pregnancy. J Matern Fetal Med. 2000;9(5):257–66.
20. Kulkarni R, Soucie JM, Lusher J, Presley R, Shapiro A, Gill J, et al. Sites of initial bleeding episodes, mode of delivery and age of diagnosis in babies with haemophilia diagnosed before the age of 2 years: a report from The Centers for Disease Control and Prevention's (CDC) Universal Data Collection (UDC) project. Haemophilia. 2009;15(6):1281–90.
21. Huq FY, Kadir RA. Management of pregnancy, labour and delivery in women with inherited bleeding disorders. Haemophilia. 2011;17 Suppl 1:20–30.

Index

© Springer Nature Switzerland AG 2020
L. V. Srivaths (ed.), *Hematology in the Adolescent Female*,
https://doi.org/10.1007/978-3-030-48446-0

Printed in the United States
by Baker & Taylor Publisher Services